OXFORD MEDICAL PUBLICATIONS

Spatial epidemiology

Spatial Epidemiology
Methods and Applications

Edited by

P. Elliott
J. C. Wakefield
N. G. Best
and
D. J. Briggs

Small Area Health Statistics Unit,
Imperial College School of Medicine, London

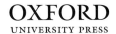

OXFORD
UNIVERSITY PRESS

OXFORD
UNIVERSITY PRESS

Oxford University Press
Great Clarendon Street, Oxford OX2 6DP

Oxford University Press is a department of the University of Oxford.
It furthers the University's objective of excellence in research,
scholarship, and education by publishing worldwide in
Oxford New York

Athens Auckland Bangkok Bogotá Buenos Aires Calcutta Cape Town
Chennai Dar es Salaam Delhi Florence Hong Kong Istanbul
Karachi Kuala Lumpur Madrid Melbourne Mexico City Mumbai
Nairobi Paris São Paulo Singapore Taipei Tokyo Toronto Warsaw

with associated companies in
Berlin Ibadan

Oxford is a registered trade mark of Oxford University Press
in the UK and in certain other countries

Published in the United States by
Oxford University Press, Inc., New York

A catalogue record for this title is available
from the British Library

Library of Congress Cataloging in Publication Data

Spatial epidemiology: methods and applications/edited by P. Elliotts *et al.*
(Oxford medical publications)
Includes index
1. Medical geography. 2. Epidemiology. I. Elliott, P. (Paul) II. Series.
RA792.S685 2000   614.4'2–dc21   00-035658

1 3 5 7 9 10 8 6 4 2
ISBN 0 19 262941 7 (alk. paper)

Typeset by
Newgen Imaging Systems (P) Ltd, Chennai, India

Printed in Great Britain on acid free paper by
Biddles Ltd, Guildford & King's Lynn

Preface

This book brings together contributions from an international group of practitioners from a wide spectrum of disciplines including epidemiologists, statisticians, geographers, demographers, and pollution modellers, with the aim of providing, a comprehensive reference volume on state-of-the-art methods and applications in the emerging discipline of spatial epidemiology. This branch of epidemiology is concerned with describing, quantifying, and explaining geographical variations in disease, especially with respect to variations in environmental exposures at the small-area scale. The recent and rapid expansion of this field looks set to continue in line with growing public, government, and media concern about environment and health issues, and a scientific need to understand and explain the effects of environmental pollutants on health.

Modelling and mapping disease and exposure relationships presents many challenges. For example, the collection of suitable data is often beset by practical and methodological problems. The models developed must acknowledge both the spatial aggregation and quality of the data used and the interpretation of the results requires care due to the ever-present problems of confounding and ecological bias. Such challenges have attracted researchers from a range of disciplines and have recently led to a number of important developments in statistical and epidemiological methods. These have been greatly facilitated by modern advances in computer software and hardware, including the development of geographical information systems (GIS) and the ability to carry out hierarchical Bayesian modelling using Markov chain Monte Carlo (MCMC) techniques.

The book is divided into four sections. Section I gives an introduction to spatial epidemiological studies and summarises data requirements and problems with respect to modelling health events, including issues of bias and confounding. Section II gives an overview of the state of the art in statistical methodology, including Bayesian approaches to disease mapping, cluster detection, analysis of point source exposures, geostatistical methods, and methods for ecological correlation studies. Section III gives examples of disease mapping and clustering studies, involving mortality data, communicable disease data, Hodgkin's disease, diabetes, and childhood leukaemias. Section IV reviews methods of exposure assessment for use in spatial epidemiological studies, and discusses possible links between exposure and health data in risk assessment, and in the effects on human health of traffic-related pollution, water quality, and climate change.

This book aims to give an authoritative account of current practice and developments in the field. As such it should be of interest to epidemiologists, public health practitioners, statisticians, geographers, environmental scientists, and others concerned with understanding the geographical distribution of disease and the effects of environmental exposures on human health. We hope that the book will be a valuable resource for undergraduate and postgraduate courses in epidemiology, medical geography, biostatistics, environmental health and environmental science, as well as a useful source of reference for health policy-makers, health economists, regulators, and others in the field of environmental health.

We thank Miss Jennifer Wells (Imperial College) for her invaluable administrative and secretarial support in realising this volume.

London   P.E.
July 2000   J.C.W.
                                                                                                     N.G.B.
                                                                                                     D.J.B.

Contents

List of abbreviations

ADMS	Atmospheric Dispersion Modelling System
AIDS	acquired immunodeficiency syndrome
ALL	acute lymphoblastic/lymphocytic leukaemia
ASR	age standardised rate
AWMN	acid waters monitoring network (UK)
BDCM	bromodichloromethane
BEAM	Bayesian ecological analysis method
BL	Burkitt's lymphoma
BOD	biological oxygen demand
CAR	conditional autoregressive
CCRG	Childhood Cancer Research Group (Oxford, UK)
CDC	Centers for Disease Control
CI	confidence interval
CMCK	covariance-matching constrained kriging
CMF	comparative mortality figure
COAD	chronic obstructive airways disease
COMARE	Committee on Medical Aspects of Radiation in the Environment
COPD	chronic obstructive pulmonary disease
CVS	census validation survey
DBCM	dibromochloromethane
DEPCAT	deprivation category
DoE	Department of the Environment (UK) (now DETR, Department of Environment, Transport and The Regions)
DH	Department of Health (England)
DHSS(NI)	Department of Health and Social Services, Northern Ireland
DNA	diribonucleic acid
EB	empirical Bayes
EC/EU	European Commission/Union
ED	enumeration district
ENSO	El Niño Southern Oscillation phenomenon
EPA	Environmental Protection Agency (USA)
EPV	extra-poisson variability
ETS	environmental tobacco smoke
FAO	Food and Agriculture Organisation (UN)
GAM	generalised additive model

GC-FID	gas chromatography flame ionisation detection
GCM	global climate model
GC-MS	gas chromatography-mass spectrometry
GHG	greenhouse gas
GIS	geographical information system
GLMM	generalised linear mixed model
GP	general practitioner
GRO(S)	General Register Office (Scotland)
HA	health authority (UK)
HBN	Hydrologic Benchmark Network (USA)
HES	hospital episode system
HIPE	Hospital In-Patient Enquiry
HIV	human immunodeficiency virus
HLA	human leukocyte antigen
HPLC	high pressure liquid chromatography
HSA	health service area
IARC	International Agency for Research on Cancer
ICD	International Classification of Diseases
ICP-MS	inductively coupled plasma-mass spectrometry
IDDM	insulin-dependent diabetes mellitus
IPCC	Intergovernmental Panel on Climate Change (UN)
ISD	Information and Statistics Division of the National Health Service in Scotland
KCW	Kensington & Chelsea and Westminster Health Authority (UK)
LA	local authority (UK)
LAD	local authority district
LL	lymphocytic leukaemia
LLTI	limiting long-term illness
L_{MO}	Monin–Obukhov length
LRS	linear risk scores
MAUP	modifiable area unit problem
MCMC	Markov chain Monte Carlo
MLE	maximum likelihood estimate
MRF	Markov random field
NASQAN	National Stream Quality Accounting Network (USA)
NCHS	National Center for Health Statistics (USA)
NCI	National Cancer Institute (USA)
NDVI	normalised difference vegetation index
NGM	National Groundwater Monitoring Network (Netherlands)
NHL	non-Hodgkin's lymphoma
NHS	National Health Service (UK)
NHSCR	National Health Service Central Register
NRC	National Research Council
NRCT	National Registry of Childhood Tumours
NRPB	National Radiological Protection Board
OCP	Onchocerciasis Control Programme

ONS	Office for National Statistics (UK) (formerly OPCS, Office for Population Censuses and Surveys)
ONS LS	Office for National Statistics Longitudinal Study
OR	odds ratio
PAH	polycyclic aromatic hydrocarbon
PCB	polychlorinated biphenyl
PES	post enumeration survey
PM	particulate matter
QDE	qualitative differential equation
RBC	red blood cells
RS	remote sensing
SAHSU	Small Area Health Statistics Unit (UK)
SAS	small area statistics
SAVIAH	small area variations in an quality and health (EU-funded research project)
SE	standard error
SEER	Surveillance, Epidemiology and End Results Program (USA)
SIDS	sudden infant death syndrome
SMR	standardised mortality/morbidity ratio
SMS	special migration statistics
SPREE	structure preserving estimate
SRR	standardised rate ratio
TB	tuberculosis
TCE	trichloroethylene
THM	trihalomethane
TNF	tumour necrosis factor
UMP	uniformly most powerful
UPA	underprivileged area
USGS	United States Geological Survey
UV-B	ultraviolet B radiation
VOC	volatile organic compound
WHCS	Welsh Health Common Services Agency
WHO	World Health Organisation
XRF	X-ray fluorescence

List of contributors

F. E. Alexander Department of Public Health Sciences, University of Edinburgh, Teviot Place, Edinburgh, EH8 9AL, UK

R. A. Arnold Statistics New Zealand, P O Box 2922, Wellington, New Zealand

P. Atkinson Public Health Laboratory Service Communicable Disease Surveillance Centre, London and School of Geography, Birkbeck College, University of London, 7-15 Gresse Street, London W1P 2LL, UK

L. Bernardinelli Dipartimento Scienze Sanitarie Applicate, Università di Pavia, Via Bassi 21, 27100 Pavia, Italy

N. G. Best Small Area Health Statistics Unit, Department of Epidemiology and Public Health, Imperial College School of Medicine, St Mary's Campus, Norfolk Place, London W2 1PG, UK

J. F. Bithell Department of Statistics, University of Oxford, 1 South Parks Road, Oxford OX1 3TG, UK

P. Boyle Division of Epidemiology and Biostatistics, European Institute of Oncology, Via Ripamonti 435, 20141 Milan, Italy

D. J. Briggs Small Area Health Statistics Unit, Department of Epidemiology and Public Health, Imperial College School of Medicine, St Mary's Campus, Norfolk Place, London W2 1PG, UK

V. Carstairs Visiting Professor, Department of Mathematics, Napier University, Edinburgh EH14 1DJ, UK

R. Colvile Imperial College of Science, Technology and Medicine, T H Huxley School of the Environment, Earth Science and Engineering, Prince Consort Road, London SW7 2BP, UK

N. Cressie Department of Statistics, 1958 Neil Avenue, The Ohio State University, Columbus OH43210-1247, USA

I. D. Diamond Department of Social Statistics, University of Southampton, Southampton SO17 1BJ, UK

P. J. Diggle Medical Statistics Unit, Department of Mathematics and Statistics, Lancaster University, Lancaster LA1 4YF, UK

P. Elliott Small Area Health Statistics Unit, Department of Epidemiology and Public Health, Imperial College School of Medicine, St Mary's Campus, Norfolk Place, London W2 1PG, UK

W. Gilks MRC Biostatistics Unit, Institute of Public Health, Robinson Way, Cambridge, UK

K. Ickstadt Department of Mathematics, Darmstadt University of Technology, 64289 Darmstadt, Germany

L. Järup Small Area Health Statistics Unit, Department of Epidemiology and Public Health, Imperial College School of Medicine, St Mary's Campus, Norfolk Place, London W2 1PG, UK

M. Kanarek Department of Preventive Medicine, University of Wisconsin-Madison, 610 N. Walnut Street, Madison, WI 53705-2397, USA

J. E. Kelsall Department of Mathematics and Statistics, Lancaster University, Lancaster LA1 4YF, UK

R. S. Kovats Department of Epidemiology and Population Health, London School of Hygiene and Tropical Medicine, Keppel Street, London WC1E 7HT, UK

S. R. Lele Department of Mathematical Sciences, University of Alberta, Edmonton AB T6G 2G1, Canada

P. Martens International Centre for Integrative Studies (ICIS), Maastricht University, P O Box 616, 6200 MD Maastricht, The Netherlands

A. J. McMichael Department of Epidemiology and Public Health, London School of Hygiene and Tropical Medicine, Keppel Street, London WC1E 7HT, UK

A. Molesworth Public Health Laboratory Service Communicable Disease Surveillance Centre, London, UK

A. Mollié Institut National de la Santé et de la Recherche Médicale (INSERM), Unité 170, 16 Avenue Paul Vaillant Couturier, Villejuif, France

C. Monfort Institut National de la Santé et de la Recherche Médicale (INSERM), Unité 170, 16 Avenue Paul Vaillant Couturier, Villejuif, France

C. Montomoli Dipartimento Scienze Sanitarie Applicate, Università di Pavia, Via Bassi 21, 27100 Pavia, Italy

S. E. Morris Small Area Health Statistics Unit, Department of Epidemiology and Public Health, Imperial College School of Medicine, St Mary's Campus, Norfolk Place, London W2 1PG, UK

M. J. Nieuwenhuijsen Imperial College of Science, Technology and Medicine, T H Huxley School of the Environment, Earth Science and Engineering, Prince Consort Road, London SW7 2BP, UK

C. Pascutto Dipartimento Scienze Sanitarie Applicate, Università di Pavia, Via Bassi 21, 27100 Pavia, Italy

L. W. Pickle National Cancer Institute, Statistical Research and Applications Branch, 6130 Executive Blvd, EPN Suite 4013, MSC 7359, Bethesda, MD 20892, USA

S. Richardson Institut National de la Santé et de la Recherche Médicale (INSERM), Unité 170, 16 Avenue Paul Vaillant Couturier, Villejuif, France

A. Staines Department of Public Health Medicine and Epidemiology, University College Dublin, Earlsfort Terrace, Dublin 2, Ireland

T. J. Vincent Childhood Cancer Research Group, University of Oxford, 57 Woodstock Road, Oxford OX2 6HJ, UK

J. C. Wakefield Small Area Health Statistics Unit, Imperial College School of Medicine, Norfolk Place, London W2 1PG and Department of Statistics, University of Washington, Box 354322, Seattle, WA 98195-4322, USA

L. Waller Department of Biostatistics, Rollins School of Public Health, Emory University, 1518 Clifton Road, N E Third Floor, Atlanta GA 30322, USA

S. D. Walter Department of Clinical Epidemiology & Biostatistics, McMaster University, Hamilton, Ontario, Canada L8N 3Z5

R. L. Wolpert Institute of Statistics and Decision Sciences, Duke University, Box 90251, Durham, NC 27708-0251, USA

The Small Area Health Statistics Unit is funded by a grant from the Department of Health, Department of the Environment, Transport and The Regions, Health and Safety Executive, Scottish Office Home and Health Department, Welsh Office, and Northern Ireland Department of Health and Social Services.

The views expressed in this publication are those of the authors and not necessarily of the funding departments.

I Introduction—health and population data

1. Spatial epidemiology: methods and applications

P. Elliott, J. C. Wakefield, N. G. Best, and D. J. Briggs

1.1 Introduction

The availability of geographically indexed health and population data, and advances in computing, geographical information systems, and statistical methodology, have enabled the realistic investigation of spatial variation in disease risk, particularly at the small-area level. Spatial epidemiology is concerned both with *describing* and *understanding* such variations. In this opening chapter we provide a general background to spatial epidemiological studies, and discuss a number of issues that are pertinent to their analysis and interpretation, including a discussion of the underlying statistical methodology. We motivate our discussion by considering the aims and use of spatial analyses in epidemiology. We distinguish between four types of study.

1. Disease mapping.
2. Geographical correlation studies.
3. The assessment of risk in relation to a point or line-source.
4. Cluster detection and disease clustering.

Disease mapping is carried out to summarise spatial and spatio-temporal variation in risk. This information may be used for simple descriptive purposes, to provide information on health needs of the population to provide context for further studies or, by comparing the estimated risk map with an exposure map, to obtain clues as to disease aetiology.

Geographical correlation studies examine geographical variations in exposure to environmental variables (that may be measured in air, water, or soil) and lifestyle factors (such as smoking and diet) in relation to health outcomes measured on a geographical (ecological) scale. While the statistical models that are used for disease mapping and geographical correlation studies may be similar (Chapters 7 and 11), the differing aims distinguish them: disease mapping studies are primarily descriptive, whilst geographical correlation studies are focused on aetiological questions.

Point and line-source studies are appropriate when increased risk close to the source is suspected, or where the source is considered to present a potential environmental hazard. The exposure may be a point-source (e.g. a chimney stack or a radio transmitter) or a linear source (e.g. a road or a powerline). In such cases, any increased exposure due to the putative source is likely to extend over a small region and only a highly localised study will have sufficient geographical resolution to provide an estimate of the associated risk.

When a well-defined biological hypothesis is driving the investigation then the interpretation of the results is most straightforward, but where the study is carried out because of a media report, or the worries of the local population, interpretation becomes much more difficult because there is no a priori hypothesis.

Finally, detection of individual disease '*clusters*' or general '*clustering*', with no associated hypothesis, may be attempted, but again interpretation is difficult. Surveillance (cluster detection) is carried out to provide early detection of raised incidence of disease when there is no specific aetiological hypothesis. More general studies of clustering, that is the tendency for disease cases to occur in a non-random spatial pattern relative to the pattern of the non-cases, have a more robust statistical formulation and again may give clues as to aetiology. For example, there is evidence of spatial clustering of Hodgkin's disease (e.g. Alexander *et al.* 1989; Chapter 15) which, along with other epidemiological evidence and laboratory studies, has suggested a possible infectious aetiology.

We note that the above characterisation of studies is convenient for our purposes but there is overlap between the categories. For example, disease mapping may provide information both on individual disease clusters and more generally on the tendency for disease cases to cluster, while a point-source of exposure may give rise to localised non-random distribution of cases. Point- and line-source exposure studies are often based on area-level summaries of exposure and health outcomes due to limitations on the geographical resolution of the available data. Exposures arising from the source are thus assumed to be constant across small areas. Such a formulation is easily extended to include geographical correlation studies and the statistical models that are utilised are often very similar.

1.1.1   A conceptual framework for spatial epidemiological studies

We now briefly describe an idealised *population/exposure/health outcome* framework within which to carry out spatial epidemiological analyses. Our focus is on studies carried out at the small-area level (small-area studies). We begin by stating an obvious fact: individuals are not uniformly distributed in space or time; they are born at a location on a particular date which depends (in probabilistic terms) on the population structure and density on that date; they then move through space as part of their daily lives or because of migration. During these movements, indexed by time, individuals will travel through numerous exposure surfaces and the integrated exposure will determine the usual biological quantity of interest: the lifelong dose (though in some instances the integrated weighted exposure or maximum dose may be more appropriate). Individual characteristics, such as age, sex and genetic factors, and lifestyle variables, such as smoking and diet, along with the lifelong dose due to an exposure of interest, all contribute to the subsequent disease experience of an individual. Statistical models may be proposed for each of the components of the idealised framework, but suitable data are required for these models to be useful.

The ideal data would consist of precise information on the population of a study region, including individual characteristics, movements, personal exposures, and subsequent health record. Of course, it is never feasible to obtain such information, and a number of simplifications to the model are imposed by the available data. In many situations, the quality of the data may seriously limit the utility of a study. This is particularly so when one considers that any increase in risk due to a putative exposure is likely to be small. However, from a public health standpoint, there is often a need to provide a view on a specific question, based on the data at hand, and with careful consideration of the aforementioned shortcomings. At the very least this will provide a qualitative answer as to whether or not there appears to be any problem. There are a number of examples in which space-time clusters of disease cases have provided clear aetiological information. For example, a cluster of malignant pleural mesothelioma cases in the small Turkish village of Karain was subsequently linked to the identification of exposure to naturally occurring erionite fibres (Baris *et al.* 1987), although this example is atypical in that it relates to an exposure that produced a high excess risk in a highly localised area.

At this point we distinguish between point data and count data. Each of the population, exposure, and health data may have associated exact spatial and temporal information (*point* data), or may be available as aggregated summaries (*count* data). Point data give the closest link to the conceptual framework outlined here but such data are rarely available routinely. Case-control studies provide point data for cases and a set of controls but are prone to selection and other biases, are expensive and time-consuming to carry out, and may not be feasible in given situations. For these reasons case-control studies are not carried out routinely but only when there is sufficient evidence/concern to warrant their use.

1.2   Health and population data

As described above, the ideal situation is when accurately recorded point data on exposures and health outcomes are available. In practice, this will rarely be the case. In this Section we describe the data that are typically available.

When a case-control study is carried out, information on the population at risk is obtained via the exact locations of the control sample. More typically, population data—at least for routine inquiries—are based on aggregated counts. In Chapter 3 the data that are available for estimating the populations of small areas is reviewed. National population registers are the gold standard but only rarely are such data available and estimates are typically based on vital registration (births and deaths) and censuses. The latter provide a snapshot of the population on a specific date, stratified by age and sex and possibly other variables. The raw census counts are themselves estimates, being subject to miscount, with the more likely error being underenumeration. Often an attempt is made to correct the raw counts: for example, the *Estimating with confidence project* in the United Kingdom provided adjustments to the 1991 census population statistics (Simpson *et al.* 1996). Such work can give valuable information on the likely discrepancy between actual and estimated population sizes, as can local registers. In particular, errors-in-variables modelling (see Chapter 5) may utilise such information.

For inter-censual years, population counts must be estimated and must take into account not only the usual demographic changes (i.e. births/deaths) but also migration. Population projections beyond the most recent census (and perhaps before the earliest usable census) will also often be required for spatial studies. The frequent lack of a common geography between censuses introduces further problems when studies span more than one census or when a set of population estimates by year is required.

In England and Wales, 70% of the censual enumeration districts (EDs) changed between the 1981 and 1991 censuses whilst the geographical units were different again in 1971. For broad-scale studies these problems are likely to be less severe but, at the small-area scale, careful attention must be given to these issues.

As with population data, health data may be available with associated point locations, or as aggregated counts, and will potentially be subject to a number of inaccuracies. For any health event there is always the potential for diagnostic error or misclassification, especially at older ages where diagnostic tests and post-mortem examinations are carried out less frequently than at younger ages. Some events may be captured poorly, if at all, in routine registers (e.g. early abortions). For others, such as cancers, case registers may be subject to double counting and under-registration as well as diagnostic inaccuracies. Some assessment of the basic quality of the data is therefore essential to inform their use in spatial analyses (see Chapter 2).

Confounding can cause major difficulties in the interpretation of all epidemiological studies and spatial studies are no exception. Confounding occurs when variables other than the environmental exposure of interest are correlated with both the exposure and the disease outcome. In spatial studies, this occurs most evidently with socio-economic variables which are strong predictors of most health outcomes and are also highly correlated with many environmental exposures (see Chapters 4 and 5). For each of the four types of study described in the Introduction it is important to take account of socio-economic variables and this is especially true of point and line-source studies. Sources of pollution tend to be in socio-economically disadvantaged areas, whilst deprivation itself is strongly linked to ill-health and health-defining behaviour such as smoking. Failure to account for social deprivation can therefore seriously bias investigation of small-area health statistics. Area-level indices of deprivation may be constructed from census variables though this may only provide a crude adjustment for the underlying variables of interest (e.g. individual-level smoking, alcohol consumption, and diet). Ideally, we would wish to have direct measures of such variables at individual or small-area scale in order to explore and account for the potential confounding. Unfortunately, such data are rarely available unless obtained as part of special surveys.

1.3   Statistical methods

In this Section we briefly describe a Poisson process framework within which small-area studies may be viewed. This framework has been considered by a number of authors including Diggle (1990), Diggle and Elliott (1995), and Wakefield and Elliott (1999). For simplicity in the following we suppress dependence of the risk on all factors apart from spatial location.

Let x denote a two-dimensional spatial location and $\lambda_0(x)$ represent the intensity function of the population at risk. For a non-infectious disease (i.e. assuming no interaction between cases) we may then assume that cases are generated by a Poisson process with intensity function $\lambda_1(x)$ where

$$\lambda_1(x) = p(x) \times \lambda_0(x)$$

and $p(x) = \Pr(\text{disease} \mid \text{location } x)$. The statistical problem then is to estimate $p(x)$.

We first consider point (i.e. case-control) data, since these provide the closest link with the Poisson framework. The controls may be a random sample from the population at risk, or be cases of another disease which has a similar age/sex profile but is unrelated to the exposure in question.

Since we do not, in general, obtain the complete set of non-cases, we are required to introduce further notation. Let $\lambda_2(x)$ denote the intensity function of the controls where

$$\lambda_2(x) = c \times [\lambda_0(x) - \lambda_1(x)] \tag{1.1}$$

and $0 < c \le 1$ represents the probability of selection for a non-case.

Spatially referenced case-control data are commonly analysed as follows. Suppose we condition on location and let Y_i denote independent Bernoulli random variables with associated locations x_i, and $\Pr(Y_i = 1 | X = x_i) = p'(x_i)$ ($i = 1, \ldots, l$ cases; $i = l+1, \ldots, l+m$ controls) where

$$p'(x) = \frac{\lambda_1(x)}{\lambda_1(x) + \lambda_2(x)}.$$

From Equation (1.1)

$$\frac{p'(x)}{1 - p'(x)} = \frac{\lambda_1(x)}{\lambda_2(x)} = \frac{p(x)}{1 - p(x)} \times \frac{1}{c}$$

providing a link between $p'(x)$ and $p(x)$. Hence, although we obviously cannot recover $\lambda_0(x)$ and $\lambda_1(x)$, we can estimate the ratio of the odds of disease at different locations.

The general approach with point data (Diggle and Rowlingson 1994) is to model the probabilities $p'(x)$ via

$$\operatorname{logit} p'(x) = \alpha + f(x; \theta)$$

where $f(x; \theta)$ represents a simple function, depending on parameters θ, which describes the effect of being at location x. For example, $f(\cdot, \cdot)$ may depend on the distance from x to the location of a putative source (see Chapter 9). Alternatively we may take $f(x; \theta) = W(x)\theta$ where $W(x)$ is a measured or modelled exposure (Chapter 10) and θ is the odds ratio. Incorporating individual-level covariates such as age and sex, and area-level covariates such as deprivation, is straightforward.

Now suppose that count data are available and let Y_i denote the observed disease count within areas A_i which contain populations N_i, $i = 1, \ldots, n$. The assumption of a Poisson process then implies $N_i \sim \text{Poisson}(\lambda_{0i})$ and $Y_i \sim \text{Poisson}(\lambda_{1i})$ where

$$\lambda_{li} = \int_{A_i} \lambda_l(x) \mathrm{d}x,$$

for $l = 1, 2$. Note that with count data we can gain no information *within* cell A_i. In particular, we do not know the form of the relationship within a cell and so we cannot evaluate these integrals. A major problem in small-area count-based studies is the possibility of ecological bias, which may arise when individual response/exposure relationships are estimated from data aggregated across groups—areas in this case (see English 1992 and Chapters 5 and 11 for a discussion).

When, as is usual, populations are statified by age and sex, with strata indexed by j say, then we have $Y_{ij} \sim$ Binomial(N_{ij}, p_{ij}) where Y_{ij} is the number of cases, N_{ij} is the population, and p_{ij} is the probability of disease, in area i and stratum j. We may then model $p_{ij} = \mu_i p_j$ where p_j is the probability of disease in stratum j (in a reference region) and μ_i is the *relative risk* (or standardised mortality/morbidity ratio, SMR) in area i, assumed constant across stratum. If the disease is rare then we may take $Y_{ij} \sim$ Poisson$(N_{ij} \times p_{ij})$ and then $Y_i = \sum_j Y_{ij} \sim$ Poisson$(E_i \theta_i)$ where the *expected number* of cases E_i, $i = 1, \ldots, n$ is given by $E_i = \sum_j N_{ij} p_j$ (see Chapter 7). Again area-level covariates such as deprivation may be incorporated in a straightforward manner.

The above framework is often implicit in many of the methods that have been proposed for the analysis of spatial epidemiological data although some non-parametric methods make minimal assumptions (see Chapters 8 and 9).

1.4   Disease mapping and clustering

The production of disease atlases has a long tradition. The maps provide a rapid visual summary of complex geographical information, and are used variously for descriptive purposes, to generate hypotheses as to aetiology, for surveillance to highlight areas at apparently high risk, and to aid policy formation and resource allocation. Increasingly, disease mapping at the small-area scale is being carried out.

Unfortunately, naive use of mapping can be highly misleading. Potential problems include data quality and completeness issues discussed in Section 1.2, distinguishing 'true' from apparent areas of disease excess, and dealing appropriately with the play of chance including the problem of multiple significance testing. Often, the raw SMRs (which are given by Y_i / E_i) are mapped. Problems are most evident in small-area disease mapping since numbers of cases tend to be small and apparent large variability across the map may merely reflect random variation. Specifically, large sparsely populated areas with few cases may predominate since the variance of the SMRs is inversely related to E_i and so small populations imply large variability in estimated rates (see Chapter 15 for further discussion).

Methods based on Bayesian statistics (Clayton and Kaldor 1987) have been used to remove the random component from the map; Chapter 7 contains a description of these methods. Such methods model the collection of 'random effects' θ_i, $i = 1, \ldots, n$ as arising from a probability (or *prior*) distribution. Assuming that these random effects are independent realisations from a distribution is known as a 'heterogeneity' prior, whilst assuming that neighbouring μ_i are correlated leads to a 'clustering' prior. Clustering *and* heterogeneity may also be considered jointly (Besag *et al.* 1991).

A putative disease cluster may first be identified by concerned members of the public, be reported by the media, or perhaps come to light following concerns about a pollution source in the vicinity. In any event, the local public health department often finds itself compelled to respond, if only to allay public anxiety. Note that as areas at apparent 'low' risk do not come to the attention of the authorities, there is built-in bias towards reporting disease excess (Chapter 5). Apparent clusters may appear purely as a chance finding, particularly for rare events such as many cancers. Often in the investigation of an apparent disease cluster, reassurance is all that is required since, for rare diseases in small areas, the excess may depend crucially on only one or two cases—and these may not stand detailed scrutiny during an initial case-by-case review (CDC 1990). Such a review deals only with the numerator (cases) of the risk estimate, whereas a proper epidemiological enquiry is concerned also with the denominator (population) and the time-frame over which the 'cluster' is assumed to occur. Decisions taken at this stage may be critical as apparent 'clusters' may depend crucially on the boundaries chosen in time or space: 'The more narrowly the underlying population is defined, the less will be the number of expected cases, the greater will be the estimate of the excess rate, and often the more pronounced will be the statistical significance' (Olsen *et al.* 1996).

The statistical problem is to estimate the risk surface $\lambda_1(x)/\lambda_0(x)$ (Section 1.3). Locations x may be highlighted as the location of a 'cluster' if they exceed a given threshold of risk. In this way an observed collection of cases is replaced by an estimated risk surface. As Alexander and Cuzick (1992) point out, identifying a cluster or clustering based on a mathematical definition is far more straightforward than a definition based on an empirical set of data.

The existence of large geographically referenced health datasets inevitably raises the questions of surveillance for cluster detection; this topic is discussed in Chapter 8.

If a cluster detection system is to be considered then a number of issues must be addressed:

• in the surveillance of large databases an assessment of data quality is vital,
• for chronic diseases the excess relative risk is likely to be low,
• on considering the available choices of age, sex, disease, space, and time, there is clearly the potential for large multiple testing difficulties,
• the problems of confounding described in Section 1.2 are clearly relevant, and
• sensitivity/specificity needs to be considered: what elevated risk is detectable given the spatial extent and temporal persistence?

As noted in Section 1.1 above, conceptually more satisfying than dealing with reports of individual 'clusters' is the study of disease clustering, which if present may give clues as to possible causes of the disease (e.g. an infectious aetiology, Alexander *et al.* 1989). The study of clustering has much in common with disease mapping and the same cautionary notes apply.

1.5   Exposure modelling and mapping

Accurate estimation and mapping of exposures is clearly vital if valid inferences are to be drawn either about the spatial distribution of risk factors, or about their geographical relationship with health outcome. In this context, we will use the term 'exposure' to refer to all explanatory variables which may be considered to have a putative association with disease status. Therefore, it includes confounders, such as social deprivation and genetic characteristics of the population, as well as other social and environmental factors.

Obtaining reliable exposure data is problematic—and in many cases represents the weakest link in epidemiological investigation. Exposures often vary markedly both between individuals, and for any individual over time, making it difficult to derive valid exposure assessments even for small geographical areas. Where suitable measures (e.g. biomarkers) exist, individual exposure sampling or biological monitoring potentially offer the most accurate methods (Chapter 20), but these tend to be both costly and invasive. For many exposures of interest, suitable measures or monitoring devices are also unavailable or of doubtful quality. Direct, individual exposure data are therefore only rarely available. Alternatively, exposure estimates may be made on the basis of environmental monitoring, either using data from pre-existing monitoring networks or through purpose-designed surveys. Because routine monitoring is usually undertaken for reasons other than exposure assessment, however, existing networks tend to provide an inadequate basis for exposure assessment: few sites may be available, the distribution of the sites is not likely to reflect the population distribution, and relevant pollutants may not be measured. Purpose-designed surveys may help to overcome these limitations, but available technologies are limited and intensive or prolonged surveys are expensive. Where suitable monitoring data are available, some form of spatial interpolation may need to be carried out in order to model the pollutant surface (where this can be conceived as a continuous surface), or to estimate individual exposures at unsampled locations (e.g. the place of residence of cases and controls) (Chapters 19 and 22). The availability of geographical information systems (GIS) has greatly enhanced the capability for spatial interpolation of exposure data (Briggs and Elliott 1995): Chapter 23 provides several examples. Kriging (Cressie 1993; Chapter 10), in particular, provides a set of powerful techniques for this purpose. The method of construction of such maps is, however, crucial, and the quality of the mapping clearly depends on the accuracy and representativeness of the available input data, as well as the inherent validity of the interpolation method used.

A further alternative is to model pollutant concentrations using dispersion models (Chapter 21). In the case of atmospheric pollution, a wide range of models have been developed—though relatively few have as yet been used for exposure assessment. For other environmental media—for example, food and drinking water (Chapter 24)—dispersion modelling is much less evolved, and the principles are more difficult to apply because of the highly complex and non-diffusive pathways involved. The modelling of pathways of exposure to foodborne contaminants in the context of modern, international food distribution systems is, for example, an urgent and challenging research problem. Whatever the medium, modelling is also constrained by the availability of reliable data on both the source activity and emissions, and the environmental conditions affecting dispersion. Modelled results also need to be validated against independent monitored data, wherever possible.

In the light of these difficulties, many epidemiological studies have traditionally used simpler, proxy measures of exposure, such as distance from source (Elliott *et al.* 1996a; Livingstone *et al.* 1996), level of source activity (Wjst *et al.* 1993; Brunekreef *et al.* 1997), or land use (Barbone *et al.* 1995; Sainsbury *et al.* 1996). These may be related either to individual residences (point data) or to the population centroid of, for example, a small census area (count data). Such measures are, however, often highly uncertain. Relationships with actual exposures are commonly unknown, and may be expected to be strongly non-linear due to the pattern of pollutant concentrations with distance from the source. Whilst concentrations of traffic-related pollution away from a roadway in relatively flat terrain may show a more-or-less exponential distance-decay, for example, emissions from a high level point-source (e.g. a chimney stack) may result in peak ground-level concentrations at some distance from the source, resulting in a skewed Gaussian distribution.

It is also important to recognise that all exposures estimates, based on point measurements of environmental pollution, pollution models or simple proxy measures, tend to imply gross approximations of actual exposures, in that they do not take direct account of the movement of people within the pollution field. Without a knowledge of time activity and behavioural patterns (Chapter 19), exposure assessment is inherently flawed. Where strong aetiological hypotheses do not exist for the exposures and health outcome of interest, uncertainties may also exist in defining the most appropriate exposure measure. This problem is exemplified by the continuing debate about atmospheric particulate pollution and respiratory health: which size fraction should be measured, whether concentrations should be determined in terms of mass measurements or particle counts, and what averaging periods should be used are all-important questions both for epidemiological studies and for policy. Much yet has to be learned, therefore, to provide a sound basis for exposure assessment.

1.6   Combining health and exposure data

There are numerous examples of geographical studies, at various scales, in which health and exposure data are combined. At the broadest scale, international differences in disease occurrence may be exploited to gain important clues as to aetiology. For example, Keys (1970) described large differences in population saturated fat intakes, which were predictive of population differences in the occurrence of coronary heart disease. The INTERSALT study (Elliott *et al.* 1996*b*) found cross-population variation in average differences in blood pressure with age that were positively associated with average levels of salt intake (measured by urinary sodium excretion); a positive relationship was also found between urinary sodium excretion and blood pressure at the individual-level. Other examples include the incidence of malignant melanoma and multiple sclerosis, both of which are strongly related to latitude. For melanoma there is a tendency for higher rates near the equator, reflecting greater exposure to sunlight (English 1992), while for multiple sclerosis there tends to be low incidence in countries near the equator (Kurtzke 1985).

At the medium geographical scale, various exposures involving air, water, soil, and radiation have been examined via geographical studies. The 'six cities' study (Dockery *et al.* 1993) examined mortality in relation to particulate matter in six US cities, while Pope *et al.* (1995) examined the same relationship in 151 US metropolitan areas. Shaper *et al.* (1980) investigated the relationship between water hardness and cardiovascular disease in towns in Great Britain. Maheswaran *et al.* (1999) also assessed the hard water story using an ecological correlation study across water zones in northwest England. In this study, water hardness variables and potential confounders were measured in the water supply and related to mortality from acute myocardial infarction. Staessen *et al.* (1999) examined the relationship between exposure to cadmium and bone density in ten districts of Belgium (including six that bordered on three zinc smelters). A number of ecological and case-control studies have investigated the relationship between radon and lung cancer; for a discussion of these see Brownson and Alavanja (1997).

At a small geographical scale, a number of studies by the UK Small Area Health Statistics Unit have investigated exposures in air, water and soil. Chapter 9 describes the approach used in such studies in relation to pre-specified sources. Another example is the study by Elliott *et al.* (2000) to investigate the association between mortality, cancer incidence, and stroke in the village of Shipham which had high levels of cadmium in the soil. For some exposures, such as non-ionising radiation from powerlines, the potential harmful effects may operate over a very small distance (up to 50–100 metres from the power line) so that only a highly localised study may investigate the issue.

The advantage of small-area studies is that the potential for ecological bias (Chapters 5 and 11) is reduced (although other problems, such as migration, are likely to be more pronounced than when larger areas are considered). The 'six cities' air pollution study and the hard water study in the northwest of England are mixed-level analyses in the sense that, although the ecological level at which the exposure was measured is at one (larger) level, adjustment for confounders is carried out at another (finer) level.

1.7   Conclusions

When a spatial epidemiological study is envisaged to investigate the relation between exposure and health there are a number of important considerations. Ideally, one will have exposure variation across the study population but, in the case of ecological studies, little variation within areas. The availability of confounder information is also vital. Without these basic requirements advanced statistical methods are unlikely to aid the analysis. Such methods are most important for small-area studies into rare diseases since, in this case, sampling variability is likely to dominate and spatial dependence between health events will also need to be dealt with. These problems, together with many of the other methodological and interpretational issues raised in this chapter, are discussed throughout the remainder of this volume.

References

Alexander, F. and Cuzick, J. (1992). Methods for the assessment of disease clusters. In *Geographical and environmental epidemiology: methods for small-area studies* (P. Elliott, J. Cuzick, D. English, and R. Stern ed.), 238–50. Oxford University Press.

Alexander, F. E., Williams, J., Cartwright, R. A., and Ricketts, T. J. (1989). A specialist leukaemia/lymphoma registry in the UK. 2: clustering of Hodgkin's disease. *British Journal of Cancer*, **60**, 948–52.

Barbone, F., Bovenzi, M., Cavallieri, F., and Stanta, G. (1995). Air pollution and lung cancer in Trieste, Italy. *American Journal of Epidemiology*, **141**, 1161–9.

Baris, Y. I., Simonato, L., Atrinli, M., Pooley, S., Saracci, R., Skidmore, J. *et al.* (1987). Epidemiological and environmental evidence of the health effects of exposure to erionite fibres: a four year study in the Cappodocian region of Turkey. *International Journal of Cancer*, **39**, 10–17.

Besag, J., York, J., and Mollié, A. (1991). Bayesian image restoration with two applications in spatial statistics. *Annals of the Institute of Statics and Mathematics*, **43**, 1–59.

Briggs, D. J. and Elliott, P. (1995). GIS methods for the analysis of relationships between environment and health. *World Health Statistics Quarterly*, **48**, 85–94.

Briggs, D. J., Collins, S., Elliott, P., Fischer, P., Kingham, S., Lebret, E. *et al.* (1997). Mapping urban air pollution using GIS: a regression-based approach. *International Journal of Geographical Information Science*, **11**, 699–718.

Brownson, R. C. and Alavanja, M. C. R. (1997). Radiation I: Radon. In *Topics in environmental epidemiology* (K. Steenland and D. Savitz ed.), 269–94. Oxford University Press, New York.

Brunekreef, B., Janssen, N. A. H., de Hartog, J., Harssema, H., Knape, M. *et al.* (1997). Air pollution from truck traffic and lung function in children living near motorways. *Epidemiology*, **8**, 298–303.

CDC (Centers for Disease Control) (1990). *Guidelines for investigating clusters of health events.* CDC, Atlanta, GA.

Clayton, D. G. and Kaldor, J. (1987). Empirical Bayes estimates of age-standardized relative risks for use in disease mapping. *Biometrics*, **43**, 671–82.

Cressie, N. (1993). *Statistics for Spatial Data* (rev. edn). Wiley, New York.

Diggle, P. (1990). A point process modelling approach to raised incidence of a rare phenomenon in the vicinity of a prespecified point. *Journal of the Royal Statistical Society, Series A*, **153**, 340–62.

Diggle, P. and Elliott, P. (1995). Disease risk near point sources: statistical analyses for analyses using individually or spatially aggregated data. *Journal of Epidemiology and Community Health*, **49**, S20–S27.

Diggle, P. J. and Rowlingson, B. S. (1994). A conditional approach to point process modelling of raised incidence. *Journal of the Royal Statistical Society, Series A*, **157**, 433–440.

Dockery, D. W., Pope, C. A. III, Xu, X., Spengler, J. D., Ware, J. H., Ray, M. E. *et al.* (1993). An association between air pollution and mortality in six US cities. *New England Journal of Medicine*, **329**, 1753–9.

Elliott, P., Shaddick, G., Kleinschmidt, I., Jolley, D., Walls, P., Beresford, J. *et al.* (1996*a*). Cancer incidence near municipal solid waste incinerators in Great Britain. *British Journal of Cancer*, **73**, 702–7.

Elliott, P., Stamler, J., Nichols, R., Dyer, A. R., Stamler, R., Kesteloot, H. *et al.* (1996*b*). Intersalt revisited: further analyses of 24 hour sodium excretion and blood pressure within and across populations. *British Medical Journal*, **312**, 1249–53.

Elliott, P., Arnold, R., Cockings, S., Eaton, N., Jarup, L., Jones, J. *et al.* (2000). Risk of mortality, cancer incidence and stroke in a population potentially exposed to cadmium. *Occupational and Environmental Medicine*, **57**, 94–7.

English, D. (1992). Geographical epidemiology and ecological studies. In *Geographical and environmental epidemiology: methods for small-area studies* (P. Elliott, J. Cuzick, D. English, and R. Stern ed.), 3–13. Oxford University Press.

Keys, A. (ed.) (1970). *Coronary heart disease in seven countries*, American Heart Association Monograph 29. American Heart Association, New York.

Kurtzke, J. F. (1985) Neurological system. In *Oxford textbook of public health.* Vol. 4, 203–49. Oxford University Press.

Livingstone, A. E., Shaddick, G., Grundy, C., and Elliott, P. (1996). Do people living near inner city main roads have more asthma needing treatment? Case control study. *British Medical Journal*, **312**, 676–7.

Maheswaran, R., Morris, S., Falconer, S., Grossinho, A., Perry, I., Wakefield, J. *et al.* (1999). Magnesium in drinking water supplies and mortality from acute myocardial infarction in North West England. *Heart*, **82**, 455–60.

Olsen, S. F., Martuzzi, M., and Elliott, P. (1996). Cluster analysis and disease mapping—why, when and how? A step by step guide. *British Medical Journal*, **313**, 863–86.

Pope, C. A., Thun, M. J., Namboodiri, M. M., Dockery, D., Evans, J., Speizer, F. *et al.* (1995). Particulate air pollution as a predictor of mortality in a prospective study of US adults. *American Journal of Respiratory Critical Care Medicine*, **151**, 669–74.

Richardson, S. (1992). Statistical methods for geographical correlation studies. In *Geograpical and environmental epidemiology: methods for small-area studies* (P. Elliott, J. Cuzick, D. English, and R. Stern ed.), 181–204. Oxford University Press.

Sainsbury, P., Hussey, R, Ashton, J., and Andrews, B. (1996). Industrial atmospheric pollution, historical land use patterns and mortality. *Journal of Public Health Medicine*, **18**, 87–93.

Shaper, A. G., Packham, R. F., and Pocock, S. J. (1980). The British regional heart study: cardiovascular mortality and water quality. *Journal of Environmental Pathology and Toxicology*, **143**, 456–62.

Simpson, S., Diamond, I., Tankin, P., and Tyre, R. (1996). Updating small area population estimates in England and Wales. *Journal of the Royal Statistical Society, Series A*, **159**, 235–47.

Staessen, J. A., Roels, H. A., Emelianov, D., Kuznetsova, T., Thijs, L., Vangronsveld, J. *et al.* (1999). Environmental exposure to cadmium, forearm bone density, and risk of fractures: prospective population study. *Lancet*, **353**, 1140–4.

Wakefield, J. C. and Elliott, P. (1999). Issues in the statistical analysis of small area health data. *Statistics in Medicine*, **18**, 2377–99.

Wjst, M., Reitmeir, P., Dold, S., Wulff, A., Nicolai, T., Freifrau von Loeffelholz-Colberg, E. *et al.* (1993). Road traffic and adverse effects on respiratory health in children. *British Medical Journal*, **307**, 596–600.

2. Health event data

A. Staines and L. Järup

2.1 Introduction

Epidemiologists are accustomed to collecting and working with data of limited quality. Many epidemiological studies use information collected for other purposes, for example, exposure information from occupational work records and disease information from medical records. It is not usually the investigating researchers who collect routinely available health data. The data quantities are often extensive, and files containing several millions of records are not unusual. While each data source is different, there are some common problems and pitfalls. The objective of this chapter is to serve as guidance to those setting out to analyse large health-related datasets. Specific problems, only arising in spatial analyses of health event data, are discussed. The focus in this chapter is mainly European systems, especially in the UK and the Scandinavian countries, although many of the issues are applicable to other industrialised countries.

2.2 Data availability and quality

2.2.1 Sources of data

Data for spatial analysis often arise from several different sources, and have seldom been gathered with the interests of the geographical epidemiologist in mind. A detailed knowledge of the various sources of data is vital. Simply to accept the data as presented may introduce fatal errors into the analyses. Even if a data source is known to be complete and of excellent quality, subtle differences in coding practice, in data entry systems, or a host of other factors may need to be considered before firm conclusions can be drawn from the results of analyses.

There are several different types of data source which are commonly made available for spatial analysis. Sources of routine health and vital statistics data available in the UK are summarised in Table 2.1.

While there are important, and occasionally vast, differences between countries in these systems, nonetheless there are some common points which are worth commenting on. Censuses are of fundamental importance for spatial epidemiology, and are covered in detail in the next chapter.

This chapter concerns records of specific health-related events at the individual-level. Such event data comes from three main kinds of data source; statutory, or effectively statutory registration systems, administrative systems of many different types, and disease registers or special surveys. These systems have important common features, and can be discussed under these broad headings.

Table 2.1 Examples of routine health and vital statistics data available in the United Kingdom (adapted from Elliott and Briggs 1997)

Data	Source*	Comment
Mortality	ONS GROS(S) DHSS(NI)	Complete, but diagnostic accuracy and coding of underlying cause of death may vary
Births	ONS GRO(S) DHSS(NI)	Complete. Provides individual data on birth weights, and postcoded denominator data for early childhood events
Stillbirths	ONS GRO(S) DHSS(NI)	Data on stillbirths complete, but data on early and late abortions not routinely available
Cancer incidence	ONS ISD	Various degrees of underascertainment and duplication, both between registries and at sub-regional level. The quality of the national register has improved in recent years.
Congenital malformations	ONS ISD	Major problems of underascertainment in national registers. Some specialised local registries have much higher levels of ascertainment. A high quality linked database is being produced in Scotland.
Hospital admissions data: Hospital Episode Statistics (England), Patient Episode Database for Wales, Scottish Morbidity Record, and Hospital Inpatient System (N Ireland)	DH WHCSA ISD DHSS(NI)	Huge database (approx. 10 million records/year in England). Episode-based, not person-based, in England and Wales. Diagnostic accuracy, coding, etc. varies between hospitals. Linked individual database available in Scotland.

*Some of these data may also be available from local sources (e.g. district health authorities, regional offices, and regional cancer registries).

ONS	Office for National Statistics
GRO(S)	General Register Office, Scotland
DHSS(NI)	Department of Health and Social Services, Northern Ireland
ISD	Information and Statistics Division of the National Health Service in Scotland
DH	Department of Health (England)

2.2.2 Statutory registration systems

For historical and practical reasons most states operate a small common core of registration systems. These registers frequently contain the best quality data available for spatial epidemiology work. However, they have been designed to serve the interests and needs of the state, and it is essential to have an intimate knowledge of their procedures and practices before using such data.

Mortality recording

Some form of recording of deaths is nearly universal amongst modern states. In developed countries the fact of death is usually very well recorded, although there may be gross systematic errors between specific causes of death. There are international standards specifying which items of information should be recorded, and a majority of states adhere to these (Ashley and Devis 1992).

Records of location at death can be surprisingly inaccurate, and rules may not be uniformly applied. For example, Williams *et al.* (1990) in a study from rural Minnesota found that almost one in four reported cases of cancer were not actually resident in the area to which they had been allocated based on their death certificates. This had the effect of abolishing a striking excess of reported cancer mortality in these areas. In the UK, the Office for National Statistics (ONS) has a rule that the place of death should not be given as the institution in which death occurred, unless the deceased had been resident there for at least six months.

Errors in coding pose a wider range of problems. While standard death certificates provide space for several codes, in many countries only one code is captured and recorded: in principle, the underlying cause of death as determined from the coding rules provided with the International Classification of Diseases (currently ICD-10) (WHO 1992). These rules are complex, and unless coding staff are carefully trained and regularly supervised, substantial errors in coding may occur. The vagaries of the causes recorded by individual medical practitioners have also been extensively studied, as have temporal shifts in fashionable diagnoses. Lopez (1992) gives a concise review of these issues.

There may also be substantial differences between countries in the way in which these rules are applied. A recent and striking example of this is the adoption by the English ONS of an automated cause of death coding system of American design (Birch 1993). This allocated a significantly higher number of deaths to pneumonia, and produced a distinct break in the time series for this condition. An extensive series of studies on death certification and diabetes has shown that over a third of the between-country variation in diabetes as a cause of death is due to different practices of physicians (Jougla *et al.* 1992; Balkau *et al.* 1993; Fuller 1993). These differences are large enough to render comparisons of international mortality for this diagnosis meaningless. Other cause of death diagnoses may be more reliable, but great care should always be exercised. This issue is also discussed in Chapter 12 where an example of a European atlas is presented (see Plate 2).

An example of a coding change which is of particular interest to epidemiologists is the shift from coding Sudden Infant Death Syndrome (SIDS) as respiratory disease to using the specific SIDS code, which came into use in 1979 (Khoury *et al.* 1984). This shift seems to have been due to an increasing awareness of SIDS amongst coders, as well as among doctors, and less reluctance to admit that for these children the cause of death was unknown.

Mortality data from routine sources can be a useful adjunct to other data sources. McClain *et al.* (1993) studied child abuse and neglect by merging death certificate data with data from other studies, to estimate by age, sex, and code group what proportion of recorded deaths in selected groups were likely to be due to intentional child abuse. This general approach, using several sources of data to complement each other, is likely to be widely applicable. A similar approach was used by Johansen *et al.* (1992) who studied asthma amongst children in Manitoba, and used several sources of data to conclude that an apparent increase in hospital admissions for this condition was probably real.

Birth recording

Again, for historical reasons, most states register births. Like death recording, the fact of birth is unambiguous. However, rules on what should be counted as births vary greatly.

There are rules based on gestational age and rules based on birthweight. There are also different rules for live births and stillbirths. Furthermore, small changes in the rules, or in their interpretation, could have important effects on certain groups of births. Definition of low birthweight is a case in point, for example whether it is defined as births less than 2500 g or 2500 g and under (Edouard and Senthilselvan 1997). For this reason international comparisons of birth records may be difficult. Several investigators have studied international comparability in birth registration practices (Alberman *et al.* 1989; Cole *et al.* 1989; Evans *et al.* 1989). These studies have confirmed the presence of substantial variation. For example, Ireland and the United Kingdom have separate systems for birth registration and birth notification, and these two systems may give different results (Hilder and Alberman 1998). Some countries have sophisticated birth registration systems (e.g. in Sweden a lot of maternal data is recorded, including information on maternal smoking). Despite the comprehensive data collection, the register has had some deficiencies, mainly concerning erroneous information on previous pregnancies and lack of diagnoses during pregnancy and for the newborn child. A persisting problem is the variability in the use of diagnoses (Cnattingius *et al.* 1995).

Infectious disease recording

Many countries have a statutory infectious disease notification system. Typically, these are based on reports from primary care and hospital practitioners. In some cases these systems are fairly complete, but in most countries it seems likely that they capture only a small proportion of infectious diseases (Barrett and Lau 1997; Finger and Auslander 1997; Seneviratne *et al.* 1997). Systems of registration vary from country to country (Anonymous 1996, 1997). Furthermore, the incompleteness of reporting varies enormously between different infections: HIV reporting is probably far more reliable than food poisoning reports, for example. For the purposes of spatial epidemiology these systems are of limited use. It may be possible to conduct some analyses for restricted areas or for specific diseases: Staines and Schweiger (1995), for example, studied ward-level variation in infectious disease notifications in Leeds, England, while Bhopal *et al.* (1992) investigated clustering of Legionnaires disease in Scotland (Bhopal *et al.* 1992). It is encouraging to note that a relatively modest intervention can produce significant improvements in reporting from physicians (Squires *et al.* 1998).

2.2.3 Administrative systems

Unlike the registration systems described above, administrative systems are created to facilitate the day-to-day running of a service (e.g. in-patient audit or Accident and Emergency attendances). These systems are often good at tracking bed use or payments, but relatively poor at anything else. All too often, the defects of these systems are discussed in reports that were produced for internal use, and never reach medical and scientific indexing systems. The very valuable reports of the NHS Clinical Coding Standards Group are a good example.

Hospital admissions

Many industrialised countries now have well-developed and elaborate systems for capturing hospital activity. England was one of the first countries to establish these

(Ashley 1972). Problems with the English systems have, however, given hospital data a poor reputation. This appears to have improved in recent years, since these data are now used for payment to hospitals. Other European countries are still said to have better systems, although very little comparative work appears to have been published.

The Irish system, known as the hospital in-patient enquiry (HIPE), typifies many of the problems of such systems. When this system was first established it was voluntary, and for many years fewer than 70% of all admissions to state-funded hospitals were recorded. Coding staff were poorly paid, and coding was viewed as unimportant both by clinical staff and by hospital managers. A decision by the Irish Department of Health to base hospital funding on HIPE returns has produced a transformation in the last six years. HIPE is now believed to be very complete, and coding staff are well-trained, and quite closely supervised from a single central office. Unpublished assessments suggest that HIPE coding is now quite reliable, and should provide a solid base for further work in the future. A similar decision by the English Department of Health had a similar impact on the English equivalent, the Hospital Episode System (HES).

The major problem with these systems is the degree of inter-hospital variation in coding practice. This can be substantial, and only regular and detailed hospital-by-hospital reviews can detect it. In England, these are carried out by the NHS Coding Centre in Loughborough, and regular reports are published for NHS regions. It remains disturbingly easy to identify changes in coding staff hospital-by-hospital, and misunderstandings of some of the fundamental rules by coding staff can produce substantial differences between hospitals in HES results. When conducting spatial analyses the only real defence against making very serious errors of inference is a detailed knowledge of the coding rules, and a keen awareness of common misunderstandings. In addition, some sort of statistical correction for differences between hospitals (i.e. 'hospital effects') is required (Bottle *et al.* 1999).

Some examples may help to clarify this point. Some errors are obvious, such as the miscoding of chest infections in small children as chronic obstructive airways disease (COAD), surprisingly common in the English HES data (Staines *et al.* unpublished observations). Other errors are less likely to be detected, unless it is possible to check routine data against hospital charts directly. During the late 1980s, for example, several hospitals in Yorkshire miscoded enuresis (bed-wetting) consistently as insulin-dependent diabetes (Staines *et al.* unpublished observations).

Retraining of coders can produce quite large shifts in diagnostic categories. Coders working on the Irish HIPE system were carefully instructed in how to apply ICD-9 rules for COAD, as opposed to bronchitis and pneumonia. This resulted in a marked decline in COAD admissions, with a concomitant rise in those due to bronchitis and pneumonia (Ann Clifton, personal communication). While precise codes may have poor validity, broader categories, for example three-digit ICD codes, are likely to be much more reliable (Dixon *et al.* 1998).

In Sweden, the *Patient Register* records all completed hospital admissions, with personal identification number included for the periods 1978–83 and from 1992 onwards for somatic care, and for 1973–83 as well as from 1992 onwards for psychiatric care. The personal identification number allows linkage to be made to other health and vital statistics data, and to population registers (see Section 2.4.3). The reason for the missing data for 1984 to 1991 was a political decision based on a public debate on confidentiality. It was later decided, however, that the benefits from having personal identification numbers in the register outweighed the disadvantages. The missing data have since been entered into the register. The Patient Register has also suffered from problems associated with data collection over long periods of time, mainly because of changes in administrative boundaries (Thomas Gunnarsson, Statistics Sweden, personal communication). Further- more, some additional problems have occurred because of mismatching between the hospital records and the population records. This mismatching was caused by some individuals' failure to give notice of changed residence.

Despite the caveats, hospital admissions data can be very valuable. They may be used as an adjunct to other sources of data, both to improve and to estimate completeness of ascertainment (Staines *et al.* 1993; Hook and Regal 1995; Shevchenko *et al.* 1995). They may be used as the principal data source for a study as, for example, in a series of studies of air pollution and health (Johansen *et al.* 1992; Anderson *et al.* 1995; Schwarz 1995). Nonetheless, hospital admissions data require considerable care if they are to be used properly. A careful choice of the disease groups and the codes for inclusion in a study, selection of appropriate reference rates, proper treatment of possible 'hospital effects', and a detailed understanding of the biases involved will help to ensure that valid inferences can be drawn.

Prescription systems

In countries where many prescriptions are paid for by the state, and where the regulation of drug sales is effective, prescription systems may be valuable sources of information. In practice, while they have been extensively used at national and regional levels in the pursuit of limiting prescribing costs, studies using them for spatial analysis are rare. The English NHS Prescription Pricing Authority system, for example, could be used for small-area analysis by using practice locations as a proxy for patient locations, but this seems not to have been done.

General practice

Primary care services, unlike hospital services, are variably developed in different countries. They are a valuable source of data about morbidity in the population. In principle, spatial, temporal, and other variations in general practice activity could be the most powerful epidemiological tools for the detection of weak environmental hazards. Unfortunately, a multitude of factors conspire to prevent this.

General practice computer systems have, quite often, been designed with epidemi- ological uses in mind. Unfortunately, there are many different systems in use, many practices use no system at all, and there is no quality control of the data. The English Read code system (O'Neil *et al.* 1995) was a valiant, but so far unsuccessful, attempt to provide a uniform and pragmatic coding system for general practice. Existing coding systems, such as ICD-9, ICD-9CM and ICD-10 (WHO 1977; Commission on Professional and Hospital Activities 1978; WHO 1992), are almost useless for general practice coding. Until these problems are solved, general practice data will only be useful as a supplement to other data, and even then only at a coarse level of geographical resolution. This is a serious limitation for geographical epidemiology. An example of mapping of infectious disease data from general practice is given in Chapter 14.

2.2.4 Specialised registers

A large number of specialised registers have been established to study various diseases. The commonest registers appear to be cancer and congenital malformation registers, and specialised disease registers such as for insulin-dependent diabetes mellitus (IDDM). This is partly for historical reasons and partly for reasons of convenience. Cancer has often been registered because it is common and has been seen as a mysterious and frightening disease. Registration of congenital malformations in the UK was started following the thalidomide disaster. IDDM has often been registered, perhaps because it is the easiest of the serious chronic diseases to register (Green *et al.* 1992). As a result, there is a great deal of published information about the design and conduct of registers for these conditions. For work on cancer in particular, the volumes of the Cancer Incidence in Five Continents series (Parkin *et al.* 1997) are indispensable.

In principle, specialist registers are no different from other sources of routine data, but in practice the quality of the data is often considerably higher. This is due to a combination of the focus of the register, and of the larger resource available per health event in a typical register, compared with, for example, hospital admissions data. For spatial analysis, where often only small differences in risk are expected, register data are usually superior to other kinds of routine data.

There are some conditions where registration has had problems. Congenital anomaly registers are an interesting example (Lechat and Dolk 1993). For several reasons it is hard to notify congenital anomalies. Many are not obvious, and some are not even detectable at birth. This is especially true for congenital cardiac defects, which have seldom been well registered by national or regional systems. Children tend to be born in one facility, and diagnosed elsewhere. For example, ONS in England runs a national system for reporting congenital anomalies. Despite extensive effort by ONS staff, this register, like many other such registers (Johnson *et al.* 1985), has been relatively incomplete (Cuckle *et al.* 1991; Mutton *et al.* 1991; Hey *et al.* 1994). However, it remains invaluable as a supplement to local registers, and as coverage gradually improves it will become an even more valuable resource for epidemiological enquiry.

Leukaemias and lymphomas are another example. For several reasons, including the deficiencies of ICD-9 and the differences between the ways in which haematological and pathological specimens are handled in hospital, the regional cancer registers in England have found it difficult to obtain acceptably complete registration of these conditions (Cartwright *et al.* 1990). This only became apparent when a large specialised register was established. This serves to emphasise the importance of detailed knowledge of the rules and procedures of sources of health data, before using them.

A rather different approach to linking health events, areas and people is carried out in some Scandinavian countries. These person-based health information systems have been widely used for epidemiological work including many studies on perinatal events, IDDM and a range of other diseases (Vågerö and Norell 1989; Lund *et al.* 1990; Cnattingius and Haglund 1992; Dahlquist and Källen 1992; Cnattingius *et al.* 1995; Jakobsson *et al.* 1997; Jiang *et al.* 1997; Rydstroem 1998).

In Sweden, for example, several registers are maintained at the Centre for Epidemiology, National Board of Health and Welfare in Stockholm. The *Cancer Register* started in 1958 and all primary cancers are reported to the register. The number of cases is around 40 000 yearly and so far 1 290 000 malignant and benign tumours have been registered. The completeness and accuracy of the register are high. The *Cancer Environment Register* includes persons who can be found in the 1960 as well as the 1970 census. The register has data on gender, place of residence, clinical diagnoses, occupation, socio-economic group, etc., as well as the cancer diagnoses. At present, there are 845 000 cancer cases registered. The *Malformation Register* contains data on newborn children with serious malformations that are diagnosed during infancy and that are reported within six months from birth. Around 1500 cases a year are reported.

The *Ischaemic Heart Disease Register* in Sweden contains data from 1987. All hospital admissions with the ICD code 410 are included. This register exemplifies some of the difficulties in gathering this type of routine data. It is believed that about 10–20% of the admissions recorded do not meet standard diagnostic criteria for acute myocardial infarction, and that only 70–75% of all acute myocardial infarctions which do occur are included.

2.3   Common problems

A number of issues related to data availability and quality will affect the ability to carry out and interpret epidemiological studies over space and time. We have already mentioned problems of diagnostic fashion and changes in diagnosis over time. Here, we discuss specific problems related to coding issues and geographical boundaries.

2.3.1   Coding differences and changes with time

A large number of different coding systems are in current use. ICD-9 (WHO 1977) is probably the most widely used system for mortality and morbidity recording. However, ICD-7 (WHO 1955) and ICD-8 (WHO 1967) are still in use, and some countries are beginning to use ICD-10 (WHO 1992). For recording procedures most countries use ICD-9-CM, the clinical modification of ICD-9, developed separately by workers in the USA and Australia. Unlike ICD-9 itself, ICD-9-CM includes codes for procedures and operations. This system is amended each year, and different countries vary in the time-liness with which they apply their upgrades. In the UK, the third and fourth modifications of the ONS procedure codes are in use. In addition several special versions of ICD-9 (and now of ICD-10) exist. Among others there are versions for paediatrics, for psychiatry, for oncology, and for dentistry. ICD-O, the oncology version, is particularly widely used, encoding both site and tumour morphology. Site codes are related to ICD-9 and now to ICD-10, and morphology codes are derived from a heavily modified version of the older SNO-MED systems. Some centres in the UK are using Read codes. Read codes are not really a classification system but rather an attempt to create a standardised medical vocabulary.

Researchers may thus need to be familiar with several different systems, and with the implications for health event rates, to which changes between systems will inevitably lead. There are some bridge-coding exercises between various versions of ICD, for example, OPCS (1983) and Registrar General (1967). If it is planned to do analyses including time periods which were coded using more than one version of ICD, it will be necessary to identify suitable local bridge codings, and use the information contained in them.

2.3.2 Boundary changes

Administrative boundaries are almost always used in studies of spatial epidemiology. In part, this is due to the relative ease with which addresses can be allocated to administrative areas in many countries, as compared with the difficulty of getting good quality point locations for people. Exceptions to this rule are provided by the Scandinavian countries. For example, in Sweden registered health event data can be linked to geographical coordinates using personal identification numbers assigned to all Swedes (see Section 2.4.3). Furthermore, many covariates of interest in ecological studies are collected for administrative areas, and make little or no sense as attributes of points. While sophisticated schemes of modelling and interpolation can estimate covariates for points (Chapters 10 and 19), the precision with which this can be done is often uncertain (Chapter 5).

Nevertheless, administrative boundaries can and do change. For some purposes (e.g. drawing thematic maps), minor changes are irrelevant. For others, including small-area population estimation and correct allocation of point data to area level, even very small changes may need to be taken into account. Since few administrative bodies use electronic mapping systems, and fewer make such maps routinely available, deciding what area is represented by a given administrative area name at a given time poses difficulties.

If it is decided to track all boundary changes in detail, it becomes necessary to have a procedure for allocating events to areas which takes account of the year-by-year changes. This is a substantial practical problem, and it is expensive to solve even with the advent of geographical information systems (GIS). However, as boundaries are often changed to reflect changes in population, it may be necessary.

For studies extending over any long period of time it may be necessary to decide on a fixed set of boundaries, and convert all individual and area level data to this common boundary. This inevitably involves a great deal of work and the exercise of considerable judgement. It is a crucial decision for any reasonably large project.

2.3.3 Boundary selection

Boundary selection arises as a problem whenever there is a range of levels at which data can be mapped and analysed. For example, in the United Kingdom, census data are available at enumeration district, ward, district, county, region and country level, among others. While the choice of area for analysis may be forced by limitations in existing data, or by computational considerations, it is important to be aware that this is not an insignificant choice, and that it is possible to get different results at different levels. This is discussed further in Chapter 5.

2.4 Georeferencing of health data

For spatial analysis, health event data must be spatially located. In general, administrative systems based on address are used. For most studies, the address chosen is the residence of the individual at the time of diagnosis. There is little published work using information on previous residences, although some interesting work on radon exposure and lung cancer has recently been carried out using such data (Darby *et al.* 1998).

It is important to be clear which residence is recorded in the data source used for a particular study. For example, what is recorded as the residence at birth might in fact be the residence at registration of the birth (up to six weeks after birth in the UK). Given the high mobility of families around the time of birth, this address might be a poor proxy for the residence at the time of conception, or during early pregnancy. Residence at death is also prone to errors, notably the tendency for elderly people to migrate after retirement, and the tendency for sick or frail elderly people to enter nursing homes. It should be noted that length of residence in an area can be determined directly in case-control studies, and where continuous population registers are available (e.g. the Scandinavian countries).

2.4.1 Area codes

Typically some link between address and a set of area codes is available. In the United Kingdom, postcodes (Raper *et al.* 1992) have been extensively used for this purpose. Similar systems exist in several other countries. The main practical problem when linking postcodes and areas has been the extraordinary proliferation of different area codes. At one time there were three different sets of codes for United Kingdom wards in use within the then Office of Population Censuses and Surveys (OPCS). Resolving this is mainly a data-processing problem, but the potential for error is clearly considerable.

In addition to errors due to the use of multiple codes, postcodes are prone to significant error (Raper *et al.* 1992). Reading and Openshaw (1993) studied the linking of postcodes to enumeration districts (EDs) in Northumberland. They found that this put 53% of postcodes in the wrong ED. In most cases the ED to which the postcode was allocated had similar socio-demographic characteristics to the correct ED, but this cannot be relied on in general.

2.4.2 Point codes

Allocating health events to points is also problematic. Postcodes, widely used in the UK, may be surprisingly inaccurate as described earlier. The grid references associated with postcodes are also inaccurate. This is partly because of the complex mixture of manual allocation, machine interpolation, and changes over time, which have led to the current postcode system. While postcodes are advertised as being accurate on average to ±100 m, manually imputed grid references, still a significant proportion of the total, have a nominal accuracy of ±400 m in each direction. This is large enough to put some postcodes in the wrong ward, and occasionally the wrong district, or even the wrong county. Fortunately, such gross errors can often be detected. Examining postcode centroids shows that they fall on a regular grid, as one would expect, and this might produce some artefacts in certain types of analysis.

In the UK, a system (AddressPoint) exists with nominal 1 m precision, although it is not currently available for routine analyses. In Sweden, address databases are available commercially, covering most urban areas. Again, these databases are expensive to obtain and the cost often prohibits the use of them for research purposes. Pending the availability of such systems at affordable prices, point-based analyses should be conducted with caution, and allocated points should be inspected visually before analyses are undertaken.

A further source of problems is the use of digitised boundary data. In England, ward level maps seem to be of good quality, at least for ward boundaries at census time. ED level maps in our experience are far harder to use, and require extensive cleaning to make them workable (Parslow *et al.* 1997). Again from our own experience, we have found that there are some discrepancies between digitised ward and county boundaries. The effect of these potential mismatches on the reliability of statistical inference is unknown.

Since covariate information is rarely available for point data except in purpose-designed case-control studies, such analyses have mostly been of disease clustering (Alexander 1991). As described above, typical methods of allocation of events to points are prone to error. Standard methods for the analysis of point data assume that point locations are known without error. It is possible, in principle, to use Bayesian methods to address this issue, and methods using fuzzy algebra have also been proposed (Jacquez 1996).

2.4.3 Disease registers in the Scandinavian countries

The basis of the Scandinavian system is the unique personal identifier. For example, all Swedes have a personal identification number consisting of 10 digits. The first 6 digits are the date of birth and the next 3 digits make up a birth number. The last digit is a check digit derived from the first 9 digits. In principle, all Swedish registers using the personal identification number can also identify the address at which a person lives. All such addresses can be georeferenced through a computerised linking to the property register, maintained by a government agency. It should be noted, however, that the coordinates thus assigned to a person represent the mid-point of the property. If the person lives in a large block of flats, the mid-point coordinate may not be a very good estimate of the exact location of that person's apartment.

Statistics Sweden (the National Office for Statistics in Sweden) maintains a number of registers with personal identification numbers: the *Demographic Register* contains all Swedes and includes personal identification number, name, address, citizenship, income, marital status, etc. Swedish researchers may use the register to gain background information on study subjects in epidemiological studies. Again, since the register is based on the personal identification number, all data could easily be georeferenced. *Census Registers* have been available in five-year spans since 1960. The contents vary slightly with time, but essentially there are data on both individuals and households including number of individuals per household, number of children, and cramped housing accommodation. There is detailed information on the type and standard of the housing as well as car ownership. The *Education Register* contains information on all Swedes, 15 to 74 years old. The highest as well as the most recent education level attained is available and the register is updated yearly. In contrast with what is possible in the UK and many other countries, these data would allow point-based spatial analyses including individual covariate information.

2.5   Implications for analysis

The problems with data sources have many implications for the design, analysis and interpretation of routine health data at a small-area level. The fundamental decision which must be taken before analyses are begun is simply stated: 'What kind of questions can be sensibly asked of these data?' In other words, given all of the problems described above, can the research question be addressed using these sources of data? If the answer to this question is no, then either the research should proceed no further or supplementary data (e.g. from special surveys) are required. For example, hospital admissions data may not be of much use in answering questions about the incidence of, say, aplastic anaemia, at least on their own. The disease is so rare that even minor coding errors or diagnostic transfers could completely obscure the real pattern, and the difficulty of identifying multiple admissions by the same patient to different facilities would be considerable.

A UK project sought to examine the spatial distribution of respiratory diseases in various parts of the country. At first glance there were many doubtful records. However, a careful examination showed that by using very broad groups of codes, some reasonable approximation could be obtained (Bottle *et al.* 1999). A register of childhood IDDM used HES data to supplement cases identified from chart review, and from questionnaires delivered to general practitioners. This was a valuable contribution to what was a very complete register of this relatively rare condition (Bodansky *et al.* 1992; Staines *et al.* 1993).

2.5.1 Methods for data-checking

Methods for the cleaning of data are well known. It is important not to skimp on checks just because the dataset is enormous, or because it is believed to come from a very reliable source. Simple internal consistency checks, simple tabulations, counts of missing values, histograms, probability plots, and all of the usual methods for data-cleaning and exploratory data analysis are readily applicable to health event data.

For spatial data a number of other checks are important. Such data are often analysed using indirect standardisation (Alexander *et al.* 1990; Clayton and Hills 1993). It will not be feasible to examine age-incidence curves for each small-area, unless the condition being studied is quite common. However, it is only common sense to examine a range of plots of incidence by age, by sex and age, and for larger aggregations of areas. Simple thematic maps of the data, including maps of covariates, maps of incidence by age and sex, and maps of other suitable functions of incidence should be examined closely to detect subtle, and not-so-subtle errors. When analysing spatial data it is necessary to think spatially.

2.6 Conclusions

A wide range of spatial data sources are available for epidemiological analysis. New and powerful methods of handling spatial data, including GIS and Bayesian multi-level modelling, have made very sophisticated and complex analyses possible. It is essential, if effective use is to be made of these new approaches, that epidemiologists are aware of the details of the data with which they propose to work, and of the specific problems and limitations of the routinely collected health data which so often form the core of a spatial analysis.

If these problems are considered carefully and addressed correctly, spatial analysis will be a valuable addition to the toolbox of the working epidemiologist, and an immense help in unravelling the pressing scientific and managerial questions which face providers of health services everywhere. If not, abuse of these tools will lead to invalid and uninteresting studies, and will damage both the professional credibility of epidemiology, and the provision of health care to our populations.

References

Alberman, E., Bergsjo, P., Cole, S., Evans, S., Hartford, R., Hoffman, H. *et al.* (1989). International Collaborative Effort (ICE) on birthweight; plurality; and perinatal and infant mortality. I: Methods of data collection and analysis. *Acta Obstetricia et Gynecologica Scandinavica*, **68**, 5–10.

Alexander, F. E. (1991). Investigations of localised spatial clustering, and extra-Poisson variation. In *The geographical epidemiology of childhood leukaemia and non-Hodgkin lymphomas in Great Britain, 1966–83* (G. Draper ed.), 69–76. Studies on medical and population subjects 53. HMSO, London.

Alexander, F. E., Ricketts, T. J., McKinney, P. A., and Cartwright, R. A. (1990). Community lifestyle characteristics and risk of acute lymphoblastic leukaemia in children. *Lancet*, **336**, 1461–5.

Anderson, H. R., Limb, E. S., Bland, J. M., Ponce de Leon, A., Strachan, D. P., and Bower, J. S. (1995). Health effects of an air pollution episode in London, December 1991. *Thorax*, **50**, 1188–93.

Anonymous (1996). Notifiable disease surveillance and notifiable disease statistics—United States, June 1946 and June 1996. *Morbidity and Mortality Weekly Report*, **45**, 530–6.

Anonymous (1997). (New arrangements for processing notifications of infectious disease returns. *Communicable Disease Report CDR Weekly*, **7**, 1.

Ashley, J. and Devis, T. (1992). Death certification from the point of view of the epidemiologist. *Population Trends*, **67**, 22–8.

Ashley, J. S. A. (1972). Present state of statistics from hospital in-patient data and their uses. *British Journal of Preventive and Social Medicine*, **26**, 135–7.

Balkau, B., Jougla, E., and Papoz, L. (1993). European study of the certification and coding of causes of death of six clinical case histories of diabetic patients. EURODIAB Sub-area C Study Group. *International Journal of Epidemiology*, **22**, 116–26.

Barrett, P. and Lau, Y. K. (1997). Incompleteness of statutory notification of bacterial gastro-intestinal infection. *Public Health*, **111**, 183–5.

Bhopal, R. S., Diggle, P., and Rowlingson, B. (1992). Pinpointing clusters of apparently sporadic cases of legionnaires' disease. *British Medical Journal*, **304**, 1022–7.

Birch, D. (1993). Automatic coding of causes of death. *Population Trends*, **73**, 36–8.

Bodansky, H. J., Staines, A., Stephenson, C., Haigh, D., and Cartwright, R. (1992). Evidence for an environmental effect in the aetiology of insulin dependent diabetes in a transmigratory population. *British Medical Journal*, **304**, 1020–2.

Bottle, A., Aylin, P., Wakefield, J., Järup, L., and Elliott, P. (1999). Use of hospital admissions data as a measure of morbidity for residents near cokeworks. *Epidemiology*, **10**(Suppl. 4), S145.

Cartwright, R. A., Alexander, F. E., McKinney, P. A., and Ricketts, T. J. (1990). *Leukaemia and lymphoma. An atlas of distribution within areas of England and Wales 1984–1988*. Leukaemia Research Fund, London.

Clayton, D. and Hills, M. (1993). *Statistical methods in epidemiology*. Oxford University Press.

Cnattingius, S. and Haglund, B. (1992) Socio-economic factors and feto-infant mortality. *Scandinavian Journal of Social Medicine*, **20**, 11–13.

Cnattingius, S., Zack, M. M., Ekbom, A., Gunnarskog, J., Kreuger, A., Linet, M. *et al.* (1995). Prenatal and neonatal risk factors for childhood lymphatic leukaemia. *Journal of the National Cancer Institute*, **87**, 908–14.

Cole, S., Hartford, R. B., Bergsjo, P., and McCarthy, B. (1989). International collaborative effort (ICE) on birthweight, plurality, perinatal, and infant mortality. III: A method of grouping underlying causes of infant death to aid international comparisons. *Acta Obstetrica Gynecologica Scandinavica*, **68**, 113–17.

Commission on Professional and Hospital Activities (1978). *International classification of diseases, 9th revision, clinical modification ICD-9-CM*. Commission on Professional and Hospital Activities, Ann Arbor, Michigan.

Cuckle, H., Nanchahal, K., and Wald, N. (1991). Birth prevalence of Down's syndrome in England and Wales. *Prenatal Diagnosis*, **11**, 29–34.

Dahlquist, G. and Källén, B. (1992). Maternal-child blood group incompatibility and other perinatal events increase the risk for early-onset type 1 (insulin-dependent) diabetes mellitus. *Diabetologia*, **35**, 671–5.

Darby, S., Whitley, E., Silcocks, P., Thakrar, B., Green, M., Lomas, P. *et al.* (1998). Risk of lung cancer associated with residential radon exposure in south-west England: a case-control study. *British Journal of Cancer*, **78**, 394–408.

Dixon, J., Sanderson, C., Elliott, P., Walls, P., Jones, J., and Petticrew, M. (1998). Assessment of the reproducibility of clinical coding in routinely collected hospital activity data: a study in two hospitals. *Journal of Public Health Medicine*, **20**, 63–9.

Edouard, L. and Senthilselvan, A. (1997). Observer error and birthweight: digit preference in recording. *Public Health*, **111**, 77–9.

Elliott, P. and Briggs, D. J. (1997). Recent developments in the geographical analysis of small area health and environmental data. In *Progress in public health* (G. Scally ed.), 101–25. Royal Society of Medicine Press, London.

Evans, S., Alberman, E., Pashley, J., and Hampton, B. (1989). International Collaborative Effort (ICE) on birthweight; plurality; and perinatal and infant mortality. II: Comparisons between birthweight distributions of births in member countries from 1970 to 1984. *Acta Obstetricia et Gynecologica Scandinavica*, **68**, 11–17.

Finger, R. and Auslander, M. B. (1997). Results of a search for missed cases of reportable communicable diseases using hospital discharge data. *Journal of the Kentucky Medical Association*, **95**, 237–9.

Fuller, J. H. (1993). Mortality trends and causes of death in diabetic patients. *Diabete et Metabolisme*, **19**, 96–9.

Green, A., Gale, E. A., and Patterson, C. C. (1992). Incidence of childhood-onset insulin-dependent diabetes mellitus: the EURODIAB ACE Study. *Lancet*, **339**, 905–9.

Hey, K., O'Donnell, M., Murphy, M., Jones, N., and Botting, B. (1994). Use of local neural tube defect registers to interpret national trends. *Archives of Disease in Childhood: Fetal and Neonatal Edition*, **71**, F198–202.

Hilder, L. and Alberman, E. (1998). *Journal of Epidemiology and Community Health*, **52**, 253–8.

Hook, E. B. and Regal, R. R. (1995). Capture-recapture methods in epidemiology: methods and limitations. *Epidemiologic Reviews*, **17**, 243–64.

Jacquez, G. M. (1996). Disease cluster tests for imprecise space-time locations. *Statistics in Medicine*, **15**, 873–85.

Jakobsen, R., Gustavsson, O., and Lundberg, I. (1997). Increased risk of lung cancer among male professional drives in urban but not rural areas of Sweden. *Occupational and Environmental Medicine*, **54**, 189–93.

Jiang, G. X., Cheng, Q., Link, H., and de Pedro-Cuesta, J. (1997). Epidemiological features of Guilllain-Barré syndrome in Sweden, 1978–1993. *Journal of Neurology, Neurosurgery and Psychiatry*, **62**, 447–53.

Johansen, H., Dutta, M., Mao, Y., Chagani, K., and Sladecek, I. (1992). An investigation of the increase in preschool-age asthma in Manitoba, Canada. *Health Reports*, **4**, 379–402.

Johnson, K. M., Huether, C. A., Hook, E. B., Crowe, C. A., Reeder, B. A., Sommer, A. *et al.* (1985). False-positive reporting of Down syndrome on Ohio and New York birth certificates. *Genetic Epidemiology*, **2**, 123–31.

Jougla, E., Papoz, L., Balkau, B., Maguin, P., and Hatton, F. (1992). Death certificate coding practices related to diabetes in European countries—the 'EURODIAB Subarea C' Study. *International Journal of Epidemiology*, **21**, 343–51.

Khoury, M. J., Erickson, J. D., Adams, M. J. Jr. (1984). Trends in postneonatal mortality in the United States. 1962 through 1978. *Journal of the American Medical Association*, **252**, 367–72.

Lechat, M. F. and Dolk, H. (1993). Registries of congenital anomalies: EUROCAT. *Environmental Health Perspectives*, **101**(Suppl. 2), 153–7.

Lopez, A. D. (1992). Mortality data In *Geographical and Environmental Epidemiology: Methods for Small-Area Studies* (P. Elliott, J. Cuzick, D. English, and R. Stern ed.), 37–50. Oxford University Press.

Lund, E., Arnesen, E., and Borgan J. K. (1990) Pattern of childbearing and mortality in married women—a national prospective study from Norway. *Journal of Epidemiology and Community Health*, **44**, 237–40.

McClain, P. W., Sacks, J. J., Froehlke, R. G., and Ewigman, B. G. (1993). Estimates of fatal child abuse and neglect, United States, 1979 through 1988. *Pediatrics*, **91**, 338–43.

Mutton, D. E., Alberman, E., Ide, R., and Bobrow M. (1991). Results of first year (1989) of a national register of Down's syndrome in England and Wales. *British Medical Journal*, **303**, 1295–7.

O'Neil, M., Payne, C., and Read, J. (1995). Read Codes Version 3: a user led terminology. *Methods of Information in Medicine*, **34**, 187–92.

OPCS (1983). *Mortality Statistics. Comparison of 8th and 9th Revisions of the ICD*. Series DH1 10. HMSO, London.

Parkin, D. M., Whelan, S. L., Ferlay, J., Raymond, L., and Young, J. (ed.). (1997). *Cancer incidence in five continents*. Vol. VII, International Agency for Research on Cancer. Scientific Publication 143. IARC, Lyon.

Parslow, R. C., McKinney, P. A., Law, G. R., Staines, A., Williams, R., and Bodansky, H. J. (1997). Incidence of childhood diabetes mellitus in Yorkshire, northern England, is associated with nitrate in drinking water: an ecological analysis. *Diabetologia*, **40**, 550–6.

Raper, J., Rhind, D., and Shepherd, J. (1992). *Postcodes: The new geography*. Chapman and Hall, London.

Reading, R. and Openshaw, S. (1993). Do inaccuracies in small area deprivation analyses matter? *Journal of Epidemiology and Community Health*, **47**, 238–41.

Registrar General (1967). *The Registrar General's statistical review of England and Wales. Part III*. HMSO, London.

Rydstroem, H. (1998). No obvious spatial clustering of twin births in Sweden between 1973 and 1990. *Environmental Research*, **76**, 27–31.

Schwartz, J. (1995). Short term fluctuations in air pollution and hospital admissions of the elderly for respiratory disease. *Thorax*, **50**, 531–8.

Seneviratne, S. L., Gunatilake, S. B., and de Silva, H. J. (1997). Reporting notifiable diseases: methods for improvement, attitudes and community outcome. *Transactions of the Royal Society of Tropical Medicine and Hygiene*, **91**, 135–7.

Shevchenko, I. P., Lynch, J. T., Mattie, A. S., and Reed Fourquet, L. L. (1995). Verification of information in a large medical database using linkages with external databases. *Statistics in Medicine*, **14**, 511–30.

Squires, S. G., Aronson, K. J., Remis, R. S., and Hoey, J. R. (1998). Improved disease reporting: a randomized trail of physicians. *Canadian Journal of Public Health* (*Revue Canadienne de Santé Publique*), **89**, 66–9.

Staines, A. and Schweiger, M. (1995). The geography of food-poisoning and infectious disease in Leeds. In *Report of the Director of Public Health, Leeds Healthcare* (E. Wain ed). Leeds Healthcare, Leeds.

Staines, A., Bodansky, H. J., Lilley, H. E. B., Stephenson, C., McNally, R. J. Q., and Cartwright, R. A. (1993). The epidemiology of diabetes mellitus in the United Kingdom: The Yorkshire Regional Childhood Diabetes Register. *Diabetologia*, **36**, 1282–7.

Vågerö, D. and Norell, S. E. (1989). Mortality and social class in Sweden—exploring a new epidemiological tool. *Scandinavian Journal of Social Medicine*, **17**, 49–58.

WHO (World Health Organisation) (1955). *Manual of the international statistical classification of diseases, injuries and causes of death*. Vol. 1. WHO, Geneva.

WHO (World Health Organisation) (1967). *Manual of the international statistical classification of diseases, injuries and causes of death*. Vol. 1. WHO, Geneva.

WHO (World Health Organisation) (1977). *Manual of the international statistical classification of diseases, injuries and causes of death*. Vol. 1. WHO, Geneva.

WHO (World Health Organisation) (1992). *ICD-10: International statistical classification of diseases and related health problems*. Vol. 1. WHO, Geneva.

Williams, A. N., Johnson, R. A., and Bender, A. P. (1990). Use of coded mortality data to assess area cancer rates: impact of residence reporting and coding errors. *American Journal of Epidemiology*, **132**, S178–82.

3. The use of population data in spatial epidemiology

R. A. Arnold, I. D. Diamond, and J. C. Wakefield

3.1 Introduction

The calculation of area-specific disease risk summaries requires an accurate estimate of the population at risk. Proportional mortality studies (e.g. Breslow and Day 1987) may be carried out to estimate relative risks, and although they do not require population estimates they suffer from their own difficulties and are not routinely carried out. Similarly, case-control studies incorporate the information on the population at risk through a set of control locations. Such studies are not routinely performed, however, due to expense, logistical difficulties, and problems of selection bias. In this chapter we consider the use of population counts in spatial epidemiological studies; it is traditional to consider the population counts (i.e. the *denominators*) as known quantities often with only a qualitative statement of the effects of inaccuracies appearing in the discussion (e.g. Elliott *et al.* 1996). Ideally, population estimates should be based on continuously updated counts of the population such as those found in population registers. However, as such registers are relatively rare, it is typical for studies to rely on censuses and/or vital registrations. In addition, estimates may be improved ancillary information from large surveys, although it is rare for surveys to be large enough to provide accurate adjustment of population counts at a fine level of aggregation. Unfortunately, the census does not provide true counts, in particular *underenumeration* typically occurs. One is also faced with the problem of how to deal with inter-censual years, including the incorporation of migration. For spatial studies in which large areas are considered the implications of inaccuracies are likely to be less serious since the under- and overestimation of the counts in small areas will tend to cancel out. Also it is much more likely in larger areas that migration will occur *within* the area of interest and so will not be relevant to risk estimation. In small-area studies, however, the effects will be far more acute. As Richardson (1992) points out there is a trade-off when one considers the size of the constituent study areas to be studied. In small areas the problems of inaccuracies in denominators will be largest but there is less chance of ecological bias (see Chapter 11), since exposures of interest will be more constant within areas.

We note that the adequacy of the estimates will be judged relative to the study objective. In general the person-time at risk in each of the areas is the quantity of interest though this is frequently approximated by the population estimate at some point (e.g. the mid-point of the study period) multiplied by the length of the study period. All other things being equal, studies for which the latency period is shortest (e.g. exposures *in utero*) will be the most easily carried out from a population estimation point of view, since a single set of population counts in the relevant period is all that is required. For diseases with a long latency such as mesothelioma it will be very difficult to obtain an accurate estimate of the person-years at risk (Chapter 5).

The outline of this chapter is as follows. In Section 3.2 we review the data available for estimating the populations of small areas and in Section 3.3 consider a number of methods of estimation. Section 3.4 concerns the implications of inadequacies in population estimates under various models describing the relationship between the 'true' and estimated counts. A number of approaches that may be used to address the sensitivity of relative risk estimates are also described. In Section 3.5 a simple example is presented that illustrates both the sensitivity of inference to the choice of counts and a method by which inter-censual counts may be estimated.

3.2   Data sources

3.2.1   Population registers

Population registers are continuously updated records of the population of some area. They usually contain basic demographic information, such as age, sex, place of birth, and marital status. Sometimes they include occupation and, for those still in education, current educational status. These registers are updated by data from vital registration and by notifications of change of address which residents are obliged to report to the registration authorities. These registers are primarily compiled for administrative purposes such as taxation, health, and social services, or electoral registration but, where available, they have great potential for epidemiologists. A good overview can be found in Redfern (1989).

Table 3.1 summarizes the availability of population registers in much of Western Europe. Local registers have a long history in many countries—dating back to the seventeenth century in Finland and Sweden—but the development of national registers that link the data from local sources is largely confined to the past forty years.

A notable exception in Table 3.1 is the UK. Although permanent registers have been proposed a number of times (e.g. Mallett 1929), they have never found favour outside of the periods of the First and Second World Wars. The last National Register in the UK was abandoned in 1952, as Redfern (1989) describes: 'in a post war spirit of "set the people free"'.

It has been suggested that the National Health Service Central Register (NHSCR) serves as a register. This includes all residents of the UK except a small percentage who were born abroad and have never registered with a doctor in the UK. However, it serves only the National Health Service and cannot be exploited by other agencies. In addition, it suffers from major drawbacks which limit its potential use for epidemiologists. These drawbacks include the following.

1. Addresses are only changed when an individual moves to a new doctor, which will typically preclude detection of moves over a short distance. Furthermore, moves to a new doctor often take a long time to reach the register.

2. Information on a woman's change of name on marriage (or divorce) only reaches the NHSCR by chance (e.g. when she registers her new name with a different doctor).

However, it will be seen later that these data can provide important information on internal migration and on which to update census based estimates.

Table 3.1 Availability of population registers in Western
Europe (adapted from Redfern 1989)

	Local population registers	Central population register
Belgium	X	X
Denmark	X	X
Finland	X	X
Luxembourg	X	X
Norway	X	X
Sweden	X	X
France	–	X
Netherlands	X	–
Portugal	–	X
Spain	X	X
Federal Republic of Germany	X	X
Greece	X	X
Italy	X	X
Ireland	–	–
UK	–	–

One further source worthy of mention, although as yet little used for geographical epidemiology, is the Office for National Statistics *Longitudinal study* (LS: Hattersley and Creeser 1995). This is a 1% sample of the population which was started with the 1971 census and has been updated using the 1981 census data, death records, births to female members of the sample, subsequent infant mortality, and cancer registrations. This dataset is similar to the French Panel Demographique and has been used widely to study topics such as occupational differentials in mortality (e.g. see Fox and Goldblatt 1982). For epidemiologists interested in estimating the size of small socio-economic groups such sources are increasingly useful. However, for reasons of preserving anonymity it is not possible to use the LS to estimate the populations of geographically small areas in the UK.

In summary, registers are potentially the most valuable source of small-area population data, and—where they exist—their use is strongly recommended. However, in countries such as the UK and the USA alternative sources are required.

3.2.2 Census data

Any population estimate requires a base population as a starting point. In many countries the most reliable base population is the decennial census. Censuses have been held throughout Western Europe and North America since the late eighteenth/early nineteenth century and consist of a count of the population on a particular day. Increasingly, census data are becoming available throughout the rest of the world and form the base for most, if not all, population projections and estimates.

Census data are necessarily restricted to demographic characteristics and basic socio-economic information. This is due both to financial restrictions and to the need to ask questions which are relevant to the majority of the population and which will be answered fully and accurately. In the UK, cost considerations have led to a large reduction in the size of the census questionnaire in both 1981 and 1991 relative to those of 1961 and 1971. In addition, the large mid-censual population survey introduced in 1966, which gave important information on internal migration, seems likely never to be repeated. It is expected that in 2001 the census will be a similar length to that in 1991.

The major advantage of census data is that population counts are available at low levels of aggregation. In the UK the basic enumeration district consists, on average, of around 180–200 households. These can then be progressively aggregated to larger geographical areas. Data are published in the UK at electoral ward level (around 5000 persons) and below that census data are available electronically—the small-area statistics (SAS) comprise around 9000 variables available for all enumeration districts. The SAS contain information on residents by age, sex, marital status, household composition, and ethnic group plus a range of social, economic, and housing characteristics. It is expected that in 2001 there will be new questions on relationship status, religion, and health.

The census is also tremendously important as a source of data on migration. These are obtained by asking individuals about their usual address some time before the census. In the UK there used to be two questions—on place of residence 1 year and 5 years before the census, respectively. Unfortunately, the question on residence 5 years before the census has been left out of UK censuses since 1981.

Censuses are always subject to underenumeration which is typically measured by a post-enumeration survey (PES). In the 1991 census underenumeration in England and Wales was around 2% although this was not exceptional by international standards. A problem arose when the census validation survey (CVS), as the PES was known, provided an estimate of the underenumeration which was not commensurate with estimates produced using demographic techniques. Moreover, the CVS did not give a geographical disaggregation of underenumeration.

In the UK, age and sex stratified population estimates are made each year at the scale of Local Authority Districts (LADs) by the Office for National Statistics (Chappell 1999). The LAD estimates made for 1991 were used by the Estimating with Confidence project to make estimates of underenumeration (Simpson *et al.* 1997*b*), and to produce adjusted population estimates at electoral ward and enumeration district level. These estimates all allocate *underenumeration* disproportionately: the highest rates of under-count occuring for men and women in their twenties, the very elderly, and those in inner-city areas. For example, it was estimated that 20% of men aged 20–24 in inner-city areas were missed.

For the 2001 census, the Office for National Statistics has developed a new strategy to allocate underenumeration down to very small areas such as postcodes. This strategy, the 'One Number Census', is based around a very large PES, and is described in Brown *et al.* (1999).

Census data are also subject to inaccuracy in areas where there are special populations; in particular, students, the armed forces, or other mobile groups present problems and much effort is put into overcoming enumeration problems in these areas. Despite these drawbacks it should be stressed that the census is the most valuable (and best) source for small-area population counts and, for non-censual years, as a base for estimates and that in the UK it is an extremely reliable source.

3.2.3 Vital registration data

Outside the census year it is necessary to estimate the populations of small areas. There are many approaches, which we describe in Section 3.3, and these often use vital registration data (births, marriages, and deaths.). Vital registration data are published at a small-area level in most countries, although they do not contain many socio-economic data and are therefore mainly used simply to adjust census counts.

3.2.4 Administrative records

A number of administrative records are used to update small-area statistics in post-census years. The most common of these are electoral rolls and housing data. While these are, by their very nature, only proxies, they do permit trends to be assessed. It has been shown (Simpson *et al.* 1997*a*) that methods based on these data are better than relying on the census alone in post-censual years.

3.2.5 Special surveys

Small-area population counts may be inferred from data available from large-scale sample surveys which are routinely undertaken for other purposes. For example, in all European Community (and many other) countries labour force surveys are taken regularly. These surveys do not normally provide population estimates below regional level, but they can be used to give an idea of trends in population size. Ratio methods (discussed in the next section) can then be used to adjust census distributions in order to estimate population size.

However, there are many situations when important data are simply not available from standard sources. For example, in noise pollution studies the population exposed to particular levels of noise may not be known and special acoustical surveys will be required. Again, when estimating the number of households exposed to some risk factor, specially commissioned social surveys may be the only sensible strategy. However, the cost of such surveys means that they should only be used when all other possibilities have been exhausted. For an example of a study linking social and acoustical surveys, see Diamond *et al.* (1989). In ecological studies (Chapter 11) it is vital to obtain information on the intra-area distribution of exposures of interest and risk factors in order to reduce ecological bias. Surveys provide one source of such information.

3.3 Small-area population estimates and projections

A number of strategies have been proposed for making small-area estimates. These fall into two main groups: (1) those based on regression models and which typically use ancillary data, perhaps from a large surveys, and (2) those based on more deterministic strategies. Both methods are outlined below. It should be noted that for small areas, say, electoral wards, it is rare that standard government national surveys are large enough to permit efficient estimation.

3.3.1 Regression estimates

Regression models have, for many years, been widely used for making small-area estimates (e.g. Morrison and Relles 1976). A good review is provided by Purcell and Kish (1979), the comprehensive set of papers by Platek *et al.* (1987) and Ghosh and Rao (1994). The basic equation is

$$\hat{\boldsymbol{P}}_2 = f(\boldsymbol{X}_1, \boldsymbol{X}_2, \hat{\boldsymbol{P}}_1), \tag{3.1}$$

where $\hat{\boldsymbol{P}}_1 = (\hat{P}_{11}, \ldots, \hat{P}_{1N})^{\mathrm{T}}$ is the population at time t_1, in N small areas; $\hat{\boldsymbol{P}}_2 = (\hat{P}_{21}, \ldots, \hat{P}_{2N})^{\mathrm{T}}$ is the estimated population at time t_2; and $\boldsymbol{X}_1$, $\boldsymbol{X}_2$ are vectors of characteristics of the N small areas at times t_1 and t_2, respectively. One may also have a separate $f(\cdot)$ for each subgroup.

Regression models can take on varying degrees of complexity, but they have to conform to a number of conditions, the most fundamental of which is that

$$\sum_{i=1}^{N} \hat{P}_{2i} = \sum_{i=1}^{N} P_{2i},$$

that is, that the estimated populations of the small areas should add to the true overall population size P_2. The latter can often be estimated very accurately. A good review of these conditions is provided by McCullagh and Zidek (1987). The simplest form of regression model is to estimate a rate of growth for each small area based on the characteristics $\boldsymbol{X}_t = (x_{t1}, \ldots, x_{tN})^{\mathrm{T}}$ that can be observed. This can be carried out by defining

$$r_i = \frac{x_{2i}}{x_{1i}},$$

so that the population at time t_2 in small area i can be estimated by

$$P_{2i} = P_{1i} r_i^{\beta}, \tag{3.2}$$

where β is a regression coefficient which must be estimated.

In general, there will be $M(>1)$ characteristics in the regression equation and Equation (3.2) will become

$$P_{2i} = P_{1i} \prod_{j=1}^{M} r_{ij}^{\beta_j}. \tag{3.3}$$

This is the basic form of the model proposed by Morrison and Relles (1976) and is described by Swanson and Tedrow (1984). Good practical examples of these models are provided by Ericksen and Kadane (1987) and Lundström (1987).

One final approach should be mentioned. This is a synthetic method which assumes that small areas have the same characteristics as given larger areas that contain them. Purcell (1979) proposed a sophisticated synthetic method, using a categorical data approach known as structure preserving estimates (SPREE). Here one has data (e.g. from a census), which can be categorized into a multiway contingency table. A subsequent survey, say a labour force survey, gives marginal totals at a higher level of aggregation, such as region. Purcell (1979) assumes a superpopulation model for the relationship between the distribution of the number of individuals in each small area over time; SPREE estimates are then calculated by adjusting the data from t_1 to t_2 subject to the new marginals and maintaining the structure in the multiway table at t_1. The estimation is made using iterative proportional fitting. This approach, although not used widely, has been shown to work well by Feeney (1987), Lundström (1987), and Pujadas (1983).

3.3.2 Local estimates

In the UK there are many producers of inter-censual small-area estimates. These include central and local government, health authorities, and commercial companies, although the geographical area differs between producers. Central government (the Office for National Statistics) produce estimates to local authority district level (there are over 400 local authorities in England and Wales—LADs contain an average of 24 wards). For very small areas (such as electoral wards) estimates are made by many local authorities. These local authorities use methods which fall into five main groups which are described below using the following notation: Census (C), Population (N), Proxy Indicator (E), age group (a), small areas (w) and time (t). Time $t = 0$ is the most recent census year, and the subscript $+$ indicates a sum over the index it replaces.

Apportionment allocates ONS local authority projections in proportion to a proxy indicator of current population, say the electoral roll or housing estimates (essentially a simple ratio estimate). This can be expressed as

$$N_{wat} = N_{+at} \frac{E_{wat}}{E_{+at}}.$$

Ratio change adjusts the census population of the area by the proportionate change in some ancillary count, say the electoral roll. This can be expressed as

$$N_{wat} = N_{wa0} \frac{E_{wat}}{E_{wa0}}.$$

Additive Change adds (or subtracts) an estimate of change from an ancillary source to the census population. This can be expressed as

$$N_{wat} = N_{wa0} + (E_{wat} - E_{wa0}).$$

Cohort Survival provides a component projection which is based on the standard demographic balancing Equation. Here the population estimate at time t is calculated by adjusting the census count N_0 by

$$N_t = N_0 + B - D + M,$$

where B, D, M are births, deaths, and net migration in the periods between the census and the estimate.

Local census is an estimate based on a census undertaken by the local authority in conjunction with, say, the annual electoral roll update.

Fuller descriptions of the above strategies are given in Simpson (1998), Simpson *et al.* (1996) and Simpson *et al.* (1997*b*). Other reviews, particularly of the multitude of projection strategies, include Joshi and Diamond (1990) and Diamond *et al.* (1990).

Simpson *et al.* (1997*a*) give a breakdown of the frequency of use of each of these methods among 46 producers of population estimates in Great Britain: apportionment (13); ratio change (16) additive change (8); cohort survival (4); local census (5). In addition, a number of local authorities rely simply on the previous census estimate. Simpson *et al.* (1997*a*) and Lunn *et al.* (1998) point out that the accuracy of the estimates depends to a large extent on the effort put into making them. For example, the local census is the most accurate but also costs much more money. All are better than doing nothing. Over the 7267 small areas considered by Simpson *et al.* (1997*a*) the mean absolute percentage inaccuracy of the total population count was 4.3%. Age-specific estimates were rather more inaccurate, as were areas with large numbers of recent movers, students, armed forces, or high levels of multi-occupancy.

In summary there are, in many countries, large numbers of producers of small-area estimates. It is also the case that local-area knowledge is extremely useful in producing small-area estimates and so those small-area estimates made by local producers tend to be most accurate. Therefore, the advice to epidemiologists is that one should only make small-area population estimates if one really needs to!

3.4   Implications of population inaccuracies

As noted in the previous sections, there is a degree of inaccuracy associated with small-area counts, which depends on both the methods of data collection and estimation used and the type and size of area. In this Section we consider the effects of this inaccuracy on epidemiological studies. Let Y_j and N_j^t denote the number of disease counts and the 'true' population in stratum j of a generic small area. For rare and non-infectious diseases the basic assumption (see Chapter 7) is that

$$Y_j \sim \mathrm{Po}(N_j^t p_j \theta),$$

where p_j is the reference rate (which we assume is known) and θ the relative risk which is assumed constant across strata. Summing over strata we obtain

$$Y \sim \mathrm{Po}(E^t \theta),$$

where $E^t = \sum_j p_j N_j^t$. The implications of data inaccuracies can be qualitatively determined by consideration of the effect on the SMR ($\theta = Y/E$). For example, census underenumeration in the study region but not in the reference region will lead to underestimation of E and hence an overestimate of relative risk. This problem will be most acute when underenumeration occurs in a stratum with a high disease probability. Luckily, the strata within which underenumeration is greatest (e.g. men in the age range 20–24) tend to have a low risk of most non-infectious diseases.

By assuming individuals have a fixed location, and so ignoring local day-to-day movements, we will overestimate the exposure of individuals who are close to sources of pollution. It may be that an elevated risk of disease only occurs after an individual has had a sufficiently long exposure to an environmental factor, or it may be that the disease in question has a long latent period. In either case, high rates of migration into and out of the study area can bias relative risk estimates. A similar bias also occurs where there is non-uniform exposure across the area of interest, where only a fraction of the population of the area is actually exposed.

3.4.1 Errors-in-variables models

The term *errors-in-variables* (e.g. Carroll *et al.* 1995; see also Chapter 5) is used to describe any non-response variable which is measured inaccurately. Within the Poisson framework we have $E[Y|E^t] = E^t\theta$ but if instead the estimated expected numbers $E^o = \sum_j p_j N_j^o$ are used, then the distribution of $Y|E^o$ is no longer Poisson but the mixture of Poisson distributions:

$$p(Y|E^o) = \int p(Y|E^t) \times p(E^t|E^o) dE^t. \tag{3.4}$$

In particular, this will yield counts Y that display overdispersion. Proceeding beyond this general formulation requires information on the relationship between the true and observed counts. The so-called *Berkson* errors-in-variables model considers the distribution $p(E^t|E^o)$ whilst a *classical* errors-in-variables model requires $p(E^o|E^t)$ and $p(E^t)$.

Wakefield and Wallace (1999) consider a disease mapping context and the simple model

$$\log E^o = \log E^t + \varepsilon, \tag{3.5}$$

with $\varepsilon \sim N(0, \sigma_1^2)$ and $\log E^t \sim N(\mu, \sigma_2^2)$. This model leads to

$$\log E^t | \log E^o \sim N(w\mu + (1 - w)\log E^o, w\sigma_2^2),$$

with $w = \sigma_1^2/(\sigma_1^2 + \sigma_2^2)$, which may be used in Equation (3.4). Although the integral (3.4) is not analytically tractable, a Markov chain Monte Carlo implementation (see Chapter 7) is possible. This approach has a number of drawbacks. Unless additional data are available the values of μ, σ_1^2 and σ_2^2 must be specified a priori; this highlights a major difficulty with determining the implications of the use of population estimates, since no gold standard exists. Estimates of μ and σ_2^2 may be obtained approximately from the distribution of the estimated expected numbers but the value of σ_1^2 (i.e. the variance of the measurement error between estimated and expected counts) is far more difficult to determine. For this reason the approach may be viewed as a sensitivity analysis. More realistically we would also like to extend (3.5) to

$$\log E^o = a + b \log E^t + \varepsilon,$$

where, as before, $\varepsilon \sim N(0, \sigma_1^2)$ and a and b represent respectively additive and multiplicative bias terms. Again specification of these values is likely to be difficult and must be informed by local knowledge of the region under consideration (see Section 3.2). Finally since (3.4) is not analytically available little insight into the effect of using estimated counts is possible. We now describe an approach that offers a closed form solution.

Berkson errors-in-variables for the expected counts

When one examines (3.4) we see that one approach that allows this integral to be evaluated analytically is to consider a Berkson model with the true expected counts following a Gamma distribution. Specifically, we may assume $E^t|E^o$ follows the gamma distribution $Ga(E^o(1+b)h, h)$ with b and h specified a priori, which results in

$$E[E^t|E^o] = E^o(1+b) \quad \text{and} \quad Var(E^t|E^o) = \frac{E[E^t|E^o]}{h}. \tag{3.6}$$

Hence the parameter b controls the amount of proportional bias in the expected counts with $b > 0$ corresponding to underenumeration in the population estimates that give rise to E^o. Since $E^o = \sum_j N_j^o p_j$ this factor may be thought of as acting upon all of the original population estimates. The parameter h controls the variance about the expectation with large values corresponding to a distribution of expected counts that is tight about the mean of the distribution. Again the spirit of this model is to assess the sensitivity of the inference to plausible errors in the population estimates.

With the gamma model just described the calculation of (3.4) is straightforward and results in a negative-binomial distribution for Y given E^o

$$Y|E^o \sim \text{NegBin}\left(E^o(1+b)h, \frac{h}{\theta} \right),$$

with

$$E[Y|E^o] = \theta E^o(1+b) \quad \text{and} \quad Var(Y|E^o) = E[Y|E^o]\left[1 + \frac{\theta}{h} \right].$$

Hence, we see that the parameter h introduces *overdispersion*. This approach has the same flavour as the introduction of random effects for θ that follow a gamma distribution which also results in a negative-binomial distribution for Y (see Chapter 7).

Recall that for the conventional Poisson model the MLE for θ is given by $\tilde{\theta} = Y/E^o$ and the variance of this estimator is θ/E^o. In the negative-binomial model just derived we obtain an MLE of

$$\hat{\theta} = \frac{Y}{E^o(1+b)} = \frac{\tilde{\theta}}{(1+b)}, \tag{3.7}$$

with

$$Var(\hat{\theta}) = \frac{\theta}{E^o(1+b)}\left(1 + \frac{\theta}{h}\right) = \frac{Var(\tilde{\theta})}{(1+b)}\left(1 + \frac{\theta}{h}\right), \tag{3.8}$$

and $b > 0$ reduces the overdispersion. The values of b and h may be difficult to determine in practice, but data from the census PES will allow estimates of the bias term (b) and migration flows measured at the census will constrain h.

Effect of migration

The uncertainties in the expected counts in a particular stratum j can arise either from errors in the determination of the reference rate p_j, or from the study area population N_j^t. We now assume that the errors in the reference rates are negligible and concentrate on the effect of uncertainty in N_j^t.

The interest in an epidemiological study centres on the relative risk θ of disease of individuals exposed to some risk factor compared to unexposed individuals. However, it may be that only some fraction ϕ_j of individuals in stratum j in a given area have been sufficiently exposed to be considered at heightened risk. Here we assume that this variation in exposure is caused by migration, though non-uniform exposure across the study area will produce a similar analysis. Thus the stratum specific model for disease counts should be

$$Y_j \sim \text{Po}\{p_j N_j^t (1 - \phi_j + \theta \phi_j)\}, \tag{3.9}$$

reflecting the fact that only some of the population is at elevated risk of disease, despite being exposed to the risk factor. Note that $\phi_j = 1$ produces the usual situation in which everyone in the area is assumed not to migrate. As before, we ignore the risk factor and define the expected counts as $E^t = \sum_j p_j N_j^t$. If we form a weighted average of the stratum specific exposure fractions

$$F = \frac{\sum_j \phi_j p_j N_j^t}{\sum_j p_j N_j^t} = \frac{1}{E^t} \sum_j \phi_j p_j N_j^t,$$

then the model for the total disease counts summing over j in (3.9) becomes simply

$$Y \sim \text{Po}\{E^t(1 - F + \theta F)\}.$$

Note that $0 \leq F \leq 1$, and $F = 1$ corresponds to no migration. Under this model the MLE is given by

$$\hat{\theta} = \frac{Y}{FE^t} - \frac{1}{F} + 1,$$

and is related to the naïve estimate of the relative risk by

$$\tilde{\theta} = \hat{\theta} - (\hat{\theta} - 1)(1 - F). \tag{3.10}$$

Since $F \leq 1$ the naïve estimator is always *attenuated* towards the null ($\theta = 1$). The variance of $\hat{\theta}$ is given by

$$\text{Var}(\hat{\theta}) = \frac{1 - F + F\theta}{E^t F^2} = \text{Var}(\tilde{\theta}) \frac{1}{F} \left(1 + \frac{1 - F}{F\theta}\right), \tag{3.11}$$

and so is always inflated. The values of the ϕ_j can be estimated from migration studies such as the UK *Longitudinal study* (e.g. Hattersley and Creeser 1995; Armstrong *et al.* 1996).

Polissar (1980) and Kliewer (1992) have quantified the effects of neglecting migration on the estimated relative risks for a number of cancer sites and disease latency periods, using estimates of age-dependent migration flows for various geographical scales in the USA. In general, the bias increases with latency time, decreases with age (older people move less frequently) and decreases at higher levels of spatial aggregation (most migration is over small distances). The scale of the bias varies strongly by disease latency period, migration rate, geographical scale, and true underlying relative risk. Biases of 0.5 or more in a true relative risk of 2.0 are not uncommon, leading to observed relative risks of 1.5 or less (see table 2 in Polissar 1980).

The formulation above can be extended to a Berkson errors-in-variables model for the observed population counts N_j^o conditional on the true populations N_j^t. In such a model, the relative risk estimate may be biased by underenumeration and attenuated by migration, with the variance inflated by the additional uncertainty associated with the observed counts.

3.4.2   Apportionment model

Best and Wakefield (1999) consider the situation in which census counts are available every 10 years and, in between, the counts are only available for larger areas than those at which the study is being carried out. As a concrete example they consider a (small-area) ward-level disease mapping study over the period 1981–91 in the Thames region of the UK. Counts are available over the period 1982–90 only at the (large-area) level of LAD.

In the Thames region, LADs contain between 8 and 45 wards with a median of 22. The problem is therefore to apportion counts to the wards with each LAD, by stratum. The approach of Best and Wakefield is to assume that within each year and stratum the constituent ward-level counts N_i, $i = 1, \ldots, I$ (removing dependence on year t and stratum j for notational convenience) are multinomially distributed given the LAD count N_+ and a vector of apportionment probabilities $\boldsymbol{p} = (p_1, \ldots, p_I)^T$, where I denotes the number of wards. The probabilities $\boldsymbol{p}$ may be found via a simple linear interpolation between the censuses. They also extend this model to allow for uncertainty in these probabilities by assuming the vector arises from a Dirichlet distribution, leading to an overdispersed multinomial distribution for the counts. In an illustrative study, Best and Wakfield found that the relative risk estimates were little changed under the apportionment models considered, but the lack of a gold standard for the true counts in each ward made the specification of the uncertainties in the model difficult.

3.5   An illustrative example

We consider the effects of population estimates on inference in the context of a recent study carried out by the UK Small Area Health Statistics Unit (SAHSU). The study was carried out in the village of Shipham which is in southwest England and has very high levels of cadmium in the soil (Elliott *et al.* 1999). For illustration we will consider all-cause mortality for all ages in the period 1981–91 for the Shipham ward (Arnold 1999). The population of Shipham as recorded in the census was 1066 in 1981 and, from the *Estimating with confidence project*, 1094 in 1991.

In the next section we carry out initial analyses of the data based on readily available population counts. In Section 3.5.2 we construct a set of population estimates using sources of data that are available across the whole of the UK. Finally, in Section 3.5.3 we present a sensitivity analysis to demonstrate the scale of the expected effects of population bias and uncertainty on relative risk estimates.

3.5.1 Initial analyses

Table 3.2 presents expected counts using regional reference rates and based on four different methods of constructing population estimates. The step change and interpolation methods are simple to implement and have traditionally been used by SAHSU; in the next section a more refined procedure is described.

Also presented are relative risk estimates (SMRs) and associated 95% confidence intervals. A lower relative risk of all cause mortality is obtained when the 1981 populations are used. This is because there were more people in Shipham over the age of 70 in 1991 than in 1981, leading to an overestimate of the expected mortality.

For small-area (e.g. enumeration districts) studies in general, population estimates are required by five-year age bands (0–4, 5–9, . . . , 80–84, 85+), sex, and calendar year. For interpretation we would also ideally have measures of the uncertainty in each of the estimates so that sensitivity and/or errors-in-variables analyses may be performed. The rates of migration would also in aid exposure assessment. In the next section we describe some of the issues that are relevant to the construction of a set of population estimates, with particular emphasis on the ward of Shipham.

3.5.2 Constructing a set of counts

In general, studies carried out by SAHSU require a set of national population estimates at small-area level (census enumeration district or ward), covering a range of years (from 1981 onwards). The datasets available to us for this purpose are the Office for National

Table 3.2 Observed and expected counts and relative risks for all cause mortality in the ward of Shipham during 1981–91 using four different population estimation methods

Population estimation method	Observed counts Y	Expected counts E	Relative risk estimate θ	95% confidence interval
1981 populations	133	145.9	0.91	0.77, 1.08
Step change at 1986	133	154.7	0.86	0.73, 1.02
Interpolation between 1981 and 1991	133	154.8	0.86	0.72, 1.02
1991 populations	133	165.4	0.80	0.68, 0.95

Statistics annual local authority district populations, the 1991 census counts adjusted for underenumeration (Simpson *et al.* 1997*a*), and vital registration.

Establishing a common geography

The frequent lack of a common geography between censuses introduces further problems when a set of population counts by year is required. In England and Wales, 70% of the censual enumeration districts (EDs) changed between the 1981 and 1991 censuses, whilst the geographical units were different again in 1971. Although it is possible to proceed with population areas where the boundaries change with time, it is far more straightforward to establish a single common geography for all years.

The geography of the 1991 census has been chosen as the standard geography for SAHSU studies. The first step in the calculation of non-census year populations is the estimation of 1981 populations within 1991 ED boundaries. Using published tables matching postcodes and enumeration districts, various methods of mapping populations from 1981 to 1991 geography have been investigated. Each method was tested by comparing the populations predicted with the published census figures in a subset of areas where the boundaries had not changed between 1981 and 1991. The method that produced the smallest errors was based on the approximate link table between 1991 EDs and 1981 wards created by Atkins *et al.* (1993; see also Dorling and Atkins 1995). The 1981 census populations were mapped to 1991 EDs as follows. The 1981 population of the 1981 ward was split across the 1991 EDs which match to it in the link table. Each ED was allocated a fraction of the ward population identical to the fraction it held in 1991. This method therefore replicates the 1991 geographical distribution of populations within each ward, and replicates the age-sex structure of the 1981 ward population in each of the EDs. In order to allow for underenumeration in the 1981 census counts, the final step is to rescale the populations inside each local authority district to the more accurate published mid-year estimate for 1981.

At the end of this procedure population estimates for 1981 and 1991 are available in the same geography, both constrained to add up to the published annual LAD population estimates.

Population estimation

The next step is to form population estimates for non-censual years. For the years between 1981 and 1991 a simple method is to linearly interpolate between the censuses, and to scale so that the populations sum to the annual LAD estimates.

Extrapolation to later years requires some knowledge of the behaviour of the population in each small area, because there are no nationally available small area data after the 1991 census. In Section 3.3 several methods for extrapolating a population from a base year to later times are reviewed. As mentioned above, SAHSU is constrained to use nationally available datasets, and does not have easy access to routine data at small-area level (e.g. number of dwellings, numbers of electors) to form population estimates. The method of cohort survival *is*, however, a feasible approach, since postcoded birth and death registrations from 1981 onwards are available, as are the 1991 census special migration statistics (SMS) which provide estimates of ward level migration flows in the year before the 1991 census.

We seek to estimate at mid-year in year t and for age group a the population $p(t, a)$, for males and females separately. In the cohort survival approach we need to know for each small area in the 12 months following mid-year in year t:

- $b(t)$ = the total births,
- $d(t, a)$ = the total deaths of people dying at age a,
- $m(t, a)$ = the net flow into the small area of people of age a.

From the census we already know $p(1981, a)$ and $p(1991, a)$, and the birth and death registrations give us $b(t)$ and $d(t, a)$. The migration flows $m(y, a)$ are however unknown, and must be estimated.

The population $p(t, a)$ at each successive year can be calculated from the year before by (i) shifting the members of each age group up by one year of age, (ii) adding the births, (iii) subtracting the deaths, and (iv) correcting for migration:

$$p(t, a) = m(t, a) + \begin{cases} b(t-1) & a = 0 \\ p(t-1, a-1) - d(t-1, a-1) & 1 \le a \le 88 \\ p(t-1, a-1) - d(t-1, a-1) & \\ \quad + p(t-1, a) - d(t-1, a) & a = 89 \end{cases} \tag{3.12}$$

For computational convenience no one ages beyond 89 years in this model. Since the age of death is used, rather than the age at mid-year, it is effectively assumed that everyone shares a birthday immediately before the date of each population estimate. This minor approximation means that all babies who are born and die between successive mid-years are still counted at the first mid-year estimate after their birth.

We do not have sufficient data to estimate a time varying migration flow $m(t, a)$, so instead we assume that the net migration flow is the same every year, $m(a)$. Under this assumption it is possible, using the 1981 and 1991 populations, to solve uniquely for $m(a)$. However, this solution varies unrealistically from age band to age band.

An alternative approach is to use the interpolated populations in the period 1981–91 to determine a migration function which can then be used to roll the population forwards beyond 1991. Figure 3.1 shows the year by year interpolated populations for Shipham ward. Using (3.12) we can deduce the migration function $m(t, a)$ *implied* by the changes from year to year. These functions are the combination of the effects of migration, and the residual uncertainty associated with the base population estimates (1981 and 1991) and the birth and death counts. The mean of these yearly migration functions $m(a)$, averaged over the 10-year period, is the best estimate of the migration patterns for each area. These estimates are compared with the migration levels from the SMS in Fig. 3.2, after being appropriately grouped to the same five age bands. The SMS relate to the single year before the 1991 census, and may not be typical of migration during the 1980s for several reasons. First, where a ward has undergone large changes during the 10 years 1981–91 no single year can be expected to be typical of the whole period. Second, it is known that the 1991 census suffered from underenumeration (Simpson *et al.* 1997*a*), especially among young males who are typically the group with the highest migration rates. Third, the British economy was in a recession at the time of the census, and migration is likely to have been lower at that time than in the mid 1980s when the economy was more active.

Although the SMS may be unreliable in absolute terms, the ratio of net (in − out) to total (in + out) migration informs estimates of the levels of in and out migration.

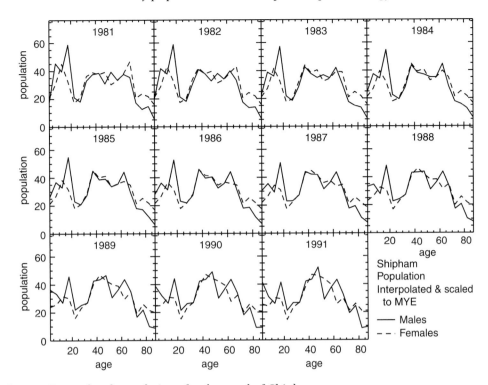

Fig. 3.1 Interpolated populations for the ward of Shipham.

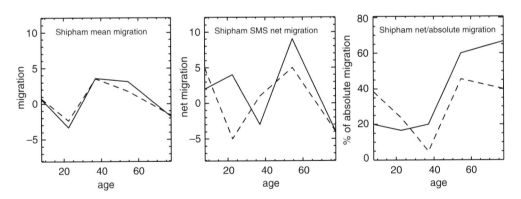

Fig. 3.2 Migration functions for the ward of Shipham. The first panel shows our estimate of the mean net migration function $m(a)$, the second is the net migration function from the SMS, and the third shows the ratio of net (in − out) to total (in + out) SMS migration. (In each panel the solid line is for males and the dashed line for females.)

We need to know the scale of such migration because of its potential attenuating effects on observed rates of disease.

Figure 3.3 shows the populations rolled forwards from 1991 in Shipham using the mean migration functions, and using estimated birth and death rates for years after 1992.

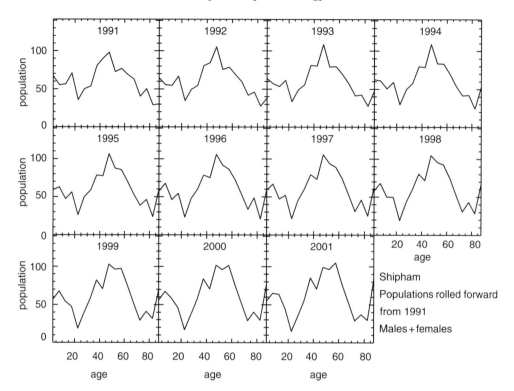

Fig. 3.3 Populations in Shipham aged forwards from 1991 to 2001 using the mean migration function from 1981 to 1991.

The use of a migration correction in combination with ageing the population preserves the expected behaviour of this ward in the age groups over 50: overall the population continues to age.

In the absence of annual data at small-area level, radical changes in any small-area populations cannot be tracked. In particular, inner-city areas with a high proportion of highly mobile young people will always be difficult to estimate. However, we expect in many cases that migration functions calculated as above may allow us to estimate the manner in which the population profile evolves after a census.

Until and unless other sources of data become available, our choices are simply to use the *Estimating with confidence* populations unchanged for the years following the 1991 census, or to use a method, such as cohort survival, with appropriately estimated migration probabilities. Using unchanged census populations will do well where population profiles reproduce themselves over time, as opposed to areas where the population does not migrate and simply ages. Some hybrid of these two approaches should be optimal, although it requires appropriate classification of each area as an ageing or static population.

Whichever method we use, it is important to estimate our level of confidence in the population counts that it provides. A rough-and-ready estimate of the error comes from the difference between the populations measured at 1981 and 1991. In addition, there is the internal measurement error in the census estimates themselves. These lack a gold standard against which they can be compared, although the work from the Estimating with Confidence project suggests that their ward totals have absolute errors less than 1.5% (with 95% confidence; see Lunn *et al.* 1998).

The most useful addition to the data that are available would be a further postcoded or, preferably, census-linked dataset (i.e one which is complied at small-area level), which tracks population either directly or by some proxy measure. Examples of such measures include registers of dwellings, electors, school rolls, or registers of patients from which detailed population and migration data can be extracted (Scott 1999).

3.5.3 Further analyses

In Section 3.4.1 an analytically tractable gamma Berkson model was introduced for the true expected counts with the first two moments given by Equation (3.6). This resulted in the MLE (3.7) with variance given by (3.8). The MLE and variance of a model incorporating migration are given by (3.10) and (3.11). Here we briefly investigate the sensitivity of inference to different specifications of b (the proportional bias in the observed count), h (the precision of the observed count) and ϕ_j (the fraction of the population at risk in stratum j), $j = 1, \ldots, J$.

Table 3.3 shows the effect of varying b, h, and ϕ_j on the estimation problem of the relative risk shown in Table 3.2. In all cases we have an observed total of 133 cases and

Table 3.3 Bias corrected relative risks for all cause mortality in the ward of Shipham under various assumptions. In each block of the table we have $b = 0$, $\varepsilon = 0$ and $\phi_j = 1$ (for all j) unless stated otherwise. The naive SMR in all cases is 0.86 with 95% interval (0.72, 1.02), and the estimates given are corrected for the stated assumption

Assumption	Relative risk estimate θ_c	95% confidence interval	Confidence interval width
Underenumeration b			
$b = -0.10$	0.95	0.81, 1.13	0.33
$b = 0.00$	0.86	0.72, 1.02	0.29
$b = 0.05$	0.82	0.69, 0.97	0.28
$b = 0.10$	0.78	0.66, 0.93	0.27
$b = 0.20$	0.72	0.60, 0.85	0.24
Relative measurement error ε			
$\varepsilon = 0.00$	0.86	0.72, 1.02	0.29
$\varepsilon = 0.10$	0.86	0.66, 1.11	0.45
$\varepsilon = 0.20$	0.86	0.56, 1.32	0.76
Fraction of population at risk ϕ_j			
$\phi_j = 1.00$	0.86	0.72, 1.02	0.29
$\phi_j = 0.90$	0.84	0.70, 1.02	0.33
$\phi_j = 0.80$	0.82	0.66, 1.03	0.37
$\phi_j = 0.70$	0.80	0.62, 1.04	0.42
$\phi_j = 0.60$	0.77	0.56, 1.05	0.49
$\phi_j = 0.50$	0.72	0.48, 1.08	0.60

an expected of 154.8, leading to a raw relative risk estimate of 0.86 with 95% confidence interval (0.72, 1.02). For ease of interpretation we have reparameterised the precision h as the relative error ε in the expected counts, by defining $h^{-1} = \varepsilon^2 E^o(1 + b)$. For example, a value of $\varepsilon = 0.10$ corresponds to an uncertainty of the order of 10% in the expected counts.

As expected, underenumeration ($b > 0$) increases the observed relative risk, whereas overenumeration decreases it. An underenumeration fraction of 10% or more is quite plausible in inner-city areas or areas which are otherwise hard to count, and it can be seen from the table that large differences in relative risks can result. Random errors in the population measurement, as measured by the relative error in the expected counts ε, do not have a great effect, however. The inflation of the variance induced is only slight for realistic levels of uncertainty.

Over a decade, migration may result in a replacement of the majority of the population. If 10% of the population moves in any one year, then after 10 years we can expect 70% of the population to have moved at least once. Even allowing for the fact that people who move once may be more likely to move again, we can always expect that large fractions of the population of an area will have changed during a study over a long time period.

The effect of migration is always to attenuate the observed relative risk, so that for an affluent area such as Shipham where the true relative risk of all cause mortality is apparently less than 1, both underenumeration and migration will increase the observed estimate. In areas where the relative risk is greater than one, underenumeration and migration will operate in opposite directions.

3.6   Concluding remarks

An epidemiological study restricted to a disease with a short latency period in an area in which the migration rates are low, and where the population has been measured accurately, will not suffer seriously from any of the biases discussed in this chapter. However, since almost always one or more of these conditions will fail to be met, some kind of bias is to be expected. Where information on migration rates and population measurement error is available, however, Equations (3.7), (3.8), (3.10), and (3.11) provide a simple means of estimating the likely scale of these biases, and are an appropriate caution against the simple interpretation of raw relative risks.

The existence of a reliable denominator is an important consideration in the planning of an epidemiological study. Often, the census is a convenient routinely available source of data, but information on the accuracy and, in particular, the level of underenumeration is vital. Such information can be used to assess informally the sensitivity via simple summaries such as the standardised mortality/morbidity ratio (SMR), or more formally via the methods of Section 3.4. Data on the level of migration is also important for determination of inter-censual counts and for exposure assessment. The main difficulty is that there rarely exists a 'gold standard' with which sets of counts can be compared.

Acknowledgements

This work is based on data provided with the support of the ESRC and JISC and uses census and boundary material which are copyright of the Crown, the Post Office, and the

ED-LINE Consortium. The Small Area Health Statistics Unit is funded by a grant from the Department of Health, Department of the Environment, Transport and the Regions, Health and Safety Executive, Scottish Office Home and Health Department, Welsh Office and Northern Ireland Department of Health and Social Services. This work was supported, in part, by an equipment grant from The Wellcome Trust (0455051/Z/95/Z).

References

Armstrong, B. G., Gleave, S., and Wilkinson, P. (1996). The impact of migration on disease rates in areas with previous environmental exposures. Abstract T280, 1996 Annual Conference ISEE. *Epidemiology*, 7(Suppl.), S88.

Arnold, R. A. (1999). Small Area Health Statistics Unit procedures for estimating small area populations. In *Population counts in small area studies: implications for studies of environment and health* (R. Arnold, P. Elliot, J. Wakefield, M. Quinn ed.). ONS Publication Series *Studies on medical and population subjects*. HMSO, London, pp. 10–24.

Atkins, D., Charlton, M., Dorling, D., and Wymer, C. (1993). *Connecting the 1981 and 1991 Censuses*. North East Regional Research Laboratory Research Report 93/9. Department of Geography, University of Newcastle upon Tyne.

Breslow, N. E. and Day, N. E. (1987). *Statistical methods in cancer research*. Vol. II: *the design and analysis of cohort studies*. IARC Scientific Publications. International Agency for Research on Cancer, Lyon.

Best, N. G. and Wakefield, J. C. (1999). Accounting for inaccuracies in population counts and case registration in cancer mapping studies. *Journal of the Royal Statistical Society, Series A*, **162**, 363–82.

Brown, J. J., Diamond, I. D., Chambers, R. L., Buckner, L. J., and Teague, A. D. (1999). A methodological strategy for a one number census in the UK. *Journal of the Royal Statistical Society, Series A*, **162**, 247–67.

Carroll, R. J., Ruppert, D., and Stefanski, L. A. (1995). *Measurement error in nonlinear models*. Chapman and Hall, London.

Chappell, R. (1999). ONS procedures for compiling population estimates at sub-national levels. In *Population counts in small-area studies: implications for studies of environment and health* (R. Arnold, P. Elliot, J. Wakefield, M. Quinn ed). ONS Publication Series *Studies on medical and population subjects*. HMSO, London, pp. 36–41.

Diamond, I. D., Ollerhead, J. B., Bradshaw, S. A., Walker, J. G., and Critchley, J. B. (1989). *A study of disturbance due to general and business aviation*. Department of Transport, London.

Diamond, I. D., Tesfaghiorghis, H., and Joshi, H. (1990). The uses and users of population projection in Australia. *Journal of the Australian Population Association*, **7**, 151–70.

Dorling, I. D. and Atkins, D. J. (1995). *Population density, change and concentration in Great Britain 1971, 1981 and 1991*. OPCS Publication Series *Studies on medical and population subjects* 58. HMSO, London.

Elliott, P., Shaddick, G., Kleinschmidt, I., Jolley, D., Walls, P., Beresford, J. *et al.* (1996). Cancer incidence near municipal solid waste incinerators in Great Britain. *British Journal of Cancer*, **73**, 702–7.

Elliott, P., Arnold, R., Cockings, S., Eaton, N., Jarup, L., Jones, J. *et al.* (1999). Risk of stroke and genitourinary cancers in a population potentially exposed to cadmium. *Occupational and Environmental Medicine*, **57**, 94–7.

Ericksen, E. P. and Kadane, J. B. B. (1987). Sensitivity analysis of local estimates of undercount in the 1980 US Census. In *Small area statistics* (R. Platek *et al.* ed.), 23–45. Wiley, New York.

Feeney, G. A. (1987). The estimation of the number of unemployed at the small area level. In *Small area statistics* (R. Platek *et al.* ed.), 198–218. Wiley, New York.

Fox, A. J. and Golblatt, P. O. (1982). *Socio-demographic differentials in mortality 1971–75*. OPCS Series LS 1. HMSO, London.

Ghosh, M. and Rao, J. N. K. (1994). Small area estimation: an appraisal. *Statistical Science*, **9**, 55–93.

Hattersley, L. and Creeser, R. (1995). *Longitudinal study 1971–1991. History, organisation and quality of data.* OPCS Series LS 7. HMSO, London.

Joshi, H. and Diamond, I. (1990). Demographic projections: who needs to know. In *Population projections: trends, methods and uses.* OPCS occasional paper 38, 1–22. HMSO, London.

Kliewer, E. V. (1992). Influence of migrant on regional variations of stomach and colon cancer in the western United States. *International Journal of Epidemiology*, **111**, 175–82.

Lundström, S. (1987). An evaluation of small area estimation methods: the case of estimating the number of nonmarried cohabiting persons in Swedish municipalities. In *Small area statistics* (R. Platek *et al.* ed.), 198–218. Wiley, New York.

Lunn, D., Simpson, S., Diamond, I., and Middleton, L. (1998). The accuracy of age-specific population estimates for small areas in Britain. *Population Studies*, **52**, 327–44.

McCullagh, P. and Zidek, J. V. (1987). Regression methods and performance criteria for small area population estimation. In *Small area statistics* (R. Platek *et al.* ed.), 198–218. Wiley, New York.

Mallett, Sir Bernard (1929). Reform of vital statistics: outline of a system of national registration. *Eugenics Review*, **21**, 87–94.

Morrison, P. A. and Relles, D. A. (1976). A method of monitoring small area population change in cities. *Public Data Use*, **3**, 10–15.

Platek, R., Rao, J. N. K., Sarndal, C. E., and Singh, M. P. (ed.) (1987). *Small area statistics: an international symposium.* Wiley, New York.

Polissar, L. (1980). The effect of migration on comparison of disease rates in geographic studies in the United States. *American Journal of Epidemiology*, **111**, 175–82.

Pujadas, L. (1983). Small area estimation. Unpublished M.Sc. thesis University of Southampton, UK.

Purcell, N. J. and Kish, K. (1979). Estimation for small domains. *Biometrics*, **35**, 365–84.

Purcell, N. J. (1979). Efficient domain estimation: a categorical data approach. Unpublished Ph.D. thesis. University of Michigan, Ann Arbor.

Redfern, P. (1989). Population registers: some administrative and statistical pros and cons. *Journal of the Royal Statistical Society, Series A*, **152**, 1–41.

Richardson, S. (1992). Statistical methods for geographical correlation studies. In *Geographical and environmental epidemiology: methods for small-area studies* (P. Elliott, J. Cuzick, D. English, and R. Stern ed.), 181–204, Oxford University Press.

Scott, A. (1999). Population estimation using routine patient registration data. In *Population counts in small area studies: implications for studies of environment and health* (R. Arnold, P. Elliot, J. Wakefield, M. Quinn ed.). ONS Publication Series *Studies on medical and population subjects.* HMSO, London, pp. 42–6.

Simpson, S. (ed.) (1998). *Making local population statistics: a guide for practitioners.* Local Authorities Research and Intelligence Association, 2 Turnstile Close, Winnersh, Wokingham RG41 5LQ, UK.

Simpson, S., Diamond, I., Tonkin, P., and Tye, R. (1996). Updating small area population estimates in England and Wales. *Journal of Royal Statistical Society, Series A*, **159**, 235–47.

Simpson, S., Cossey, R., and Diamond, I. (1997*a*). 1991 population estimates for areas smaller than districts. *Population Trends*, **90**, 31–9.

Simpson, S., Diamond, I., Middleton, L., and Lunn, D. (1997*b*). Methods for making small area population estimates in Britain. *International Journal of Population Geography*, **3**, 265–80.

Swanson, D. A. and Tedrow, L. M. (1984). Improving the measurement of temporal change in regression models for county population estimates. *Demography*, **21**, 373–89.

Wakefield J. C. and Wallace, C. (1999). Implications of estimated counts for small area studies of environment and health. In *Population counts in small area studies: implications for studies of environment and health* (R. Arnold, P. Elliott, J. Wakefield, M. Quinn ed.). ONS Publication Series *Studies on medical and population subjects.* HMSO, London, pp. 63–74.

4. Socio-economic factors at areal level and their relationship with health

V. Carstairs

4.1 Introduction

Mapping of disease or exposure implies examination of data from a geographical perspective. This chapter adopts that perspective, although much of the analysis that documents the associations between socio-economic factors and health has been based on data collected at the level of the individual. In Britain, for instance, well-known differentials in mortality by social class were recognised in the last century, once occupation (as a basis for social class) appeared as an item on the death certificate.

The need to interrogate the routine health databases has acted as a spur to the development of area methods of analysis to identify areas with high rates of disease. Growing interest in 'inequalities in health' in the United Kingdom (Department of Health 1995, 1998a) and elsewhere has focused attention particularly on socio-economic, among other, differentials. This chapter is mainly concerned with the development and application of area methods to examine socio-economic differentials and their effects on health in the UK. The situation in other countries, where the methodology has tended to be less developed (mainly for historical reasons including data availability), is reviewed briefly in Section 4.4.

4.2 Data and methods

4.2.1 The postcode basis

Area analysis is facilitated by the use of a residence code that permits the allocation of a dwelling or an event to a small geographical level, and such events can then be aggregated to a larger geographical level to provide a sufficient volume for analysis. In the UK, the basis for this approach is provided by the postcode system, with a 'unit' postcode being common to about 14 households (see Chapter 14). Most routine health records now use the postcode system of area referencing. A Postcode Directory permits the allocation of the unit postcode to a wide range of areas of differing size (Table 4.1). In addition, using a map grid reference, postcodes may be grouped to give an arbitrarily constructed area such as a circle around a point source of pollution, a method of value in assessing possible environmental effects on health (see Chapter 9).

4.2.2 The area basis

Census material provides population denominator data to allow rates to be calculated, for example at the level of individual ward or postcode sector. Identifying areas with

Table 4.1   Areas used in analyses (England and Wales)

	Number
Local Authority counties	55
and districts	403
Health Authorities areas	8
and districts	190
Local Education Authority areas	107
Wards	9930
Postcode sectors	*c.* 7700
Enumeration districts	*c.* 110 000
Total population	*c.* 51 million

high rates of morbidity or mortality may in itself prove of value in planning the delivery of health care, and the mapping of such data will allow the pattern of variation to emerge more clearly (Gordon and Womersley 1997). Rates for such areas also commonly provide the basis for calculating the correlation between the health events and the area (socio-economic) characteristics, the latter of which are often provided by census variables (see Section 4.2.3).

At the lowest level of census output, that is at enumeration district (ED) level (Table 4.1), the smaller populations (around 140 households) result in fewer events and rates cannot reliably be computed, although statistical methods can be used to smooth out random fluctuations (Chapter 7). When used in health studies, EDs will often be grouped together on the basis of their census characteristics to provide a more robust measure (Reading *et al.* 1990), and rates can be calculated by summing over the events and populations at various levels of area characteristics (although this will not of course provide a geographical base). Since postcodes may span ED boundaries in England and Wales, some errors may occur in matching individual addresses (postcode units) to EDs via the Postcode Directory (Collins *et al.* 1998; Chapter 2).

Data for larger areas such as administrative, health, and education authorities are more readily available and feature in some analyses. These larger areas present much less diversity than emerges at a lower level: low numbers of events present a problem at smaller area level. Aggregation over years, however, can help to reduce this problem.

The area-based approach has the advantage that most events/persons can be allocated to an area by means of the postcode, and linking to the socio-economic characteristics for that area permits the analysis of records that do not carry social information. Area analysis has thus become a popular means not only of characterising differences between populations, but also of identifying inequalities in health through the analysis of socio-economic data and their relationships with health.

Using an area approach invites the criticism of the 'ecological fallacy' (see Chapter 11), that is the implication that all individuals living in an area share the characteristics of that area, which is clearly not the case; although others take a different view (Krieger 1992; Bartley 1994). Individual characteristics may appear more specific, but they do not avoid this problem as social categories are by no means homogeneous. Social class, for instance, provides a crude measure of social status, with individuals within a category exhibiting very different attitudes and lifestyles. Classification aims to group together individuals/households that, on balance, are more like one another than those in other groups or classes.

4.2.3 Construction of deprivation indices in the UK

Both single variables and composite measures have been utilised to define the socio-economic characteristics of an area and come in the main from census sources. Data from local authority sources are also used in some composite measures, and social security benefits data from the Department of Social Security at small-area level have recently been reported in a study from Northern Ireland (O'Reilly and Stevenson 1998). Census data have the advantage of capturing information on a uniform basis for (nearly) all members of the population, although there are limitations to their ability to encompass the totality of both individual and environmental circumstances.

The composite measures in general use, labelled as deprivation indices, combine data from a number of census variables and are designed to place an area on a dimension from affluence to poverty. This construct underlies two indices in common use—Carstairs (1995) and Townsend (1987)—with '(lack of) material resources' providing a basis for measurement (Table 4.2).

The Jarman Underprivileged Area (UPA) score (Jarman 1983, 1984) was developed mainly in the context of need for primary care services, but has been adopted as an index of socio-economic circumstances in general by some researchers. While contextual information relating to the actual area (e.g. transport/leisure/health facilities) has been reported in some small-scale local studies (Sooman and Macintyre 1995), such information needs to be assembled specially, and is not part of any national database.

An example of mapping of deprivation at the level of electoral ward is given in Fig. 4.1, which shows a map of Greater London with each ward shaded accorded to quintiles of scores based on Jarman's UPA index for the 1991 census. It clearly demonstrates areas of relative deprivation in Inner London with areas of relative affluence in the surrounding suburbs.

The construction of the deprivation indices rests on the assumption that some life circumstances are preferential to others, such as being employed rather than unemployed, having a car, living in spacious rather than crowded conditions, or having all housing amenities. Other characteristics may be viewed as a means of achieving these (and other) ends, or of conferring access to various opportunities in life: income as well as wealth, social class (with its implications in relation to level of income), and educational attainment. Material deprivation denies individuals opportunities through 'lack of goods

Table 4.2 Definitions: What are indices trying to measure?

Carstairs:	Material deprivation: access to material resources—a dimension from affluence to poverty; reflects wealth and income
Jarman: (UPA score)	Need for primary care services: factors affecting demand for GP services
Townsend:	Material deprivation: 'the material apparatus, goods, services, resources, amenities, physical environment, and location of life'
DoE:	Needs for local authority services: factors relevant to allocation of resources

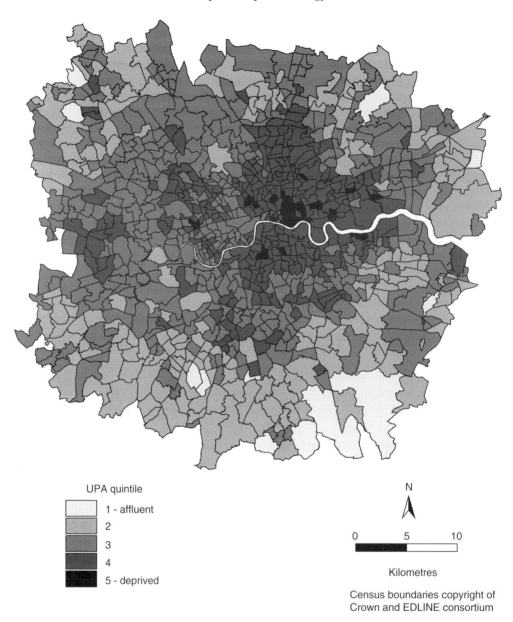

UPA quintile

1 - affluent

2

3

4

5 - deprived

N

0   5   10

Kilometres

Census boundaries copyright of
Crown and EDLINE consortium

Fig. 4.1 Underprivileged area (UPA) score quintiles for wards within the M25 boundary.

and services, resources and amenities and of a physical environment that are customary
in society' (Townsend 1987). One commentator has suggested that 'the concept of deprivation covers the various conditions, independent of income, experienced by people who
are poor, while the concept of poverty refers to the lack of income and other resources
which makes those conditions inescapable or at least highly likely' (Gordon 1995). While
financial circumstances would appear to underpin 'access to material resources', information

on incomes is not readily accessible in the UK, since it has not been included in the census. Both car and home ownership are included in deprivation indices in the UK as a proxy for wealth in the absence of better data, although as car ownership, in particular, is becoming more widespread, its ability to discriminate between areas is likely to lessen over time.

Indices that are in common use in relation to health analyses in the UK contain a wide range of individual indicators (Table 4.3). Carstairs (Carstairs and Morris 1991) and Townsend (Townsend *et al.* 1988) agree on three of the four variables included in their indices: unemployment, overcrowding, and no car access. Carstairs includes a measure of social class (percentage of individuals in households with head in social class IV/V) while Townsend uses 'households not owner-occupied', a circumstance that could fail to discriminate between large sections of the population in areas with high levels of public housing. The Jarman score has only three of its eight variables in common with these two indices (Jarman 1983, 1984), and has been criticised with respect to its lack of a sound methodological basis, and the inclusion of demographic variables with strong weights (Davey Smith 1991; Senior 1991).

Although many of the individual variables in these three indices appear similar, definitions differ. Townsend, for instance, defines three of the component variables in terms of households whereas all of those in Carstairs relate to individuals. The 'unskilled' variable in Jarman uses 'Socioeconomic Group 11', whereas in Carstairs it is 'Social

Table 4.3   Variables and weights included in indices

	CAR	JAR	TOWN	DoE
Unemployment (M + F)		3.34	X	X
male	X			
No car	X	X	X	
Low social class (IV/V)	X			
Unskilled (SEG11)		3.74		
Overcrowding	X	2.88	X	X
Not owner-occupied			X	
Lacking amenities				X
Single parent household		3.01		
Under age 5 years		4.64		
Pensioner living alone		6.62		
Moved in past year		2.68		
Ethnic minorities		2.50		
Children in unsuitable accommodation				X
Children in low earner households				X
Age 17/not in education				X
Non-census variables				
SMR < 75				X
Unemployed more than 1 year				X
Income support recipients				X
Low education level (GCSE D or less)				X
Derelict land				X

CAR, Carstairs; JAR, Jarman; TOWN, Townsend; DoE, Department of the Environment, 1991.

Class IV/V'. While the Jarman index tends to be used as originally defined, some experiment has taken place in relation to Carstairs and Townsend: for example, an amalgam of the two, omitting 'overcrowded housing', was used in a study of health events from the Longitudinal Study (Sloggett and Joshi 1998), a national study that links census data for the individual with vital statistics and the reporting of health events (see Section 4.3).

An index that originates from a government department, the Department of the Environment (DoE 1995), makes use of many other housing and demographic indicators from the census, with the latest (1991) index containing variables that are not census-based (Table 4.3). These do not focus specifically on a concept of deprivation, but may reflect circumstances relevant to the distribution of resources. Six indicators are for use at enumeration district level, another (age 17, not in full-time education) at ward level, and six non-census indicators (an Index of Local Conditions) at district level (DoE). The attraction of these latter variables lies in the possibility of updating them for inter-censual years, thus overcoming one of the shortcomings of census-based indices that are available only at ten-year intervals. Although the DoE measure has featured in at least one national health study (Drever and Whitehead 1995), many of its individual variables are found to have only weak association with health measures (Table 4.4).

Table 4.4 Correlation of composite and single variables with mortality and census sickness measures (source: Morris and Carstairs 1991; Congdon *et al.* 1997; Bentham *et al.* 1995)

	SMR 0–64 M%F	Perm. sick 16+	SMR 45–64 M	LLTI 45–64 M	SMR 0–64 M	LLTI 0–64 M
Carstairs	0.75	0.83			0.87	0.81
Townsend	0.73	0.80	0.60	0.73	0.84	0.70
Jarman	0.68	0.67			0.79	0.70
DoE	0.76	0.80			0.79	0.69
Unemployment (M + F)		0.82	0.59	0.75	0.81	0.80
male	0.74	0.82			0.81	0.82
No car access	0.80	0.65	0.78			
Social class IV/V	0.62	0.70	0.46	0.67		
Crowded housing	0.65	0.73	0.37	0.41		
Tenure not owned	0.55	0.64	0.52	0.62		
Single parent family	0.53	0.57				
Large households	0.42	0.45				
Economically inactive			0.43	0.72		
Females economically inactive			−0.29	−0.54		
House lacking amenities	0.16	0.06				
Lone elderly	0.10	0.13				
Children aged under 5	0.02	−0.12				
Dependent children			−0.01	0.09		
Moved in last year	−0.16	−0.35				
Ethnic origin	−0.05	−0.16				

SMR, Standardised Mortality Ratio; LLTI, Limiting LongTerm Illness.

4.2.4 Calculation of a deprivation score

As well as differing in the selection of variables and the way these are defined, the constituent variables of deprivation indices are combined in different ways to achieve a score (Box 1).

Box 1 Approaches to deriving an area index

Indices	*Statistical treatment*
Carstairs	Z-scores, no weighting, no transformation
Jarman	Z-scores, weighting all variables, arcsine transformation
Townsend	Z-scores, no weighting, log transformation
DoE	Signed chi-square, log transformation based on absolute values not percentage

Calculating an area deprivation score (example)

	Area *EH41.3*	*Mean*	*SD*
Overcrowding	0.22	0.25	0.11
Male unemployment	0.08	0.13	0.07
Low social class	0.23	0.24	0.10
No car	0.27	0.41	0.19

NB Means and standard deviations for all Scotland postcode sectors

Deprivation score:

$$= (0.22 - 0.25)/0.11 \quad +(0.08 - 0.13)/0.07 \quad +(0.23 - 0.24)/0.10 \quad +(0.27 - 0.41)/0.19$$
$$= -0.27 \qquad\qquad\quad -0.71 \qquad\qquad\quad -0.10 \qquad\qquad\quad -0.74$$
$$= -1.82$$

This example shows that in postcode sector EH41.3, 22% of individuals were living in overcrowded accommodation (more than one person per room), compared with 25% in the total population; 8% of men were unemployed; 23% were in a household with the head in Social Class IV or V; and 27% in a household without a car, compared with 41% overall. The standard deviation indicates that most variability exists in car ownership, which in fact has a range at postcode sector level (c. 1000 sectors) from 3% to 89% in Scotland.

The total score across all sectors ranges from −7.3 to +12.3, with a minus score indicating more affluence and a positive score greater deprivation (Carstairs and Morris 1991).

For scores that incorporate a weighting system (e.g. Jarman) the appropriate term will be multiplied by the weight for the variable, resulting in a wider range in the scores: from −45 to +45 for Jarman at sector or ward level, and from −51 to +54 for EDs in three London Health Districts (Curtis 1990). At Local Authority district level the DoE scores ranged from −40 to +40 (Drever and Whitehead 1995). Scores may be calculated at any area level available in the census output; means and standard deviations will vary depending on the number of areas examined, and the range in scores on the area level used. Greatest diversity between areas is found at smaller-area level.

Variables are expressed as the percent of individuals or households in an area with the relevant characteristic, and are mostly subjected to the Z-score technique that reduces them to a standardised value with zero mean and a standard deviation of unity, so that they may be summed on a uniform basis. It may be noted that although this approach facilitates comparison of areas at any one moment in time, time-trend data need to be handled with special care, since individual area scores are affected by changes in other parts of the country. In some cases, variables that are highly skewed are first transformed to an approximately normal distribution, with a log transformation being the most popular method, although others are used. Variables in the Jarman score are additionally weighted in accordance with weights determined by general practitioners as indicators of their relative contribution to GP workload (Jarman 1984) (Table 4.3).

The unweighted basis of some indices has been questioned (Gordon 1995). An analysis that used income data for the individual from the General Household Survey for 1984, and the Family Expenditure Survey for 1983 and 1990, together with a number of household variables, found that the best predictor of income level was achieved with combinations of *weighted* variables (around 40% of variance explained), although the weights varied between the three datasets used (Davies *et al.* 1997). Modelled on that approach, a combination of individual-level and census data was used to calculate a weighted area deprivation index in a small study (Saunders 1998).

4.3   Linking deprivation and health

For reporting gradients in health outcomes, deprivation scores are commonly grouped into quintiles or deciles of the range, or use other characteristics of the distribution; Carstairs, for instance, identifies seven so-called DEPCATS. The values allow comparison of disease rates or standardised mortality (or morbidity) ratios. An example of the use of DEPCATS in Scotland (in relation to mortality from various causes) is given in Fig. 4.2.

Correlation analysis has been much used for reporting levels of association between health and deprivation variables (Table 4.4); the Pearson product-moment method is usual, but ranking methods have occasionally been used. An alternative approach is some form of multivariate analysis that seeks to identify the contribution made by each

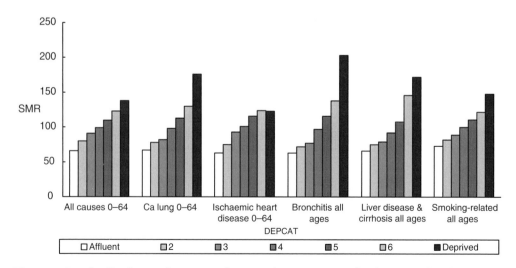

Fig. 4.2 Standardised mortality ratios for specific causes, Scotland 1980–5 by deprivation category (DEPCAT).

variable, taking into account the intercorrelation between them, and reporting the percent of variance explained, while multi-level modelling examines data at various area levels, as well as for the individual.

There is a large and growing literature on health inequalities in relation to socio-economic measures. Mortality offers a reliable base and has been extensively analysed, mostly focusing on 'premature' mortality and all causes, although cause-specific data and different age groups also feature (Townsend *et al.* 1988; Carstairs and Morris 1991; Eames *et al.* 1993; McLoone and Boddy 1994; Phillimore *et al.* 1994; Drever and Whitehead 1995). The morbidity variables of 'permanent sickness' from the 1981 census, applying mainly to the population of working age, and, in 1991 'limiting long-term illness' (LLTI), applicable to all age groups, have been extensively examined (Bentham *et al.* 1995; Haynes *et al.* 1996; Congdon *et al.* 1997). (See Table 4.5.)

A number of other end-points have also been examined: for example, the cancer register provides a valuable source of information and a selected range of specific causes of disease has recently been reported, based on first admissions to both general and mental hospitals (McLaren and Bain 1998). Many other morbidity variables appear in the literature (Table 4.5), some obtained from population surveys rather than from official statistics; see for example, Bentham *et al.* (1995). Biological variables such as height, birthweight,

Table 4.5   Health variables examined in relation to deprivation

Mortality	*Health behaviour*
by age, sex and cause	teenage pregnancies and outcomes
'premature' (i.e. < 65)	breast-feeding
potential years of life lost	participation in screening
life expectancy	cervical screening uptake
	immunisation uptake
	sickness absence
	smoking
Morbidity	*Service use*
(a) from routine data systems	GP consultations
permanent sickness	hospital admissions
limiting long-term illness	
cancer registration, and survival	
perceived general health	
tuberculosis notifications	
birthweight	
admissions to mental	
hospital × cause	
admissions to general	
hospitals × cause	
(b) from local and survey data	
perceived general health	
self-reported conditions	
Nottingham Health profile	
height/weight/BMI	
dental state	

and dental state can be objectively assessed, but some self-reported morbidity measures (including those from the census) may of course be subject to variations in people's perceptions, variations in practice, or resource use or availability (Blane *et al.* 1996, 1997). The Longitudinal Study has provided a large database for many researchers. Started in 1971, a 1% sample of the population was selected on the basis of four birth dates, and is updated by the addition of new births and new migrants, and the subtraction of deaths and outward migrants. A range of events occurring to the members of the sample is incorporated (via record linkage techniques), including marriages and births, cancer registration and death, with individual characteristics from the census records being added to the information base. Although mainly used for analysis at the individual level, a few area-based studies originate from this source (Sloggett and Joshi 1998). Health behaviour (for example, teenage pregnancies) and service use, mainly based on GP consultations and hospital admissions, provide other types of study.

With a few exceptions in respect of some specific causes of illness or death a gradient of increasing morbidity/mortality from the most affluent to the most deprived areas is invariably reported in all studies. This trend is generally linear in character (Figs 4.2 and 4.3). Levels of premature mortality (0–64), permanent sickness and limiting long-term illness (LLTI) are reported to be 1.5–2.5 times higher in deprived areas than in affluent areas. Larger differentials are found at younger ages and for some specific causes such as lung cancer: for example, a three fold difference can be observed across deprivation categories for cancer registrations (Fig. 4.3).

A clear gradient in survival is also found for some, but not all, cancer sites (Schrijvers *et al.* 1995; Pollock and Vickers 1997) The ratios quoted are, of course, influenced by the size of area (ranging from EDs, wards, and postcode sectors to local authority and health districts), the deprivation measure employed and its distribution.

The correlation of deprivation with mortality is stronger at 0–64 than at 65 and over, and generally stronger with census sickness measures than with mortality (Table 4.4)

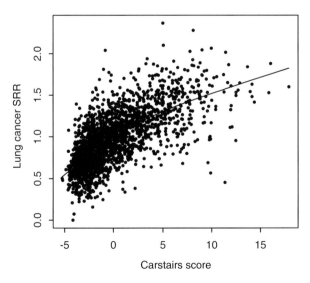

Fig. 4.3 Standardised registration ratios (SRRs) relating lung cancer incidence to Carstairs' score, Thames Region.

(Bentham *et al.* 1995; Carstairs 1995). At 0–64, both mortality and sickness measures are more strongly correlated with Carstairs and Townsend than with Jarman and DoE, probably due to the inclusion of demographic variables in those two indices (Bentham *et al.* 1995). On the other hand, Jarman is more strongly correlated with hospital admission measures (Morris and Carstairs 1991).

The relationship with the component variables of 'unemployed' and 'no car' is generally stronger than 'low social class', 'tenure not owned', and 'overcrowded housing' (Table 4.4). Others—'single parents', 'large households', 'economically inactive', and 'higher education'—show modest correlations, while for some housing and demographic characteristics the correlations are decidedly weak (Morris and Carstairs 1991; Congdon *et al.* 1997).

Analyses have not only shown the strong relationship between health and socio-economic circumstances, but have also identified a widening gap between affluent and deprived areas over the decade to 1991. Death rates fell overall over the period, but the gains were greater in affluent areas (Townsend *et al.* 1988; McLoone and Boddy 1994; Carstairs 1995). There were increases in mortality in some age groups in deprived areas, a finding also reported in an analysis of life-expectancy (at birth) between 1984–6 and 1992–4 at the level of health district authority. The gains were greatest in prosperous areas and improvements negligible in the most deprived (Raleigh and Kiri 1997).

Useful and interesting as these findings are, they inform us about the pattern of inequality but rarely add anything to our understanding of the causes of these differentials. One study in the UK has attempted to examine aspects of behaviour, considering the influence of both smoking (20 years earlier) and alcohol consumption (12 years earlier) on mortality in 1992. It concluded that differences in smoking accounted for about 85% of the excess in the most deprived decile, compared with the most affluent, deprivation for about 12% and alcohol for 6% (Law and Morris 1998). A study from the US, on the other hand, found that the income-mortality risk gradients were similar for both smokers and non-smokers and that the mortality risks associated with a $10 000 lower income still remained after adjustment for smoking and other risk factors (Davey Smith *et al.* 1996; see also Section 4.4).

The extent to which area, rather than individual, characteristics 'explain' variations in health has become a subject for debate (Macintyre *et al.* 1993), and some studies have investigated this topic using both area and individual characteristics. An anonymised sample of individual census records was used to analyse LLTI, with mortality added (Curtis 1990), while the Longitudinal Study provided a basis for examining both mortality and a range of fertility measures (Sloggett and Joshi 1998). Strong gradients were established between an area measure and all fertility measures except stillbirths, with a marked flattening of the gradient when ratios were adjusted for personal circumstances, in particular in areas of above-average deprivation. The differential between deprived and non-deprived persons was wider in non-deprived places. The study suggests that personal deprivation is not compounded by residence in a deprived place, but the authors acknowledge that 'contextual effects influencing health are not well identified by census indicators of social composition' (Sloggett and Joshi 1998). Another enquiry examining consultation rates in general practice also found the role of indices of deprivation to be considerably reduced when characteristics of individuals were taken into account (Carr-Hill *et al.* 1996). Other studies have not come to such definite conclusions, and suggest a role for the area over and above individual effects, perhaps because additional information is captured at area level (Shouls *et al.* 1996; Hart *et al.* 1997).

Insofar as deprived areas also tend to be areas with important sources of environ-mental pollution, deprivation is a potentially potent confounder of studies of environ-mental pollution and health. This is discussed farther in the next chapter.

4.4   The international scene

As noted at the beginning of the chapter, area methods for deprivation analysis appear to have been most commonly practised in the UK. Although in the US three census regions relevant to establishing area characteristics have been defined (the 'census tract', the census 'block group', and the 'Zip code'), there are few examples of the use of area data for work on socio-economic characteristics and health (Krieger *et al.* 1997). This is despite a methodological study that linked individual data from the census to those for census tracts and blocks and concluded that census-based methodology offers a valid and useful approach to overcoming the absence of socio-economic data in most US medical records (Krieger 1992). The examples that do exist have all made use of income data from the census.

Two analyses, relating to white and black men recruited to the Multiple Risk Factor Intervention Trial (MRFIT) between 1973 and 1975, have reported on mortality in a 16-year follow-up period. The median income of the Zip code area of residence correlated strongly with unemployment and education levels, the percentage of individuals in professional or managerial occupations, and the percentage below the poverty line. Both for white men (Davey Smith *et al.* 1996*a*) and black men (Davey Smith *et al.* 1996*b*) a clear gradient in mortality was observed in relation to income, with the association being continuous with no evidence of a threshold. The change in risk associated with a $10 000 lower income was reported as 1.22 for smokers and 1.18 for non-smokers in white men, and 1.29 and 1.31 in the same groups in black men, with higher relative risks identified for many specific causes. The income level for districts within the 50 states of the United States was also employed in a multi-level analysis of self-rated health to investigate the proposition that health inequalities are greater in areas with greater inequality in incomes; individuals living in states with greater inequality in incomes were 30% more likely to report poor/fair health after individual characteristics had been taken into account (Kennedy *et al.* 1998).

A few studies have emerged from Canada, with a scene-setting paper providing guid-ance on methods: data were derived for 49 census division (counties) for a number of dimensions of social and environmental characteristics (Jerret *et al.* 1998). Educational level was a strong predictor of mortality at 0–64 years for both males and females, with low income (as defined) being stronger for men than women. From 23 single socio-economic measures for 255 municipalities in Manitoba, 6 were found to explain most of the variance in the health measure, compiled from hospital admissions for four complaints plus fertility. The regression coefficients from a stepwise multiple regression procedure supplied the weights for a socio-economic risk index, composed from these 6 variables, that explained substantially more (60%) of the variance in the health measure than either household income or high-school completion rate (Frohlich and Mustard 1996). Income, from the census records at enumeration area level, was also used in a small-scale study that reported persons in the four lower decile income areas to be signifi-cantly more likely to undergo surgery for cataract (Meddings *et al.* 1998).

Studies from Europe are almost entirely based on individual data. These are either cross-sectional in nature, capturing data from population surveys—e.g. the European Union Working Group on Health Inequalities (Kunst *et al.* 1998)—or on a longitudinal design, linking individual characteristics from the census with subsequent mortality or morbidity. Scandinavian countries in particular have the benefit of population registers and unique person identifiers to facilitate such linkage (Silvonen *et al.* 1998; see also Chapter 2). Some examples using composite area measures have, however, appeared for Sweden. The Jarman UPA score was calculated, using the UK weights, for more than 8000 areas, and a wide range in deprivation identified (Bajekal *et al.* 1996). Twenty percent of the variation in mortality at 20–64 years in 284 municipalities was explained by the UPA score in a later paper (Sundquist *et al.* 1997). Nevertheless, in a subsequent enquiry, Swedish GPs weighted some of the variables quite differently from GPs in the UK (Malstrom *et al.* 1998). Also in Sweden, an inverse relationship was established between unemployment rates in counties and sickness absence rates, when adjusted for occupation (Knutsson and Gorne 1998).

A number of studies have examined the applicability of the Jarman index in Amsterdam. In relation to GP contacts for residents aged 16 and over, six out of the eight Jarman indicators were associated with differentials in contact rates, with poor quality of housing and being born in a foreign country being most important (Reijenveld 1996). The Jarman index was also used in an analysis of admissions to mental hospitals with a range of other socio-economic indicators at individual level. A significant (albeit weak) correlation with admissions, length of stay (negative) and re admissions was reported: in more affluent areas there were fewer admissions, longer stays and fewer readmissions, while a revolving door pattern was apparent for more deprived areas (Dekker *et al.* 1997). Also from Amsterdam, a range of health measures had a higher prevalence in more deprived areas, in particular for 'physical limitations' and 'poor health'; most of the poorer health could, however, be attributed to the lower socio-economic status of the residents rather than the area characteristics (Reijenveld 1998).

Deaths at age 0–74 over four 5-year periods to 1989 were examined in New South Wales, using the single variable of 'percent unskilled'. Correlations between 0.55 and 0.69 were reported for males and females, with ratios of 1.3–1.45 : 1 between areas with lower and higher educational levels for Sydney, and with no reduction found in the socio-economic differentials over time (Quine *et al.* 1995). Also for Sydney, mortality and hospital morbidity were examined using the composite Ross index (40 variables). This was found to be no more effective than the single indicators of percentage unskilled and percentage unemployed (Taylor *et al.* 1992).

4.5 Conclusion

Individual socio-economic variables and deprivation indices at area level have proved their value in allowing a socio-economic dimension to emerge from a range of routine databases over the past two decades. As the social climate changes, however, it is likely that the constituent variables in the indices will require review; car ownership is now more widespread, and overcrowding in housing has fallen to a low level. More administrative data from official sources are becoming available at small-area level—unemployment claimants, income support recipients, and participants in higher education.

If available on a continuing basis, these could offer alternatives to the use of census-based measures that are available only at 10-yearly intervals. Unemployment levels from the census have already been shown to correlate nearly as strongly with health state as with the composite indices (Table 4.4), and this indicator has been the focus of a number of studies (Haynes *et al.* 1996); educational attainment may be a potent factor in influencing attitudes and behaviour and in developing skills that can provide insulation from adverse experiences; income support data give some direct insight into the financial standing of populations. At the present time, the lack of population denominators at small-area level to transform these counts into meaningful statistics presents problems in using the data (except for the educational variable); patient information held in the primary care registers could provide a resource if it could reach a standard to fill this gap.

Socio-economic position does not, of itself, explain health state; rather it represents a complex of living experience, living and working conditions, attitudes and social orientation, income, wealth, and assets for the individual. As well as these personal attributes, 'poor places' provide socially adverse environments that strike at the health status of even the non-poor inhabitants—many residents suffer from a combination of poor opportunities, poor services, sometimes high crime, low morale and stigma which compounds the individual experience of poverty (Sloggett and Joshi 1998). Absolute poverty and impoverished environments are nevertheless not sufficient as a focus for explanation since gradients in health are found throughout the socio-economic dimension, and 'the linear nature of the association ... presents a serious challenge to any simple interpretation couched in terms of absolute poverty' (Davey Smith *et al.* 1996*a,b*). Theoretical constructs were set out in the Black Report (Black 1980) and have provided the framework for much analysis since that time (Davey Smith 1991*a,b*; Bartley 1994; Blane *et al.* 1996, 1997). Of these, 'artefactual' explanations and theories of 'natural or social selection' have been dismissed as making only a small contribution to the inequalities observed (Fox *et al.* 1985) and further progress probably resides in determining the influence of the environment, of material circumstances, cultural habits, and behaviour on health states (Davey Smith *et al.* 1994; Blane *et al.* 1997).

Current routine data sets probably cannot aid this search; the new national health surveys now appearing on the scene (Department of Health 1998*b*; Scottish Office Department of Health 1998) may make some contribution, although the determinants of health are likely to remain elusive and prove difficult to measure. Cross-sectional data are also unlikely to prove sufficient since both health state and current socio-economic state are arrived at after a lifetime of experience. Longitudinal study designs offer the best prospect for examining influences over the life-cycle, but the continuing emergence of new risk factors inevitably means that relevant information may not have formed part of the original data collection.

Area-based data will continue to have an important role to play in monitoring changes in health differentials in the population. Nevertheless, these need to be enhanced with data on the characteristics of the area, as well as those of the residents, if they are to aid understanding of the contextual effects on population health.

References

Bajekal, M., Jan, S., and Jarman, B. (1996). The Swedish UPA score: an administrative tool for identification of underprivileged areas. *Scandinavian Journal of Social Medicine*, **24**, 177–84.

Bartley, M. (1994). Unemployment and ill-health: understanding the relationship. *Journal of Epidemiology and Community Health*, **48**, 333–7.

Bentham, G., Eimermann, J., Haynes, R., Lovett, A., and Brainard, J. (1995). Limiting longterm illness and its associations with mortality and indicators of social deprivation. *Journal of Epidemiology and Community Health*, **49**(Suppl. 2), S57–64.

Black, D. (Chairman) (1980). *Inequalities in health: report of a working group*. Department of Health and Social Security, London.

Blane, D., Bartley, M., and Smith, G. D. (1997). Disease aetiology and materialistic explanations of socioeconomic mortality differentials *European Journal of Public Health*, **4**, 385–91.

Blane, D., Power, C., and Bartley, M. (1996). Illness behaviour and the measurement of class differentials in morbidity. *Journal of the Royal Statistical Society A*, **159**, 77–92.

Carr-Hill, R., Rice, N., and Rolan, M. (1996). Socioeconomic determinants of consultations in general practice based on the fourth National Morbidity Survey of general practice. *British Medical Journal*, **312**, 1008–13.

Carstairs, V. and Morris, R. (1991). *Deprivation and health in Scotland*. Aberdeen University Press, UK.

Carstairs, V. (1995). Deprivation indices: their interpretation and use in relation to health. *Journal of Epidemiology and Community Health*, **49**(Suppl. 2), S3–8.

Collins, S. E., Haining, R. P., Bowns, I. R., Crofts, D. J., Williams, T. S., and Hall, D. M. B. (1998). Errors in postcode to enumeration district mapping and their effect on small area analyses of health data. *Journal of Public Health Medicine*, **20**, 325–30.

Congdon, P., Shouls, S., and Curtis, S. (1997). A multi-level perspective on small area health and mortality: a case study of England and Wales. *International Journal of Population Geography*, **3**, 243–63.

Curtis, S. (1990). Use of survey data and small area statistics to assess the link between individual morbidity and neighbourhood deprivation. *Journal of Epidemiology and Community Health*, **44**, 62–8.

Davey Smith, G. (1991). Second thoughts on the Jarman index. *British Medical Journal*, **302**, 359–60.

Davey Smith, G., Blane, D., and Bartley, M. (1994). Explanation for socioeconomic differentials in mortality. *European Journal of Public Health*, **4**, 131–44.

Davey Smith, G., Wentworth, D., Neaton, J. D., Stamler, R., and Stamler, J. (1996). Socio-economic differentials in mortality risk among men screened for the Multiple Risk Factor Intervention Trial. I: White Men. *American Journal of Public Health*, **86**, 486–96; and (1996*b*) Trial II: Black Men. *American Journal of Public Health*, **86**, 497–504.

Davies, H., Joshi, H., and Clarke, C. (1997). Is it cash that the deprived are short of? *Journal of the Royal Statistical Society A*, **160**, 107–26.

Dekker, J., Peen, J., Gorris, A., Jeihnen, H., and Kwakman, H. (1997). Social deprivation and psychiatric admission rates in Amsterdam. *Social Psychiatry and Psychiatric Epidemiology*, **32**, 485–92.

Department of the Environment (1995). *1991 Deprivation index: a review of approaches and a matrix of results*. HMSO, London.

Department of Health (1995). *Variations in health: what can the Department of Health and the N.H.S do?* Department of Health, London.

Department of Health (1998*a*). *Independent inquiry into inequalities in health*. HMSO, London.

Department of Health (1998*b*). *Health survey for England 1995*. HMSO, London.

Drever, F. and Whitehead, M. (1995). Mortality in regions and local authority districts in the 1990s; exploring the relationship with deprivation. *Population Trends*, **82**, 19–25.

Eames, M, Ben-Shlomo, Y., and Marmot, G. (1993). Social deprivation and premature mortality: regional comparison across England. *British Medical Journal*, **302**, 1197–1202.

Fox, A. J., Goldblatt, P. O., and Jones D. R. (1985). Social class mortality differentials: artefact, selection or life circumstances? *Journal of Epidemiology and Community Health*, **39**, 1–8.

Frohlich, N. and Mustard, C. (1996). A regional comparison of socioeconomic and health indices in a Canadian province. *Social Science and Medcine*, **42**, 1273–81.

Gordon, A. and Womersley, J. (1997). The use of mapping in public health and planning health services. *Journal of Public Health Medicine*, **19**, 137–8.

Gordon, D. (1995). Census based deprivation indices: their weighting and validation. *Journal of Epidemiology and Community Health*, **49**(Suppl. 2) S39–42.

Hart, C., Ecob, R., and Davey Smith, G. (1997). People, places and coronary heart disease risk factors: a multilevel analysis of the Scottish Heart Health study archive. *Social Science and Medicine*, **45**, 893–902.

Haynes, R., Gale, S., Lovett, A., and Eimermann, J. (1996). Unemployment rate as an updatable health needs indicator for small areas. *Journal of Public Health Medicine*, **18**, 27–32.

Jarman, B. (1983). Identification of underprivileged areas. *British Medical Journal*, **286**, 1705–9.

Jarman, B. (1984). Underprivileged areas: validation and distribution of scores. *British Medical Journal*, **289**, 1587–92.

Jerrett, M., Eyles, J., and Cole, D. (1998). Socioeconomic and environmental correlates of premature mortality 0–64 in Ontario. *Social Science and Medicine*, **47**, 33–49.

Kennedy, B. P., Kawachi, I., Glass, R., and Prothrow-Smith, D. (1998). Income distribution, socioeconomic status and self-rated health in the United States: a multilevel analysis. *British Medical Journal*, **317**, 917–21.

Knutsson, A. and Gorne, H. (1998). Occupation and unemployment rates as predictors of long-term sickness absence rates in two Swedish counties. *Social Science and Medicine*, **47**, 25–31.

Krieger, N. (1992). Overcoming the absence of socioeconomic data in medical records: validation and application of a census-based methodology. *American Journal of Public Health*, **82**, 703–10.

Krieger, N., Williams, D. R., and Moss, N. E. (1997). Measuring social class in U. S. Public Health Research: concepts, methodologies and guidelines. *Annual Review of Public Health*, **18**, 342–78.

Kunst, A. E., Groenhof, F., Mackenbach, J., and the E.U. Working Group on Inequalities in Health (1998). Mortality and occupational class in 11 E.C. countries. *British Medical Journal*, **316**, 1631–5.

Law, M. R. and Morris, J. K. (1998). Why is mortality higher in poorer areas and in more northern areas of England and Wales. *Journal of Epidemiology and Community Health*, **52**, 344–52.

MacIntyre, S., MacIver, S., and Sooman, A. (1993). Area, class and health; should we be focusing on places or people? *Journal of Social Policy*, **22**, 213–34.

Malstrom, M., Sundquist, J., Bajekal, M., and Johansson, S. E. (1998). Indices of need and deprivation for primary health care. *Scandinavian Journal of Social Medicine*, **26**, 1245–30.

McLaren, G. and Bain, M. (1998). *Deprivation and health in Scotland: some insights from NHS data*. ISD Scotland Publications, Edinburgh.

McLoone, P. and Boddy, A. (1994). Deprivation and mortality in Scotland 1981 and 1991. *British Medical Journal*, **309**, 1453–4.

Meddings, D. R., Hertzman, C., Barer, M. L., Evans, R. C. E., Kazanjian, A. *et al.* (1998). Socioeconomic status, mortality and the development of cataract at a young age. *Social Science and Medicine*, **46**, 1451–7.

Morris, R. and Carstairs, V. (1991). Which deprivation? A comparison of selected deprivation indices. *Journal of Public Health Medicine*, **13**, 318–26.

O'Reilly, D. and Stevenson, M. (1998). The two communities in Northern Ireland, deprivation and ill-health. *Journal of Public Health*, **20**, 161–8.

Phillimore, P., Beattie, A., and Townsend, P. (1994). Widening inequality in the north of England 1981–1991. *British Medical Journal*, **309**, 1125–8.

Pollock, A. M. and Vickers, N. (1997). Breast, lung and colorectal cancer incidence and survival in South Thames Region, 1987–1991: the effect of social deprivation. *Journal of Public Health Medicine*, **19**, 288–94.

Quine, S., Taylor, R. and Hayes, L. (1995). Australian trends in mortality by socioeconomic status using NSW small area data 1970–90. *Journal of Biosocial Science*, **27**, 409–19.

Raleigh, V. S. and Kiri, V. A. (1997). Life expectancy in England: variation and trends by gender, health authority and level of deprivation. *Journal of Epidemiology and Community Health*, **51**, 49–58.

Reading, R., Openshaw, J., and Jarvis, N. S. (1990). Measuring child health inequalities using aggregations of enumeration districts. *Journal of Public Health Medicine*, **12**(3/4), 160–7.

Reijneveld, S. A. (1996). Predicting the workload in an urban general practice in The Netherlands from Jarman's indicators of deprivation at patient level. *Journal of Epidemiology and Community Health*, **50**, 541–4.

Reijneveld, S. A. (1998). The impact of individual and area characteristics on urban socioeconomic differences in health and smoking. *International Journal of Epidemiology*, **27**, 33–40.

Saunders, J. (1998). Weighted census-based deprivation indices: their use in small areas. *Journal of Public Health Medicine*, **20**, 253–60.

Schrijvers, C. T., Mackenbach, J. P., Lutz, J. M., Quinn, M. J., and Coleman, M. P. (1995). Deprivation, stage at diagnosis and cancer survival. *International Journal of Cancer*, **63**, 324–9.

Scottish Office Department of Health (1998). *Scottish Health Survey 1995*. HMSO, Edinburgh.

Senior, M. L. (1991). Deprivation payments to GPs: not what the doctor ordered. *Environment and Planning C: Government Policy*, **9**, 79–84.

Shouls, S., Congdon, P., and Curtis, S. (1996). Modelling inequality in reported longterm illness in the UK: combining individual and area characteristics. *Journal of Epidemiology and Community Health*, **50**, 366–76.

Silvonen, A. P., Kunst, A. E., Lahelma, E., Valkonen, T., and Mackenbach, J. (1998). Socio economic inequalities in health expectancy in Finland and Norway in the late 1980's. *Social Science and Medicine*, **47**, 303–16.

Sloggett, A. and Joshi, H. (1998). Deprivation indicators as predictors of life events 1981–1992 based on the UK ONS longitudinal study. *Journal of Epidemiology and Community Health*, **52**, 229–33.

Sooman, A. and MacIntyre S. (1995). Health and perceptions of the local environment in socially contrasting neighbourhoods in Glasgow. *Health and Place*, **1**, 15–26.

Sundquist, J., Bajekal, M., and Johansson, S. E. (1997). The UPA score and mortality in Swedish municipalities. *Scandinavian Journal of Primary Health Care*, **15**, 203–9.

Taylor, R., Quine, S., Lyle, D., and Britton, A. (1992). Socioeconomic correlation of mortality and hospital morbidity differentials by Local Government Authorities in Sydney 1985–90. *Australian Journal of Public Health*, **16**, 302–6.

Townsend P. (1987) Deprivation. *Journal of Social Policy*, **16**, 125–46.

Townsend, P., Phillimore, P., and Beattie, A. (1988). *Health and deprivation: inequalities and the north*. Croom Helm, London.

5. Bias and confounding in spatial epidemiology

P. Elliott and J. C. Wakefield

5.1 Introduction

In this chapter, we address some of the issues that affect the interpretation of spatial epidemiological studies. We separate the two concepts of bias and confounding, although in practice they are closely related. By bias, we mean that study results deviate (in either direction) from some 'true' value that the study was designed to estimate. By confounder, we refer to a variable that is not of primary interest, but which is independently associated with both the outcome and with the exposure variable under study. Failure to adjust appropriately for the confounder will lead to bias.

In general, bias and confounding are major problems affecting all observational studies, and are not special to spatial studies. However, as we will describe, there are several forms of bias that are specific to spatial studies; while some are explicitly recognised, others may not be readily apparent.

Sources of bias that we discuss here include selection effects, especially selection of particular geographical, temporal, disease, and demographic strata (e.g. in studies of disease clusters); ascertainment, numerator, and denominator bias; bias induced by the choice of the disease induction/latency period and mis-specification of the exposure-disease model; exposure inaccuracy bias and the errors-in-variables problem; spatial dependency; significance tests; and ecological bias. We also specifically discuss socio-economic confounding, as this is a major potential source of bias in spatial epidemiology.

5.2 Selection bias

In case-control studies, selection bias refers to bias that may arise due to the process by which cases and controls are selected into a study. Here, we are concerned with the mechanism by which parameters such as study areas, disease classifications, time periods, and populations at risk, are chosen for investigation. This is a particular problem in disease cluster studies which often arise in response to public or media concerns about allegedly high disease risk in the area (see Chapter 9). Several points are worthy of note. First, such clusters often do not reflect a priori concerns about specific risk factors in the area, and so there is no specific hypothesis. Rather, it appears that the risk in the area is 'high' compared with some reference value, but since this observation is generated by the data themselves, conventional test procedures are invalid. A number of questions arise: for example, 'Why was this area chosen, and not any other? Why this time period, this disease?'. Without information on this selection procedure (which is, nearly always, unobtainable) an appropriate distribution for the test statistic is unavailable: were the selection procedure to be known, then an appropriate distribution for the test statistic could be obtained (perhaps via simulation).

As a simple example, suppose there are N toxic waste sites in a country and a television company systematically calculated rates for each of K diseases over T time periods and for J age-sex groups, and then reported the rate that gave the smallest p-value. This p-value will clearly be highly significant: for example, with $N = 10$, $K = T = J = 4$ the probability that the maximum p-value will be less than 0.005 is $1 - 0.995^{640} = 0.96$. In this case a Bonferroni correction may be applied and a result significant at the 5% significance level corresponds approximately to $0.05/640 = 0.00008$ for a single test, so that only a p-value less than this value would be worthy of further investigation. This process is viewed as conservative, however (see Thomas *et al.* 1985 for a discussion of this and other procedures). In general, such a simple solution will not be available.

Usually, the answer to the first of the above questions, 'Why this area?', is that high rates of some disease have been noticed, and an investigation is initiated. No one, however, is concerned about low rates of disease, although, based on sampling variability, demographic characteristics, etc., we would expect that rates of disease will fluctuate between areas, with some areas having high rates and some low. This problem is exacerbated when one is looking at the small numbers of cases that are typically found in cluster investigations with rare diseases in small areas. It may even be that in the areas with low rates of disease an important (causal) protective factor is operating, but this will never be investigated!

This selection phenomenon is illustrated in Fig. 5.1. Here, the relative risks of a disease are shown for four hypothetical areas over a 12-year period. The population sizes, age-sex structure, and disease rates correspond to an expected number of cases in each year and each area of 0.3. For each of the four areas we then plot the estimated relative risk (Standardised mortality/morbidity ratio, SMR) versus time (in years). The cases have been generated under a model of constant relative risk, so that the only difference between the disease incidence in each of the areas is random variability. These data might lead to the instigation of an investigation in Area A where the rates appear to be rising, while the rates in Area D (in particular) would be reassuring.

A related selection problem that has beset this type of cluster investigation is what has been called 'boundary shrinkage' or the 'Texas sharpshooter' effect (Rothman 1990). Here, the boundaries (geographic, temporal, demographic, disease) are drawn tightly around the cases. Thus, while the observed number of cases is retained (the 'cluster'), the expected number is reduced, hence increasing the apparent observed/expected ratio (SMR). The boundary selection procedures may not be occurring explicitly, but may be present nonetheless. This type of phenomenon was discussed, for example, in relation to the incidence of leukaemia and lymphoma in young people near the Dounreay nuclear plant, where selection of different time periods and geographical boundaries resulted in differing estimates of risk (Wakeford *et al.* 1989).

Another problem arises when disease mapping techniques are used to find areas at apparently high risk of disease, especially when the maps relate to small areas/rare diseases, where often the picture is dominated by random variability. In this case, small numbers of cases in remote areas may predominate, and the eye is drawn to these large

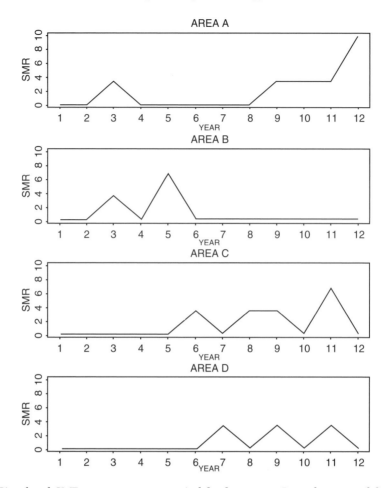

Fig. 5.1 Simulated SMRs over a 12-year period for four areas. In each year and for each area the population is such that the expected number of cases is 0.3.

geographical areas with apparently high risk. This is essentially a ranking procedure by relative risk, which may be addressed using hierarchical modelling (see Chapter 7).

These problems of area/cluster selection are in many ways analagous to the ranking of institutional performance, such as school and hospital league tables (Goldstein and Spiegelhalter 1996).

5.3   Ascertainment, numerator, and denominator bias

As discussed in Chapters 2 and 3, numerous problems affect counts of both numerator and denominator that are used in risk estimates. For the numerator (cases), there can be either under- or overascertainment, depending on diagnostic accuracy, completeness of registration, and possible duplication (Chapter 2). As an example, underascertainment is particularly acute for studies of early abortion as it is estimated that approximately 25%

of pregnancies are lost before being clinically apparent (Wilcox *et al.* 1988). For the denominator, usually, estimates are available at only certain points in time (e.g. at the decennial census) and so some sort of modelling or estimation is required to obtain counts for the unmeasured periods (Chapter 3). Migration is a serious problem since it affects both the denominator and the exposure period. The latter is particularly serious since it is very difficult to model this effect. Both numerator and denominator effects could lead to biases in either direction. Therefore, a detailed understanding of the diseases, registration systems and population data is required to interpret the likely direction and size of these effects in any given area/time period. As it is unlikely that these effects are spatially neutral, they will produce bias in risk estimates. Even where these effects are spatially neutral (i.e. they occur equally across the map), they will still bias estimates of disease incidence, though not of relative risk. In highly localised studies, perhaps the potential for systematic bias from such data problems is less, although such studies are especially prone to data aberrations that could distort the findings.

It may be that an apparent excess risk of disease in a particular area could be explained entirely by such artefactual considerations. For example, in a study of cancer incidence in Dalgety Bay in Scotland, risk estimates using census data to provide population counts were too high because of rapid population growth. Instead, data from general practitioner lists were used to obtain population estimates, and hence improved estimates of risk (Black *et al.* 1994).

5.4 Disease induction and mis-specification of the exposure-disease model

An important issue that affects epidemiological estimation of disease risk is specification of an appropriate exposure-disease model. This affects all epidemiological studies, but is included here as it needs to be addressed in spatial epidemiological enquiries. One question is what induction or latency period to allow for. Rothman and Greenland (1998) discuss the various definitions of induction and latency periods for both infectious and non-infectious diseases. If the induction period is mis-specified then bias toward the null will result. For some diseases, the induction period is very short and this can be used to advantage (e.g. for cluster detection/investigation). For example, a disease outbreak of, say, *Escherichia coli* or *Salmonella typhimurium* will occur rapidly in time and may allow rapid identification of the source of the outbreak using standard case-control methods. Other infectious diseases, such as Legionnaire's disease, with slightly longer latency, have also been shown to cluster (Bhopal *et al.* 1992).

In general, diseases with short induction and latency periods are more amenable to spatial epidemiology since there is less opportunity for bias to occur due to loss to follow-up, migration, and competing causes of disease. It is also likely that for a disease with a short induction/latency period, the variability in this period between individuals will be less and so it becomes far easier to define an appropriate study period. In particular, birth-related events, including low birthweight, congenital anomalies, and childhood cancers may be fruitful to study both for this reason and because the developing fetus and young child may be particularly susceptible to environmental insults. Here, specification of the assumed exposure-disease relationship is crucial as only a brief window of exposure may

Spatial epidemiology

be relevant, for example first trimester exposure in congenital anomalies. Examples include the investigations of malformations and leukaemias associated with contaminated water supply in Woburn, Massachusetts (Lagakos *et al.* 1986), spontaneous abortions and chlorinated by-products in the public water supply (Swan *et al.* 1998), and childhood leukaemias near high voltage overhead power lines (Feychting *et al.* 1996).

For other diseases, most notably cancers, induction/latency periods between first exposure and appearance of clinical disease of up to thirty years or more may be observed. Typical examples include lung cancer and mesothelioma. This basic biological model needs to be taken into consideration in the design of spatial epidemiological studies. For example, in a study of cancers near municipal solid waste incinerators in Great Britain, a ten-year induction/latency period was specified for solid cancers between start up of an incinerator and the inclusion of cancer in the study (Elliott *et al.* 1996).

5.5   Exposure inaccuracy bias and errors-in-variables modelling

A major difficulty in epidemiology in general, and spatial epidemiology in particular, is the lack of *accurate* exposure and confounder information. In the epidemiological literature this problem is known as exposure misclassification. Ideally, we would like to measure the lifelong biological dose due to an exposure of interest but this is never possible. In Chapters 19, 20, and 21, various alternative measures are described for air pollutants. These include, at one extreme, individual measures such as personal monitors, and at the other, simplistic indicators such as distance from a putative source. Measures interpolated from fixed-site monitor data lie in between these extremes. Individual confounder data, such as diet and levels of smoking and alcohol consumption, are also inevitably measured with error. The statistical approach to dealing with the problem is known as *errors-in-variables* (Carroll *et al.* 1995) or *measurement error* (Fuller 1987) modelling. We will use the former term and save the latter for a particular source of error. In general, errors-in-variables modelling is applicable whenever we have error in addition to that usually assumed in a statistical model. So, for example, we may also use such modelling when numerator and denominator problems are considered (see Chapter 3).

In this section we summarise some of the basic mathematical results concerning the possible effects of exposure misclassification; the Appendix contains a more detailed description. Examples of the use of errors-in-variables models in spatial epidemiology are relatively rare. Two instances of their use are Bernardinelli *et al.* (1997; see also Chapter 16) in a disease mapping study, and Jordan *et al.* (1997) in an ecological correlation study.

Consider the situation of a univariate continuous predictor in a simple linear regression. It is well known (e.g. Fuller 1987) that where a predictor is measured with error, but is an unbiased estimate of the true predictor, the resultant estimator is *attenuated* to the null. The degree of attenuation depends on the sizes of the measurement error variance across the study population; Equation (5.3) in the Appendix gives the explicit form. As the examples in the Appendix show, this phenomenon only occurs under certain circumstances. Unfortunately, for the Poisson model that is frequently used in spatial epidemiology, specification of the error terms is less straightforward than in the linear case, and few results on the effect of exposure misclassification are available.

In the environmental epidemiology context there are a number of situations involving errors-in-variables (see Wakefield and Elliott 1999), in particular:

- variables subject to measurement error,
- interpolated variables, and
- variables only available as an area-level measure.

Measurement error includes errors introduced by the instrument used to measure the variable. In small-area applications these may occur when environmental exposures are measured in air, soil, or water. In many instances it will be straightforward to model these errors since information will be available on the measurement process. Another situation in which measurement error modelling may be used is when an exposure score is derived from a deterministic formula. For example, in a study of the relationship between power lines and brain cancers the electromagnetic field strength at particular locations may be derived from the voltage and load of the line and the distance of residence from the line. This information is combined using a deterministic formula but some idea of the uncertainty in the resultant field strength is available, and may be utilised within the errors-in-variables model. Measurement error models may also be used for lifestyle variables which are measured on individual study participants (e.g. dietary variables, see Carroll *et al.* 1995 for references).

In an area-level analysis it is important to distinguish between two hypothetical exposure situations. The first occurs when the exposure within each area may be constant but measured with error. In this case an errors-in-variables approach will, theoretically at least, correct for bias. The second situation occurs when the exposure may be non-constant within an area, with different individuals receiving different exposures. If only area-level averages are available, then an errors-in-variables approach can only account for the fact that these averages are not measured exactly; the effect of within-area variability is a different problem, namely an example of ecological bias, and will be discussed in Section 5.8 (see also Chapter 11). In most studies, the true picture is likely to be a combination of these two situations.

As described in Chapter 9, a common approach to modelling the association between disease risk and the location of a point or line-source is to assume a simple relationship between risk and distance. Distances from putative sources that are used as surrogate exposures may be extracted using geographical information systems (GIS) but will not be exact, particularly for small-area centroids, but will have an associated precision (e.g. within ±10 metres). This error may also be described as measurement error.

Another errors-in-variables situation arises when a spatially varying exposure quantity is observed at a finite set of locations (e.g. an air pollution monitoring network) and we wish to *interpolate* the value at additional locations (e.g. residential addresses in a case-control study). An example in which these type of data are available, the SAVIAH study, is described in Chapter 22. Data of these kind are often referred to as 'geostatistical' data with kriging being a traditional solution; see for example Cressie (1993), Chapter 10, and Diggle *et al.* (1998). Such interpolation is ideally suited to errors-in-variables modelling since, as well as a point estimate of the exposure, a measure of the uncertainty in this estimate is typically available. In Chapter 10, Figs. 10.4 and 10.5 display, respectively, maps of the interpolated air pollution surface *and* the standard error of this surface. In fact, rather than carrying out the exposure and health modelling separately, the two may be combined; this is particularly appealing within a Bayesian framework. For health data in the form of counts, the average exposure in an areal unit may be estimated using a 'block kriging' approach (Chapter 10). We stress, however, that in this case ecological bias is a distinct possibility.

A number of important explanatory variables may only be measured at the *area level*, for example socio-economic status. To avoid ecological bias these measures must be truly area level (i.e. constant within an area). Wakefield and Stephens (2000) describe an analysis in which a socio-economic index was modelled via an errors-in-variables approach. As described in more detail in Section 5.9, such indices are complex. They may be viewed, at the individual-level, as surrogates for diet and smoking status (say); but if individual-level factors were measured, there may still be an additional effect, for example, due to access to services or to less tangible factors such as safety and quality of the environment. In many studies, ambient air pollution is assumed to be relatively constant across an area in which case an errors-in-variables approach may be adopted. Maheswaran *et al.* (1999) describe a study that investigated the relationship between acute myocardial infarction and water hardness in the northwest of England. The water constituents magnesium, fluoride, calcium, and lead were measured at locations within water company-defined water zones and this was the ecological level of the analysis. Wakefield and Morris (1999) describe an errors-in-variables approach to determining the 'true' average levels of water constituents within each water zone.

Great care must be taken when errors-in-variables modelling is carried out, particularly in the case when no gold standard exists since the analysis is driven by assumptions that are unverifiable from the data being analysed. For this reason non- and semi-parametric methods are appealing in errors-in-variables modelling. A frequentist semi-parametric approach has recently been suggested by Spiegelman and Casella (1997).

We finally note that, although recently developed Bayesian Markov chain Monte Carlo techniques (e.g. see Chapter 7) allow the routine analysis of complex data structures, they do not necessarily provide insight into the underlying structure of the problem since each application is a 'one-off'. For errors-in-variables specifically, there is a need for more theoretical work in order to determine the effects of measurement error. This would be highly desirable to inform the design of studies.

5.6   Spatial dependency

A particular issue in the analysis of spatial data is that outcomes in spatial units that are 'close' are not independent of each other (see Chapter 11). Risk estimates at locations and areas close to each other will tend to be positively correlated as the areas will share a number of characteristics, including both the social and physical environment. If all such characteristics could be measured, then in theory they could be properly accounted for in the statistical analysis as the model would be fully specified. However, in practice, this will never be the case and unmeasured factors may introduce spatial dependence. Pocock *et al.* (1982) considered ways in which this dependency could be measured in an early example in which the relationship between hard water and heart disease in towns in Great Britain was investigated. An analysis that does not take such dependencies into account may give spurious precision and potentially biased estimates of effect in the non-linear case. Methods for dealing with this problem are described in Chapters 7 and 11 (see also Richardson 1992).

5.7 Significance tests

A number of problems arise in the statistical evaluation of spatial studies, which require careful consideration in the analysis and reporting of results. Most of these are germane to all epidemiological analyses, but we mention them here as particular problems may arise in spatial statistics that may not be readily apparent to the investigator. For example, there is a general problem of multiple testing (over different areas, disease categories, time periods, age, and sex groups, etc.) but as a consequence of the selection effects mentioned in Section 5.2, it is unclear how many tests have effectively been performed. The selection of areas at apparent high risk results from a large number of 'informal' scans through the data, as has already been discussed.

Another related problem is that, where a large number of tests have been done, the most 'significant', or those with the largest apparent effects, are selectively reported. This is analagous within a given study to publication bias across different studies. A related problem is where selection procedures are used in the statistical modelling of confounders (e.g. forward selection, backward elimination, or stepwise selection), such that only the most 'significant' variables are retained. This will result in biased estimates of the main effects, and since the selection mechanism for the confounders has not been accounted for, spurious precision will result. This problem, which is common to all multiple regression modelling scenarios that use these techniques, is discussed in detail in Miller (1990). A potential solution is provided by Bayesian model averaging (Raftery and Richardson 1996) in which no single model is selected. This approach also has its drawbacks, however, since the interpretation of the coefficients is not straightforward, the computation is time-consuming, and careful thought must be given to the initial class of models to investigate.

Often in environmental epidemiological studies, the underlying biological mechanism is largely unknown, and multiple hypotheses might be studied. Some means to protect against Type I error (false positive) needs to be in place in order not to raise false alarms. In the recent study of 72 municipal solid waste incinerators in Great Britain (Elliott *et al.* 1996), a two-stage procedure was adopted to help reduce this problem. First, the incidence of 13 specific cancers, possibly associated with incineration products, was examined around a sample of 20 incinerators. The incidence of the five solid cancers, showing nominally significant associations ($p < 0.05$) with proximity to the incinerators, was then examined around the remaining 52 incinerators. A further significance test was carried out in the second stage of the study at $p < 0.05$. This is not an ideal solution (Thomas *et al.* 1985) as, in particular, it involves loss of information, although it did offer a pragmatic approach to the multiple testing problem. Other approaches that have been advocated include use of Bonferroni-type corrections. These and other alternatives are discussed in Thomas (1985) and Thomas *et al.* (1985).

The above example examined data over many incinerators and pooled incinerator-specific estimates of risk to give an overall estimate. In Elliott *et al.* (1996) a 'fixed effects' model was assumed (i.e. no allowance was made for possible between-site heterogeneity). An alternative approach, used by Dolk *et al.* (1998) in a study of congenital malformations near landfill sites in Europe, is to model a between-site effect via a 'random effects' approach. This leads to wider interval estimates and hence more conservative tests.

Maps of significance levels have been advocated in the disease mapping literature, but these tend to highlight areas with large populations as these will produce small *p*-values even for relative risks that are close to unity.

Finally, caution is required in the analysis of data with spatial dependence as discussed in the previous section. Positive dependence between nearby areas leads to loss of information and ignoring this aspect leads to anti-conservative tests. This is discussed by Richardson (1992). A related difficulty is provided by non-spatial overdispersion (e.g. extra-Poisson variability). Figure 1 of Hills and Alexander (1989) illustrates the effect of this overdispersion in terms of the level of anti-conservatism.

5.8   Ecological bias

We now consider a source of bias that occurs when an ecological (i.e. a group-level) analysis is carried out, but we wish to make inference for the individuals within the groups. In the present context we are particularly interested in the case where the groups correspond to areas. In this case, so-called *ecological bias* may occur, leading to the *ecological fallacy*. In its most extreme form the sign of regression coefficients may be reversed. We do not intend to provide a comprehensive summary here but will highlight key points. Chapter 11 discusses ecological bias in detail.

Greenland (1992) identifies several sources of ecological bias and provides a good summary; we closely follow his nomenclature here. Other key references include Richardson *et al.* (1987), Greenland and Morgenstern (1989), Piantadosi *et al.* (1988), and Greenland and Robins (1994). We now briefly discuss four of the more common sources of ecological bias.

Specification bias

Suppose that we are interested in the relationship between an outcome Y and an exposure U, with the relationship between these quantities at the individual-level being described via a probability model $p(Y|U, \beta)$, where we have a vector of unknown parameters β. We assume that $E[Y|U] = h_\beta(U)$. We now summarise work, as yet unpublished, by Salway and Wakefield (submitted).

Suppose that there are n_i individuals in area i and, rather than observe the individual responses and exposures, we instead observe averages, Y_i and U_i (i.e. $Y_i = 1/n_i \times \sum_{j=1}^{n_i} Y_{ij}$), and

$$U_i = |A_i|^{-1} \int_{A_i} U_i(\mathbf{x}) \mathrm{d}\mathbf{x}, \tag{5.1}$$

where A_i represents the two-dimensional region corresponding to area i. In practice U_i will often be the average of a number of measurements taken across each area. We suppose $U_{ij} = U(\mathbf{x}_{ij})$ denotes the exposure of an individual at location $\mathbf{x}_{ij}$. The relationship between Y_i and U_i is given by

$$E[Y_i|U_i] = \frac{1}{n_i}\sum_j E[Y_{ij}|U_i, \beta] = \frac{1}{n_i}\sum_j E_{U_{ij}|U_i}\{E[Y_{ij}|U_{ij}]\} = \frac{1}{n_i}\sum_j E_{U_{ij}|U_i}\{h_\beta(U_{ij})\}$$

$$\tag{5.2}$$

If we have a linear model, i.e. $h_\beta(U) = \beta_0 + \beta_1 U$ then (5.2) gives

$$E[Y_i|U_i] = \beta_0 + \beta_1 U_i,$$

and an ecological analysis will give an unbiased estimate of the individual-level relationship. For a non-linear model then bias will occur: for example (Chapter 11), if we have $h_\beta(U) = \exp(\beta_0 + \beta_1 U)$ then we must evaluate

$$E_{U_{ij}|U_i}[\exp(\beta_0 + \beta_1 U_{ij})],$$

in order to see the effect of aggregation. To proceed further we need to make an assumption about the form of the exposure distribution within the area. If we assume $U_{ij}|U_i \sim N(U_i, \sigma_i^2)$ then

$$E[Y_i|U_i] = \exp(\beta_0 + \beta_1 U_i + \beta_1^2 \sigma_i^2/2)$$

and so we see that the expectation has gained an additional term that depends on the within-area variability in the exposure. Note that if the exposure is constant within an area (i.e. $\sigma_i^2 = 0$) then no specification bias will result. If the model $\exp(\beta_0 + \beta_1 U_i)$ is used then bias will result and, unfortunately, the extent or direction of this bias remains unresolved, though some simulation work has been carried out (see Chapter 11, and Plummer and Clayton 1996). Diggle and Elliott (1995) discuss ecological bias, in particular in the context of the assessment of risk in relation to a point source.

A great difficulty here is that we need to know the distribution of U within each area. We have here assumed that a sufficient number of measurements have been made within each area so that U_i given by (5.1) is not subject to error.

Note that, as mentioned in the last section, we are in a different situation to the errors-in-variables scenario where uncertainty in the true level is the cause of the bias; here non-constant exposure across each area is the cause of the bias (we have assumed that U_i is known exactly). Hence, so far as ecological bias is concerned, the only thing to be gained by taking multiple measurements within an area is accurate estimates of U_i and σ_i^2 and information about the within-area distribution of the exposure; in a pure errors-in-variables situation multiple measurements will explicitly reduce the bias (see Equation (5.4) in the Appendix).

In Chapter 22, a study is described in which a linear Poisson (additive) model is assumed in order to overcome this source of bias; in general, however, a multiplicative model is preferred (e.g. see Breslow and Day 1980).

We note here that pure specification bias has no connection with confounding.

Confounding

Ecological bias may also occur due to confounding both within and between areas. This is extensively discussed in Greenland and Robins (1994). The between-area confounding is analagous to the confounding that may potentially arise in all epidemiological studies. The effects of within-area confounders are, in general, very difficult to determine and have been the subject of much recent research (see Chapter 11). To overcome this source of bias, information on the within-area distribution of confounders and exposures is required. For this reason, if it is thought that within-area confounding is possible, then it is imperative to gain some information on values of the confounder, through a survey for example (Plummer and Clayton 1996).

Mutual standardisation

A third possible source of ecological bias occurs when there is incomplete adjustment for confounding. If the disease rates are adjusted for confounders at the area level, but the exposure is left unadjusted, then bias will result. The only way to prevent bias occurring in this manner is to adjust the exposure in the same way as the disease rates were adjusted. This adjustment will rarely be possible, however, since it requires data on the within-area distribution of the exposure and confounder variables. This problem is extensively discussed in Rosenbaum and Rubin (1984).

Effect modification

Greenland (1992) also summarises problems that occur in an ecological context in which there is interaction between the exposure and a covariate (so that this covariate is an effect modifier). In this case then even for a linear model, information is required on the average exposure for each level of the effect modifier, and this will typically not be available (though approximations are available, see Greenland 1992). We note that the effect modifier need not be a confounder (see Rothman and Greenland 1998: 254 for a useful discussion of this issue).

5.9   Socio-economic confounding

As discussed briefly in Chapter 1, socio-economic confounding is a major potential source of bias in small-area epidemiological studies. This is because socio-economic variables are strongly predictive of disease occurrence (Chapter 4), and are also associated with areas that have high levels of industry and pollution. Hence, in the absence of a real effect due to pollution, one may still detect an association between industry and disease. By socio-economic variables, we refer to the totality of the experiences of a population, related to socio-economic circumstances such as housing, wealth, diet, and medical care, that are associated with the health of the population independent of the pollution effect.

   Thus, while many of the indices of deprivation at small-area scale were constructed on the basis of variables readily available at census (unemployment, overcrowding, social class, and the like), known risk factors for disease such as poor diet and smoking (Kleinschmidt *et al.* 1995) also tend to cluster together in these areas. The way that this confounding effect is commonly dealt with is to adjust for socio-economic deprivation at the small-area scale, and to examine for any residual association with proximity to an industrial site, or to some other estimate of exposure. For example, Elliott *et al.* (1996) examined proximity to incinerators having adjusted the expected numbers of cases by stratifying on quintiles of the Carstairs index of deprivation (Chapter 4) at the level of census enumeration district.

   This approach assumes implicitly that deprivation is a 'cause' of ill-health. However, different interpretations are possible. For example, if at least some of the causal pathway for the deprivation effect were reflecting the fact that deprived areas are more polluted, then adjustment for deprivation may be inappropriate in a study designed to estimate the pollution effect *per se*. Alternatively, non-causal interpretations are also available. Since poor people tend to live in poor areas, and people who become sick (and hence unemployed) may become poor, there will be a tendency for sick people to migrate toward the deprived areas. The health statistics for these areas would then reflect the fact that sick people tend to live there, rather than indicating an effect of environmental pollution (i.e. reverse causality).

In the incinerators example (Elliott *et al*. 1996), it was argued that any effect of 'over adjustment' for deprivation (potentially removing a pollution effect) was outweighed by the demographic, socio-economic, and lifestyle factors that powerfully operate in the opposite direction. This may explain why higher risk of lung cancer near incinerators was detected in areas before an incinerator was operating, even after adjustment for deprivation.

5.10 Conclusions

In this chapter we have illustrated that the sources of bias in spatial studies are both numerous and complex, and hence great care is needed in the interpretation of such studies. The bias can operate in both directions. In cluster studies, the often unspecified selection mechanisms will tend to lead to overestimates of effect (positive bias). On the other hand, migration and exposure mis-classification will tend to operate in the opposite direction. This will not always be the case, however. Brenner *et al*. (1992) describe how relative risk estimates are biased away from the null in the case in which the risk in an area is related to the percentage exposed, and this percentage is subject to error. This bias occurs for both linear and log-linear risk/exposure models. Socio-economic factors have profound effects on disease risk and are, in general, likely to dominate spatial variation in risk. This should be borne in mind when models for spatial and non-spatial over-dispersion are postulated.

At present, the approach to spatial studies is relatively naive, in that little attention has been paid either to possible interactions between environmental exposures, disease risk and confounders such as age, sex, and deprivation, or to how these are distributed both within and between areas. Proper consideration of these factors will add an extra layer of complexity into the analysis, but with the potential to reduce biases. To improve on studies in this way, however, requires considerable investment in improved data availability and quality, exposure assessment and measures of socio-economic deprivation. These measures will also need to be specific to the disease, study areas, time periods and populations in question.

Appendix: errors-in-variables modelling

Simple linear regression

This Appendix contains material that is expanded upon more comprehensively in Wakefield and Stephens (2000). The results in this Section are generally applicable to epidemiological studies where exposures are measured with error. We include them here, however, as in spatial epidemiology, exposure assessment is often one of the weakest components of the study design, and often only proxy measures of exposure (e.g. distance

from a point source) are available. We begin by discussing an often-quoted result in one
of the simplest errors-in-variables situations. To take a concrete example, suppose the
rate of disease Y across the areas of a study region is related to an exposure of interest X
in those areas through the simple linear model

$$Y = \beta_0 + \beta_x X + \epsilon_y,$$

where the ϵ_y are independent and identically distributed normal residuals with constant
variance σ_y^2, which we will denote as $\epsilon_y \sim_{i.i.d.} N(0, \sigma_y^2)$. Suppose also that across the areas
of the study region the distribution of X is normal with mean μ_x and variance σ_x^2.
Conventionally, once X is observed it is treated as a known fixed quantity with the only
randomness being associated with Y. In this case the standard (non-Bayesian) estimators
are unbiased for the true parameters. Now suppose that, instead of X, we obtain a
surrogate for the exposure W. There are two common formulations that are used to
model the relationship between X and W. In the *classical* error model, we model W given
X (denoted $W|X$) while in the *Berkson* error model we model $X|W$. We consider these
two models in more detail in the next section. For now we assume the simple classical
model

$$W = X + \epsilon_w$$

with $\epsilon_w \sim_{i.i.d.} N(0, \sigma_w^2)$. We also assume that ϵ_w and ϵ_y are independent, an assumption
that is known as *non-differential* errors.

If we now assume the model

$$Y = \beta_0^* + \beta_x^* W + \epsilon_y^*,$$

with $\epsilon_y^* \sim_{i.i.d.} N(0, \sigma_y^{*2})$, then it may be shown (e.g. Fuller 1987) that the maximum
likelihood estimator β_x^* is an unbiased estimator not of β_x, but of

$$\beta_x \times \frac{\sigma_x^2}{\sigma_x^2 + \sigma_w^2} \tag{5.3}$$

Hence if $\sigma_w^2 > 0$ (which is the case if X is measured with error) then the estimator of β_x
will be *attenuated*. The level of the attenuation depends on the ratio of the measurement
error in W and the between-area variability in X (i.e. σ_w^2/σ_x^2).

Suppose that we take m replicate measurements in each area, and that the above model
holds. Then $\hat{\beta}$ is an unbiased estimator of

$$\beta_x \times \frac{\sigma_x^2}{\sigma_x^2 + \sigma_w^2/m} \tag{5.4}$$

and so we see that the attenuation is decreased as m is increased and so the problem
may be solved by design (if the model is correct). This contrasts with ecological bias (see
Section 5.8).

This result is very clearcut but in general the situation is much more complicated.
In the next section we consider a more complex scenario.

Multiple linear regression

We now let Z denote explanatory variables that are measured without error (e.g. age or sex will often be accurately recorded in an epidemiological study). It is clear that to analyse errors-in-variables problems we must consider the relationship between the true and surrogate responses given the known covariates, i.e. $p(W, X|Z)$; this was briefly discussed in the previous section. For notational simplicity we assume that X and Z are univariate. The *classical errors-in-variables* model considers

$$p(W, X|Z) = p(W|X, Z) \times p(X|Z),$$

whereas with the *Berkson errors-in-variables* model we have

$$p(W, X|Z) = p(X|W, Z) \times p(W|Z).$$

Since W is observed, the latter approach only considers $p(X|W, Z)$.

In experimental studies, the Berkson measurement error model will often be appropriate. For example, when the level of a variable, W, is recorded from a machine setting, the true level X is then modelled as a function of W. In observational studies, the classical measurement error model is more typical though Berkson measurement errors do arise; Richardson and Deltour (1998) give as an example the situation in which ambient air pollution W is measured for a group of individuals, perhaps defined by a common area, and individual exposures X are required. A reasonable Berkson model may then be $E[X|W] = W$.

Fuller (1987) and Carroll *et al.* (1995) contain comprehensive accounts of the frequentist approach to errors-in-variables modelling (the latter also contains a chapter on Bayesian approaches).

Suppose that we have normal linear model, i.e.

$$Y = \beta_0 + \beta_x X + \beta_z Z + \epsilon_y$$

with $\epsilon_y \sim_{i.i.d.} N(0, \sigma_y^2)$ but instead we fit the model

$$E[Y|W, Z] = \beta_0^* + \beta_x^* W + \beta_z^* Z.$$

Suppose that X and W are related via the classical errors-in-variables model:

$$W = \theta_0 + \theta_1 X + \epsilon_w,$$

with $\epsilon_w \sim_{i.i.d.} N(0, \sigma_w^2)$. Here, θ_0 and θ_1 represent *additive* and *multiplicative* bias terms, respectively. Now consider the exposure model

$$X = \mu_{x|z} + \epsilon_{x|z},$$

with $\epsilon_{x|z} \sim N(0, \sigma_{x|z}^2)$ and $(\epsilon_y, \epsilon_w, \epsilon_{x|z})$ all mutually independent. We further assume that (X, Z) are bivariate normal with μ_x and μ_z and a variance/covariance matrix containing elements σ_x^2, σ_{xz}, and σ_z^2. Then, defining

$$\lambda_0 = \frac{\mu_x \sigma_w^2 - \theta_0 \theta_1 \sigma_{x|z}^2 + \mu_z \sigma_{xz} \sigma_w^2 / \sigma_z^2}{\theta_1^2 \sigma_{x|z}^2 + \sigma_w^2},$$

$$\lambda_1 = \frac{\theta_1 \sigma_{x|z}^2}{\theta_1^2 \sigma_{x|z}^2 + \sigma_w^2},$$

$$\lambda_2 = \frac{\sigma_{xz} \sigma_w^2 / \sigma_z^2}{\theta_1^2 \sigma_{x|z}^2 + \sigma_w^2}$$

we may show that

$$\beta_0^* = \beta_0 + \beta_x \lambda_0$$

$$\beta_x^* = \beta_x \lambda_1 = \beta_x \times \frac{\theta_1 \sigma_{x|z}^2}{\theta_1^2 \sigma_{x|z}^2 + \sigma_w^2}$$

$$\beta_z^* = \beta_z + \beta_x \lambda_2.$$

We note the following:

- If we have $\theta_1 = 1$ and $\sigma_w^2 = 0$ but $\theta_0 \neq 0$, then we have no estimation bias in β_x and β_z due to θ_0 since we have simply relocated the Xs and hence the slopes are unaffected.
- If $\theta_0 = 0$, $\theta_1 = 1$ (i.e. we have an unbiased surrogate) and there are no known covariates Z (and so $\sigma_{x|z}^2 = \sigma_x^2$) then

$$\beta_x^* = \beta_x \lambda_1$$

where

$$\lambda_1 = \frac{\sigma_x^2}{\sigma_x^2 + \sigma_w^2}$$

and we obtain the result of the previous section. The quantity λ_1 is sometimes referred to as the *reliability ratio*.
- If X and Z are correlated then there is bias in the estimation of β_z, as well as in β_x. By symmetry we note that if confounders are measured with error and the exposure is accurately measured then we still obtain bias in the estimation of β_x.
- If $\theta_1 \geq 1$ then we always have attenuation of β_x, for $\theta_1 < 1$ we may overestimate the size of the coefficient.
- The variance is also inflated (see Wakefield and Stephens 2000, for the exact form).

We end this section by noting that once we are outside the class of normal linear models, very few results are available to suggest the effects of errors-in-variables (though there is work on the binomial model, see Carroll *et al.* 1995). In particular the attenuation of estimated coefficients should not be assumed.

Acknowledgement

This work was supported, in part, by an equipment grant from the Wellcome Trust (0455051/Z/95/Z).

References

Bernardinelli, L., Pascutto, C., Best, N. G., and Gilks, W. R. (1997). Disease mapping with errors in covariates. *Statistics in Medicine*, **16**, 741–52.

Bhopal, R., Diggle, P., and Rowlingson, B. (1992). Pinpointing clusters of apparently sporadic cases of Legionnaires' disease. *British Medical Journal*, **304**, 1022–7.

Black, R. J., Sharp, L., Finlayson, A. R., and Hardness, E. F. (1994). Cancer incidence in a population potentially exposed to radium-226 at Dalgety Bay. *British Journal of Cancer*, **69**, 140–3.

Brenner, H., Savitz, D. A., Jockel, K.-H., and Greenland, S. (1992). Effects of nondifferential exposure misclassification in ecologic studies. *American Journal of Epidemiology*, **135**, 85–95.

Breslow, N. E. and Day, N. E. (1980). *Statistical methods in cancer research*. Vol. I: *The analysis of case-control studies*, IARC Scientific Publications 32. International Agency for Research on Cancer, Lyon.

Carroll, R. J., Ruppert, D., and Stefanski, L. A. (1995). *Measurement error in nonlinear models*. Chapman and Hall, London.

Cressie, N. A. C. (1993). *Statistics for spatial data* (rev. edn). Wiley, New York.

Diggle, P. J. and Elliott, P. (1995). Disease risk near point sources: statistical issues for analyses using individually or spatially aggregated data. *Journal of Epidemiology and Community Health*, **49**, S20–S27.

Diggle, P. J., Tawn, J. A., and Moyeed, R. A. (1998). Model-based geostatistics (with discussion). *Applied Statistics*, **47**, 299–350.

Dolk, H., Vrijheid, M., Armstrong, B., Abramsky, L., Bianchi, F., Garne, E. *et al.* (1998). Risk of congenital anomalies near hazardous-waste landfill sites in Europe: the EUROHAZCON study. *Lancet*, **352**, 423–7.

Elliott, P., Shaddick, G., Kleinschmidt, I., Jolley, D., Walls, P., Beresford, J. *et al.* (1996). Cancer incidence near municipal solid waste incinerators in Great Britain. *British Journal of Cancer*, **73**, 702–10.

Feychting, M., Kaune, W. T., Savitz, D. A., and Ahlbom, A. (1996). Estimating exposure in studies of residential magnetic fields and cancer. Importance of short-term variability, time interval between diagnosis and measurement, and distance to power line. *Epidemiology*, **7**, 220–4.

Fuller, W. A. (1987). *Measurement error models*. Wiley, New York.

Goldstein, H. and Spiegelhalter, D. J. (1996). League tables and their limitations: statistical issues in comparisons of institutional performance. *Journal of the Royal Statistical Society Series B*, **159**, 385–443.

Greenland, S. (1992). Divergent biases in ecologic and individual-level studies. *Statistics in Medicine*, **11**, 1209–23.

Greenland, S. and Morgenstern, H. (1989). Ecological bias, confounding and effect modification. *International Journal of Epidemiology*, **18**, 269–74.

Greenland, S. and Robins, J. (1994). Ecological studies-biases, misconceptions and counterexamples. *American Journal of Epidemiology*, **139**, 747–60.

Hills, M. and Alexander, F. (1989). Statistical methods used in assessing the risk of disease near a point source of possible environmental pollution: a review. *Journal of the Royal Statistical Society, Series A*, **152**, 353–63.

Jordan, P., Brubacher, D., Tsugane, S., Tsubono, Y., Gey, K. F., and Moser, U. (1997). Modelling of mortality data from a multi-centre study in Japan by means of Poisson regression with errors in variables. *International Journal of Epidemiology*, **26**, 501–7.

Kleinschmidt, I., Hills, M., and Elliott, P. (1995). Smoking behaviour can be predicted by neighbourhood deprivation measures. *Journal of Epidemiology and Community Health*, **49**, S72–S77.

Lagakos, S. W., Wesser, B. M., and Zelen, M. (1986). An analysis of contaminated well water and health effects in Woburn, Massachusetts (with discussion). *Journal of the American Statistical Association*, **81**, 583–614.

Maheswaran, R., Morris, S., Falconer, S., Grossinho, A., Perry, I., Wakefield, J. *et al.* (1999). Magnesium in drinking water supplies and mortality from acute myocardial infarction in North West England. *Heart*, **82**, 455–60.

Miller, A. J. (1990). *Subset selection in regression*. Chapman and Hall, London.

Piantadosi, S., Byar, D. P., and Green, S. B. (1988). The ecological fallacy. *American Journal of Epidemiology*, **127**, 893–904.

Plummer, M. and Clayton, D. (1996) Estimation of population exposure in ecological studies. *Journal of the Royal Statistical Society, Series B*, **158**, 113–26.

Pocock, S. J., Cook, D. G., and Shaper, A. G. (1982). Analysing geographic variation in cardiovascular mortality: methods and results. *Journal of the Royal Statistical Society, Series A*, **145**, 313–41.

Raferty, A. and Richardson, S. (1996). Model selection for generalised linear models via GLIB: application to nutrition and breast cancer. In *Bayesian biostatistics* (D. A. Berry and D. K. Stangl ed.), 321–53. Marcel Dekker, New York.

Richardson, S. (1992). Statistical methods for geographical correlation studies. In *Geographical and environmental epidemiology: methods for small-area studies* (P. Elliott, J. Cuzick, D. English, and R. Stern ed.), 181–204, Oxford University Press.

Richardson, S. and Deltour, I. (1998). Bayesian modelling of measurement error problems with reference to the analysis of atomic-bomb survivor data. In *Statistics for the environment 4: Health and the environment* (V. Barnett, A. Stein, and K. F. Turkman ed.), 259–79. Wiley, New York.

Richardson, S., Stucker, I., and Hemon, D. (1987). Comparison of relative risks obtained in ecological and individual studies: some methodological considerations. *International Journal of Epidemiology*, **16**, 111–20.

Rosenbaum, P. R. and Rubin, D. B. (1984). Difficulties with regression analyses of age-adjusted rates. *Biometrics*, **40**, 437–43.

Rothman, K. J. (1990). A sobering start for the Cluster Busters' Conference. *American Journal of Epidemiology*, **132**(Suppl.), S6–S13.

Rothman, K. and Greenland, S. (1998). *Modern epidemiology* (2nd edn). Lippincott, Williams and Wilkins, Philadelphia.

Salway, R. and Wakefield, J. C. (submitted). Issues in the analysis of ecological data. Submitted to *Journal of the Royal Statistical Society Series A*.

Spiegelman, D. and Casella, M. (1997). Fully parametric and semiparametric regression models for common events with covariate measurement error, in main study/validation study designs. *Biometrics*, **53**, 395–409.

Swan, S. H., Waller, K., Hopkins, B., Windham, G., Fenster, L., Schaefer, C. *et al.* (1998). A prospective study of spontaneous abortion: relation to amount and source of drinking water consumed in early pregnancy. *Epidemiology*, **9**, 126–33.

Thomas, D. C. (1985). The problem of multiple inference in identifying point source environmental hazards. *Environmental Health Perspectives*, **62**, 411–18.

Thomas, D. C., Siemiatycki, J., Dewar, R., Robins, J., Goldberg, M., and Armstrong, B. G. (1985). The problem of multiple inference in studies designed to generate hypotheses. *American Journal of Epidemiology*, **122**, 1080–95.

Wakefield, J. C. and Elliott, P. (1999). Issues in the statistical analysis of small area health data. *Statistics in Medicine*, **18**, 2377–99.

Wakefield, J. C. and Morris, S. (1999). Spatial dependence and errors-in variables in environmental epidemiology. In *Bayesian statistics 6* (J. M. Bernardo, J. O. Berger, A. P. Dawid, and A. F. M. Smith ed.). Oxford University Press.

Wakefield, J. C. and Stephens, D. A. (2000). Bayesian errors-in-variables modelling. *Generalised linear models: a Bayesian perspective* (D. Dey, M. Ghosh, and B. Mallick ed.). Marcel Dekker, New York, in press.

Wakeford, R., Binks, K., and Wilkie, D. (1989). Childhood leukaemia and nuclear installations. *Journal of the Royal Statistical Society, Series A*, **152**, 61–86.

Wilcox, A. J., Weinberg, C. R., O'Connor, J. F., Baird, B. D., Schlatterer, J. P., Canfield, R. E. *et al.* (1988). Incidence of early loss of pregnancy. *New England Journal of Medicine*, **319**, 189–94.

II Statistical methods

6. Overview of statistical methods for disease mapping and its relationship to cluster detection

P. J. Diggle

6.1 Introduction

Our main aim in this chapter is to describe a theoretical framework for the analysis of spatial variation in disease risk, within which different formats of epidemiological data naturally give rise to different statistical methods. A secondary aim is to discuss the similarities and differences between disease mapping problems and problems concerned with disease clustering or the detection of disease clusters. There is some degree of overlap between the issues discussed in this chapter and those considered in other parts of the book, especially the other chapters in this section.

6.2 Theoretical framework for spatial analysis of disease risk

Suppose that we wish to describe the spatial distribution of disease within a population which resides in some geographical region, A. We represent the population by a set of locations $x_i \in A$, $i = 1, \ldots, N$, such that the first n_1 are *cases* and the remaining $n_0 = N - n_1$ are *non-cases*. Our theoretical model for this problem is that cases and non-cases form a pair of independent, inhomogeneous Poisson point processes, with respective intensities $\lambda_1(x)$ and $\lambda_0(x)$. Informally, this means that the number of cases in any sub-region, B say, follows a Poisson distribution with expectation $\mu_B = \int_B \lambda_1(x) dx$ and, conditional on the number of cases in B, their locations are an independent random sample from the distribution on B with probability density proportional to $\lambda_1(x)$. A similar interpretation holds for the non-cases, with $\lambda_0(x)$ replacing $\lambda_1(x)$.

We emphasise that this is a *theoretical* model. In order to apply it to epidemiological data, we need to tackle many difficult issues, including the precise definition of the population at risk, and an appropriate convention for the reference location (e.g. place of residence at diagnosis, place of birth, place of work).

In an epidemiological setting, both $\lambda_1(x)$ and $\lambda_0(x)$ will typically be very complicated, reflecting the complexity of human settlement patterns. However, our interest will usually be confined to questions concerning spatial variation in disease risk or, equivalently, in the *spatial odds function*, $\rho(x) = \lambda_1(x)/\lambda_0(x)$, and this will often have a much simpler form. For example, if the disease strikes at random then $\rho(x) = \rho$, a constant for all locations x.

In modelling the spatial variation in $\rho(x)$ we need to be able to take account of known risk factors, and to identify the spatial variation in unknown risk factors. Because $\rho(x)$ is necessarily non-negative, a natural way to do this is through a log-linear model of the form

$$\rho(x) = \exp\left\{\alpha + \sum_{j=1}^{p} \beta_j z_j(x) + S(x)\right\}, \tag{6.1}$$

in which the $z_j(x)$ represent spatially varying known risk factors, with associated known or unknown regression parameters β_j, and $S(x)$ represents unexplained spatial variation. Philosophically, we may choose to think of $S(x)$ in Equation (6.1) either as a deterministic function of unknown form, or as a realisation of a spatial stochastic process. We shall explore later in the chapter the implications of both points of view. Note that the formulation (6.1) temporarily excludes individual-specific covariates such as age and sex.

Ostensibly, the Poisson model excludes any possibility of clustering of cases, in the sense that it formally assumes that case locations are mutually independent. However, for diseases that are environmental in origin it may be reasonable to assume that any such clustering is a by-product of spatial variation in unrecognised risk factors, which are accommodated in the model through the term $S(x)$ in (6.1). Also, in general it is difficult to make a sharp empirical distinction between a process consisting of dependent points with a constant intensity and one consisting of independent points with non-constant intensity. For example, Bartlett (1964) showed that a class of processes with constant intensity but containing clusters of dependent points is statistically indistinguishable from a class of processes with points distributed independently according to a spatially varying intensity $\lambda(x)$ which is itself the realisation of a stochastic process. Processes of this type are called *Cox processes*, following their introduction in a non-spatial setting by Cox (1955). Making $S(x)$ in (6.1) a stochastic process is consistent with using Cox processes rather than inhomogeneous Poisson processes as the underlying models for the cases and non-cases.

Our theoretical model has an alternative interpretation which is extremely useful in practice. Instead of thinking of our population as a pair of Poisson processes (conditional on the realised values of $S(x)$ for all $x \in A$ if $S(x)$ is stochastic), we can think of the whole population as a single Poisson process, with intensity $\lambda(x) = \lambda_1(x) + \lambda_0(x)$, and a set of binary labels, $Y_i = 1$ or 0 according to whether the ith member of the population is a case or a non-case, respectively. It follows that, conditional on the complete set of locations x_i, $i = 1, \ldots, N$, the N labels Y_i are mutually independent Bernoulli trials, with expectations $\mu_i = E[Y_i | x_i] = P(Y_i = 1 | x_i)$ given by

$$\mu_i = \frac{\lambda_1(x_i)}{\lambda_1(x_i) + \lambda_0(x_i)} = \frac{\rho(x_i)}{1 + \rho(x_i)} \tag{6.2}$$

which, in conjunction with (6.1), defines a logistic regression model for the Y_i. This alternative interpretation uses a standard property of the Poisson process, whose application in the present context appears to be due to Diggle and Rowlingson (1994).

Its practical importance is that it allows us to formulate and analyse models for $\rho(x)$ which require this function to be specified only at the locations x_i, not throughout the region A. In particular, we can then include in the model (6.1) explanatory variables which are not intrinsically spatial, but rather are properties of the individual members of the population which are known to be important determinants of disease risk, for example, age, sex, or socio-economic status. The binary labelling formulation is also valid under wider assumptions than the Poisson process formulation. Specifically, we could assume mutually independent labels Y_i without requiring that the population at risk can be represented as a realisation of a Poisson process. This would accommodate the obvious fact that populations typically are composed of family groups with a common location for all members of the group. The assumption of *independent* labelling conditional on $S(x)$ still formally excludes consideration of infectious diseases, or conditions which are genetic in origin. However, conditionally *dependent* labellings can be generated by including a non-spatial random effect on the right-hand side of (6.1); we return to this point in the subsection Extra-Poisson variation in Section 6.3.1.

6.3   Methodology for disease mapping

6.3.1   Individual-level data

A complete set of individual-level data would consist of the reference locations for every member of the population at risk and their corresponding binary labels, Y_i. This is seldom feasible. An alternative is to conduct a *case-control* study, in which we record the locations of all known cases, and of a random sample of non-cases, termed *controls*. Even this may not be practicable according to the strict definition of a random sample, and an important stage in any study of this kind is to define how the controls should be chosen. From a theoretical point of view, the minimal requirement is that the selection of controls should be spatially neutral: that is, with regard to their spatial locations the controls have the same statistical properties as if they were a random sample of all non-cases. Provided that this condition is satisfied, the resulting data can be used to estimate the spatial odds function up to a constant of proportionality, because the controls then constitute a realisation of an inhomogeneous Poisson process with intensity $p\lambda_0(x)$, where p is the proportion of non-cases included as controls. Since p is typically unknown, this explains why we can only estimate the spatial odds function up to an arbitrary constant of proportionality (see Section 8.2.4 of Chapter 8 for further discussion).

Note that this condition is unlikely to be satisfied in the important case of a *matched* case-control design. Matching has many desirable consequences, but invalidates the use of statistical methods derived on the assumption of a randomised case-control design. This is well known in the general epidemiological setting (for a review, see Breslow 1996), but is sometimes forgotten in the spatial setting (e.g. see Biggeri *et al.* 1996). The development of appropriate spatial statistical methods for matched case-control studies remains an open problem. Relevant work in progress includes Diggle *et al.* (2000) and Chetwynd and Diggle (1998). In what follows, we consider only randomised case-control studies.

Non-parametric estimation of a density ratio

In this section, we consider the problem of estimating the odds function $\rho(x)$ when $S(x)$ in (6.1) is a deterministic function of unspecified form and we have no information on relevant explanatory variables $z_j(x)$. This is equivalent to assuming that case and control locations are independent random samples from probability densities on A of unspecified form. Bithell (1990) proposed to use a standard method of non-parametric density estimation, the kernel method (Silverman 1986), to estimate each density and so construct a non-parametric estimate of $\rho(x)$ as the ratio of the two kernel estimates, $\hat{\rho}(x) = \hat{f}_1(x)/\hat{f}_0(x)$. The standard form of the kernel estimate of a bivariate density $f(x)$, based on data x_i, $i = 1, \ldots, n$, is

$$\hat{f}(x) = (n^{-1}h^{-2}) \sum_{i=1}^{n} k\{(x - x_i)/h\}, \tag{6.3}$$

in which $k(\cdot)$ is a *kernel function*, typically a radially symmetric bivariate probability density with a single mode at the origin, and h is a scaling constant, usually called the *bandwidth* of the estimator. Physically, (6.3) corresponds to placing a probability of n^{-1} at the location x_i and then spreading this probability over a region around x_i in a way determined by $k(\cdot)$ and, more particularly, by the value of h. For example, a common choice for $k(\cdot)$ is the product of two univariate standard Gaussian densities, in which case $h^{-2}k(x/h)$ represents a bivariate Gaussian density with circular symmetry and standard deviation h in each coordinate direction. In particular, this implies that when h is small, the kernel estimate concentrates a probability of n^{-1} tightly around each x_i, giving a very spiky estimate $\hat{f}(x)$, whereas when h is large the total probability is spread more evenly over the whole region A, giving a much smoother estimate $\hat{f}(x)$.

In the original setting of probability density estimation, it is natural to scale a kernel estimate so that it integrates to 1. In the point process setting, it is more natural to interpret a density estimate as an estimate of the mean number of points per unit area. To achieve this, we modify the definition (6.3) replacing the n^{-1} factor by $|A|^{-1}$, where $|A|$ denotes the area of A. This is equivalent to redefining our estimator for the odds function as

$$\hat{\rho}(x) = (n_1/n_0)\hat{f}_1(x)/\hat{f}_0(x). \tag{6.4}$$

Implementation of the kernel estimate therefore requires two choices to be made: of the kernel function $k(\cdot)$ and the bandwidth h. In general, the precise choice of $k(\cdot)$ is considered to be unimportant (but see below for a cautionary note) whereas the choice of the value of h is critical. There is an extensive literature on methods for choosing h, with Silverman (1986) providing an accessible review. However, there is no guarantee that values of h which are appropriate for separate estimation of $f_1(x)$ and $f_0(x)$ will be appropriate for estimating their ratio. Note in particular that small errors of estimation in the tails of $f_1(x)$ and $f_0(x)$ could easily translate into very large errors of estimation for their ratio. Other features of the epidemiological setting which should influence our approach are the following. First, we only have data on a finite region A whereas a kernel estimate defines a probability density over the whole plane. Second, and as noted earlier, we can expect the forms of $f_1(x)$ and $f_0(x)$ to be very complicated but our interest is in possibly small departures from constancy of their ratio.

Recognising these special features of the epidemiological problem, Bithell (1990) argued that the bandwidths used for estimation of $f_1(x)$ and $f_0(x)$ should be equal, irrespective of the relative numbers of cases and controls, whereas conventional theory for separate estimation of $f_1(x)$ and $f_0(x)$ suggests that the bandwidth should depend on sample size. Kelsall and Diggle (1995a,b) provided a theoretical justification for this by showing that when $\rho(x)$ is constant, the use of equal bandwidths eliminates the dominant term in the mean square error of $\hat{\rho}(x)$. Anderson and Titterington (1997) and Bowman and Azzalini (1997) focus on the difference, rather than the ratio, of kernel estimators for $f_1(x)$ and $f_0(x)$, which seems less natural in an epidemiological setting.

It is intuitively clear that any kernel estimate of $\rho(x)$ will have poor precision in areas where there are few cases or controls (i.e. in sparsely populated sub-regions of A). Also, the precise behaviour of $\hat{\rho}(x)$ in such sub-regions can depend crucially on the choice of the kernel function, $k(\cdot)$. To avoid overinterpretation of features of $\hat{\rho}(x)$ it is therefore important to estimate its precision. Kelsall and Diggle (1995a,b) give theoretical expressions for the mean square error of $\hat{\rho}(x)$. They also propose the following Monte Carlo method for assessing non-constancy of $\rho(x)$.

Let H denote the hypothesis that $\rho(x)$ is constant. Under H, the binary labelling interpretation of the Poisson process model implies that we can simulate the disease distribution conditional on the population locations and on the total number of cases in A by randomly selecting n out of the N locations as cases. From this simulated population, we then recompute $\hat{\rho}(x)$. By repeating the simulation and estimation, we construct a random sample of realisations of $\hat{\rho}(x)$ from its sampling distribution under H. By comparing the estimate $\hat{\rho}(x)$ from the original data with this random sample of realisations, we can then assess whether the data are consistent with H. For a formal, exact test of significance we define a scalar test statistic, T say, the value of which we can calculate from each estimated surface $\hat{\rho}(x)$ and which measures departure from H. For example, we could define

$$T = \int_A \{\hat{\rho}(x) - \rho_0\}^2 \mathrm{d}x,$$

where $\rho_0 = n_1/n_0$. Under H, denoting by t_0 the value of T for the original data and by $t_1, \ldots, t_s$ the values for s simulations, the probability that t_0 ranks among the k largest of the t_i, is $k/(s+1)$. Hence, the rank of t_0 defines an exact p-value for a test of significance (Barnard 1963). Less formally, if we order the simulated values of $\rho(x)$ for each x, the range covered by any specified proportion, p say, of these values estimates a tolerance interval for $\hat{\rho}(x)$, that is, an interval within which $\hat{\rho}(x)$ should lie with probability p if $\rho(x)$ is constant. For example, if we simulate $s = 1000$ times, the range covered by the central 950 values of $\hat{\rho}(x)$ at each x defines a set of estimated 95% point-wise tolerance intervals. We give an illustration below.

An inherent limitation of the density ratio approach is that it cannot easily adjust for explanatory variables.

Non-parametric binary regression

In this section, we continue to assume that $S(x)$ in (6.1) is deterministic, and that we have no information on relevant explanatory variables $z_j(x)$. However, we adopt the alternative, binary labelling formulation of our model and seek to estimate the function $\mu(x) = \rho(x)/\{1 + \rho(x)\}$ which, from (6.2), represents the probability that a member of the population would be a case, given that they were at location x. This is a non-parametric regression problem, in which the observed x_i are the values of the explanatory variable and the labels y_i are the responses. The kernel method again provides a solution to the problem. In general, for a response variable y, explanatory variable x and data (x_i, y_i), $i = 1, \ldots, N$, a non-parametric estimator for $\mu(x)$ is a weighted average

$$\hat{\mu}(x) = \sum_{i=1}^{N} w_i(x) y_i \tag{6.5}$$

in which, for each x, the $w_i(x)$ are non-negative weights which sum to one and give more weight to observations close to x. The Nadaraya–Watson kernel estimator (Nadaraya 1964; Watson 1964) constructs the weights from a kernel function $k(u)$ by defining

$$w_i(x) = k\{(x - x_i)/h\} \sum_{j=1}^{N} k\{(x - x_j)/h\}. \tag{6.6}$$

For binary y_i, the resulting estimator for $\mu(x)$ is equivalent to the kernel ratio estimator of $\rho(x)$ defined by (6.4), in the sense that $\hat{\mu}(x) = \hat{\rho}(x)/\{1 + \hat{\rho}(x)\}$. However, the binary regression interpretation gives a different rationale for choosing the bandwidth h which, as noted above, remains valid when the spatial distribution of the population at risk cannot be modelled by a Poisson process. Kelsall and Diggle (1998) explore the consequences of this, and conclude that a reasonable method of bandwidth selection is to minimise a cross-validation criterion,

$$CV(h) = \left[\prod_{i=1}^{N} \hat{\mu}_h^{-i}(x_i)^{y_i} \{1 - \hat{\mu}_h^{-i}(x_i)^{1-y_i}\} \right]^{-1/N}, \tag{6.7}$$

where $\hat{\mu}_h^{-i}(x_i)$ denotes the estimate of $\mu(x_i)$ based on all of the data except (x_i, y_i).

Note that the Monte Carlo method of assessing departure from constant $\rho(x)$ can still be used in this setting.

Generalised additive models

A limitation of the methods discussed in the previous two sections is their inability to make use of additional explanatory variables $z_j(x)$. One way round this is to use a generalised additive model (GAM, Hastie and Tibshirani 1990). For a binary response variable, the natural generalised additive model is an additive logistic model, in which

$$\log[\mu(x)/\{1 - \mu(x)\}] = \alpha + \sum_{j=1}^{p} \beta_j z_j(x) + S(x). \tag{6.8}$$

Note the similarity to (6.1). For the model (6.8), Hastie and Tibshirani's methodology allows for joint estimation of the regression parameters α and β_j and the non-parametrically specified function $S(x)$. In this semi-parametric setting, the null hypothesis of interest is usually that $S(x)$ is constant, rather than that $\mu(x)$ is constant, because the role of the $z_j(x)$ is to take account of known risk factors. Because this is not a simple hypothesis, an exact Monte Carlo test is no longer available. However, approximate

Monte Carlo tolerance intervals for $\hat{S}(x)$, and hence for $\hat{\mu}(x)$ given the observed explanatory variables, can be obtained by repeatedly re-estimating $S(x)$ in (6.8) from simulations of the fitted logistic regression model for $\mu(x)$ ignoring $S(x)$, this being equivalent to assuming that $S(x)$ is a constant and thereby absorbing it in to the parameter α in (6.8).

Kelsall and Diggle (1998) develop the application of the GAM methodology to the disease mapping problem and propose a cross-validation criterion for choosing the bandwidth parameter. They then use the method to estimate the pattern of spatial variation in cancer mortality in the Walsall District Health Authority, England, between 1982 and 1992. The data consist of the residential locations of 2015 deaths from lung cancer and of 5839 controls selected at random from the population register of June 1994. Covariate adjustments are made for sex and for age, which is fitted as a quadratic effect based on the results of a simple exploratory analysis. Note that within the modelling framework of (6.8), $\exp\{S(x)\}$ denotes the residual odds ratio of disease after adjustment for known explanatory variables. Taking logarithms to the base 2 of $\exp\{S(x)\}$ transforms the residual odds ratio so that a one unit increase corresponds to a doubling of the odds relative to baseline. Figure 6.1 shows the resulting map of the estimate of $S(x)$ scaled in this way. The overall test of departure from constant risk gives a p-value of 0.002, based on 500 simulations. The thick solid contour identifies a single, annular sub-region in which the estimates $\hat{S}(x)$ lie above the 95% upper tolerance limits, whilst the dashed contours identify two sub-regions in the south and southeast of the study region, and two small pockets in the north, where the estimates $\hat{S}(x)$ lie below the 95% lower limits.

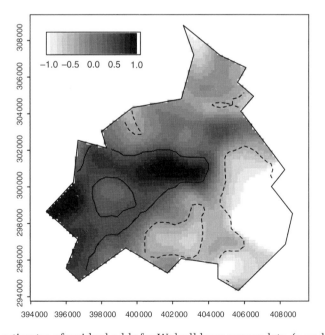

Fig. 6.1 Scaled estimates of residual odds for Walsall lung cancer data. (x and y scales in units of 1 metre.)

Model-based geostatistics

If we make $S(x)$ in (6.8) a stochastic process we define a generalised linear mixed model (Breslow and Clayton 1993) in which $S(x)$ is a spatially structured random effect. Models of this kind are used by Diggle *et al.* (1998) in what they term *model-based geostatistics* to solve spatial prediction problems involving discrete response variables. In this approach, the central idea is to define the estimate of $S(x)$ as that function of the data, y_i, $i = 1, \ldots, N$, which minimises the mean squared error, $E[\{\hat{S}(x) - S(x)\}^2]$. By a standard result in probability theory, this problem has the formal solution

$$\hat{S}(x) = E[S(x)|y_1, \ldots, y_N]. \tag{6.9}$$

The explicit evaluation of $\hat{S}(x)$ is seldom feasible, as in general it involves an N-dimensional integration. However, by adopting a Bayesian inferential framework, Diggle *et al.* (1998) were able to apply Markov chain Monte Carlo methods (Gilks *et al.* 1996) to simulate samples from the posterior distribution of $S(x)$ given y_i, $i = 1, \ldots, N$. These simulated samples can then be used to estimate the expectation, or any other required property, of this conditional distribution.

The specific models used by Diggle *et al.* (1998) specify that $S(x)$ is a stationary Gaussian process the correlation function of which, $\text{corr}\{S(x), S(x')\}$, is a function of the distance d between x and x'. In particular, they use a powered exponential model with $f(d) = \exp\{-(d/\phi)^\kappa\}$. However, the associated discussion of Diggle *et al.* (1998) points out that, whilst the simple exponential, $f(d) = \exp(-d/\phi)$, is a reasonable single-parameter model, a better choice for a two-parameter extension is a class of models based on Bessel functions, and known as the 'Matérn class' after Matérn (1986). This model is discussed in Chapter 10 in the context of exposure mapping.

Point-source problems

An important special case of the disease mapping problem concerns the estimation of disease risk in relation to a point source of environmental pollution. An example of this which has received great attention in the UK is the question of whether the risk of childhood cancer is elevated in the vicinity of nuclear power stations (e.g. see the collection of papers and associated discussion edited by Muirhead and Darby 1989). Chapter 9 reviews statistical methods for the assessment of risk in relation to point sources.

The simplest version of the point-source problem seeks to model the spatial odds function $\rho(x)$ as a function only of the distance, $d(x)$ say, between x and a pre-specified point x_0. A log-linear model, $\rho(x) = \exp\{\alpha + \beta d(x)\}$, would provide a simple solution, but is strictly inappropriate since (if β is negative, the case of likely interest) it implies that $\rho(x)$ approaches zero at large values of $d(x)$ whereas a more reasonable assumption would be that $\rho(x)$ approaches a non-zero constant level. Stone (1988) and Bithell and Stone (1989) proposed a non-parametric approach to the problem, but imposing the reasonable constraint that $\rho(x)$ should be a non-increasing function of $d(x)$. Most subsequent applications of Stone's test have been for area-level data, but in the original paper Stone also noted the possibility of adapting the method to individual-level data.

Diggle (1990) proposes a parametric model of the form $\rho(\boldsymbol{x}) = \rho_0[1 + \alpha f\{d(\boldsymbol{x})\}]$ in which $f(d)$ is a non-increasing function which approaches zero for large d. In this model, ρ_0 represents the odds corresponding to background risk, and α the proportionate increase in odds at the point source. Diggle and Rowlingson (1994) use the same model as Diggle (1990), but by fitting the model using the binary labelling interpretation they avoid the need to estimate the spatially varying intensity of the population at risk and are able to include log-linear adjustments for other known risk factors. Lawson (1993) and Lawson and Williams (1994) propose a more general class of models in which the risk depends on orientation as well as distance. They also argue that if, for example, elevation in risk is a consequence of the dispersion of an airborne pollutant, it may not be appropriate to restrict $\rho(\boldsymbol{x})$ to be non-increasing with distance from the source.

Diggle *et al.* (1997) extend Diggle and Rowlingson's model to include a plateau of constant elevated risk $1 + \alpha$ within distance δ of the point source. One motivation for this extension is to embed within the parametric modelling a representation of the simpler and well-established epidemiological method of comparing disease rates in sub-regions 'close' and 'not close' to the point source.

All of the methods described so far in this section assume that the available explanatory variables, including distance from the point source, can explain all of the spatial variation in risk. When this is not so, we need to reintroduce the function $S(\boldsymbol{x})$ to describe the residual spatial variation, either as a deterministic function of unspecified form, or as an unobserved spatial stochastic process. The latter approach would be embraced by the model-based geostatistics methodology of Diggle *et al.* (1998) and is discussed with specific reference to environmental epidemiology in Lawson (1994).

6.3.2   Area-level data

Area-level data arise when information on disease cases is presented only in a spatially aggregated form, typically as counts, Y_i, of the numbers of cases in each of a set of sub-regions A_i, $i = 1, \ldots, m$ which partition the study region A. In principle, this represents a loss of spatial information. However, the loss is counterbalanced by the much greater availability of reliable population data at the area level. For example, in the UK the ten-year national census provides information on population size, stratified by age and sex, and on a variety of relevant socio-economic measures, at the level of census *enumeration districts* (EDs), which on average contain approximately 400 individuals each. By mapping individual case information onto these same EDs, we can make a direct comparison between cases and the population as a whole without the need for a potentially expensive case-control study.

An approximate Poisson model

Using the Poisson process formulation of our theoretical model, it follows that the numbers Y_i of cases in the sub-regions A_i are mutually independent and Poisson-distributed, with means

$$\mu_i = \int_{A_i} \lambda_1(\boldsymbol{x})\mathrm{d}\boldsymbol{x} = \int_{A_i} \rho(\boldsymbol{x})\lambda_0(\boldsymbol{x})\mathrm{d}\boldsymbol{x}. \tag{6.10}$$

If we now make the assumption that all of the variables which determine $\rho(x)$ are constant within each A_i, (6.10) simplifies to

$$\mu_i = \rho_i \int_{A_i} \lambda_0(x)\mathrm{d}x, \tag{6.11}$$

and we can replace the integral by its unbiased estimator N_i, the population size within A_i. Incorporating the log-linear model (6.1) for the ρ_i, we then arrive at a simple Poisson regression model, $Y_i \sim \mathrm{Po}(\mu_i)$, with

$$\mu_i = N_i \exp\left(\alpha + \sum_{j=1}^{p} \beta_j z_{ij}\right). \tag{6.12}$$

Note that this defines a log-linear regression model for the Y_i in which $\log N_i$ is used as an offset (i.e. an explanatory variable with known regression coefficient): for non-rare diseases, a binomial approximation might be preferred, as for example in Knorr-Held and Besag (1998). A common practice in the Poisson case is to replace the N_i by standardised expectations, E_i, representing the numbers of cases expected in the separate sub-regions according to appropriate age-sex adjusted rates, for example regional rates. Diggle *et al.* (1997) use this approach to model spatial variation in disease risk in relation to a point source. The use of standardised expectations E_i in place of the population sizes N_i does not affect the status of the Poisson distributional assumption. However, the more basic assumption that all relevant covariates are constant within sub-regions is at best an approximation, but perhaps a reasonable one provided the A_i are sufficiently small. We note that this assumption may result in ecological bias; see Chapter 11. Several authors, including Cook-Mozaffari *et al.* (1989), use Poisson regression models directly, without explicit consideration of their relationship to an underlying individual-level model.

Extra-Poisson variation

One obvious source of extra-Poisson variation in area-level data is violation of the assumption that all relevant covariates are constant within each A_i. Diggle *et al.* (1997) suggest using the following standard adjustment for extra-Poisson variation (McCullagh and Nelder 1989: 200). Let $\hat{\mu}_i$ denote the fitted values corresponding to the counts Y_i, and define $X^2 = \sum_{i=1}^{m}(Y_i - \hat{\mu}_i)^2/\hat{\mu}_i$. If we relax the Poisson assumption to allow $\mathrm{Var}(Y_i) = \kappa\mu_i$ for some value of $\kappa > 1$, then an estimate of κ is $\tilde{\kappa} = X^2/r$ where r is the residual degrees of freedom from the fitted regression model. A simple quasi-likelihood adjustment for extra-Poisson variation then consists of multiplying the Poisson-based standard errors of the estimated regression parameters by $\sqrt{\tilde{\kappa}}$ (McCullagh and Nelder 1989).

A potentially more complex source of extra-Poisson variation arises through failure to recognise residual spatial variation in risk after adjustment for all known risk factors. In our model for individual-level data, this residual spatial variation is described by the term $S(x)$ in (6.1). In the setting of area-level data, models in which observations $y_1, \ldots, y_m$ are mutually independent conditional on an underlying spatial process have been proposed by Clayton and Kaldor (1987) and by Besag *et al.* (1991); see also Chapter 7. In this setting, the stochastic process $S(\boldsymbol{x})$, previously defined for all $\boldsymbol{x}$ in a continuous spatial region, is replaced by a stochastic vector $(S_1, \ldots, S_m)$ defined for each area. The authors cited above use Bayesian estimates of the latent variables S_i to solve the disease mapping problem, an approach which is similar in spirit to, but substantially pre-dates, the geo-statistical methodology of Diggle *et al.* (1998). We now summarise this approach, considering first the simplest possible example in which all of the spatial variation is described by the S_i (i.e. there are no additional covariates).

The basic model is now that counts $\boldsymbol{Y} = (Y_1, \ldots, Y_m)$ are mutually independent Poisson variates conditional on $\boldsymbol{S} = (S_1, \ldots, S_m)$, and with conditional expectations $E_i\mu_i$, where E_i again denotes the standardised expectation in the ith sub-region and

$$\mu_i | \boldsymbol{S} = \exp(\alpha + S_i). \tag{6.13}$$

To complete the (non-Bayesian) model specification we need to specify the joint distribution of $\boldsymbol{S}$. A standard assumption is that S is multivariate Gaussian, with mean zero (so that the S_i can be interpreted as fluctuations about an overall mean level α) and a variance matrix whose structure reflects our assumptions about the way in which the spatial relationships amongst the sub-regions A_i affect their associated relative risks. Given the model specification, the minimum mean square error predictor for the relative risk in sub-region A_i is then

$$\tilde{\mu} = e^{\alpha} E[\exp(S_i)|\boldsymbol{Y}]. \tag{6.14}$$

An empirical Bayes solution involves plugging in estimates of α and of the covariance matrix of $\boldsymbol{S}$ into (6.14), in effect treating these parameter estimates as if they were known constants (see Section 15.4.2 of Chapter 15). A fully Bayesian implementation treats all of the model parameters as random variables, assigns prior probability distributions to them, and leads to the solution

$$\tilde{\mu}_i = E[\mu_i|\boldsymbol{Y}]. \tag{6.15}$$

The empirical Bayes solution (6.14) and the fully Bayesian solution (6.15) often give similar point predictions, but empirical Bayes typically underestimates the associated prediction variance because it does not allow for uncertainty in the model parameters. Of course, in a Bayesian inferential framework there is no compelling reason to use the expectation to summarise the posterior distribution of the μ_i.

The simplest possible specification for the joint distribution of S would be that the S_i are mutually independent with common variance σ^2. The resulting predictions $\tilde{\mu}_i$ are non-spatial, in the sense that they make no use of the locations of the A_i. Nevertheless, they have the sensible property that they compromise between taking the data at face-value (meaning that $\tilde{\mu}_i = Y_i$) and assuming that the same risk applies in all sub-regions ($\tilde{\mu}_i = \bar{Y}$), to an extent determined by the value of the assumed between-region variance, σ^2. A non-spatial specification of this kind can be interpreted as a parametric counterpart to the quasi-likelihood adjustment described at the beginning of this section.

For an overtly spatial specification, we require a multivariate Gaussian distribution for S in which dependence between a pair of sub-regions is determined by their spatial locations. The specification of stochastic models of this kind was an important research topic in its own right during the 1970s (e.g. see Besag 1974 and the associated discussion). Besag's preferred approach, and the one which has since become the standard, is to specify a model for S via the *full conditional* distributions of each S_i given all other S_j. This imposes non-obvious constraints for self-consistency of the implied model for S which are addressed in the celebrated Hammersley–Clifford theorem. In the present context, the task of model formulation is complicated by the irregular spatial arrangement of the sub-regions A_i. The resulting models are known as *Markov random fields*.

One legitimate formulation, used by Clayton and Bernardinelli (1992) in response to criticism of an earlier suggestion in Clayton and Kaldor (1987), is the following. Define a set of constants $a_{ij}, j \neq i$, which represent the 'strength of adjacency' between A_i and A_j and let $a_i = \sum_{j \neq i} a_{ij}$. Then, we assume that the full conditional distribution of S_i is Gaussian, with expectation

$$\mathrm{E}[S_i | S_j, j \neq i] = a_i^{-1} \sum_{j \neq i} a_{ij} S_j$$

and variance

$$\mathrm{var}(S_i | S_j, j \neq i) = a_i^{-1} \gamma,$$

where $\gamma > 0$ is a parameter to be estimated. Clayton and Bernardinelli (1992) acknowledge that in practice 'it is rather difficult to decide upon a degree of adjacency' and therefore suggest using binary a_{ij}, equal to 1 or 0 according to whether sub-regions A_i and A_j do, or do not, respectively, share a common boundary.

A possible compromise between mutually independent S_i and Clayton and Bernardinelli's (1992) spatial model, suggested by Besag *et al.* (1991), is to replace S_i by the sum of two components, $S_i = S_{1i} + S_{2i}$, in which the S_{1i} follow the independence model and the S_{2i} follow the spatial model. By adjusting the relative sizes of the variances of the two components, we can then explore the consequences of assuming a range of strengths of spatial dependence. This model is discussed by Mollié (1996) and in Chapters 7 and 15.

Markov random field models are very natural to describe local dependence in regular spatial layouts, and are widely used in fields of application such as image analysis (Geman and Geman 1984; Besag 1986). In epidemiology, as indicated above, a potential difficulty associated with them is the need to specify the strength of adjacency coefficients a_{ij} in a way which acknowledges the potentially complicated shapes and sizes of the sub-regions, A_i, for which data are available. Put another way, it is an unattractive feature that politically determined regional boundaries can affect the scientific interpretation of public health data in a potentially arbitrary manner (which is *not* saying that politics is irrelevant to public health!).

Geostatistical models recognise the continuous nature of geographical space but, at least as implemented by Diggle *et al.* (1998), require the health outcome data to be associated with well-defined point locations. Application of geostatistical methods to epidemiological data at the areal level typically ascribes each count Y_i and its associated covariate information to a reference location within the corresponding sub-region A_i (e.g. its geometric centroid). Kelsall and Wakefield (1999) describe an interesting alternative approach, in which a stochastic process $S(x)$ in continuous space is used to derive

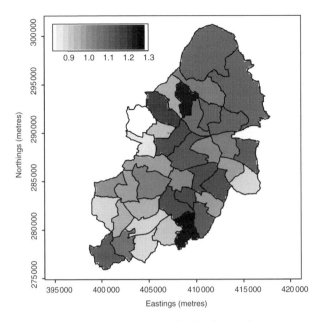

Fig. 6.2 Estimated spatial variation in relative risk of colorectal cancer in Birmingham, using the model of Clayton and Bernardinelli (1992).

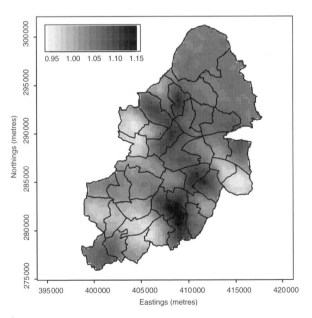

Fig. 6.3 Estimated spatial variation in relative risk of colorectal cancer in Birmingham, using the model of Kelsall and Wakefield (submitted).

approximations to the relevant statistical properties of the spatially aggregated counts Y_i, resulting in the estimation of a smoothly varying surface $\hat{S}(x)$.

Figure 6.2 shows the result of applying the Clayton and Bernardinelli (1992) model to data on counts of colorectal cancer cases recorded for each of 36 electoral wards in the UK city of Birmingham. The example is taken from as yet unpublished analysis by Kelsall and Wakefield (submitted), who calculate expected numbers of cases based on the population sizes of the wards, stratified by age and sex. The map shows discontinuities at ward boundaries as a consequence of the spatial discretisation of the model. For comparison, Fig. 6.3 shows the result of applying Kelsall and Wakefield's approach. The two maps have some broad features in common, but are very different in detail. In particular, the model used to produce Fig. 6.3 allows the estimates to vary smoothly over the whole study region. Note also that the range of the estimates is narrower in Fig. 6.2 than in Fig. 6.3. A partial explanation is that the two models differ in the strength of their assumed spatial dependence. The appearance of the map can be affected by adjustment of the prior distributions assumed for the model parameters, which serves to underline that these methods are not amenable to full automation but require the investigator to exercise their judgement in 'tuning' the model to the data. An alternative approach to modelling aggregated counts, again in terms of a smooth underlying function, is described by Wolpert and Ickstadt (1998); see also Chapter 22.

6.4   Clusters, clustering, or spatial variation in risk?

Within spatial epidemiology, cluster detection, clustering, and spatial variation in risk should properly be regarded as separate problems, but the distinctions among them are often blurred. One possible reason for this is that words like 'cluster' are used either without a formal definition, or with a definition which is neither mathematically precise nor compatible with its associated statistical method of analysis. For example, Knox (1989) defines a *cluster* as *a geographically bounded group of occurrences of sufficient size and concentration to be unlikely to have occurred by chance*. As a non-mathematical definition, this is unexceptionable, but how should we then operationalise the detection of such clusters? The reference to 'unlikely to have occurred by chance' in Knox's definition has obvious connotations of significance testing, and many of the proposed methods of cluster detection consist, either explicitly or implicitly, of testing (perhaps repeatedly) the observed disease distribution against a null hypothesis, H say, of complete spatial randomness, meaning in the current context that:

(1) cases occur independently of each other;

(2) all members of the population are at equal risk.

Further discussion is provided by, for example, Openshaw *et al.* (1988), Cuzick and Edwards (1990), Besag and Newell (1991), and in Chapter 8. Translated to the theoretical framework of Section 6.2, the hypothesis H is equivalent to the independent Bernoulli labelling model (6.2), together with the assumption that $\rho(x_i) = \rho_0$, a constant for all x_i. A possible extension is to insist only that (2) above should hold after adjustment for known risk factors, corresponding to a specification of the form

$$\rho(x_i) = \exp\left\{ \alpha + \sum_{j=1}^{p} \beta_j z_j(x_i) \right\},$$

where the explanatory variables $z_j(x_i)$ represent the known risk factors. However, under this model it is possible that a *single* case of disease at a location within a sparsely populated sub-region would represent strong statistical evidence against *H*, violating Knox's requirement of 'sufficient size'. The same applies to a modest but consistent excess of cases over a very large sub-region, violating the requirement of 'concentration'. The point here is not that there is necessarily anything wrong with Knox's definition, but that it is inherently difficult to translate it into a formal statistical prescription, and this is a recipe for confusion if we try to apply a formal statistical method to a given set of data and use the result as an answer to the question: 'is this a cluster?'.

A second reason for confusion is that all three problems can initially be addressed via a test of the *same* null hypothesis, *H*. They are distinguished by the implied alternative hypothesis and by the scientific purpose of the analysis. From this point of view, it is easy to articulate the distinction between clustering and spatial variation in risk:

- *clustering* is departure from assumption (1) of *H*, in the direction of positive dependence, meaning that conditional on the existence of a case at *x*, the probability of a case at a location *x'* sufficiently close to *x* is greater than the unconditional probability of a case at *x'*, and
- *spatial variation in risk* is departure from assumption (2) of *H*.

If we seek to go beyond a test of the null hypothesis *H*, a natural progression is to the fitting of stochastic models the parameters of which are scientifically interpretable. Clustering invites an interpretation in terms of genetic susceptibility or infectious transmission. Spatial variation in risk invites an environmental interpretation, with point-source modelling as a special case. Note that clustering and spatial variation in risk are not mutually exclusive, and that both are statements about the process generating the data, rather than about the observed data themselves. The same distinction is made by Alexander and Cuzick (1992).

Cluster detection, in contrast, *is* concerned with classifying features of the observed spatial distribution of disease. In the author's opinion, a better name for this activity would be *anomaly detection*, or *surveillance*. Having identified a stochastic model which broadly fits the available data, any residual spatial structure represents unexplained, and therefore potentially interesting, variation and becomes a candidate for further investigation (which may or may not involve formal statistical methods). In work of this kind, an important role for statistics is to guard against the danger of following too many false positive trails. This is a difficult balance to strike. Inevitably, random mechanisms do throw up anomalous patterns from time to time, and there is both an economic and a social cost to the follow up of such anomalies, not least the concern caused by the raising of what might prove to be a false alarm. Conversely, there is an obvious cost of failure to follow up a real effect. An important unsolved problem for spatial epidemiology is to resolve this conflict in a manner which is both scientifically rigorous and socially realistic.

References

Alexander, F. E. and Cuzick, J. (1992). Methods for the assessment of disease clusters. In *Geographical and environmental epidemiology: methods for small area studies* (P. Elliott, J. Cuzick, D. English, and R. Stern ed.), 238–250. Oxford University Press.

Anderson, N. H. and Titteringotn, D. M. (1997). Some methods for investigating spatial clustering with epidemiological applications. *Journal of the Royal Statistical Society, Series A*, **160**, 87–105.

Barnard, G. A. (1963). Contribution to the Discussion of Professor Bartlett's paper. *Journal of the Royal Statistical Society, Series B*, **25**, 294.

Bartlett, M. S. (1964). The spectral analysis of two-dimensional point processes. *Biometrika*, **51**, 299–311.

Besag, J. (1974). Spatial interaction and the statistical analysis of lattice systems (with discussion). *Journal of the Royal Statistical Society, Series B*, **36**, 192–225.

Besag, J. (1986). On the statistical analysis of dirty pictures (with discussion). *Journal of the Royal Statistical Society, Series B*, **48**, 259–302.

Besag, J. and Newell, J. (1991). The detection of clusters in rare diseases. *Journal of the Royal Statistical Society, Series A*, **154**, 143–55.

Besag, J., York, J., and Mollié, A. (1991). Bayesian image resoration, with two applications in spatial statistics (with discussion). *Annals of the Institute of Statistical Mathematics*, **43**, 1–59.

Biggeri, A., Barbone, F., Lagazio, C., Bovenzi, M., and Stanta, G. (1996). Air pollution and lung cancer in Trieste, Italy: spatial analysis of risk as a function of distance from source. *Environmental Health Perspectives*, 104, 750–4.

Bithell, J. F. (1990). An application of density estimation to geographical epidemiology. *Statistics in Medicine*, **9**, 691–701.

Bithell, J. F. and Stone, R. (1989). On statistical methods for analysing the geographical distribution of cancer cases near nuclear installations. *Journal of Epidemiology and Community Health*, **43**, 79–85.

Bowman, A. and Azzalini, A. (1997). *Applied smoothing techniques for data analysis*. Oxford University Press.

Breslow, N. E. (1996). Statistics in epidemiology: the case-control study. In *Advances in Biometry* (P. Armitage and H. A. David, ed.), 287–318. Wiley, New York.

Breslow, N. E. and Clayton, D. G. (1993). Approximate inference in generalized linear mixed models. *Journal of the American Statistical Association*, **88**, 9–25.

Chetwynd, A. G. and Diggle, P. J. (1998). Investigation of spatial clustering from matched and stratified case-control studies. Lancaster University, Statistics Technical Report.

Clayton, D. and Bernardinelli, L. (1992). Bayesian methods for mapping disease risk. In *Geographical and environmental epidemiology: methods for small area studies*. (P. Elliott, J. Cuzick, D. English, and R. Stern ed.), 205–20. Oxford University Press.

Clayton, D. and Kaldor, J. (1987). Empirical Bayes estimates of age-standardised relative risks for use in disease mapping. *Biometrics*, **43**, 671–81.

Cook-Mozaffari, P., Darby, S., Doll, R., Forman, D., Hermon, C., and Pike, M. C. (1989). Geographical variation in mortality from leukaemia and other cancers in England and Wales in relation to proximity to nuclear installations, 1969–78. *British Journal of Cancer*, **59**, 476–85.

Cox, D. R. (1955). Some statistical methods related with series of events (with discussion). *Journal of the Royal Statistical Society, Series B*, **17**, 129–57.

Cuzick, J. and Edwards, R. (1990). Spatial clustering for inhomogeneous populations (with discussion). *Journal of the Royal Statistical Society, Series B*, **52**, 73–104.

Diggle, P. J. (1990). A point process modelling approach to raised incidence of a rare phenomenon in the vicinity of a pre-specified point. *Journal of the Royal Statistical Society Series A*, **153**, 349–62.

Diggle, P. J. and Rowlingson, B. S. (1994). A conditional approach to point process modelling of raised incidence. *Journal of the Royal Statistical Society, Series A*, **157**, 433–40.

Diggle, P., Elliott, P., Morris, S., and Shaddick, G. (1997). Regression modelling of disease risk in relation to point sources. *Journal of the Royal Statistical Society, Series A*, **160**, 491–505.

Diggle, P. J., Moyeed, R. A., and Tawn, J. A. (1998). Model-based geostatistics (with discussion). *Applied Statistics*, **47**, 299–350.

Diggle, P. J., Morris, S., and Wakefield, J. (2000). Point-source modelling using matched case-control data. *Biostatistics*, **1**, 89–105.

Geman, S. and Geman, D. (1984). Stochastic relaxation, Gibbs distributions and the Bayesian resoration of images. *I.E.E.E. Transactions on Pattern Analysis and Machine Intelligence*, **6**, 721–41.

Gilks, W. R., Richardson, S., and Spiegelhalter, D. J. (ed.) (1996). *Markov chain Monte Carlo in practice*, Chapman and Hall, London.

Hastie, T. J. and Tibshirani, R. J. (1990). *Generalized additive models*. Chapman and Hall, London.

Kelsall, J. E. and Diggle, P. J. (1995*a*). Kernel estimation of relative risk. *Bernoulli*, **1**, 3–16.

Kelsall, J. E. and Diggle, P. J. (1995*b*). Nonparametric estimation of spatial variation in relative risk. *Statistics in Medicine*, **14**, 2335–42.

Kelsall, J. E. and Diggle, P. J. (1998). Spatial variation in risk: a nonparametric binary regression approach. *Applied Statistics*, **47**, 559–573.

Kelsall, J. E. and Wakefield, J. C. (submitted). Modelling spatial variation in disease risk. Submitted to *Journal of the American Statistical Association*.

Knorr-Held, L. and Besag, J. (1998). Modelling risk from a disease in time and space. *Statistics in Medicine*, **17**, 2045–60.

Knox, E. G. (1989). Detection of clusters. In *Methodology of enquiries into disease clustering* (P. Elliott ed.), Small Area Health Statistics Unit, London.

Lawson, A. (1993). On the analysis of mortality events associated with a prespecified fixed point. *Journal of the Royal Statistical Society, Series A*, **156**, 363–77.

Lawson, A. (1994). Using spatial Gaussian priors to model heterogeneity in environmental epidemiology. *The Statistician*, **43**, 69–76.

Lawson, A. (1995). McMC methods for putative pollution source problems in environmental epidemiology. *Statistics in Medicine*, **14**, 2473–85.

Lawson, A. B. and Williams, F. L. R. (1994). Armadale: a case-study in environmental epidemiology. *Journal of the Royal Statistical Society, Series A*, **157**, 285–98.

McCullagh, P. and Nelder, J. A. (1989). *Generalized linear models* (2nd edn). Chapman and Hall, London.

Matérn, B. (1986). *Spatial variation* (2nd edn). Springer, Berlin.

Mollié, A. (1996). Bayesian mapping of disease. In *Markov chain Monte Carlo in practice* (W. R. Gilks, S. Richardson, and D. J. Spiegelhalter ed.), 359–79. Chapman and Hall, London.

Muirhead, C. and Darby (ed.) (1989). Royal Statistical Society Meeting on Cancer Near Nuclear Installations, *Journal of the Royal Statistical Society, Series A*, **152**, 305–84.

Nadaraya, E. A. (1964). On estimating regression. *Theory of Probability and its Applications*, **10**, 186–90.

Openshaw, S., Craft, A. W., Charlton H., and Birch, J. M. (1988). Investigation of leukaemia clusters by the use of a geographical analysis machine. *Lancet*, **i**, 272–3.

Silverman, B. W. (1986). *Density estimation for statistics and data analysis*. Chapman and Hall, London.

Stone, R. A. (1988). Investigations of excess environmental risks around putative sources: statistical problems and a proposed test. *Statistics in Medicine*, **7**, 649–60.

Watson, G. S. (1964). Smooth regression analysis. *Sankhya, Series A*, **26**, 359–72.

Wolpert, R. L. and Ickstadt, K. (1998). Poisson/gamma random field models for spatial statistics. *Biometrika*, **85**, 251–67.

7. Bayesian approaches to disease mapping

J. C. Wakefield, N. G. Best, and L. Waller

7.1 Introduction

Disease mapping may be defined as the estimation and presentation of areal summary measures of health outcomes, and has a long history in epidemiology (see e.g. Chapter 12 and the references in Smans and Esteve 1992). The aims of disease mapping include simple description, hypothesis generation, allocation of health care resources, assessment of inequalities, and estimation of background variability in underlying risk in order to place epidemiological studies in context. Unfortunately, there are well-documented difficulties with the mapping of raw estimates since, for small areas and rare diseases in particular, these estimates will be dominated by sampling variability. The most common summary measure is the standardised morbidity/mortality ratio (SMR) which is defined, for area i, by Y_i/E_i where Y_i and E_i denote the observed and expected number of counts in area i, respectively. The variance of this estimate is proportional to E_i^{-1} and so for areas with small populations there will be high sampling variability. To overcome this variability it is now commonplace to carry out 'smoothing' of the raw rates via hierarchical modelling. Although this approach may also be justified in a likelihood *random effects* context, or via a minimum mean squared error argument (e.g. Lindley and Smith 1972; Clayton and Kaldor 1987), in this chapter we describe the hierarchical smoothing model from a fully Bayesian perspective.

Good review papers on Bayesian methods for disease mapping have been published by Clayton and Bernardinelli (1992) and Mollié (1996). In this chapter, our aim is to examine more fully the underlying assumptions of the approach and provide more discussion of the mathematical details. The structure of the chapter is as follows. In Section 7.2 we describe a three-stage hierarchical model within which disease mapping data may be viewed. Historically the use of fully Bayesian methods has been hindered by computational consideration and, in Section 7.3, we consider implementation and, in particular, simulation-based techniques. In Section 7.4 we provide two illustrative examples of the use of Bayesian disease mapping models. Section 7.5 considers some extensions and alternative approaches to the models presented here, and Section 7.6 provides a concluding discussion. The two appendices contain more detailed developments of specific aspects.

7.2 Statistical formulation

In general, health outcomes may be available as area-level aggregated *count data*, or each case may have an associated exact location (e.g. from a case-control study), giving rise to *point data*. Count data are more typically used for disease mapping studies (often arising from routinely available sources for example, see Chapter 2); we therefore focus on methods for modelling count data in this chapter. Methods for the estimation and mapping of disease relative risk using point data are described in Chapter 6.

In this section we will describe a three-stage hierarchical model for disease counts. At the first stage we model the observed counts as a function of area-level summaries such as the risk or the relative risk. At the second stage, a joint distribution is specified for the collection of these risks or relative risks, possibly as a function of area-level explanatory variables. These first two stages constitute a generalised linear mixed model (Clayton 1996). The second stage distribution depends on unknown parameters and these are assigned a (hyper) prior distribution at the third stage of the model. The models of this section are closely related to those described in Chapter 11 for ecological correlation studies.

7.2.1 First-stage model

Let Y_{ij} and N_{ij} represent the number of cases and the number of individuals at risk in stratum j, $j = 1, \ldots, J$, and area i, $i = 1, \ldots, n$. As in all epidemiological studies, stratification by known risk factors (e.g. age and sex) is important since different areas will, in general, contain different proportions of individuals within each stratum and ignoring this information may lead to spurious conclusions. For example, Knorr-Held and Besag (1998) analysed lung cancer data in Ohio, USA for 1968–88 and showed that if the age structure of each county is ignored then it appears that the risk for white women is greater than for non-white women. However, when the age structure is accounted for, this conclusion is reversed. In this chapter, we assume that both the cases and the populations at risk are measured without error (though see Appendix I). The effects of relaxing these assumptions are considered more fully in Chapter 3, where the issue of inaccuracies in population counts is considered; and in Best and Wakefield (1999), where errors in both the numerators (cases) and denominators (populations) are considered.

Binomial model

With known populations and for non-infectious diseases, the starting point for analysis is the binomial model

$$Y_{ij}|p_{ij} \sim \text{Bin}(N_{ij}, p_{ij}), \tag{7.1}$$

where p_{ij} is the risk (probability) of disease in area i and stratum j. The maximum likelihood estimates (MLEs) for the stratified area-specific risks are given by $\hat{p}_{ij} = Y_{ij}/N_{ij}$ but, in general, the data will be too sparse to obtain robust estimates of each of these $n \times J$ quantities and so some simplifying assumptions are required. It is usual to make the proportionality assumption

$$\frac{p_{ij}}{1 - p_{ij}} = \theta_i \times \frac{p_j}{1 - p_j}, \tag{7.2}$$

so that the effect of being in area i is to multiply each of the strata-specific *reference odds* $p_j/(1 - p_j)$ by the common *odds ratio*, θ_i, for that area. In this way we have reduced the number of quantities to estimate per area from J to 1. However, the proportionality assumption is clearly very strong and must be checked. For example, simple graphical plots of $\hat{p}_{ij}/(1 - \hat{p}_{ij})$ versus $\hat{p}_j/(1 - \hat{p}_j)$ may be constructed to assess proportionality or, more formally, logistic regression models containing area × stratum interactions may be fitted. If non-proportionality is found then separate analyses of collections of strata within which proportionality holds may be carried out.

The reference odds may be estimated simultaneously with the θ_i (e.g. Clayton 1996), or be fixed using either a set of odds from a reference area (external standardisation), or the overall odds for the study region

$$\frac{\hat{p}_j}{1 - \hat{p}_j} = \frac{\sum_i Y_{ij}}{\sum_i (N_{ij} - Y_{ij})},$$

(internal standardisation). In the case where the $\hat{p}_j$ are treated as known, the MLEs of the odds ratios θ_i may be estimated via the logistic regression model

$$\text{logit } p_{ij} = \log \theta_i + \hat{\gamma}_j \tag{7.3}$$

where the $\hat{\gamma}_j = \log\{\hat{p}_j/(1 - \hat{p}_j)\}$ are known offsets. We note that this model does not acknowledge uncertainty in the γ_j, which may be a problem if these quantities are not estimated from extensive data.

In some situations (e.g. hypothesis generation studies, see Chapter 11), the relative risks θ_i will be regressed on a $k \times 1$ vector of area-specific explanatory variables, X_i, via the model

$$\log \theta_i = \alpha + X_i^T \beta, \tag{7.4}$$

where β is a $k \times 1$ vector of regression coefficients. The use of internal standardisation with known offsets, (i.e. Equation (7.3)), requires care since the a priori estimation of γ_j may remove some of the effect of the exposure X_i. For example, older individuals may tend to live in areas with large values of X_i. These and other issues are discussed in Breslow and Day (1987, Chapter 4).

The model (7.1)–(7.4) does not acknowledge overdispersion in the data (i.e. $\text{var}(Y_{ij}) > N_{ij} p_{ij}\{1 - p_{ij}\}$) which may have both spatial and non-spatial components and arises from, for example, unmeasured risk factors and inaccuracies in the numerator and denominator. Appendix I develops models for overdispersion via the consideration of unknown risk factors and data anomalies. The models that we describe in the next section explicitly model this overdispersion.

With the binomial formulation it is not possible to aggregate the data Y_{ij} across stratum $j = 1, \ldots, J$, since the sum of binomial random variables $Y_i = \sum_j Y_{ij}$ is not of convenient form, and in particular is not binomial except in the uninteresting case where $p_{ij} = p_i$. In principle, this lack of data reduction is not a problem. However, it may create computational difficulties due to memory requirements if n and/or J are large and, in practice, numerical estimation problems may also arise if there are large numbers of (i, j)

cells containing zero cases since in this case the likelihood is likely to be very flat and hence contain little information.

Poisson model

For rare diseases we may approximate the binomial distribution (7.1) by the Poisson distribution:

$$Y_{ij} \sim \text{Po}(N_{ij} \times p_{ij}).$$

The proportionality assumption corresponding to (7.2) is then expressed as

$$p_{ij} = \theta_i \times p_j, \tag{7.5}$$

where θ_i now corresponds to the *relative risk* of disease in area i with respect to the reference rate in each stratum. A great advantage of the Poisson approximation is that, when combined with the proportionality assumption (7.5), we may collapse over strata to obtain

$$Y_i \sim \text{Po}(E_i \times \theta_i) \tag{7.6}$$

where $Y_i = \sum_j Y_{ij}$ and $E_i = \sum_j N_{ij} p_j$ denotes the *expected number* of cases in area i with strata-specific references rates p_j. The MLE $\hat{\theta}_i = Y_i/E_i$ corresponds to the SMR. In general, the use of SMRs corresponds to *indirect standardisation*. Care must be taken with such an approach (e.g. see Breslow and Day 1987), essentially because, if the proportionality assumption (7.5) is not valid, then inappropriate summary relative risks θ_i will be obtained (see Chapter 9 for a fuller discussion).

For the Poisson model, we may specify a log-linear model for the relative risk as a function of area-specific risk factors X_i

$$\log \theta_i = \alpha + X_i^T \beta. \tag{7.7}$$

The use of (7.6) and (7.7) will often suffer from the same problems of overdispersion ($\text{var}(Y_i) > E_i \theta_i$) that were present for the binomial model, see Appendix I.

7.2.2 Second-stage model

In general, and for small areas in particular, the MLEs of odds ratios or relative risks, $\hat{\theta}_i$, will be highly unstable due to sparse data. To provide more robust estimation one may specify a joint model for $\boldsymbol{\theta} = (\theta_1, \ldots, \theta_n)^T$ which allows the estimate of each θ_i to 'borrow strength' from the remaining estimates $\theta_{i'}$, $i' \neq i$. This is achieved by specifying a multivariate probability distribution for $\boldsymbol{\theta}$. There are many possibilities for this distribution with an important choice being on the form of the variability in the θ_i. We may believe that the θ_i vary across the map without spatial pattern (so-called unstructured variability), display spatial dependence (structured variability), or exhibit a combination of the two. In particular, this choice will determine the level of global and local smoothing (corresponding to unstructured and structured variability, respectively) that is carried out. There are various decisions corresponding to each of these possibilities.

Unstructured variability

We first consider models that produce global smoothing across the study region. In the case of binomial data and no stratification (i.e. $Y_i|p_i \sim \text{Bin}(N_i, p_i)$), a distribution for p_i that is analytically tractable is the beta distribution (see Appendix I for details). This case is not of great interest, however, since we would almost always want to stratify the disease counts by age and sex. Such stratification may be carried out with reference odds evaluated via internal or external standardisation, and incorporated in (7.3). A natural approach then is to model the logarithm of the odds ratios, θ_i, in (7.2) as

$$\log \theta_i = \alpha + X_i^T \beta + V_i, \qquad (7.8)$$

where V_i is the *residual log odds ratio* in area i, relative to the reference region (after adjustment for known stratification risk factors and X_i).

The vector $V = (V_1, \ldots, V_n)^T$ is often assumed to arise from the n-dimensional normal distribution

$$V \sim N_n(\mathbf{0}_n, \sigma_v^2 I_n),$$

where $\mathbf{0}_n$ denotes the $n \times 1$ vector of zeros, I_n the $n \times n$ identity matrix and $\sigma_v^2 > 0$ controls the between-area variability of the V_i. Various models for overdispersion are discussed in Appendix I but the most natural interpretation of V_i in (7.8) is of an unmeasured risk factor that is common to all individuals in area i, and does not display a spatial pattern. Note that for small V_i, σ_v reflects, approximately, the standard deviation of the residual odds ratios.

The model (7.8) may be used when we have (7.2) with known reference probabilities p_j. Knorr-Held and Besag (1998) consider the more general case in which both θ_i and p_j are simultaneously estimated via the model

$$\text{logit } p_{ij} = \alpha + X_i^T \beta + V_i + \gamma_j,$$

with $V_i \sim_{\text{i.i.d.}} N(0, \sigma_v^2)$, as before, and $\gamma_j = \text{logit } p_j$.

For the Poisson model (7.6), an analytically tractable second stage distribution for the unstructured variability is the gamma distribution. In the following, $\text{Ga}(a, b)$ denotes the gamma distribution with mean a/b and variance a/b^2. This choice is natural since the gamma is conjugate to the Poisson and so the marginal distribution of Y_i can be calculated in closed form as negative binomial. In general, a and b are treated as unknown and the posterior distribution for these parameters is not of closed form (e.g. Clayton and Kaldor 1987). The marginal variance $\text{var}(Y_i|a, b)$ can take a variety of forms depending on the gamma formulation that is chosen. Table 7.1 summarises three possibilities.

Case I results in a variance function that is proportional to the mean and is the closest to the conventional quasi-likelihood approach (McCullagh and Nelder 1989) that has been used in spatial epidemiological context by Diggle *et al.* (1997). Case II was used by Clayton and Kaldor (1987) in a disease mapping context and Case III allows the variance to be a quadratic function of the mean. Distinguishing between these cases, via residuals for example, is likely to be difficult unless the range of the expected number of cases is large (see Wakefield and Morris 1999). When the expected number of cases is not large

Table 7.1 Marginal variances for the data Y_i following from different gamma specifications in the model $Y_i|\theta_i \sim \text{Po}(E_i\theta_i)$. In each case $\text{E}[\theta_i] = a_i$ and $\text{E}[Y_i|a_i, b] = E_i a_i$ where $a_i = \exp(\alpha + X_i^T \boldsymbol{\beta})$

Case	Assumption	var(θ_i)	var($Y_i|a_i, b$)
I	$\theta_i \sim \text{Ga}(E_i a_i b, E_i b)$	$a_i/(E_i b)$	$\text{E}[Y_i|a_i, b](1 + 1/b)$
II	$\theta_i \sim \text{Ga}(a_i b, b)$	a_i^2/b	$\text{E}[Y_i|a_i, b](1 + E_i/b)$
III	$\theta_i \sim \text{Ga}(b, b/a_i)$	a_i^2/b	$\text{E}[Y_i|a_i, b](1 + \text{E}[Y_i|a_i, b]/b)$

the forms of the variance will not be so different and hence it will be difficult to distinguish between them.

Although the gamma distribution is natural for incorporating unstructured over-dispersion, it does not extend to allowing structured variability with positive spatial correlations (but see Chapter 22 for a variation of this model which does allow for spatial dependence via a gamma *mixture* distribution). Instead, a normal distribution is often used for both the structured and the unstructured components. For the unstructured component we may again assume

$$\log \theta_i = \alpha + X_i^T \boldsymbol{\beta} + V_i, \tag{7.9}$$

where α is an intercept term representing the overall log relative risk of disease in the study region compared to the reference rate, and V_i is the residual log relative risk in area i compared with the study region. As before, $\boldsymbol{V} = (V_1, \ldots, V_n)^T$ is assumed to arise from the n-dimensional normal distribution

$$\boldsymbol{V} \sim N_n(\boldsymbol{0}_n, \sigma_v^2 \boldsymbol{I}_n). \tag{7.10}$$

Note that the marginal distribution of Y_i is not available in closed form for the Poisson-log normal model; the mean and variance may be derived, however. For the model given by (7.6), (7.10), and (7.10) this is

$$\text{var}(Y_i|\mu_i, \sigma_v^2) = \text{E}[Y_i|\mu_i, \sigma_v^2]\{1 + \text{E}[Y_i|\mu_i, \sigma_v^2](\exp(\sigma_v^2) - 1)\},$$

where

$$\text{E}[Y_i|\mu_i, \sigma_v^2] = E_i \exp(\mu_i + \sigma_v^2/2),$$

and $\mu_i = \alpha + X_i^T \boldsymbol{\beta}$. Hence the variance is a quadratic function of the mean (Case III in Table 7.1). For the normal distribution, the different assumptions analogous to those in Table 7.1 all lead to the same marginal variance function for the data. We note that the marginal median of Y_i is given by $E_i \exp(\mu_i)$.

Note, that as pointed out by Wolpert and Ickstadt (1998), the Poisson-log normal model does not aggregate consistently. What this means is that if we specify a lognormal distribution for each of the relative risks and then combine two areas (say) and specify a log normal distribution for the relative risk of the combined area, then these distributions are inconsistent (because the sum of log normal distributions is not log normal). This issue is related to the problem of pure specification ecological bias (see Chapter 5) in which risk relationships do not remain constant across levels of aggregation. Provided the user remains aware of these issues, this does not seem such a great disadvantage, however, particularly since a normal second-stage distribution has been observed empirically to provide a good model for log relative risks over a range of aggregations, and is convenient in a number of other respects such as model flexibility and ease of computation.

A number of tests of heterogeneity have been proposed to assess departures from constant relative risk across the map (see Alexander and Cuzick 1992 and Chapter 8). However, we note that heterogeneity in area-level estimates of risk will almost always be present; the question of interest is whether this heterogeneity is of epidemiological significance. As pointed out above (and in Appendix I) the unstructured residual odds ratios or relative risks, $\exp(V_i)$, may be interpreted as corresponding to unknown or unmeasured risk factors that are *shared* by all individuals within area i. Hence between area heterogeneity in risk may indicate the absence of an important ecological (area-level) risk factor from the model (Appendix I). Theoretically, if these risk factors were observed then they could be included in the model and we would no longer need the V_i.

Spatial variability

We now consider the modelling of spatially structured variability in the log relative risks. The first stage model is identical to that with unstructured variability, but we model the log odds ratios (binomial data) or log relative risks (Poisson data) via

$$\log \theta_i = \alpha + X_i^T \beta + U_i \tag{7.11}$$

where U_i, $i = 1, \ldots, n$ denote spatially structured area-specific random effects, in contrast to the unstructured random effects V_i considered previously. The problem is to model the n-dimensional random variable $U = (U_1, \ldots, U_n)^T$, allowing for dependence between U_i and U_j, $i \neq j$. Due to the multitude of possibilities for this dependence, the modelling at this stage is fundamentally more difficult than in the unstructured case. Modelling may proceed either by specifying the *joint distribution* of U, or via the univariate *conditional distributions* $U_i | U_j = u_j$, $j \neq i$, $i = 1, \ldots, n$.

First, suppose

$$U \sim N_n\left(\mathbf{0}_n, \sigma_u^2 \Sigma\right), \tag{7.12}$$

where $N_n(\cdot, \cdot)$ denotes the n-dimensional normal distribution and Σ is an $n \times n$ positive definite correlation matrix. The parameter $\sigma_u^2 > 0$ controls the overall variance of the U_i. Let $Q \stackrel{.}{=} \Sigma^{-1}$ and Q_{ij} denote element (i,j) of this matrix, $i, j = 1, \ldots, n$. As reviewed in Besag and Kooperberg (1995), standard properties of the multivariate normal distribution (e.g. Johnson and Kotz 1972; Searle *et al.* 1991) produce the set of conditional distributions

$$U_i | U_j = u_j, j \neq i \sim N\left(\sum_{j=1}^{n} W_{ij} u_j, \sigma_u^2 D_{ii}\right), \tag{7.13}$$

where $W_{ii}=0$, $W_{ij}=-Q_{ij}/Q_{ii}$ and $D_{ii}=Q_{ii}^{-1}$. This derivation is described in detail in Appendix II. The specification (7.13) is sometimes referred to as an *autonormal* model (Besag 1974). From the symmetry of Q we have that

$$W_{ij}D_{jj} = W_{ji}D_{ii}. \tag{7.14}$$

From a modelling perspective, use of the joint formulation requires specification of the elements of the covariance matrix Σ, while use of the conditional formulation reduces to specification of the matrix W of weights W_{ij} and D_{ii} in (7.13). The approaches are related through the relationship $Q=D^{-1}(I-W)$, where D is an $n \times n$ diagonal matrix containing elements D_{ii}, $i=1,\ldots,n$. As we describe in more detail below, however, convenient choices for W and D do not lead to a joint model that is a well-defined probability density since they lead to a Q that is singular (and consequently the mean of each U_i is undefined and the variances are infinite).

Conditional modelling

Besag (1974) argued that modelling the conditional distributions will often be more straightforward than the joint distribution in problems in which random variables are defined spatially. The majority of approaches incorporating a conditional model for spatial dependence proceed by first specifying a set of spatial weights for use in (7.13). These weights traditionally define a set of 'neighbours' that contribute positive weight to the conditional expectation of U_i with $W_{ij}=0$ for the remaining regions, and $W_{ii}=0$. This is in the same spirit as Markovian models in time series. The set of conditional distributions given by (7.13) defines a Markov random field (MRF) model.

In the Gaussian conditional autoregression (CAR) the specification (7.13) with a positive definite Q leads to

$$U \sim N_n(\boldsymbol{0}_n, \sigma_u^2(I_n - W)^{-1}D).$$

Cressie and Chan (1989) proposed taking $D_{ii}=E_i^{-1}$ and $W_{ij}=\rho(E_j/E_i)^{1/2}$ for $j\in\partial i$, where ∂i denotes the set of labels of the 'neighbours' of area i, and $W_{ij}=0$ otherwise. Letting $W=\rho C$, a positive definite Q requires ρ to lie in the interval $(\rho_{\min}, \rho_{\max})$ where $\rho_{\min}^{-1}<0$ and $\rho_{\max}^{-1}>0$ are, respectively, the smallest and largest eigenvalues of $D^{-1/2}CD^{1/2}$. If we expect the spatial dependence to be positive, then we may take $\rho\in(0,\rho_{\max})$. The parameter ρ may be interpreted as measuring the strength of spatial dependence in the data since $\operatorname{corr}(U_i, U_j|U_k, k\neq i,j)=\rho$. This interpretation is appealing but the conditional mean is given by

$$E[U_i] = \frac{\rho}{E_i^{1/2}}\sum_{j\in\partial i} E_j^{1/2},$$

which does not seem a natural choice. Cressie and Chan (1989) also give alternatives in which the spatial dependence depends on the distance between area centroids.

A common MRF model is the *intrinsic Gaussian autoregression* prior considered by Besag *et al.* (1991) and given by

$$U_i|U_j = u_j, j \neq i \sim N\left(\bar{u}_i, \frac{\omega_u^2}{m_i}\right), \tag{7.15}$$

where $\bar{u}_i = \frac{1}{m_i}\sum_{j\in\partial i} u_j$ and m_i is the number of neighbours. Comparison with (7.13) reveals that we have $D_{ii} = m_i^{-1}$ and $W_{ij} = m_i^{-1}$ for neighbouring areas $W_{ij} = 0$ otherwise. This specification seems natural, the conditional mean of U_i is the average of the neighbouring U_j's, but does not yield a positive definite precision matrix $\boldsymbol{Q}$. To see this, note that in the ith row of $\boldsymbol{I} - \boldsymbol{W}$ we have a single one and m_i entries with values $-m_i^{-1}$ and so the row sums are all zero indicating the matrix $\boldsymbol{Q}$ only has rank $n-1$ and so is not invertible. The variance, ω_u^2, in (7.15), is no longer proportional to a marginal variance (since the latter no longer exists), to emphasise this we have changed our notation from σ_u^2 to ω_u^2; the latter is only interpretable conditionally.

The joint specification corresponding to (7.15) is given by

$$f(\boldsymbol{U}) \propto \exp\left\{-\frac{1}{2\omega_u^2}\sum_{i<j}(U_i - U_j)^2\right\}.$$

It is again clear that the joint distribution does not exist since we may have an arbitrary mean level for each U_i. Besag and Kooperberg (1995) note that, if we take $E[U_i|U_j = u_j, j \neq i] = \lambda\bar{u}_i$ with $0 < \lambda < 1$, then the joint distribution is well defined. Unfortunately, to obtain reasonable levels of dependence, λ has to be very close to one and hence the *non-stationary* version (7.15) may be preferred (see Chapter 10 for a discussion of non-stationarity). A great advantage of a non-stationary model is that the form of the spatial dependence may vary across the study region.

When, as we have specified in (7.11), there is an intercept in the model we require an additional constraint on the prior specification (7.15) to allow identifiablity. Besag and Kooperberg (1995) suggest constraining the U_i to have zero mean and specifying a uniform prior on the whole of the real line for the intercept α. Equivalently, the unconstrained prior (7.15) may be used if we do not include an intercept term in (7.11); we use the latter parameterisation in the applications of Section 7.4.

One difficulty with the conditional approach is that it is often unclear how to choose the weights W_{ij} and the neighbourhood ∂i. To define *neighbours*, a number of authors (e.g. Clayton and Kaldor 1987; Besag *et al.* 1991; Richardson *et al.* 1995; Bernardinelli *et al.* 1997; Waller *et al.* 1997) have taken areas i and j to be neighbours if they share a common boundary. This is reasonable if all regions are of similar size and arranged in a regular pattern (as is the case for pixels in image analysis where these models originated), but is not particularly attractive otherwise. Various other neighbourhood/weighting schemes are possible (e.g. see Cliff and Ord 1981) though such formulations should be considered in the light of the symmetry constraint (7.14). Cressie and Chan (1989) take the neighbourhood structure to depend on the distance between area centroids and determine the extent of the spatial correlation (i.e. the distance within which regions are considered neighbours) via an exploratory analysis using the variogram (Cressie 1993; Chapter 10). Cressie and Chan (1989), Best *et al.* (1999), and Conlon (1999) consider distance-based weights with weights decreasing with increasing inter-centroid distances.

For the Gaussian CAR, if the neighbourhood criterion (i.e. ∂i, $i = 1,\ldots,n$) is specified along with var(U_i) and cov(U_i, U_j) for neighbouring i and j (with $Q_{ij} = 0$ for non-neighbouring i and j), then Besag and Kooperberg (1995) describe a procedure (based on the Dempster (1972) algorithm) by which $\boldsymbol{Q}$ may be determined. For the intrinsic Gaussian autoregression this approach may be modified so that, along with the neighbourhood criterion, the quantities $\text{var}(U_i - U_j)$ for neighbouring i and j, are specified. In this case W_{ij} and D_{ii} in (7.13) are then determined. Besag and Kooperberg (1995) report that this approach has been used in the examples of Besag *et al.* (1991), but apart from this the approach has not so far been used in a spatial epidemiological context.

In addition to the choice of spatial weights and neighbourhood structures required for the conditional approach, one could also consider the use of non-Gaussian forms for the conditional distributions. For example, Besag *et al.* (1991) and Best *et al.* (1999) consider the Laplacian distribution which leads to a second-stage spatial model based on the median rather than the mean of neighbouring rates. This may be more appropriate when discontinuities in disease rates are expected between areas.

We finally note that whether the conditional model defines a proper or an improper joint distribution the interpretation of the variances (σ_u^2 or ω_u^2) requires care since they depend on the neighbourhood structure. The specification of equal prior variances is most easily accommodated in the joint specification that we now describe.

Joint modelling

Our description of joint modelling is based on the multivariate normal distribution $N_n(\mathbf{0}_n, \sigma_u^2 \mathbf{\Sigma})$. The $n \times n$ positive definite correlation matrix $\mathbf{\Sigma}$ contains elements Σ_{ij}, $i, j = 1, \ldots, n$ with the off-diagonal terms Σ_{ij}, $i \neq j$ describing the correlation between U_i and U_j (i.e. the residual log odds ratios or residual log relative risks in areas i and j). Various structured forms may be assumed for $\mathbf{\Sigma}$. A common choice is to assume that the dependence is a function of the distance, d_{ij}, between the population-averaged centroids (say) of areas i and j, that is, $\Sigma_{ij} = f(d_{ij}, \boldsymbol{\phi})$ where $\boldsymbol{\phi}$ represents a vector of parameters defining the particular structural form chosen. This assumption of *isotropy* is common but can be weakened to allow, for example, directional components. For ease of development, we will limit attention to formulations assuming isotropy. Such joint modelling is described by Raftery and Banfield (1991), and naturally assumes that distance is an appropriate metric for defining spatial associations (Besag *et al.* 1991: 52).

An obvious choice for $f(d_{ij}, \boldsymbol{\phi})$ is the family

$$f(d_{ij}, \boldsymbol{\phi}) = \exp\left\{ -\left(\frac{d_{ij}}{\phi_1}\right)^{\phi_2} \right\}, \tag{7.16}$$

where $\phi_1 > 0$, $\phi_2 \in (0, 2]$ and $\boldsymbol{\phi} = (\phi_1, \phi_2)$. Note that $\phi_2 = 2$ produces a covariance matrix that has both theoretical and practical drawbacks (see the discussion in Diggle *et al.* 1998). Devine *et al.* (1996) and Wakefield and Morris (1999) use model (7.16) with $\phi_2 = 1$ and investigate the extent of the spatial dependence using a variogram. A number of correlation functions are available as alternatives to (7.16). A two-parameter family that may be preferable (see the discussion in Diggle *et al.* 1998) is the Matérn class (Matérn 1986). In this case we have a scale parameter $\phi_1 > 0$ and a smoothness parameter $\phi_2 > 0$ and

$$f(d_{ij}, \boldsymbol{\phi}) = \frac{1}{2^{\phi_2 - 1}\Gamma(\phi_2)} \left(\frac{d_{ij}}{\phi_1'}\right)^{\phi_2} B\left(\frac{d_{ij}}{\phi_1'}\right),$$

where $\phi'_1 = \phi_1/(2\sqrt{\phi_2})$ and $B(\cdot)$ is the modified Bessel function of order ϕ_2. Handcock and Stein (1993) use this class in a kriging context.

Combining spatial and unstructured variability

Besag *et al.* (1991) propose to combine unstructured and structured variability via the model

$$\log \theta_i = \alpha + X_i^T \beta + U_i + V_i, \tag{7.17}$$

which they term a *convolution* prior. The U_i and V_i represent spatially structured and unstructured contributions respectively to the log odds ratio or log relative risk, and are assumed to be independent.

7.2.3 Third-stage model

We let ψ denote the parameters of the distributions that we have specified for the random effects U and/or V. At the final stage of the model we specify hyperpriors for these parameters, the intercept α, the regression coefficients β. For α and β, improper uniform or normal priors with large variance are often specified to represent vague beliefs.

Considerable care is required when specifying hyperpriors for ψ. Gamma distributions are typically chosen for the inverses of variances (i.e. σ_v^2, σ_u^2, and ω_u^2), a common choice being $\text{Ga}(\varepsilon, \varepsilon)$ with ε very small (say 10^{-2} or 10^{-3}). However, Kelsall and Wakefield (1999) point out that even a diffuse prior such as this can be highly informative. In particular these priors are not consistent with very small levels of variability in the random effects. As an alternative they suggest using a $\text{Ga}(0.5, 0.0005)$ prior for the inverse variance parameters since, in many contexts, this will give a plausible range of relative risks across the map. Mollié (Chapter 15) and Bernardinelli *et al.* (Chapter 16) suggest alternative strategies for choosing the hyperpriors of the conditional model. Experience of choosing appropriate hyperpriors for the parameters of the joint covariance model is limited and sensitivity of the resulting inference to different specifications should be carefully assessed.

7.3   Implementation

We define $\delta = (\delta_1, \ldots, \delta_n)^T$ where $\delta_i = \log \theta_i$, $i = 1, \ldots, n$. We are then interested in the posterior distribution

$$p(\delta, \alpha, \beta, \psi | Y) \propto p(Y|\delta) \times p(\delta|\alpha, \beta, \psi) \times p(\alpha, \beta, \psi). \tag{7.18}$$

This distribution is analytically intractable; in this section we describe how implementation may be achieved.

Posterior estimation can proceed via either an empirical Bayes or fully Bayesian approach. The principle behind empirical Bayes methods is to replace the unknown third-stage hyperparameters α, β, and ψ by point estimates based (say) on the maximised likelihood of the hyperparameters given the data $\hat{\alpha}$, $\hat{\beta}$, and $\hat{\psi}$. Maximisation may be achieved using the EM-algorithm (Dempster *et al.* 1977). The posterior distribution of the vector of log relative risks, δ, given the data Y and point estimates $\hat{\psi}$, is then considered. Further details may be found in Clayton and Kaldor (1987), Devine *et al.* (1996), and Chapter 15. Devine *et al.* (1996) also describe the use of a constrained empirical Bayes technique that modifies the risk estimates to correct for the fact that the sample variance of the collection of empirical Bayes estimates underestimate the true variance. See Carlin and Louis (1996) for a general discussion of empirical Bayes methods.

Unfortunately, empirical Bayes methods suffer from a number of limitations. In particular, the estimates of disease risk/relative risk fail to reflect the uncertainty associated with the hyperparameter estimates $\hat{\alpha}$, $\hat{\beta}$, and $\hat{\psi}$ and are thus overprecise. These problems are avoided by implementing a fully Bayesian approach in which the *joint* posterior distribution (7.18) is investigated. Inference about the relative risks θ requires integration of the joint posterior with respect to (α, β, ψ) and, after this integration is carried out, the posterior uncertainty associated with these hyperparameters is acknowledged.

The intractability of the posterior distribution has led to the use of Markov chain Monte Carlo (MCMC) simulation methods to generate *samples* from the joint posterior distribution. As pointed out by Smith and Gelfand (1992) there is a duality between a probability density function and samples from that density. Given the former we may generate samples, and given the latter we may reconstruct the former. The principle is best understood by imagining a histogram constructed from a set of values sampled at random from a probability distribution: given a large enough sample, the histogram can provide virtually complete information about the distribution from which these samples were drawn. In particular, the mean, variance, percentiles, and other summaries of the distribution can be estimated by calculating the corresponding statistics from the sample. In a disease mapping context we may, for example, calculate the probability that the odds ratio or relative risk in a particular area exceeds a given threshold by counting the number of simulated values which are larger than the threshold.

MCMC algorithms proceed by simulating values of subsets of parameters *conditional* on the remaining parameters. The approach is particularly appealing for hierarchical models in which the conditional independencies indicated in (7.18) may be exploited. In particular, great simplifications of the algorithms may be achieved when we proceed with the conditional spatial specification. In contrast, for the joint model, for unknown ϕ we must, at each iteration evaluate Σ^{-1} and its determinant. Hence, this model requires far more computer time for implementation.

A strategy that avoids this computation within the algorithm is a discretisation of the prior distribution for ϕ (e.g. Kelsall and Wakefield, submitted). In this way, the matrix inversions corresponding to each prior choice may be carried out before beginning the MCMC iterations.

Details of the computational algorithms used for MCMC simulation are provided elsewhere (e.g. Gilks *et al.* 1996; Brooks 1998). These methods are implemented in the WinBUGS statistical software package (Spiegelhalter *et al.* 1996), which includes specific functions to fit conditional and joint models discussed in this chapter; it is this software we use for the examples of Section 7.4.

It is important to be aware of the potential practical problems of using MCMC methods for disease mapping analyses. All MCMC algorithms generate a sequence of *dependent* values which will *eventually* resemble a sample from the required posterior distribution: that is, the frequency with which values in an interval appear in the sample is equal to the probability content of the posterior probability content of the interval. However, early samples (called the 'burn-in') should be discarded since they are not representative of the posterior distribution. Various methods exist for determining how many samples to discard, although none are foolproof and most require the benefit of experience and judgement (see Mengersen *et al.* 1999, for a review). The number of samples generated after the discard phase will affect the accuracy of the posterior inference. Although MCMC methods allow estimation of the full posterior, the finite size of the simulation will introduce a degree of approximation error, known as the Monte Carlo standard error. Samples which are large and are nearly independent (i.e. have low auto-correlations between consecutively sampled values) will have a relatively low Monte Carlo standard error. Unfortunately, models used in a mapping context may exhibit high correlations between model parameters and include terms which are only weakly identi-fied; this tends to result in highly autocorrelated samples and hence the MCMC simula-tion must be run for a large number of iterations in order to generate a sample of sufficient accuracy for posterior inference. Further discussion of these and other potential implementation problems relating to CAR models are discussed by Best *et al.* (1999).

7.4   Illustrative example

In this section we provide a short example to illustrate the practical application of Bayesian methods for disease mapping. Specifically, we compare the conditional and joint approaches to modelling spatial correlation between small-area disease rates. More detailed applications of these methods are provided in Chapters 15 and 16.

The study region of interest comprises the 144 electoral wards of the Mersey and West Lancashire districts of northwest England. We consider incidence of two cancers with contrasting aetiology: (i) lung cancer—the most common tumour, known to be related to smoking and socio-economic deprivation; and (ii) brain cancer—a less common tumour whose aetiology is largely unknown. Observed ward-level counts Y_i, $i = 1, \ldots, 144$, were obtained for each tumour site from the cancer registration data held by the UK Office for National Statistics. For brain cancer, the number of cases per ward ranged from 0 to 17 (median $= 6$) over the 11-year period 1981–91. For lung cancer, we used data for a single year (1991) to provide a more comparable number of cases per ward (range $= 0$–60; median $= 20$). Ward-level population counts by five-year age group and sex were obtained from the 1991 UK census. We note that these examples should be viewed as illustrative only. In particular, the examination of lung cancer rates when no information on smoking behaviour (or an approximate proxy for it) is available, is not an informative epidemiological enterprise.

Cancers are relatively rare diseases, and so it is convenient to assume a Poisson distribution for the observed counts Y_i, as in Equation (7.6). Expected counts E_i for each cancer were internally standardised for age and sex with the risks for each stratum being calculated a priori, as described in Section 7.2.1. Figure 7.1 shows maps of the maximum likelihood estimators $\hat{\theta}_i = Y_i/E_i$ corresponding to the observed ward-specific SMRs for each cancer. Interpretation is difficult due to the sampling variability that is inherent in such estimates.

Bayesian smoothed estimates of the area-specific relative risks were then estimated using both the conditional and joint modelling approaches described in Section 7.2.

(a)   (b)

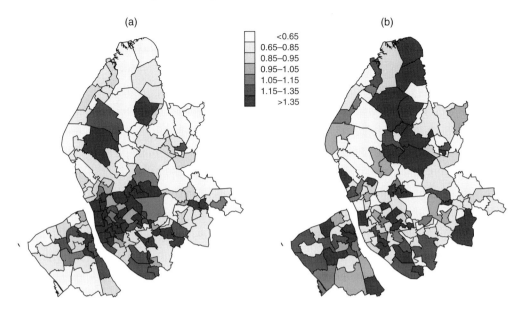

	<0.65
	0.65–0.85
	0.85–0.95
	0.95–1.05
	1.05–1.15
	1.15–1.35
	>1.35

Fig. 7.1 Maximum likelihood estimates of the relative risks (SMRs) for (a) lung cancer; (b) brain cancer.

Under the conditional approach, we fitted the convolution model given by Equation (7.17). We used simple adjacency weights ($W_{ij} = m_i^{-1}$ for $j = \partial_i$ and $W_{ij} = 0$ otherwise) as in (7.15) to specify the conditional distributions of the spatial random effects U_i. Independent Ga(0.5, 0.0005) hyperprior distributions were assumed for the inverse variance parameters ω_u^{-2} and σ_v^{-2}.

Under the joint approach, we fitted the second stage model $\log \theta_i = \alpha + U_i$, where the vector of spatial random effects $U = (U_1, \ldots, U_{144})^T$ was modelled using the multivariate normal prior given in (7.12) with $\Sigma_{ij} = \exp(-\lambda d_{ij})$ which corresponds to (7.16) with $\lambda = \phi_1^{-1}$ and $\phi_2 = 1$. We do not include separate unstructured random effects V_i in this model since the parameter λ, which is estimated along with the other model parameters, controls the degree (or lack of), spatial dependence between the random effects. We note, however, that it is feasible to include a set of non-spatial random effects in this model. A Ga(0.01, 0.01) hyperprior distribution was assumed for the inverse variance parameter σ_u^{-2} and a uniform distribution on the range (0.001, 10) was chosen for λ. The upper limit of the latter prior corresponds to a correlation matrix Σ which is approximately equal to the identity matrix since $\Sigma_{ii} = \exp(-10 \times d_{ii}) = 1$ when $d_{ii} = 0$ and $\Sigma_{ij} = \exp(-10 \times d_{ij}) \approx 0$ for all d_{ij}, $i \neq j$ where d_{ij} ranges from 1.55 km to 49.5 km across the study region. The lower bound of the prior leads to off-diagonal elements of Σ_{ij} in the range $\exp(-0.001 \times 1.55) = 0.998$ to $\exp(-0.001 \times 49.5) = 0.952$, representing very strong spatial dependence.

Model fitting was carried out using MCMC simulation methods implemented in the WinBUGS software. Two separate chains starting from different initial values were run for each model. Convergence was checked by visual examination of 'time series' style plots of the samples for each chain, and by computing the Gelman and Rubin (1992)

Table 7.2 Posterior means (95% credible intervals) of the variance components for each model and cancer site

	Lung cancer		Brain cancer	
	Conditional	Joint	Conditional	Joint
Unstructured variance, σ_v^2	0.007 (0.0002, 0.037)	–	0.003 (0.001, 0.017)	–
Spatial conditional variance, ω_u^2	0.202 (0.096, 0.323)	–	0.0008 (0.0001, 0.003)	–
Spatial marginal variance, σ_u^2	–	0.148 (0.072, 0.347)	–	0.015 (0.003, 0.042)
Distance decay, λ	–	0.236 (0.078, 0.509)	–	4.956 (0.202, 9.739)

diagnostic based on the ratio of between to within chain variances for each model. On this basis, the first 3000 samples of each simulation were discarded as 'burn-in'; each chain was run for a further 20 000 iterations, and posterior estimates were based on pooling the $2 \times 20\,000$ samples for each model. This gave Monte Carlo standard errors $< 1\%$ of the posterior standard deviation for all parameters except the variance components σ_v^2 and ω_u^2 for which the Monte Carlo standard errors were about 8% of the standard deviation.

Table 7.2 shows the posterior mean and 95% credible intervals for the variance components for each dataset and model. Comparison of the equivalent parameter estimates for each cancer site shows that there is considerably more variability in the relative risks of lung cancer than of brain cancer. This excess variability is largely attributed to spatially structured effects: under the conditional model, the variance of the spatial components, ω_u^2, is over two orders of magnitude greater for lung cancer than for brain cancer, while the unstructured variance, σ_v^2, is negligible for both cancers. Under the joint model, the overall variance parameter σ_u^2 is one order of magnitude greater for lung cancer than for brain cancer, and λ is much smaller, indicating greater variability in the random effects among ward-level risk of lung cancer compared with brain cancer. In terms of interpretation we may calculate the distance at which the correlations drop to 0.5 which is given by $\log 2/\lambda$. For lung and brain cancers, respectively, the distances are approximately 2.9 km and 0.14 km indicating far greater spatial dependence for the former.

Figures 7.2(a) and (b) show the smoothed estimates of the relative risk of lung cancer, θ_i, for the conditional convolution model and the joint model, respectively. Corresponding maps for brain cancer are shown in Figs 7.3(a) and (b). Although the estimates for lung cancer look similar under both models, the estimates for brain cancer show a different spatial pattern under the conditional model. This pattern may be explained by noting the following: (i) the conditional model is non-stationary; (ii) the posterior distribution for the conditional spatial variance parameter ω_u^2 is close to zero for brain cancer, suggesting that the risk in any given ward is very similar to that in neighbouring wards; (iii) the observed SMRs for brain cancer tend to be higher in the southwest (median $= 1.1$, interquartile range $= 0.90$–1.30) versus the rest of the study region

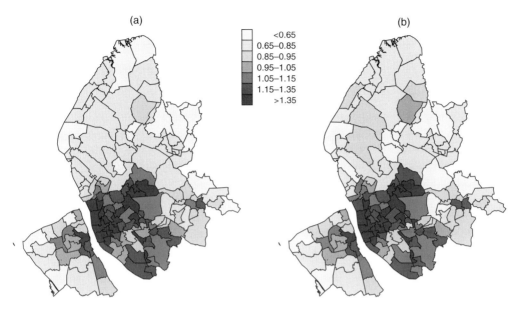

Fig. 7.2 Posterior mean relative risk of lung cancer, θ_i, estimated using (a) the conditional formulation; (b) the joint formulation.

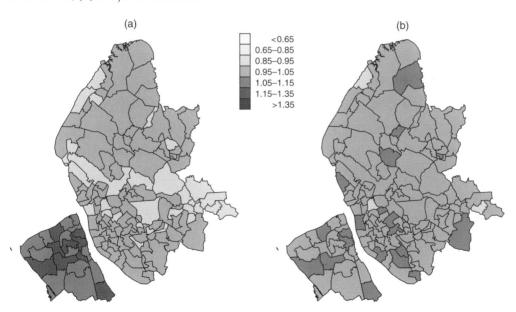

Fig. 7.3 Posterior mean relative risk of brain cancer, θ_i, estimated using (a) the conditional formulation; (b) the joint formulation.

(median $= 0.85$, interquartile range $= 0.68$–1.21); (iv) the River Mersey separates wards in the southwest from the rest of the region and thus acts as a boundary under the adjacency-based conditional weighting scheme (i.e. the 21 wards southwest of the Mersey are not considered to be neighbours of any wards across the river). This combination of factors effectively leads to the risk estimates in all wards southwest of the river being smoothed towards one 'local' mean, while the risk estimates of all wards northeast of the river are smoothed towards a different (and lower) 'local' mean. We found that nearly identical estimates of relative risk were obtained by fitting a model with unstructured random effects only, but allowing a separate intercept term for wards to the southwest and for wards to the northeast of the river.

The southwest to northeast trend in relative risk is less pronounced for lung cancer under the conditional model because the risks in the two regions are more comparable. The phenomenon does not occur for either cancer under the joint formulation since the distance-based correlation structure allows cross-river dependence of the U_i.

This example clearly demonstrates that considerable care is needed when specifying, estimating, and interpreting Bayesian disease mapping models! Further analyses of these data are presented in Chapter 8.

7.5   Extensions and alternative approaches

7.5.1   Spatio-temporal models

Let $\theta_i(t)$ denote the log relative risk/log odds ratio in area i at time t. Then Bernardinelli *et al.* (1995) propose the following model:

$$\log \theta_i(t) = \alpha + \delta_{i1} + \beta t + \delta_{i2} t.$$

They allow δ_{i1} and δ_{i2} to be both either structured or unstructured random effects. This model therefore allows for a temporal trend that is allowed to vary across areas. In order to investigate whether regional spatial patterns change over time, Waller *et al.* (1997) consider an extension, nesting spatial effects within time (i.e. the model includes a set of n unstructured random effects V_{it} and n spatially structured random effects U_{it} for each time period t). The prior variances may also vary with time period. Using such a formulation, Waller *et al.* (1997) found increasing residual clustering in annual lung cancer mortality for counties in Ohio, USA, across the years 1968–88. Knorr-Held and Besag (1998) analyse the same data, adding age-adjustment and using a binomial model in their analysis, and summarise spatial pattern across time.

Knorr-Held and Besag (1998) note that models with independent time and space effects offer ease in interpretation (U_i and V_i offer adjustments to relative risk, while U_{it} and V_{it} offer adjustments to relative risk within time period), but Bernardinelli *et al.* (1995) stress that space-time interactions may be expected in disease incidence data. Knorr-Held (1999) has recently implemented a model incorporating spatio-temporal interactions with a temporally evolving spatial structure.

7.5.2   Non-parametric mixture models

Various authors have proposed a mixture model approach to disease mapping (e.g. Clayton and Kaldor 1987; Schlattmann *et al.* 1996). The basic idea is that the population under investigation consists of an unknown number of homogeneous sub-regions with different levels of risk. Within each sub-region, the disease counts are assumed to follow a Poisson distribution, whilst the distribution of risk parameters across sub-regions is specified as a non-parametric mixture with an unknown number of components. Each component has an uncertain mixing weight and associated relative risk parameter. Knorr-Held and Raßer (1999) use a fully Bayesian approach based on a reversible jump MCMC algorithm (Green 1995). Unlike the models described in Section 7.2, such non-parametric models make no assumptions concerning the form of spatial or unstructured variation in disease risk, and are qualitatively useful in that they provide a method of classifying areas into one of a small number of risk categories which can be advantageous for display/exploratory purposes. However, it is not possible to incorporate the uncertainty in the mixing distribution in inference via maximum likelihood approaches and Bayesian non-parametric models are subject to difficulties with both implementation and prior specification.

7.5.3   Methods based on Poisson processes

Another approach to modelling aggregate counts of events (cases and non-cases) in geographical areas is to view the events as realisations of a heterogeneous Poisson process integrated over small areas (e.g. Wakefield and Elliott 1999; Section 6.3.2 in Chapter 6). In this case the expected number of cases is given by

$$\int_{A_i} \lambda_1(x)\, dx$$

where A_i denotes the ith area, x is the spatial location in A_i, and $\lambda_1(x)$ is the intensity function of the process that generates the cases. The latter is usually modelled as

$$\lambda_1(x) = \rho(x)\lambda_0(x)$$

where $\lambda_0(x)$ is an intensity function representing the population density and $\rho(x)$ can be specified as a function of spatially referenced covariate effects. This approach is very natural since one is modelling the underlying risk surface, rather than the discrete set of risks corresponding to the areas that are arbitrarily imposed by the data collection procedure.

Best *et al.* (Chapter 22) describe a related model in which the intensity function is modelled explicitly as a function of spatial location and environmental covariates. Kelsall and Wakefield (submitted) assume that the underlying logarithm of the relative risk is modelled by a Gaussian process in continuous space and then derive the correlation between areas i and j, $i \neq j$, calculating the average correlation between locations within each of the areas. They choose a correlation function that is a cubic function of distance but many others are possible (Wackernagel 1998).

7.6   Concluding remarks

There are a number of unresolved issues in the hierarchical modelling of disease risk across geographical areas, and in the display and interpretation of disease maps. Modelling the spatial dependence in particular is a difficult problem since there are few areas and the form may change across the study area. The form of the spatial dependence should, if possible, be related to potential exposures. For example, distance-based models may be more likely to be more realistic for air pollution that varies smoothly.

The strategy for modelling spatial dependence depends on the sensitivity of inference to the choice of form assumed and, to an extent, on the aim of the analysis. In some studies the form of the spatial dependence may be of interest in itself since it may suggest the type of exposure that is (at least partially) responsible for the variability in relative risk. In ecological studies the estimate of the regression coefficient is of principle importance and so the residual spatial dependence is a nuisance parameter (though a sensitivity analysis should be carried out). There may also be confounding between the exposure and unmeasured risk factors that are being picked up by the spatial random effects.

Summarising the results of a mapping study will, in general, not be straightforward and a number of summaries may be presented. For example, maps showing point estimates of the relative risks, and the precision of such estimates, are informative. The posterior probability of the exceedance of a threshold of interest will also often be useful. As can be seen from the examples presented here, it will often be necessary to run a variety of models with differing assumptions to explore the robustness of any particular inference. Where inconsistencies are found, these need to be explained. Too often a single map, or a small number of maps are presented (with potentially great visual impact) among the potentially large number that could be selected. Choice of cut-points, colours, and shading schemes are also important (Smans and Esteve 1992; Chapter 14). These aspects of presentation must be considered and addressed with great care.

As always in spatial epidemiological studies the necessity for high quality data should not be forgotten, and proposed modelling approaches should acknowledge the possible existence of data anomalies.

Appendix I: models for overdispersion

In Section 7.2.2, random effects were introduced in order to acknowledge that there may be both errors in the numerator and denominator data, and risk factors that are unmeasured. These models lead to excess variation in the observed counts. In this section we discuss this overdispersion in more detail. Bernardinelli *et al.* (1995: 2436) motivate the use of random effects by stating that, 'A cluster size bigger than the area size leads to a [spatially structured] *clustering* model, while a cluster size smaller than the area size leads to a *heterogeneity* model'. In this section we expand on this statement, and attempt to make it more precise, by considering various modelling scenarios.

Binomial case

We begin with the binomial model and let Y_i and N_i denote the number of cases and the population at risk in area i, $i = 1, \ldots, n$. If the risk is constant within each area, and independent between areas, then we have $Y_i|p_i \sim_{i.i.d.} \text{Bin}(N_i, p_i)$. This model follows immediately when there is no variability in risk within the area but an alternative derivation has been described by Knorr-Held and Besag (1998). Suppose that within each area, there are K strata corresponding to different risk factors, and that, for area i, the disease probability in stratum k is given by p_{ik}, with the probability of an individual falling in stratum k being ν_{ik}, $k = 1, \ldots, K$. If it is assumed that the collection of stratum counts within each area $(N_{i1}, \ldots, N_{iK})$ follow a multinomial distribution $\text{Mult}_K(N_i, \boldsymbol{v}_i)$ where $\boldsymbol{v}_i = (v_{i1}, \ldots, v_{iK})^T$, then (without knowledge of which stratum individuals are contained within) the response of each of the N_i individuals in area i is Bernoulli with constant probability of disease $p_i = \sum_k v_{ik} p_{ik}$. Each of the outcomes is independent (due to the multinomial sampling) and so Y_i is $\text{Bin}(N_i, p_i)$. This multinomial formulation is appropriate provided individuals in the K risk groups are randomly distributed within the area. When we have clustering of risk factors within each area (as would be the case if the stratum referred to genetic risk factors, say), then dependence is induced which will increase the variance and hence invalidate the binomial assumption.

We now consider the use of random effects in the binomial model. Specifically suppose that $p_i \sim_{i.i.d.} f(q, \tau^2)$ where $f(\cdot, \cdot)$ represents a probability density function with $\text{E}[P_i] = q$ and $\text{var}(P_i) = \tau^2 q (1-q)$. This leads to a marginal distribution for Y_i that is no longer binomial but for which

$$\text{E}[Y_i] = N_i q \quad \text{and} \quad \text{var}(Y_i) = N_i q (1-q) \sigma_i^2,$$

where $\sigma_i^2 = 1 + \tau^2(N_i - 1)$ (which is greater than one if $N_i > 1$). Note also that marginally we have $\text{cov}(Y_i, Y_{i'}) = 0$ for $i \neq i'$ since p_i and $p_{i'}$ are independently drawn from f. With regard to the above quote of Bernardinelli *et al.*, this model, literally interpreted, is based on *each area* corresponding to a *single cluster*. We may therefore interpret such a model as accounting for unmeasured area-level covariates that do not display spatial structure.

As an aside we note that McCullagh and Nelder (1989: 125) develop a model for overdispersion that is closely related to that just described. Letting $Y = \Sigma_i Y_i$ and $N = \Sigma_i N_i$ denote the total number of cases and the total population of the study region, their model gives $\text{E}[Y] = Nq$ and $\text{var}(Y) = Nq(1-q)\sigma^2$ where $\sigma^2 = 1 + \tau^2(c-1)$ with $c = \Sigma_i N_i^2 / N \geq 1$. To obtain the marginal distribution of Y_i a specific form is required for f. The conjugate choice is the beta distribution $\text{Be}(\alpha, \beta)$ with $q = \alpha/(\alpha + \beta)$ and $\tau^2 = (\alpha + \beta + 1)^{-1}$. This choice allows the probabilities $\Pr(Y_i = y) = \text{E}_p[\Pr(Y_i = y | p)]$ to be evaluated analytically and leads to a beta-binomial marginal distribution. Again, such a model may be interpreted as accounting for unmeasured, spatially unstructured area-level covariates. If these unknown covariates are spatially correlated, or are associated with spatial regions larger than the areas $i = 1, \ldots, n$ used in the analysis, an alternative form is required for f which allows for spatial dependence (for example joint or conditional models, specified on the logistic scale, see Section 7.2.2).

Note that none of the above models explicitly arise from a scenario involving a cluster size *smaller* than the area size. Since we would not expect clusters to follow areas boundaries that are defined (usually) for administrative reasons, random effects models should be viewed as rough approximations to the 'true' data-generating mechanism.

Poisson case

We proceed as with the binomial case. Consider $Y_i | \theta_i \sim_{i.i.d.} \text{Po}(E_i \theta_i)$ and suppose that known risk factors have been accounted for within the expected numbers. We then assume that the relative risks θ_i are drawn from a distribution $f(\phi, \tau'^2)$ with $\text{E}[\theta_i] = \phi$ and $\text{var}(\theta_i) = \phi \tau'^2$. This leads to $\text{E}[Y_i] = E_i \phi$ and $\text{var}(Y_i) = E_i \phi \sigma_i^2$ where $\sigma_i^2 = 1 + \tau'^2 E_i$. As described in Section 7.2.2, the conjugate choice for f is the gamma distribution. The above description is consistent with Case II of Table 7.1 with $\phi = \exp(\alpha)$ (i.e. no area-level covariates) and $\tau'^2 = b^{-1}$. Similar developments are possible for the other two cases in Table 7.1. Again the interpretation is that individuals within each area consist of a single cluster with a cluster-specific relative risk. As before, cluster sizes larger than the area size may be approximated by choosing a form for f incorporating spatial dependence.

We now give another development of random effects models in which we directly show how such models may be interpreted in terms of an unobserved covariate. Suppose that the 'true' model is given by

$$Y_i|\theta_i \sim \text{Po}(E_i\theta_i) \tag{7.19}$$

with

$$\log \theta_i = \alpha' + Z_i\beta \tag{7.20}$$

and where Z_i is a risk factor whose levels are independently distributed across the areas of the study region via some distribution f. If we do not observe Z_i then we may view the random effects that we introduce as acting as surrogates for the unmeasured covariate. For example, suppose that f corresponds to a normal distribution with μ_z and variance σ_z^2. Then suppose we assume the model

$$\log \theta_i = \alpha + V_i \tag{7.21}$$

with $V_i \sim_{i.i.d.} N(0, \sigma_v^2)$. Then this model corresponds exactly to (7.19) and (7.20) with $\alpha = \alpha' + \beta\mu_z$, $\sigma_v^2 = \beta^2\sigma_z^2$ and $V_i = \beta(Z_i - \mu_z)$, directly relating the random effect to an unmeasured risk factor. Obviously spatially dependent random effects may be justified in exactly the same way by assuming that the exposures across areas have spatial pattern.

Finally, we show how the random effects may be interpreted as accounting for data anomalies. We begin with denominator errors. Let E_i' denote the 'true' expected number and E_i the observed expected number in area i, and assume that the inaccuracies in area i may be modelled using the simple Berkson errors-in-variables model (see Chapter 3):

$$\log E_i' = \log E_i + V_i$$

with $V_i \sim_{i.i.d.} N(0, \sigma_v^2)$. Finally, we assume that there is no between-area variability in the relative risks so that $\log \theta_i = \alpha$. Then we again obtain a model equivalent to (7.19) and (7.21) that is Y_i follows the distribution $\text{Po}(E_i e^\alpha e^{V_i})$ with $V_i \sim_{i.i.d.} N(0, \sigma_v^2)$. In a similar vein, $\exp(V_i)$ may be viewed as accounting for numerator errors in area i (e.g. case under- or overascertainment). For both types of error the assumption of independent errors across areas may be reasonable. In practice the random effects are accounting for the combined effect of both unmeasured risk factors and for numerator and denominator data anomalies.

Appendix II: properties of the normal distribution

Suppose we have $U = (U_1, \dots, U_n)^T$ and assume

$$U \sim N_n(\mathbf{0}_n, \sigma_u^2 \Sigma),$$

where $N_n(\cdot, \cdot)$ denotes the n-dimensional normal distribution, $\mathbf{0}_n$ an $n \times 1$ vector of ones, $\sigma_u^2 > 0$ and $\mathbf{\Sigma}$ is an $n \times n$ positive definite matrix. Let $\mathbf{Q} = \mathbf{\Sigma}^{-1}$ and suppose now that $\mathbf{U}^T = (\mathbf{U}_1, \mathbf{U}_2)$ where $\mathbf{U}_1$ is $m \times 1$ ($1 \leq m < n$) and $\mathbf{U}_2$ is $(n-m) \times 1$. Then (e.g. Searle *et al.* 1991) we have

$$\mathbf{U}_2 | \mathbf{U}_1 = \mathbf{u}_1 \sim N_{n-m}(-\mathbf{Q}_{22}^{-1} \mathbf{Q}_{21} \mathbf{U}_1, \sigma_u^2 \mathbf{Q}_{22}^{-1}), \tag{7.22}$$

where

$$\mathbf{Q} = \begin{bmatrix} Q_{11} & Q_{12} \\ Q_{21} & Q_{22} \end{bmatrix}.$$

We now explicitly consider a disease mapping context and use (7.22) to derive the CAR model given by (7.13). We first let $\mathbf{W} = \{W_{ij}, i, j = 1, \dots, n\}$ denote the matrix of weights and $\mathbf{D}$ an $n \times n$ diagonal matrix containing elements $D_{ii}, i = 1, \dots, n$, such that $\mathbf{D}^{-1}(\mathbf{I} - \mathbf{W})$ is symmetric and positive definite. Writing $\mathbf{Q} = \mathbf{D}^{-1}(\mathbf{I} - \mathbf{W})$ we then have

$$\mathbf{U} \sim N_n(\mathbf{0}_n, \sigma_u^2 \mathbf{Q}^{-1}). \tag{7.23}$$

Taking $\mathbf{U}_2$ to be U_i and $\mathbf{U}_1$ to be the $(n-1) \times (n-1)$ matrix obtained from $\mathbf{U}$ by deleting the ith row and the ith column, we may use (7.22) to yield (7.13), as required. From (7.22) it also follows that the partial correlation between U_i and U_j is given by $\text{corr}(U_i, U_j | U_k = u_k, k \neq i, j = \text{sgn}(W_{ij})(W_{ij}W_{ji})^{1/2}$.

Acknowledgement

This work was supported, in part, by an equipment grant from The Wellcome Trust (0455051/Z/95/Z).

References

Alexander, F. and Cuzick., J. (1992). Methods for the assessment of disease clusters. In *Geographical and environmental epidemiology: methods for small-area studies* (P. Elliott, J. Cuzick, D. English, and R. Stern, ed.), 238–50. Oxford University Press.

Bernardinelli, L., Clayton, D., Pascutto, C., Montomoli, C., Ghislandi, M., and Songini, M. (1995). Bayesian analysis of space-time variation in disease risk. *Statistics in Medicine*, **14**, 2433–43.

Bernardinelli, L., Pascutto, C., Best, N. G., and Gilks, W. R. (1997). Disease mapping with errors in covariates. *Statistics in Medicine*, **16**, 741–52.

Besag, J. E. (1974). Spatial interaction and the statistical analysis of lattice systems. *Journal of the Royal Statistical Society, Series B*, **36**, 192–236.

Besag, J. and Kooperberg, C. (1995). On conditional and intrinsic autoregressions. *Biometrika*, **82**, 733–46.

Besag, J., York, J., and Mollié, A. (1991). Bayesian image restoration with two applications in spatial statistics. *Annual of the Institute of Statistics and Mathematics*, **43**, 1–59.

Best, N. G. and Wakefield, J. C. (1999). Accounting for inaccuracies in population counts and case registration in cancer mapping studies. *Journal of the Royal Statistical Society A*, **162**, 363–82.

Best, N. G., Arnold, R. A., Thomas, A., Waller, L. A., and Conlon, E. M. (1999). Bayesian models for spatially correlated disease and exposure data. In *Bayesian Statistics 6* (J. M. Bernardo, J. O. Berger, A. P. Dawid, and A. F. M. Smith ed.), 131–56, Oxford University Press.

Breslow, N. E. and Day, N. E. (1987). *Statistical methods in cancer research*. Vol. II: *The analysis of cohort studies*, IARC Scientific Publications 82. International Agency for Research on Cancer, Lyon.

Brooks, S. P. (1998). Markov chain Monte Carlo method and its application. *The Statistician*, **47**, 69–100.

Carlin, B. P. and Louis, T. A. (1996). *Bayes and empirical Bayes methods for data analysis*, Chapman and Hall, London.

Clayton, D. G. (1996). Generalised linear mixed models. In *Markov chain Monte Carlo in practice* (W. R. Gilks, S. Richardson, and D. J. Spiegelhalter ed.), 279–301. Chapman and Hall, London.

Clayton D. G. and Bernardinelli L. (1992). Bayesian methods for mapping disease risk. In *Geographical and environmental epidemiology: methods for small-area studies* (P. Elliott, J. Cuzick, D. English, and R. Stern ed.), 205–20. Oxford University Press.

Clayton, D. G. and Kaldor, J. (1987). Empirical Bayes estimates of age-standardised relative risks for use in disease mapping. *Biometrics*, **43**, 671–82.

Cliff, A. D. and Ord, J. K. (1981). *Spatial processes: models and applications*. Pion, London.

Conlon, E. M. (1999). *Estimation and flexible correlation structures in spatial hierarchical models of disease mapping*. Unpublished PhD thesis, Division of Biostatistics, School of Public Health, University of Minnesota.

Cressie, N. A. C. (1993). *Statistics for spatial data* (rev. edn). Wiley, New York.

Cressie, N. and Chan, N. H. (1989). Spatial modelling of regional variables. *Journal of the American Statistical Association*, **84**, 393–401.

Dempster, A. P. (1972). Covariance selection. *Biometrics*, **28**, 157–75.

Dempster, A. P., Laird. N. M., and Rubin. D. B. (1977). Maximum likelihood from incomplete data via the EM algorithm. *Journal of the Royal Statistical Society, Series B*, **39**, 1–38.

Devine, O. J., Louis, T. A., and Halloran, M. E. (1996). Identifying areas with elevated disease incidence rates using empirical Bayes estimators. *Geographical Analysis*, **28**, 187–99.

Diggle, P. J., Morris, S. E., Elliott, P., and Shaddick, G. (1997). Regression modelling of disease risk in relation to point sources, *Journal of the Royal Statistical Society, Series A*, **160**, 491–505.

Diggle, P. J., Tawn, J. A., and Moyeed, R. A. (1998). Model-based geostatistics. *Applied Statistics*, **47**, 299–350.

Gelman, A. and Rubin, D. B. (1992). Inference from iterative simulation using multiple sequences. *Statistical Science*, **7**, 457–511.

Gilks, W. R., Richardson, S., and Spiegelhalter, D. J. (1996). *Markov chain Monte Carlo in practice*. Chapman and Hall, New York.

Green, P. J. (1995). Reversible jump Markov chain Monte Carlo computation and Bayesian model determination. *Biometrika*, **82**, 711–32.

Handcock, M. S. and Stein, M. L. (1993). A Bayesian analysis of kriging. *Technometrics*, **35**, 403–10.

Johnson, N. L. and Kotz, S. (1972). *Distributions in statistics: continuous multivariate*. Wiley, New York.

Kelsall, J. E. and Wakefield, J. C. (1999). Discussion of 'Bayesian models for spatially correlated disease and exposure data', by Best *et al*. In *Bayesian Statistics 6* (J. M. Bernardo, J. O. Berger, A. P. Dawid, and A. F. M. Smith ed.), **151**, Oxford University Press.

Kelsall, J. E. and Wakefield, J. C. (submitted). Modelling spatial variability in disease risk. Submitted to *Journal of the American Statistical Association*.

Knorr-Held, L. (1999). Bayesian modelling of inseparable space-time variation in disease risk. University of Munich Institute of Statistics Technical Report.

Knorr-Held, L. and Besag, J. (1998). Modelling risk from a disease in time and space. *Statistics in Medicine*, **17**, 2045–60.

Knorr-Held, L. and Raßer, G. (1999). Bayesian detection of clusters and discontinuities in disease maps. University of Munich Institute of Statistics Technical Report.

Lindley, D. V. and Smith, A. F. M. (1972). Bayes estimates for the linear model (with discussion). *Journal of the Royal Statistical Society, Series B*, **34**, 1–41.

Matérn, B. (1986). *Spatial variation* (2nd edn). Springer, Berlin.

McCullagh, P. and Nelder, J. A. (1989). *Generalised linear models* (2nd edn). Chapman and Hall, London.

Mengersen, K. L., Robert, C. P., and Guihenneuc-Jouyaux, C. (1999). MCMC convergence diagnostic: A 'review'. In *Bayesian Statistics 6* (J. M. Bernardo, J. O. Berger, A. P. Dawid, and

A. F. M. Smith, ed.), 415–40. Oxford University Press. (See also http://www.maths.qut.edu.au/mengersen/McDiag)

Mollié, A. (1996). Bayesian mapping of disease. In *Markov chain Monte Carlo in practice* (W. R. Gilks, S. Richardson, and D. J. Spiegelhalter ed.), 359–79. Chapman and Hall, London.

Raftery, A. E. and Banfield, J. D. (1991). Stopping the Gibbs sampler, the use of morphology, and other issues in spatial statistics (discussion of Besag, York and Mollié). *Annals of the Institute of Statistical Mathematics*, **43**, 32–43.

Richardson, S., Montfort, C., Green, M., Draper, G., and Muirhead, C. (1995). Spatial variation of natural radiation and childhood leukaemia incidence in Great Britain. *Statistics in Medicine*, **14**, 2487–501.

Schalttmann, P., Dietz, E., and Bohning, D. (1996). Covariate adjusted mixture models and disease mapping with the program Dismap Win. *Statistics in Medicine*, **15**, 919–29.

Searle, S. R., Casella, G., and McCulloch, C. E. (1991). *Variance components*. Wiley, London.

Smans, M. and Esteve, J. (1992). Practical approaches to disease mapping. In *Small area studies in geographical and environmental epidemiology* (J. Cuzick, P. Elliott, D. English, and R. Stern ed.), 141–50. Oxford University Press.

Smith, A. F. M. and Gelfand, A. E. (1992). Bayesian statistics without tears: a sampling-resampling perspective. *The American Statistician*, **46**, 84–8.

Spiegelhalter, D. J., Thomas, A., Best, N. G., and Gilks, W. R. (1996). *BUGS: Bayesian inference using Gibbs sampling, Version 5.0*. Medical Research Council Biostatistics Unit, Cambridge.

Stern, H. S. and Cressie, N. (1999). Small-area and point-level Bayesian models for inference on extremes in disease maps. In *Disease mapping and risk assessment for public health*, (A. B. Lawson, D. Boehning, E. Lesaffre, A. Biggeri, J. F. Viel, and R. Bertollini ed.), 63–84. Wiley, Chichester.

Wackernagel, H. (1998). *Multivariate geostatistics* (2nd edn). Springer, New York.

Wakefield, J. C. and Elliott, P. (1999). Issues in the statistical analysis of small-area health data. *Statistics in Medicine*, **18**, 2377–99.

Wakefield, J. C. and Morris, S. E. (1999). Spatial dependence and errors-in-variables in environmental epidemiology. In *Bayesian Statistics 6* (J. M. Bernardo, J. O. Berger, A. P. Dawid, and A. F. M. Smith, ed.), 657–84, Oxford University Press.

Waller, L. A., Carlin, B. P., Xia, H., and Gelfand, A. (1997). Hierarchical spatio-temporal mapping of disease rates. *Journal of the American Statistical Association*, **92**, 607–17.

Wolpert, R. L. and Ickstadt, K. (1998). Poisson/gamma random field models for spatial statistics. *Biometrika*, **85**, 251–67.

8. Clustering, cluster detection, and spatial variation in risk

J. C. Wakefield, J. E. Kelsall, and S. E. Morris

8.1 Introduction

The detection and investigation of disease 'clusters' has a long and controversial history in epidemiology. In this chapter we will discuss issues relating to, and review methods proposed for, *cluster detection* and *clustering*. We will not be concerned with *cluster investigation* with respect to putative hazards; this topic is considered in Chapter 9. We will also concentrate on non-infectious diseases; there is a large literature on infectious diseases but the methods of analysis, though related, have a different flavour and are beyond the scope of this chapter. Much of the controversy surrounding 'clusters' stems from the difficulty in giving a definition of a 'cluster'. Clustering refers to the pattern of the location of disease cases, relative to the pattern of the non-cases. Differences between the two patterns may occur because the cases are more 'clumped' than the non-cases and, informally, we refer to this as 'clustering'. A more formal definition follows below. In terms of mechanisms, clustering may occur due to (a) an infectious agent or a genetic susceptibility, and/or (b) risk factors, measured and unmeasured. Here we are particularly concerned with *unmeasured* risk factors, that is, residual (spatial) clustering, since known risk factors have been taken into account (Alexander and Cuzick 1992). We note that cause (a) is more in line with a mathematical definition of clustering in terms of non-independence of cases. A more mathematically rigorous consideration of clustering may be carried out using the theory of point processes (Diggle 1983; Cressie 1993). For example, the spatial point processes underlying the distribution of cases and non-cases may be modelled as Poisson processes with inhomogeneous intensity functions (see Section 8.2.4). Infection (also known as contagion) may be modelled by having 'parent cases' arising from a Poisson process with a random number of 'offspring cases' being generated and distributed about the original parent via some bivariate probability density function. Such *Poisson cluster processes* were introduced by Neyman and Scott (1958).

In recognition of the usual epidemiological use, we prefer to allow the term clustering to extend beyond simple non-independence of cases, in contrast to some authors (e.g. Section 6.4 in Chapter 6). We say that a disease exhibits (spatial) clustering if there is *residual spatial variation* in risk. Diseases have many causes and we never have information on all of the relevant risk factors and hence, for all diseases, even after consideration of known risk factors some degree of residual spatial variation in risk, and hence clustering, will be present. The important consideration is whether this clustering is epidemiologically significant, and whether the data allow this variation to be detected.

This definition of clustering does not therefore distinguish between (a) and (b) above (i.e. infectious and genetic agents and risk factors). We note that these two causes are mathematically indistinguishable (Bartlett 1964) but in terms of interpretation it is important to distinguish between them.

If a disease exhibits clustering then the areas of high residual risk will lead (in expectation) to an 'excess' of cases in those areas. Such a collection of cases is what we define as a *cluster*. Note again that this definition is in terms of the underlying risk surface. With this definition a cluster may be over a very large geographical area—the usual epidemiological definition of a cluster is in terms of a realisation of cases that are close in space (e.g. Knox 1989). We view *cluster detection* as the identification of areas of high residual risk though historically, statistical techniques reflect a definition in terms of an excess of cases (see Section 8.2).

In some instances, the investigation of clustering and cluster detection may be viewed as part of the same undertaking; since if multiple clusters are detected this is equivalent to clustering. A number of methods begin with the former and proceed to the latter (if clustering has been found). Cluster detection implies an early-warning system, however, which is reflected in it often being referred to as *surveillance*. It is vital to assess the sensitivity/specificity (with respect to the spatial and temporal extent, and size of the elevated risk) of any proposed surveillance methods. We note that such methods may also be used retrospectively to gain clues as to aetiology. When clusters are found, clues may be obtained by comparing exposures in areas of elevated (residual) risk. In terms of the spatial residual risk surface we note that it may also be profitable to compare areas of low risk since these may correspond to protective factors or areas within which exposures are at low levels. When clustering of a disease is detected the implication is that a cause of the clustering should be sought. Often, a clustering analysis or cluster detection will be carried out as a first stage; if clustering is detected then a more comprehensive case-control or ecological study may follow.

When methods proposed for the detection of clustering are considered, it is useful to take into account the specific mechanisms that may cause clustering, and the reasons for estimating the level of clustering that a disease exhibits. Unfortunately, only very rarely have aetiological insights been made as a result of investigations into clustering and clusters (Alexander and Cuzick 1992) which has led Rothman (1990) to call this endeavour into question. Neutra (1990), in a response to Rothman, agreed with a number of his conclusions but believed that investigation of putative clusters was a necessary part of the public health response. He also described situations in which *detailed* epidemiological investigation was appropriate; there should be at least five cases in the cluster and the relative risk should be high (e.g. 20 or more). The disease should be one for which a unique and detectable class of agents have been found to be responsible in the past, and the agent should be rare in general, detectable and persistent over time in the study area. Heterogeneity of exposure within the study area is also desirable. It is interesting that Table 2 in Neutra (1990) lists 35 agents for which the International Agency for Research on Cancer believe there is sufficient evidence of carcinogenicity in humans. Of these, only one (the mineral erionite), was discovered as a result of a cluster in a particular area (a Turkish village), the remainder were classified as medical or occupational clusters.

As discussed above we may distinguish between non-independence of cases and unknown risk factors as being responsible for clustering and clusters. Some of the methods that we review were explicitly designed to detect non-independence (though this is not to say that they may not be of use in other situations). So far as unknown risk factors are concerned these may be of various types including areal-level environmental factors and individual-level factors. This distinction is important as the nature of the clustering will clearly be dependent on the risk factor(s) that are responsible. The nature of risk factors responsible will suggest the appropriate scale at which methods should be implemented. For example, in Section 8.2 we describe methods that examine the number of cases in areas defined to have constant area, or to contain either a constant population at risk or a constant number of cases. Environmental risk factors are commonly hypothesised to be responsible for clustering and may act through a variety of media (e.g. air, water, or soil). Point sources of air pollution produce exposures that may be approximated by a circular region (see Chapter 21). In this case a distance-based method may be appropriate to detect the local-scale clustering that may result. The scale of clustering due to waterborne contaminants in the water supply is more difficult to hypothesise but if treatment plants supply areas of constant population a measure of clustering based on population density may be appropriate. Soilborne exposures (arising, for example, from pesticide use) may not produce clustering on a constant distance scale, but an urban/rural indicator of exposure may perhaps be appropriate. It is desirable to have a clustering hypothesis available a priori in which case (data availability notwithstanding) a model-based approach may be adopted in which disease risk is related to the suggested risk factor (e.g. distance from putative hazard, levels of exposure in water/soil, urban/rural indicator). Unfortunately, as noted by Rothman (1990) (see also Chapter 19) many environmental exposures are very poorly measured, reducing the power of statistical methods to detect associations. Possible clustering of leukaemias due to extremely low frequency electromagnetic radiation from overhead powerlines may be difficult to detect with isotropic distance methods, though if field strength is available this may be used within a model-based approach. So far as individual risk factors, such as smoking and diet (or socio-economic status), are concerned we may expect that these will lead to broader-scale variability (under the assumption that levels of these factors will vary smoothly geographically). Rothman (1990) notes that we are not interested in clustering of the cases *per se* but the clustering of the risk factors that lead to the cases. Diseases have multiple causes, however, and disentangling the complex multi-factorial disease-risk associations will be difficult. Risk factors that are associated with a short latency period are also far more readily identified. Longer latencies dilute the effect in specific time periods, even before one considers the effects of migration (see Chapter 3). For example, we may expect that congenital malformations may be due to exposures received *in utero* and the resultant clusters will be more amenable to detection than diseases such as mesothelioma for which the latency period may be thirty years or more.

As with all spatial epidemiological studies it is vital to assess data quality when a study is envisaged. This topic is extensively discussed in this volume (in particular see Chapters 2, 3, and 5). In the context considered here individual clusters or clustering in general may simply be the result of data anomalies (Besag *et al.* 1991*a*). This issue is relevant to each of the exposure, population, and health data. In terms of the health data, case ascertainment is a serious problem. Underascertainment will lead to a loss of power but perhaps more seriously may not be spatially neutral and so may induce clustering. This clustering may occur on a broad geographical scale (e.g. defined by the catchment area of a cancer registry) or may be more local (e.g. reflecting coding practices in individual hospitals). Diagnostic inaccuracies may also lead to apparent spatial variation in risk, possibly at a relatively local scale (corresponding to a local pathology laboratory for example). This problem may be reduced to some extent by only choosing those diagnoses that are less prone to error, for example, cancer incidence in children and young people where ascertainment is high (Draper 1991) or severe cases only. So far as the population data are concerned the effects of inaccuracies may be reflected at various scales. For example, a small-scale 'cluster' of congenital malformations or childhood leukaemia in a region with a recently built housing estate may simply be due to an inappropriate denominator from a previous census that does not allow for the influx of new families. A number of the methods that we describe make use of case-control data. The locations of cases and controls may not be known exactly and so may be taken as the centroid of the area (e.g. postcode or census enumeration district) within which the residential addresses of the cases and controls lie. This loss of accuracy may lead to attenuation of clustering. It is clearly important that the accuracy of the locations is the same for both cases and controls.

The interest in methods for, and the philosophy behind, the investigation of clusters and clustering is evidenced by the number of papers devoted to the topic. In 1989 there was a national conference on the clustering of health events held in the USA, with a special issue of the *American Journal of Epidemiology* dedicated to its proceedings appearing in 1990. Draper (1991) also contains an investigation into the spatial epidemiology of childhood leukemia and non-Hodgkin's lymphoma in Great Britain, with a number of authors applying their methodology. These diseases often exhibit clustering and have provided the stimulus for a number of the proposed methods, including space-time approaches. Three issues of *Statistics in Medicine* have been dedicated to methods in spatial epidemiology (Jacquez 1993, 1996; Lawson *et al.* 1995). Recently, an extensive set of methods were tested on a large number of simulated datasets (Alexander and Boyle 1996). In addition, numerous journal articles have appeared; we highlight a number of the key references but do not present an extensive review.

The structure of this chapter is as follows. In Section 8.2 we provide a review of methods; we also give examples of the use of some of the methods in spatial epidemiology. In Section 8.3 we provide illustrative examples of a number of the methods described in the previous Section, based on real epidemiological data; in particular we analyse a set of case-control data and two sets of disease count data. Section 8.4 contains a concluding discussion.

8.2   Review of methods

In this section we describe a number of the approaches that have been proposed for assessing the level of clustering in a set of data, and for cluster detection. We separate the methods into four groups. We first consider methods that primarily detect *overdispersion* in a series of counts. Suppose we have count data and we have adjusted for the effect of known risk factors through the calculation of expected numbers or through regression modelling. Then, in our terminology overdispersion can reflect:

- *heterogeneity*, that is, independent counts with $\mathrm{var}(Y_i) > \mathrm{E}[Y_i]$ for $i = 1, \ldots, n$, and/or
- *spatial dependence*, that is, dependence between Y_i and Y_j that depends on a spatial distance measure between areas indexed by i and j, $i, j = 1, \ldots, n$, $i \neq j$.

This spatial dependence is assumed to be positive from this point onwards (i.e. responses that are geographically close are assumed to be similar). The second set of methods that we describe assess the spatial dependence in a set of data and produce a single summary statistic that describes this dependence. The third set of methods were developed from the mid 1980s onwards, and were designed to assess whether the number of cases within areas defined through various measures, are in excess of that expected by chance alone. In the final section we describe a number of approaches, most of which have been developed recently, for estimating the residual spatial risk surface. Here, the emphasis is less on hypothesis testing and more on estimation, with an underlying model being specified for the unknown risk surface. Throughout we also comment on the ability of methods to adjust for known risk factors.

We only briefly comment on the large number of methods that have been suggested for investigating space-time clustering; much of the literature concerns the detection of contagion. Mathematically speaking the modelling of space-time processes is more difficult than the modelling of a spatial process but a number of space-time methods appeared early in the clustering literature. For example, Knox (1964) proposed a method by which all pairs of cases were characterised as 'close' or 'not-close' in space and time, leading to a 2×2 table. This approach is simple but has a number of disadvantages; for example, the definitions of close and not-close are somewhat arbitrary and the method is unsuitable for a disease with a long latency period. The method is still widely used, however (e.g. Morris *et al.* 1998). To address these and other concerns the basic method has been extended by a number of authors (e.g. Mantel 1967; Pike and Smith 1974; Knox and Gilman 1992*a*). Smith (1982) gives a discussion of space-time clustering and provides a review of a number of methods. Diggle *et al.* (1995) describe a '*K*-function' (see Section 8.2.2) approach for the detection of space-time clustering.

The available data may be in the form of counts or points, or a combination of the two (e.g. point data for the cases and counts for the population at risk). Some methods can deal with both while others were developed specifically for one type. We first establish some notation for count data. We suppose the study region is divided into n non-overlapping areas and let Y_{ij} and N_{ij} denote the number of disease cases and population at risk in area i and age-sex (say) stratum j, $i = 1, \ldots, n; j = 1, \ldots, J$, and p_j denote a set of reference disease probabilities (see Chapters 7 and 9). Then for rare and non-infectious diseases we may make the assumption that the effect of living in area i is to multiply all of the area-specific rates by a relative risk θ_i, so that

$$Y_i \sim \text{Po}(E_i\theta_i), \tag{8.1}$$

where $Y_i = \Sigma_j Y_{ij}$ and we have expected numbers $E_i = \Sigma_j p_j N_{ij}$. We assume that internal standardisation has been carried out (i.e. we have $p_j = \Sigma_i Y_{ij}/\Sigma_i N_{ij}$, in which case $Y_+ = \Sigma_i Y_i = \Sigma_i E_i = E_+$. In this case the null hypothesis is given by

$$H_0 : \theta_1 = \cdots = \theta_n = 1.$$

8.2.1 Traditional methods

In this section, we describe two methods which assess the null hypothesis via examination of the set of Y_i and E_{ij}. No indication of the location of clusters is formally obtained.

Pearson's chi-squared statistic

A simple approach is to calculate the statistic

$$T = \sum_i \frac{(Y_i - E_i)^2}{E_i}.$$ (8.2)

Under H_0, T follows, asymptotically, a chi-squared distribution on $n-1$ degrees of freedom (one degree of freedom is lost because $E_+ = Y_+$). Large values of T will result if there is heterogeneity. As with all the methods of this section the significance of the test statistic may also be assessed by randomly simulating observations Y_i under the null hypothesis and calculating the test statistic under each simulation. Comparison with the observed statistic leads to a *Monte Carlo test*. Increases in, and access to, computing power mean that such an approach is now straightforward and explain the trend towards less reliance on asymptotic arguments.

The use of Equation (8.2) is straightforward but the power of the test against realistic alternatives is not clear. As with all classical hypothesis testing procedures the null hypothesis will be rejected for large sample sizes even for slight departures from H_0. Hence, it is statistical, and not epidemiological, significance that is being judged. Large positive values of $Y_i - E_i$ may be examined for clues to the location of a cluster.

Potthoff and Whittinghill's method

Potthoff and Whittinghill (1966*b*) consider the uniformly most powerful (UMP) test for departure from H_0 with respect to the alternative that the relative risks θ_i are random effects and drawn from the conjugate gamma distribution (see Chapter 7). They are unable to derive a UMP test in this case so instead use the fact that $Y_1, \ldots, Y_n | Y_+$ follows a multinomial distribution and appeal to the results of Potthoff and Whittinghill (1966*a*) in which the UMP test for a multinomial distribution versus the multinomial-Dirichlet alternative is derived. This leads (Potthoff and Whittinghill, 1966*b*, eqn 13) to the test statistic

$$T = E_+ \sum_i \frac{Y_i(Y_i - 1)}{E_i}.$$ (8.3)

The term $Y_i(Y_i - 1)$ is the observed number of (unordered) pairs of cases in area i. Large values of (8.3) indicate heterogeneity. Under H_0, T has mean $Y_+(Y_+ - 1)$ and variance $2(n-1)Y_+(Y_+ - 1)$. Asymptotic normality may then be appealed to though it is straightforward (and preferable) to carry out a Monte Carlo test. Again, large positive values of $Y_i(Y_i - 1)/E_i$ give an indication of clusters.

The method of Potthoff and Whittinghill is specifically designed for detecting heterogeneity but Muirhead and Butland (1996) consider the use of the method to detect 'clustering' by considering the statistic for different levels of aggregation. It is not clear how the results should be interpreted, however, since, for example, the tests are not independent.

In general, the assumption that the θ_i arise from a probability distribution provides a mechanism for inducing various forms of overdispersion. In particular, if the θ_i are assumed to be an *independent* sample from a probability density function (the so-called random effects distribution) then heterogeneity, as defined in the introduction to this section, is recovered. The section on disease mapping below briefly describes such models, and also the spatial versions; for more details see Chapter 7. Dean (1992) presents a general description of score tests for heterogeneity in Poisson and binomial data. In particular, various forms of overdispersion are considered through the specification of the first two moments of the random effects distribution.

8.2.2   Distance/adjacency methods

In this section, we consider methods that were explicitly designed for detecting spatial dependence between counts (or points for the *K*-function method). Again the methods do not, in general, pinpoint the location of clusters.

Autocorrelation statistics

A number of approaches have been suggested for measuring spatial autocorrelation. There are various ways of measuring the 'closeness' of two areas. Let $Z_i = Y_i/E_i$ denote the standardised mortality/morbidity ratio (SMR) of area i and denote by W_{ij} a measure of the closeness of areas i and j. In the simplest case we can take $W_{ij} = 1$ if areas i and j are adjacent (i.e. have a boundary in common) and 0 otherwise. Cliff and Ord (1981) describe various other possibilities; another common choice is the inverse distance between the area centroids. The choice of weights depends on the type of spatial dependence that one is trying to detect. For example, a distance-based measure will be appropriate if a smoothly varying environmental pollutant is thought to be responsible for the clustering. We now describe three statistics that have been proposed: Moran's *I*, Geary's *c* and a non-parametric rank-based method, denoted *D*. Walter (1993) describes these statistics in detail. Moran's *I* statistic (Moran 1948) is given by

$$I = \frac{n\Sigma_i\Sigma_j W_{ij}(Z_i - \bar{Z})(Z_j - \bar{Z})}{\left(\Sigma_i\Sigma_j W_{ij}\right)\Sigma_k(Z_k - \bar{Z})^2}. \tag{8.4}$$

This statistic has some similarity with the conventional correlation coefficient and is measuring the similarity between close (as measured by W_{ij}) areas. If there is no spatial dependence *I* will be close to zero, with values close to one indicating clustering. Geary's *c* statistic (Geary 1954) is closely related and is given by

$$c = \frac{(n-1)\Sigma_i\Sigma_j W_{ij}(Z_i - Z_j)^2}{2\left(\Sigma_i\Sigma_j W_{ij}\right)\Sigma_k(Z_k - \bar{Z})^2}. \tag{8.5}$$

If there is spatial dependence, terms in the numerator will be small (similar SMR's in 'close' regions) and the value of the statistic will be close to zero; the absence of spatial dependence leads to *c* close to one. The means and variances of *I* and *c* are available theoretically (Cliff and Ord 1981) and asymptotic normality may be appealed to in order to obtain the observed significance level. Again a Monte Carlo test may be used. Letting Z_i^* denote the ranks of the Z_i we may calculate a non-parametric measure of spatial dependence

$$D = \frac{\Sigma_i \Sigma_j W_{ij} |Z_i^* - Z_j^*|}{\Sigma_i \Sigma_j W_{ij}}, \tag{8.6}$$

with small values of D implying positive dependence. Again significance may be judged through a Monte Carlo test. A major problem with these statistics (Besag and Newell 1991) is that the unequal variances of the Z_is are not allowed for. Strictly, therefore, these methods are inappropriate for SMRs unless they are based on equal expected numbers. High values of Z_i will tend to occur in areas with small populations (i.e. in rural areas), and these are likely to be close together, inducing positive dependence. This was borne out by the simulations of Walter (1993).

Commenges and Jacqmin-Gadda (1997) describe a family of score tests for overdispersion in the case of correlated outcomes. A special case of their general family is closely related to Moran's test and one of their examples concerns a spatial epidemiology setting.

Whittemore's method

Whittemore *et al.* (1987) proposed a distance-based statistic for the detection of clustering. Let $r = [Y_1/Y_+, \ldots, Y_n/Y_+]^T$ denote the vector of the observed proportion of cases that lie in each of the n areas and D an $n \times n$ matrix containing the distances, d_{ij}, between the centroids of areas i and j, $i, j = 1, \ldots, n$. Then Whittemore *et al.* (1987) suggested that the null hypothesis of constant risk may be tested using the mean distance between all pairs of cases as a statistic. This is given by

$$T = \frac{n}{n-1} \times r^T D r. \tag{8.7}$$

Conditioning on Y_+, and under H_0, the sampling distribution of $Y^T = [Y_1, \ldots, Y_n]$ is multinomial with $E[Y] = Y_+ \times p$ where $p_i = E_i/E_+$, $i = 1, \ldots, n$ which allows the mean and variance of T in (8.7) to be derived. This statistic has been criticised by a number of authors. Turnbull *et al.* (1990) note that since distance between cases is considered, clustering in urban (rural) areas will produce lots of small (large) distances; see also Tango (1995). Again, Monte Carlo simulation can be used to perform the test.

Tango's method

Tango (1995) suggests the use of the statistic

$$T = (r - p)^T A (r - p), \tag{8.8}$$

where r and p are defined as above and A denotes an $n \times n$ matrix with elements a_{ij}, $i, j = 1, \ldots, n$, measuring the 'closeness' between areas i and j. Tango (1995) suggests the form

$$a_{ij} = \exp(-d_{ij}/\phi), \tag{8.9}$$

with $\phi > 0$ chosen a priori to reflect the expected extent of spatial dependence. The matrix A can be viewed as a correlation matrix and it may be useful to think in terms of the reparameterised $\phi' = \log 2 \times \phi$ which gives the distance at which the correlation between the residual relative risk in two areas is 0.5. The form (8.9) is often used in geostatistics to describe the correlation structure of a Gaussian process (Diggle *et al.* 1998; Chapter 6), and also in disease mapping when spatial random effects are assumed to follow a multivariate normal distribution (see Chapter 7). To locate the position of 'clusters' Tango (1995) suggests using a version of the test designed for assessing clusters around a pre-defined point source.

In an approach which also uses distance between cases and controls Knox and Gilman (1992*b*) examine spatial clustering in cases of leukaemia, and controls, by comparing the frequency distributions of distance between pairs of cases and controls.

K-*functions*

In the introduction we briefly described the spatial point process formulation of clustering; in the context considered here, the so-called *K*-function approach describes the second-moment structure of the processes that give rise to the cases and controls. The method has been used in a spatial epidemiological context by Diggle and Chetwynd (1991); our description closely follows that in Diggle and Morris (1996). The expected number of points in a unit area describes the first-moment structure of a stationary process; let λ_1 denote this quantity for the cases and λ_2 for the controls. These quantities are not of intrinsic interest in the clustering context. For example, if the controls constitute all of the non-cases then $\lambda_1/(\lambda_1 + \lambda_2)$ across the region as whole describes the *prevalence* of the disease. Hence, it is natural to consider the second-moment structures of cases and controls.

For an isotropic spatial point process of intensity λ points per unit area, the *K*-function at distance s, $K(s)$, is such that $\lambda K(s)$ gives the expected number of further events of the process within a distance s of an arbitrary event of the process (Ripley 1977). For a completely random process (i.e. a homogeneous planar Poisson process), $K(s) = \pi s^2$. For an aggregated process $K(s) - \pi s^2$ is greater than zero and monotone non-decreasing in s. Let $K_1(s)$ and $K_2(s)$ represent the *K*-functions of the case and control point processes, respectively. The difference $D(s) = K_1(s) - K_2(s)$ may be taken as a measure of the extra clustering amongst cases compared to the clustering amongst the controls. By examination of this statistic it is clear that clustering is being examined in a cumulative distance rather than a population sense. In practice, the statistic $\hat{D}(s)$ is calculated (based on estimators in Ripley 1977) for a range of values of s. For pre-selected values, $s_1, \ldots, s_m$, an overall clustering test statistic is given by

$$D = \sum_{k=1}^{m} w_k \hat{D}(s_k), \tag{8.10}$$

with weights $w_k = [\text{var}\{\hat{D}(s_k)\}]^{-1/2}$. The variance in this expression is evaluated under the null hypothesis of random relabelling of cases and controls. Under the null hypothesis, Monte Carlo methods may be used to evaluate w_k and the sampling distribution of D. A plot of $\hat{D}(s)$ versus s (with tolerance limits under random labelling imposed) is useful for assessing at which distances departures from random labelling are seen. Care must be taken when such plots are interpreted, however, since $\hat{D}(s_1)$ and $\hat{D}(s_2)$ for $s_1 \neq s_2$ are not independent. The range of distance to examine is also, to some extent, arbitrary and likely to be important in the overall significance of D. We note that the K-function approach is invariant to random case underascertainment (though this assumption is unlikely to be true over a large study region).

Diggle *et al.* (1995) extend the method to the investigation of space-time clustering and Bhopal *et al.* (1992) apply that methodology to Legionnaires' disease in Scotland.

8.2.3 Moving window and related methods

In this section we describe methods that superimpose a number of circular regions on to the study region and then determine the significance of the number of cases that fall within each circle. Different methods define the circles in terms of distance (Openshaw), the number of cases (Besag and Newell), and the population size (scan statistics). These methods may be described as cluster detection approaches and are screening devices by which particular regions may be highlighted and subsequently investigated. We also include in this section the method of Cuzick and Edwards. The methodology of this section may also be applied to the point-source problem (see Chapter 9).

Openshaw's method

Openshaw *et al.* (1987) proposed a 'geographical analysis machine' method in which a regular grid is superimposed on the study region and circles of constant radius are drawn on the intersections of the grid lines. The spirit of the method has remained unchanged but various refinements have been made (for a summary see Openshaw 1996). Typically, a range of radii are constructed based on the scale at which clustering is expected and the grid lines are such that adjacent circles overlap by 80%. A common geography for populations and cases is established (census enumeration districts are recommended for the UK) and then 'jagged' circles are formed containing the area centroids. Circles are 'flagged' if they attain a certain level of significance, under the assumption that cases within circles follow a Poisson distribution. The *p*-value is small to address the multiple testing problem but there is no theoretical development of a particular size; $p = 0.005$ has often been used in applications. Obviously the size of p is crucial to the sensitivity and specificity of the method and the lack of guidelines for this choice remains a major drawback.

Openshaw's method has been heavily criticised in the literature. In particular, there is clearly a huge multiple testing problem; there are not only a large number of tests, the tests are dependent also. The original version of the method, at least, was also highly computer-intensive. Since the different circles contain different numbers of cases and different populations at risk the power to detect clusters will vary across circles. As an informal procedure that is straightforward to code, the method has its merits, however.

Besag and Newell's method

The method of Besag and Newell (1991) was developed to rectify some of the problems of Openshaw's method. The first step in applying the method is to select a cluster size k. For each case in turn a circle is drawn, centred on that case, with radius such that the kth nearest neighbouring case is included. As with Openshaw's method the expected number of cases is calculated for each circle and those circles with a statistically significant excess of cases are highlighted. Unlike Openshaw's method the circles are now comparable since they are all based on k cases. The choice of k is clearly vital and several values are typically selected. By defining the cluster in terms of the number of cases the method has a greater chance of detecting small rural clusters than the distance-based method of Openshaw. The question of whether there is clustering over the study region may be answered via a Monte Carlo test, which accounts for the multiple non-independent tests, but Besag and Newell (1991) stress that the method is not designed for this task but rather to flag areas for further investigation. Newell and Besag (1996) note that the method is designed to detect 'data anomalies' which may reflect the data quality issues discussed in Section 8.1.

Scan statistics

Scan statistics were originally developed to 'scan' across a time region of interest with the statistic being taken as the maximum number of events to occur within windows of constant size (Naus 1965). Subsequently, a considerable amount of literature on scan statistics, in both temporal and spatial contexts, has appeared (e.g. see Naus 1988; Wallenstein *et al.* 1993). In the spatial setting the approach is closely related to those of Openshaw and Besag and Newell. The fixed window of the original formulation makes it clear that the statistic is being compared to an underlying intensity that is uniform; in a spatial context this is clearly unreasonable.

Turnbull *et al.* (1990) suggested an approach by which the 'windows' are defined to contain a constant population, N^* (say), and are centred on each area centroid. The maximum number of cases across the windows may then be used as a test statistic, that is

$$M = \max_j Y_j(N^*), \tag{8.11}$$

where j indexes the areas as defined via the population N^*. A Monte Carlo test is then performed under random distribution of cases across windows. The approach therefore differs from others in this section since the most significant circle over the whole study region is searched for instead of all circles 'significant' at a certain level. Since only a single test is carried out it is straightforward to determine the correct statistical properties of the procedure. However, in practice, the statistic is repeated using various values of the population size upon which circle construction is based, thus producing a set of non-independent tests. The original method was illustrated using leukaemia incidence in upstate New York. Using this same set of data, Waller *et al.* (1994) compare the Turnbull methods, with a variety of other procedures including those of Openshaw, Besag and Newell and Whittemore.

Hjalmars *et al.* (1996) and Kulldorff *et al.* (1997) apply a closely related method to childhood leukaemia in Sweden, and breast cancer cases in the northeastern United States, respectively. They choose the population within each circle to be less than a specified fraction of the total population of the study region. Let Y_i and E_j denote the observed and expected number of deaths in circle j. Then the test is based on the maximum likelihood ratio statistic across all circles

$$L = \max_j \left(\frac{Y_j}{E_j}\right)^{Y_j} \left(\frac{Y_+ - Y_j}{Y_+ - E_j}\right)^{Y_+ - Y_j} I(Y_j > E_j). \tag{8.12}$$

The indicator function $I(\cdot)$ takes the value 1 if the observed number of cases in the circle under consideration exceeds the expected number and 0 otherwise. This indicator is present because we are not interested in windows containing less cases than expected, only those containing an excess of cases. Once the window with the greatest exceedance is identified, the sampling distribution of L is evaluated using a Monte Carlo test. Further details on the exact methodology may be found in Kulldorff and Nagarwalla (1995) and Kulldorff (1997).

There are a number of difficulties with this method. The choice of population size is somewhat arbitrary and there are no clear guidelines for a choice, Hjalmars *et al.* (1996) use 10% of the total population to define the windows while Kulldorff *et al.* (1997) use 50%. In practice, the method is not just used to indicate a single cluster but a number of potential clusters are highlighted. Once this is done the properties of the procedure become unknown (in common with the methods of Openshaw and Besag and Newell). The circles are also not completely comparable since it is populations and not expected numbers that are defining the choice of radii (although it is straightforward to use expected numbers). A related scan statistic is described by Anderson and Titterington (1997).

Cuzick and Edwards' method

Cuzick and Edwards (1990) proposed a number of statistics for examining clustering in a case-control situation. Suppose there are n_1 cases and let $m_i(k)$ denote the number of cases amongst the k nearest neighbours of case i, so that $0 \leq m_i(k) \leq k$ $i = 1, \ldots, n_1$. Then one may examine clustering via the statistic

$$T_k = \sum_{i=1}^{n_1} m_i(k). \tag{8.13}$$

In the so-called inverse sampling method the suggested statistic is

$$T_k^{\text{inv}} = \sum_{i=1}^{n_1} m_i'(k), \tag{8.14}$$

where $m_i'(k)$ denotes the number of cases that are nearer to case i than the kth nearest control. The first two moments of T_k and T_k^{inv} may be derived (though for the latter the variance is unwieldy) and asymptotic normality appealed to. Although a Monte Carlo test is available, Cuzick and Edwards (1996) use the asymptotic version in an extensive simulation study.

When population data are available a modification of T_k is the statistic

$$U_k = \sum_{j=1}^{n_1} (Y_j - E_j), \tag{8.15}$$

where circular regions are centred on each case, the radii are chosen so that E_j is taken to be as close to k as possible (by analogy with the two-sample k nearest neighbour approach), and Y_j is the number of cases within each of these regions. Under the null hypothesis $E[U_k] = 0$ and the variance may be calculated (see Cuzick and Edwards 1996). This has the flavour of a scan statistic, in particular it may be compared with (8.11) and (8.12).

In all of the above the choice of k is clearly of great importance. Cuzick and Edwards (1996) suggest that various values be taken with the overall significance level being adjusted via an improved Bonferroni-type adjustment due to Simes (1986), though this does not fully adjust for the positive correlation of the tests.

They also describe an informal procedure for locating clusters by which, for a given value of k, cases with $m_i(k)$ greater than a threshold value are flagged and then a cluster is indicated when such cases occur close to each other.

Dolk *et al.* (1998) investigates localised clustering of anopthalmia via the Cuzick and Edwards and the K-function methods; little evidence of clustering was found.

8.2.4   Risk surface estimation

In this section we consider methods that explicitly estimate the underlying spatial residual risk (or odds) surface. These methods offer potentially more information on the nature of clusters and clustering at the expense of a greater statistical understanding and (often) specialised software. The advantage of the methods previously described is their simplicity which allows them to be routinely applied to large databases. The methods of this section will usually be applied as part of a thorough analysis within well-planned studies.

Kernel methods

A number of authors (Bithell 1990, 1992; Lawson and Williams 1993; Kelsall and Diggle 1995*a,b*) have considered the use of kernel methods (Silverman 1986; Bowman and Azzalini 1997) in spatial epidemiology.

Let x_i, $i = 1, \ldots, n_1$ denote the locations of n_1 cases, and x_i, $i = n_1 + 1, \ldots, n_1 + n_2 = n$ the locations of n_2 controls in the study region A. We suppose that the cases and controls represent randomly sampled proportions q_1 and q_2 of all cases and non-cases and view these points as observations from Poisson processes, with intensity $\lambda_1(x)$ for the cases and $\lambda_2(x)$ for the controls. The log odds function, up to an additive constant (since we do not have the complete set of non-cases), is given by

$$\rho(x) = \log\{\lambda_1(x)/\lambda_2(x)\} \tag{8.16}$$

and we wish to investigate the spatial variation in $\rho(x)$ over A.

Conditioning on n_1 and n_2 we may view the case and control locations as independent samples from the densities $f_1(x)$ and $f_2(x)$ where

$$f_j(x) = \alpha_j^{-1}\lambda_j(x) \quad \text{and} \quad \alpha_j = \int_A \lambda_j(x)\, dx,$$

for $j = 1, 2$. Letting $r(x)$ denote the log ratio of densities, we have

$$r(x) = \log\{f_1(x)/f_2(x)\} = \rho(x) - c_1,$$

where $c_1 = \log(\alpha_1/\alpha_2)$. Hence if

$$\hat{f}_j(x) = n_j^{-1} \sum_{i=1}^{n_j} K_h(x - x_i),$$

represent kernel density estimates of $f_j(x)$, $j = 1, 2$, where $K_h(u) = h^{-2} K(h^{-1} u)$ and K represents a radially symmetric kernel function, we have

$$\hat{r}(x) = \log\{\hat{f}_1(x)/\hat{f}_2(x)\}.$$

Kelsall and Diggle (1995a, b) show how the bandwidth h may be chosen via a cross-validation technique designed to (approximately) minimise $\int_A \{\hat{r}(x) - r(x)\}^2 \, dx$.

As an alternative to kernel density estimation, Kelsall and Diggle (1998) have reformulated the problem to one of binary regression. Binary labels $y_1, \ldots, y_n$ are attached to the points $x_1, \ldots, x_n$ where $y_i = 1$ for the cases ($i = 1, \ldots, n_1$) and $y_i = 0$ for the controls ($i = n_1 + 1, \ldots, n$). Conditional on x_i, the y_i are realisations of mutually independent Bernoulli random variables Y_i with $P(Y_i = 1 | X_i = x) = p(x)$, where

$$p(x) = \frac{q_1 \lambda_1(x)}{q_1 \lambda_1(x) + q_2 \lambda_2(x)}.$$

It follows that

$$\mathrm{logit}\{p(x)\} = \rho(x) + c_2,$$

where $c_2 = \log(q_1/q_2)$.

The kernel regression is then given by

$$\hat{p}(x) = \sum_{i=1}^{n} K_h(x - x_i) y_i \bigg/ \sum_{i=1}^{n} K_h(x - x_i). \tag{8.17}$$

Kelsall and Diggle (1998) note that $\hat{r}(x)$ and logit $\{\hat{p}(x)\}$ are equivalent (up to an additive constant) but prefer the latter since a cross-validatory estimate of h is readily available. In practice, individual covariate information will often be available; in the kernel density estimation approach it is not possible to incorporate this information, the kernel regression approach may be extended, however, as illustrated in the next section.

Generalised additive models

Kelsall and Diggle (1998) describe how a generalised additive model (GAM, Hastie and Tibshirani 1990) approach may be taken in the spatial context when covariates are available. Let the Bernoulli variable, Y, again indicate case-control status and u denote a vector of l individual-specific covariates. Then let $P(Y = 1 | X = x, U = u) = p(x, u)$ denote the probability that the individual at location x with covariates u is a case, and define the GAM

$$\mathrm{logit}\{p(x, u)\} = u^T \beta + g(x), \tag{8.18}$$

where $\boldsymbol{\beta}$ is a l-dimensional vector of regression coefficients and $g(\cdot)$ is a smooth function in $\boldsymbol{x}$. Kelsall and Diggle (1998) describe how $g(\boldsymbol{x})$ may be estimated using kernel regression within the GAM framework. The residual risk surface $\hat{g}(\boldsymbol{x})$ (with associated tolerance regions) may be examined for evidence of residual spatial variation in risk and a Monte Carlo test of constant residual risk overall may also be performed.

There are a number of open questions concerning this approach including the choice of smoothing parameter and the incorporation of the uncertainty in $\hat{g}(\boldsymbol{x})$ into the overall procedure. The method that we next describe provides an attempt to solve these problems.

Geostatistical methods

Diggle *et al.* (1998) suggested a framework within which applications such as that considered here may be handled. The approach is similar in spirit to the GAM methodology just described but is fully parametric. For point data the model takes the form

$$\text{logit}\{\,p(\boldsymbol{x}, \boldsymbol{u})\} = \boldsymbol{u}^T \boldsymbol{\beta} + S(\boldsymbol{x}), \tag{8.19}$$

where $S(\boldsymbol{x})$ is the realisation of a process; a Gaussian process is chosen by Diggle *et al.* (1998). The relationship with (8.18) is clear. The implementation of this model is most natural from a Bayesian perspective though the Markov chain Monte Carlo (MCMC) algorithm. This is computationally expensive and requires experience, both to implement and to assess convergence.

In principle, a version of the variogram (see Chapter 10) could be used to assess the spatial correlation structure of the processes that gave rise to the case and control points.

Disease mapping

Disease mapping models and applications are described extensively elsewhere in this volume (Chapters 6, 7, 15, 16) and so we do not go into much detail here. We note, however, that the model proposed by Besag *et al.* (1991*b*) may be used to investigate components of variability due to heterogeneity and clustering. Specifically, the relative risk in (8.1) may be modelled via

$$\log \theta_i = \boldsymbol{u}^T \boldsymbol{\beta} + v_i + w_i, \tag{8.20}$$

where the residuals v_i and w_i model heterogeneity and spatial dependence, respectively.

Martuzzi and Hills (1995) describe a method for investigating the extent of heterogeneity by examining the profile likelihood of the variance parameter in a Poisson/ gamma model (see Chapter 7). Knorr-Held and Raßer (1999) propose a method for cluster detection in which areas within a region of interest are partitioned into groups containing contiguous areas within which the relative risk is assumed constant. The numbers and positions of the groups are estimated along with the associated relative risks. The approach is computationally intensive and the algorithm, which utilises reversible jump MCMC (Green 1995), is not straightforward to implement. The prior distribution on the numbers of clusters also requires careful consideration.

8.3   Illustrative examples

In this section we consider two examples, one with point data, and the other with count data. The analyses we present should not be viewed as definitive, we merely wish to illustrate features of the methods.

Point data

The data for this example consist of the residential locations of 467 cases of larynx cancer and 9191 cases of lung cancer that, for the purposes of illustration, will be considered as a set of controls. These data were collected in the Chorley–Ribble area of Lancashire over the period 1974–83. These data have been analysed by a number of authors (for a description of previous analyses see Kelsall and Diggle 1995*b*), often with the aim of investigating the relationship between risk in relation to an industrial incinerator. We, however, will ignore this aspect and treat the data as an example by which we can investigate evidence for clustering of larynx cancer. The study region is approximately 150 km^2.

Figure 8.1(a) shows the locations of the cases and controls and Fig. 8.1(b) a perspective view of a kernel density estimate of the controls alone. The non-uniform distribution of residences is clearly the major source of variation in the distribution of cases and controls.

Cuzick and Edwards' method

We calculated the statistic (8.13) for values of k between 1 and 50. Figure 8.1(c) shows the unadjusted (i.e. no correction for multiple testing) *p*-values. There is no evidence of clustering.

K-functions

The K-function approach was applied here with distances between 0 and 3 km. The observed significance level of (8.10) was 0.93 using a normal approximation to the sampling distribution of D and 0.98 using a Monte Carlo test based on 99 simulations under the null hypothesis. This indicates some evidence of anti-clustering (i.e. more clustering in the controls than in the cases). Figure 8.1(d) indicates that any clustering in the controls is at a distance of up to approximately 500 m but the evidence is very weak.

Kernel estimation

We used the kernel regression estimate (8.17) suggested by Kelsall and Diggle (1998). Figure 8.1(e) shows a plot that may guide the choice of the smoothing parameter h; on the vertical axis the value of a cross-validation objective function $CV(h)$ is plotted. The value of h is chosen to minimise $CV(h)$ with the latter scaled so that when $h = \infty$ (which corresponds to a flat residual risk surface) it equals unity. In this way, if h is such that $CV(h) < 1$ then it is identified as a value that produces a better estimate of relative risk than that under the null hypothesis of constant residual risk. Since on Fig. 8.1(e) $CV(h) \geq 1$ for all values of h considered, this suggests that there is not a great deal of variability in risk. This is confirmed by examination of Fig. 8.1(f) which displays the

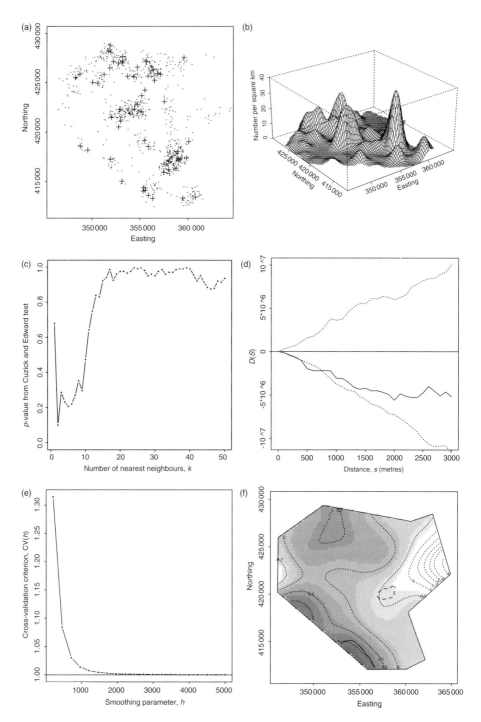

Fig. 8.1 Point data in the Chorley–Ribble area: (a) larynx cancer (+) and controls (·), (b) perspective view of kernel density estimate of control data, (c) Cuzick and Edwards' *p*-values for various choices of cluster size *k*, (d) *K*-function plot of $\hat{D}(s)$ versus distance *s*, (e) choice of smoothing parameter *h* for kernel regression estimate, (f) kernel regression estimate of risk surface. All distance axes are in metres.

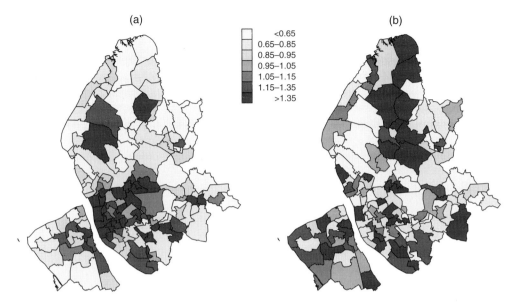

Fig. 8.2   Count data: SMRs for (a) lung cancer, and (b) brain cancer data.

estimated risk surface along with 95% tolerance contours. There is a slight suggestion of elevated risk in the bottom left corner of the study region but when such contours are interpreted we should recall that for small h we would expect approximately 2.5% of the region to be highlighted. The Monte Carlo test of constant residual risk gave a significance level of 0.41.

   Hence, for these data all approaches indicate little evidence of clustering.

Count data

As a representative set of count data we consider the disease mapping example presented in Chapter 7. The data consist of cases of lung and brain cancer diagnosed during the period 1981–91 in the Mersey and West Lancashire districts of northwest England. There are 1512 and 918 cases of lung and brain cancer, respectively, in 144 electoral wards. Expected numbers were calculated using internal standardisation with adjustment for age and sex and population counts from the 1991 census. Figure 8.2 shows the SMRs for (a) lung cancer, and (b) brain cancer. From these maps lung cancer appears to display a greater degree of clustering than brain cancer, though interpretation is not straightforward. The study region is approximately 40 km × 40 km and is split by the Mersey estuary.

Traditional methods

For all methods the (one-sided) significance level is based on 999 simulations under H_0. Table 8.1 presents the results of a number of tests. The Pearson and Potthoff and Whittinghill statistics measure general homogeneity and we see that each of the statistics for lung cancer is highly significant while there is no evidence to reject H_0 for brain

Table 8.1 Summary of test statistics for the lung and brain cancer data

	Value of statistic (p-value)			
Statistic	Lung cancer		Brain cancer	
Pearson	487.5	(0.001)	145.8	(0.388)
Potthoff and Whittinghill	1.1×10^7	(0.001)	8.7×10^5	(0.489)
Moran	0.36	(0.0001)	−0.01	(0.510)
Geary	0.656	(0.001)	0.967	(0.246)
Rank (D)	37.4	(0.001)	47.9	(0.467)
Whittemore	14,526	(0.001)	13,353	(0.174)
Tango	0.0044	(0.001)	0.001	(0.103)

cancer. We may calculate the quasi-likelihood measure of extra-Poisson variability (McCullagh and Nelder 1989; Chapter 9) by dividing the statistic (8.2) by the degrees of freedom. For lung and brain cancer we obtain 3.41 and 1.02, indicating substantial overdispersion for lung cancer. This is consistent with the analyses of Chapter 7. For example, in model (8.20) the non-spatial random effects had standard deviations 0.08 (lung) and 0.05 (brain), and the spatial random effects standard deviations 0.33 (lung) and 0.06 (brain).

Distance/adjacency methods

Table 8.1 also presents statistics for a number of methods that were designed to detect spatial dependence. For the method of Tango a value of $\phi = 5$ km was used in (8.9). We also evaluated Tango's statistic for ϕ in the range 0.5–12.5 km; for lung cancer the statistics were all significant at the 0.001 level while for brain cancer $\phi = 12.5$ km was the only statistic to produce a p-value that was significant at the 5% level (0.045). Each of the statistics indicate strong evidence of spatial dependence for lung cancer and no evidence for brain cancer. Again, these results are consistent with the disease mapping analysis in which the model (8.9) was used to measure the correlation between different areas; the distance-decay parameters ϕ' (distance at which correlations dropped to 0.5) were estimated as approximately 3 km and 0.14 km for lung and brain indicating strong spatial dependence for the former.

Moving window methods

Each of the analyses that we now report were carried out at the ED level; there are 3141 EDs in the study region.

   We implemented Openshaw's method with circle sizes of 1–5 km in 0.5 km intervals, and a significance level of 0.005. Figure 8.3 displays the resultant 'significant' circles; 1080 out of a possible 19 506 circles are drawn, giving a proportion of 0.0567. Unfortunately, it is not straightforward to evaluate the distribution of the number of significant tests under the null hypothesis due to the dependence between the tests but the expected number is equal to the p-value and so we have far more rejections than we would expect. The information provided by Fig. 8.3(a) is limited since approximately

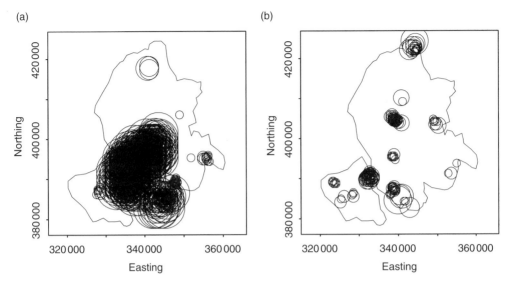

Fig. 8.3 Results of Openshaw's geographical analysis machine for (a) lung cancer, and (b) brain cancer data. Axes labels are in metres.

half of the study area is highlighted. For brain cancer (Fig. 8.3(b)) 154 out of 18 165 circles are drawn giving a proportion 0.0085 which is closer to the nominal 0.005. It is interesting to compare this plot with Fig. 7.3(b) in Chapter 7 since the clusters indicated by Openshaw lie in almost exactly the same locations that have slightly elevated relative risks.

We implemented Besag and Newell's method with cluster sizes $k = 4, 8, 16, 32$. With a significance level of 0.005 the resulting significant circles are shown in Fig. 8.4. For lung cancer there are 1512 cases and hence 1512 potential circles. Proportions 0.127, 0.110, 0.011, and 0.180 were highlighted for cluster sizes of $k = 4, 8, 16, 32$, respectively. Examination of Fig. 8.4 reveals a number of areas that may be worthy of further investigation. For brain cancer, as expected, far fewer areas are highlighted; the proportions of significant circles as a function of k are 0.063, 0.037, 0.023, and 0.003. Figure 8.4 is far more informative than the equivalent summary of Openshaw since the clusters are more precisely highlighted.

The statistic (8.11) of Turnbull, the scan statistic (8.12), and the Cuzick and Edwards one-sample statistic (8.15) were evaluated for these data. For each statistic proportions 0.10, 0.05, and 0.01 of the total population were included in the moving windows. For the lung cancer data all three of the statistics were significant at the 0.01 level (with 99 Monte Carlo simulations) for each of the three proportions. Some indication of the areas that caused the excess may be obtained by looking at the most significant circles; these were found to be to the north side of the estuary in the study region. For brain cancer, the significance levels were all in the range 0.46–0.57 except for the Turnbull statistic with 1% of the population which had significance level 0.16.

Maps of smoothed relative risks appear in Figs. 7.2 and 7.3.

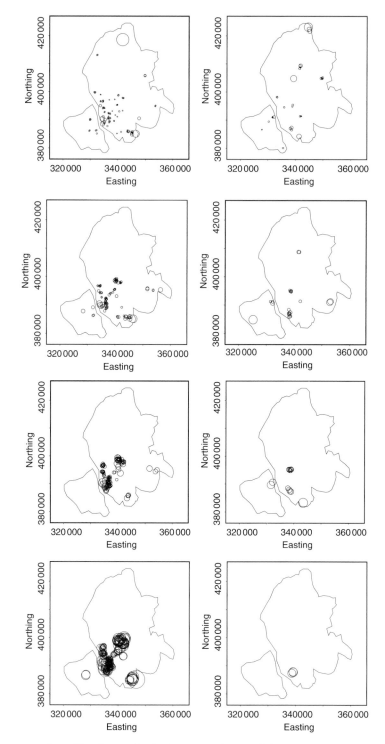

Fig. 8.4 'Clusters' found by the method of Besag and Newell, lung cancer on the left and brain cancer on the right, cluster size k is 4 (row one), 8 (row two), 16 (row three), 32 (row four). Axes labels are in metres.

8.4 Discussion

In Section 8.2 of this paper we described a number of methods that have been suggested for the related aims of cluster detection and the detection of clustering. Certain points are worth stressing. Given the nature of disease incidence (and the usual form in which data become available), it is vital that any proposed method can adjust for covariate information (either through the expected numbers or via regression). This is especially true for count data. For point (case-control) data, *matched* cases and controls may be available but great care must be taken when point-based methods are utilised since, in general, the basic method for unmatched data will not be directly applicable and some adjustment of the procedure will be required.

We view the methods of Sections 8.2.1–8.2.3 as useful initial observations of the data. The statistical properties of many of the suggested procedures are not clearly understood making interpretation difficult, however. As far as the moving window methods are concerned, multiple testing with non-independent tests is a serious problem and the choice of significance level is likely to be crucial. This being the case we believe that the basic approaches, particularly for count data that are routinely available, have some merit as exploratory tools to highlight areas of interest; in fact, this was the rationale for their construction. The continual refinement of procedures that are intrinsically flawed (as has been carried out by some authors) is not a strategy that is likely to be beneficial, however. In all cases, great care must be paid to the presentation and interpretation of results to avoid unnecessary and unwarranted alarm among the local residents.

The risk surface estimation methods of Section 8.2.4 clearly provide the most information, though they are not without their drawbacks. In particular, they are more computationally expensive and more difficult to implement (as opposed to the exploratory methods that may be computationally expensive but are straightforward to implement). They are also more dependent on assumptions which must be assessed (via diagnostics) before any faith can be placed in inferential summaries. It is likely that these and related methods will continue to be developed and will become more and more sophisticated. In particular, we envisage that methods based on modelling the risk surface will see greater use in spatial epidemiology in the future. An important consideration in such a development is whether the data are of sufficient quality (this is especially relevant to count data), and sufficiently informative, to support the use of refined methods. It is clear that in both the development, application and interpretation of the results of any method, epidemiological input is of vital importance.

Acknowledgement

This work was supported, in part, by an equipment grant from the Wellcome Trust (0455051/Z/95/Z).

References

Alexander, F. E. and Boyle, P. (1996). *Methods for investigating localized clustering of disease.* IARC Scientific Publications 135. International Agency for Research on Cancer, Lyon.

Alexander, F. and Cuzick, J. (1992). Methods for the assessment of disease clusters. In *Geographical and environmental epidemiology: methods for small-area studies*. (P. Elliott, J. Cuzick, D. English, and R. Stern ed.), 238–50. Oxford University Press.

Anderson, N. H. and Titterington, D. M. (1997). Some methods for investigating spatial clustering with epidemiological applications. *Journal of the Royal Statistical Society, Series A*, **160**, 87–105.

Bartlett, M. S. (1964). The spectral analysis of two-dimensional point processes. *Biometrika*, **51**, 299–311.

Besag, J. and Newell, J. (1991). The detection of clusters in rare diseases. *Journal of the Royal Statistical Society, Series A*, **154**, 143–55.

Besag, J., Newell, J., and Craft, A. (1991a). The detection of small-area anomalies in the database. In *The geographical epidemiology of childhood leukaemia and non-Hodgkin lymphoma in Great Britain 1966–83* G. Draper ed. 101–8. HMSO, London.

Besag, J., York, J., and Mollié, A. (1991b). Bayesian image restoration with two applications in spatial statistics. *Annals of the Institute of Statistics and Mathematics*, **43**, 1–59.

Bhopal, R., Diggle, P., and Rowlingson, B. (1992). Pinpointing clusters of apparently sporadic cases of Legionnaires' disease. *British Medical Journal*, **304**, 1022–7.

Bithell, J. F. (1990). An application of density estimation to geographical epidemiology. *Statistics in Medicine*, **9**, 691–701.

Bithell, J. F. (1992). Statistical methods for analysing point-source exposures. In *Geographical and environmental epidemiology: methods for small-area studies* (P. Elliott, J. Cuzick, D. English, and R. Stern ed.), 221–30. Oxford University Press.

Bowman, A. W. and Azzalini, A. (1997). *Applied Smoothing Techniques For Data Analysis*. Oxford University Press.

Breslow, N. E. and Day, N. E. (1980). *Statistical methods in cancer research*. Vol. 1: *The analysis of case-control studies*, IARC Scientific Publications 32. International Agency for Research on Cancer, Lyon.

Cliff, A. D. and Ord, J. K. (1981). *Spatial processes: models and Applications*, Pion, London.

Commenges, D. and Jacqmin-Gadda, H. (1997). Generalized score test of homogeneity based on correlated random effects. *Journal of the Royal Statistical Society, Series B*, **59**, 157–71.

Cressie, N. A.C. (1993). *Statistics for spatial data* (rev. edn). Wiley, New York.

Cuzick, J. and Edwards, R. (1990). Spatial clustering for inhomogeneous populations. *Journal of the Royal Statistical Society, Series B*, **52**, 73–104.

Cuzick, J. and Edwards, R. (1996). Cuzick–Edwards one-sample and inverse two-sampling statistics. In *Methods for investigating localized clustering of disease* (F. E. Alexander and P. Boyle ed.), 200–2, IARC Scientific Publications 135. International Agency for Research on Cancer, Lyon.

Dean, C. B. (1992). Testing for overdispersion in Poisson and binomial regression models, *Journal of the American Statistical Association*, **87**, 451–7.

Diggle, P. J. (1983). *Statistical analysis of spatial point patterns*. Academic Press: London.

Diggle, P. J. and Chetwynd, A. C. (1991). Second-order analysis of spatial clustering for inhomogeneous populations. *Biometrics*, **47**, 1155–63.

Diggle, P. J. and Morris, S. (1996). Second order analysis of spatial clustering. In *Methods for investigating localized clustering of disease* (F. E. Alexander and P. Boyle ed.), 207–14, IARC Scientific Publications 135. International Agency for Research on Cancer, Lyon.

Diggle, P. J., Chetwynd, A. G., Haggkvist, R., and Morris, S. E. (1995). Second order analysis of space-time clustering. *Statistical Methods in Medical Research*, **4**, 124–36.

Diggle, P. J., Tawn, J. A., and Moyeed, R. A. (1998). Model-based geostatistics (with discussion). *Applied Statistics*, **47**, 299–350.

Dolk, H., Busby, A., Armstrong, B. G., and Walls, P. H. (1998). Geographical variation in anopthalmia and micropthalmia in England, 1988–1994. *British Medical Journal*, **317**, 905–10.

Draper, G. J. (ed.) (1991). *The geographical epidemiology of childhood leukaemia and non-Hodgkin lymphoma in Great Britain 1966–1983*. HMSO: London.

Geary, R. C. (1954). The contiguity ratio and statistical mapping. *The Incorporated Statistician*, **5**, 115–45.

Green, P. J. (1995). Reversible jump Markov chain Monte Carlo computation and Bayesian model determination. *Biometrika*, **82**, 711–32.

Hastie, T. J. and Tibshirani, R. J. (1990). *Generalised additive models*. Chapman and Hall, London.

Hjalmars, U., Kulldorff, M., Gustafsson, G., and Nagarwalla, N. (1996). Childhood leukaemia in Sweden: using GIS and a spatial scan statistic for cluster detection. *Statistics in Medicine*, **15**, 707–15.

Jacquez, G. M. (ed.) (1993). Proceedings of workshop on statistics and computing in disease clustering. *Statistics in Medicine*, **12**, 1751–1968.

Jacquez, G. M. (ed.) (1996). Proceedings of conference on statistics and computing in disease clustering. *Statistics in Medicine*, **15**, 681–952.

Kelsall, J. E. and Diggle, P. J. (1995*a*). Kernel estimation of relative risk. *Bernoulli*, **1**, 3–16.

Kelsall, J. E. and Diggle, P. J. (1995*b*). Non-parametric estimation of spatial variation in relative risk. *Statistics in Medicine*, **14**, 2335–42.

Kelsall, J. E. and Diggle, P. J. (1998). Spatial variation in risk: a nonparametric binary regression approach. *Applied Statistics*, **47**, 559–73.

Knorr-Held, L. and Raßer, G. (1999). Bayesian detection of clusters and discontinuities in disease maps. University of Munich Institute of Statistics Technical Report.

Knox, G. (1964). The detection of space-time interactions. *Applied Statistics*, **13**, 25–9.

Knox, E. G. (1989). Detection of clusters. In *Methodology of enquiries into disease clustering* (P. Elliott ed.). Small Area Health Statistics Unit, London.

Knox, E. G. and Gilman, E. (1992*a*). Leukaemia clusters in Great Britain. 1: Space-time interactions. *Journal of Epidemiology and Community Health*, **46**, 566–72.

Knox, E. G. and Gilman, E. (1992*b*). Leukaemia clusters in Great Britain. 2: Geographical concentrations. *Journal of Epidemiology and Community Health*, **46**, 573–6.

Kulldorff, M. (1997). A spatial scan statistic. *Communications in Statistics: Theory and Methods*, **26**, 1481–96.

Kulldorff, M. and Nagarwalla, N. (1995). Spatial disease clusters: detection and inference. *Statistics in Medicine*, **14**, 799–810.

Kulldorff, M., Feuer, E. J., Miller, B. A., and Freedman, L. S. (1997). Breast cancer clusters in the Northeast United States: a geographical analysis. *American Journal of Epidemiology*, **146**, 161–70.

Lawson, A. B. and Williams, F. L.R. (1993). Applications of extraction mapping in environmental epidemiology. *Statistics in Medicine*, **12**, 1249–58.

Lawson, A. B., Waller, L., and Biggeri, A. (ed.) (1995). Spatial disease patterns. *Statistics in Medicine*, **14**, 2289–2502.

Mantel, N. (1967). The detection of disease clustering and a generalised regression approach. *Cancer Research*, **27**, 209–20.

Martuzzi, M. and Hills, M. (1995). Estimating the degree of heterogeneity between event rates using likelihood. *American Journal of Epidemiology*, **141**, 369–74.

McCullagh, P. and Nelder, J. A. (1989). *Generalized linear models* (2nd edn). Chapman and Hall, London.

Moran, P. A.P. (1948). The interpretation of statistical maps. *Journal of the Royal Statistical Society, Series B*, **10**, 243–51.

Muirhead, C. R. and Butland, B. K. (1996). Testing for over-dispersion using an adapted form of the Potthoff-Whittinghill method. In *Methods for investigating localized clustering of disease* (F. E. Alexander and P. Boyle ed.), 40–52, IARC Scientific Publications 135. International Agency for Research on Cancer, Lyon.

Morris, J. K., Alberman, E., and Mutton, D. (1998). Is there evidence of disease clustering in Down's syndrome? *International Journal of Epidemiology*, **27**, 495–8.

Naus, J. I. (1965). The distribution of the size of the maximum cluster of points on a line. *Journal of the American Statistical Association*, **60**, 532–8.

Naus, J. I. (1988). Scan statistics. In *Encyclopedia of statistical sciences*, Vol. 8 (S. Kotz, N. L. Johnson, and C. B. Read ed.), 281–5, Wiley, New York.

Neutra, R. R. (1990). Counterpoint from a cluster buster. *American Journal of Epidemiology*, **132**, 1–8.

Newell, J. N. and Besag, J. E. (1996). The detection of small-area database anomalies. In *Methods for investigating localized clustering of disease* (F. E. Alexander and P. Boyle ed.), 88–100, IARC Scientific Publications 135. International Agency for Research on Cancer, Lyon.

Neyman, J. and Scott, E. L. (1958). Statistical approach to problems of cosmology. *Journal of the Royal Statistical Society, Series B*, **20**, 1–29.

Openshaw, S. (1996). Using a geographic analysis machine to detect the presence of spatial clustering and the location of clusters in synthetic data. In *Methods for investigating localized clustering of Disease* (F. E. Alexander and P. Boyle ed.), 68–86, IARC Scientific Publications 135. International Agency for Research on Cancer, Lyon.

Openshaw, S., Charlton, M., Wymer, C., and Craft, A. W. (1987). A mark I geographical analysis machine for the automated analysis of point data sets. *International Journal of Geographical Information Systems*, **1**, 335–58.

Pike, M. C. and Smith, P. G. (1974). A case-control approach to examine diseases for evidence of contagion, including diseases with long latent periods. *Biometrics*, **30**, 263–79.

Potthoff, R.F and Whittinghill, M. (1996*a*). Testing for homogeneity in the binomial and multinomial distributions, *Biometrika*, **53**, 167–82.

Potthoff, R. F. and Whittinghill, M. (1996*b*). Testing for homogeneity in the Poisson distribution. *Biometrika*, **53**, 183–90.

Ripley, B. B. (1977). Modelling spatial patterns (with discussion). *Journal of the Royal Statistical Society, Series B*, **39**, 172–212.

Rothman, K. J. (1990). A sobering start for the Cluster Busters' Conference. *American Journal of Epidemiology*, **132**(Suppl.), S6–S13.

Silverman, B. N. (1986). *Density estimation for statistics and data analysis*. Chapman and Hall, London.

Simes, R. J. (1986). An improved Bonferroni procedure for multiple tests of significance. *Biometrika*, **73**, 751–4.

Smith, P. G. (1982). Spatial and temporal clustering. In *Cancer epidemiology and prevention* (D. Schottenfeld, J. F. Fraumeni ed.), 391–407. W. B. Saunders, Philadelphia.

Tango, T. (1995). A class of tests for detecting 'general' and 'focussed' clustering of rare diseases. *Statistics in Medicine*, **14**, 2323–5.

Turnbull, B. W., Iwano, E. J., Burnett, W.S, Howe, H. L., and Clark, L. C. (1990). Monitoring for clusters of disease: application to leukaemia incidence in upstate New York. *American Journal of Epidemiology* **132**(Suppl. 1), S136–S143.

Wallenstein, S., Naus, J., and Glaz, J. (1993). Power of the scan statistic for detection of clustering. *Statistics in Medicine*, **12**, 1829–43.

Waller, L. A., Turnbull, B. W., Clark, L. C., and Nasca, P. (1994). Spatial pattern analyses to detect rare disease clusters. In *Case studies in biometry*, (N. Lange and L. Ryan ed.), 3–23. Wiley, New York.

Walter, S. D. (1993). Assessing spatial patterns in disease rates. *Statistics in Medicine*, **12**, 1885–94.

Whittemore, A. S., Friend, N., Byron, W., Brown, J. R., and Holly, E. A. (1987). A test to detect clusters of disease. *Biometrika*, **74**, 631–5.

9. Assessment of disease risk in relation to a pre-specified source

S. E. Morris and J. C. Wakefield

9.1 Introduction

Awareness of the potential adverse health outcomes of environmental pollutants has led to a large literature on the investigation of disease 'clusters'. In this chapter we critically review the specific problem of the assessment of disease risk in relation to a *pre-specified* source, (or focus); we will not consider general clustering or the examination of putative disease clusters without reference to a specific source, these are discussed in Chapter 8. The types of investigation upon which we concentrate may be concerned with a single source, or with multiple sources of the same type. The putative source of hazard may consist of 'point' sources (such as incinerators or nuclear installations) or 'line' sources (such as railway lines, power lines or main roads). Obviously, these sources are not strictly points or lines and in some cases, for example, landfill sites, 'points' may cover a large geographical area. This is a consideration when, say, distance from source is used as a surrogate for exposure.

We concentrate on statistical methods that have been proposed and only briefly comment on issues that influence interpretation, such as data quality and control of confounding; discussion of these issues may be found in Elliott *et al.* (1995), Wakefield and Elliott (1999), and Chapter 5. The need for careful examination of the data cannot be overemphasised since a large proportion of the apparent spatial variability in observed risk may be the result of data collection anomalies. Methods for the assessment of risk in relation to a point source are also discussed in a number of general spatial epidemiological review papers, for example, Hills and Alexander (1989), Marshall (1991), and Elliott *et al.* (1995). Besag and Newell (1991) provide a good discussion of the pitfalls of cluster investigation.

The structure of this chapter is as follows. In the next section we provide a context for point-source studies and then describe a general statistical framework. Section 9.3 describes a number of conventional epidemiological techniques and Section 9.4 semi-parametric statistical approaches to modelling. In Section 9.5 we review regression methods and in Section 9.6 illustrate a number of the methods using data on the incidence of stomach cancer in the proximity of a municipal incinerator. Section 9.7 contains concluding remarks.

9.2 Background and context

9.2.1 General issues

An investigation into risk with respect to a pre-defined source may be carried out for a number of reasons. Often the investigation will be as a result of media or public interest; a well-publicised example (which provided the stimulus for a number of methodological developments) is the 'cluster' of childhood leukaemia cases around the Sellafield reprocessing plant (Gardner 1992). Alternatively a study may be carried out to investigate a well-defined epidemiological hypothesis. These two types of enquiry may lead on from each other as in the investigation of Dolk *et al.* (1997*a,b*) in which excess incidence of leukaemia was found close to a radio and TV transmitter in Sutton Coldfield in the United Kingdom. This led to a study of all such transmitters in the UK which did not reveal increased risk. Although the methods reviewed in this chapter are generally appropriate for both types of enquiry, the interpretation will often be very different and we note that, in general, the distinction between the two types will not be clear-cut.

When the media or public generate the enquiry, the *p*-values associated with a conventional hypothesis test are inappropriate since the data both generate and test the hypothesis. It is very difficult to adjust significance levels to account for the selection mechanism since the form of this mechanism is almost always unknown. Before proceeding with the analysis the study parameters should be carefully defined. These include the disease classification, study region, time period, and population (e.g. age-sex groups) of interest. Clusters may appear or disappear on the basis of these choices. These parameters are far easier to specify in the case of an epidemiologically motivated study. The size of the study region must be large enough to contain the effects of the pollution and, more generally, to provide an exposure contrast across the population within the region while, if possible, keeping constant the other risk factors that act upon the population. Too large a region may include other sources of pollution (or a different degree of urbanisation) which will make interpretation more difficult. The study will also be more time-consuming and expensive to carry out since more data will need to be collected, checked, and analysed. In terms of a suitable time period, epidemiological information will be required to determine a suitable latency period. For example, Elliott *et al.* (1996) allowed a ten-year lag period in a study of cancers around municipal incinerators. It is also desirable to cover time periods 'before' and 'after' the operation of the putative source of pollution; in this way unmeasured confounders (those which are constant over time) may be eliminated since the study population act as their own controls. Even when the selection mechanism difficulty does not apparently arise, the interpretation of *p*-values is not straightforward due to the multiple tests, corresponding to selection of different diseases (e.g. cancer sites) and population sub-groups, that are performed. It is clear that the easiest interpretation occurs when there are a small number of tests. Obviously, these should be chosen a priori. These issues are discussed more extensively in Chapter 5.

An important practical issue is the geographical scale at which the study is carried out; often the health, population, and exposure data will be available at different scales. These scales could also change over time as, for example, administrative boundaries change (e.g. differing census geographies).

As with all epidemiological investigations, the potential for confounding is an important consideration, both when a study is envisaged and carried out. This is particularly true in the context considered here where the effects of environmental pollutants tend not to be large (relative risks less than two are typical) and the distribution of confounder variables is not spatially neutral. Hence, the probability of a case within a specific area depends not only on the population density in that area, but also on the confounder variables of the population (e.g. the age and sex distribution; smoking prevalence). While information on the age and sex of health and population data is usually straightforward to obtain, that on other risk factors such as smoking, dietary information, and socio-economic status is more difficult to determine. The relationship between health, pollution, and socio-economic 'deprivation' is complex (see Chapter 5) but for many diseases there is a strong link between health and deprivation, and pollution sources tend to be in deprived areas (Jolley *et al*. 1992). Hence, deprivation is a confounder and so must be controlled for during the analysis.

We emphasise the important distinction between point data and count data. Each of the population, exposure and health data may have associated exact spatial and temporal information (*point* data) or be available as aggregated summaries (*count* data). Point data, if accurate, are optimal but such data are rarely available routinely. We also note that even with point data we are still making the huge simplification that individuals do not move from their residential address, for example, we do not account for daily movement. Routine health and population statistics are generally held at the area level: for example in the UK health data are often available at the postcode and population data at enumeration district (ED) level (e.g. Elliott *et al*. 1992*a*). While case-control studies provide point data for cases and a set of controls, they require epidemiological expertise to minimise difficulties of selection and other biases, are expensive and time-consuming to carry out, and may not be feasible in given situations. For these reasons case-control studies are not usually carried out in immediate response to media or public concerns about environmental health risks, but only when there is sufficient evidence or scientific concern to warrant their use (i.e. in the case of an a priori epidemiological hypothesis). A case-control study may be essential for investigations into risk factors that are associated with a source that produces exposures acting on a small spatial/temporal scale. For example, the electromagnetic waves produced by powerlines reach background levels at distances that are relatively close to the lines; most studies use distances of 30–300 metres from the line to define the exposed population (Li *et al*. 1996). In general, point data are far more amenable to modelling than count data since they consist of exact locations and are less likely to contain inaccuracies. In practice, the choice between case-control and aggregated data studies is seldom made by statistical considerations alone.

There are a number of difficulties associated with the use of aggregated data. The areas at which data are aggregated are often defined for electoral or census purposes and not at a scale that is appropriate for exposure assessment. The usual approach to the assessment of risk with aggregated data is to define an area-level measure of exposure (leading to an *ecological* study). As such, the analysis is open to ecological bias (Greenland and Morgenstern 1989; Diggle and Elliott 1995; Chapter 11) since only under very strict conditions concerning the form of the risk/exposure relationship and confounders do group- and individual-level analyses produce identical inference. There are also a number of difficulties with both the health and population data that are typically used for such analyses (Wakefield and Elliott 1999). In general, for any health event there is always the potential for diagnostic error or misclassification (Chapter 2). For cancers in particular, case registries may be subject to double counting and under-registration, in addition to diagnostic inaccuracies. Population data are typically obtained from the census which is subject to problems of underenumeration. Populations for the inter-censual years must also be estimated with the need to consider migration, as well as births and deaths (Chapter 3). Additional information, for example local information, is invaluable for interpretation. Best and Wakefield (1999) discuss models that may be used to assess numerator and denominator errors. We note that, with point data, problems of census counts do not arise but there may still be inaccuracies in the health data (though it is likely that more checking has been carried out).

A general issue is whether the assessment of the health effects of a putative source should be via hypothesis testing or via estimation. When an investigation of a 'cluster' is carried out, the configuration of cases relative to the 'at risk' population is examined, and a null hypothesis that may be informally stated as: 'the cases are randomly distributed amongst the population at risk', is tested. In contrast, the emphasis may be on the estimation of the underlying risk surface that gave rise to the cases; methods with this emphasis tend to depend on a greater number of assumptions than test-based alternatives. An advantage of estimation is that one is not faced with the ambiguity of the 'evidential content' (the probability of the null hypothesis *given* the data) of classical hypothesis tests (e.g. Berger and Sellke 1987). An estimated risk surface is also likely to be far more informative in a public health context than the result of a hypothesis test. We return to this issue in the discussion.

A major problem with investigations with respect to a pre-specified point source is that an acceptable measure of exposure, either at the individual or area level, must be available (see Chapter 19). Ideally, exposure data should be collected at the individual level (e.g. using personal monitors) but this is rarely possible (and will never be available routinely). Instead, the distance from the source to the centroid of the area is frequently used as a proxy for exposure. The exact specification of the source is also important. In the case of Sellafield, Bithell (1992) presented analyses in which a point in the centre of the site gave stronger evidence of increased risk than analyses in which the postcode location of the site was taken.

The study may consider multiple point sources of the same type under two different scenarios: a single study area may contain more than one focus, or the study may consider multiple areas (as in the transmitter example above). In the former case a simple approach is to take the exposure of an individual or area to be that associated with the closest source (with respect to the measure used, e.g. distance or rank). This method may be followed with the majority of the methods that we describe. A preferable approach is to take the exposure variable as the direct contribution from the totality of sites, but this will require modelling of the pollution surface, via dispersion modelling, for example (see Chapter 21).

In the remainder of this section we describe the basic models that are used for aggregated and point data. It is possible to motivate these models using a point process formulation; we briefly mention this approach in Section 9.4, further details may be found elsewhere (e.g. Diggle 1990; Diggle and Rowlingson 1994; Wakefield and Elliott 1999).

9.2.2   Poisson model for aggregated data

The basic formulation for data collected at the areal level is as follows. Let the study region, A, be partitioned into n disjoint regions and the observed number of cases in stratum j falling in the ith region in the study period of interest be denoted Y_{ij}, $i = 1, \ldots, n, j = 1, \ldots, J$. Often, stratification will be taken over age, sex and calendar year, and perhaps across a discrete measure of deprivation also. Similarly, let N_{ij} be the total population at risk in region i and stratum j. For rare and non-infectious diseases, the counts Y_{ij} may then be considered as independent Poisson random variables, i.e.

$$Y_{ij} \sim \text{Po}(N_{ij}p_{ij}),$$

where p_{ij} is the probability of disease in region i and stratum j. For non-rare diseases, con-ditional on N_{ij}, we may instead assume that the Y_{ij} is binomially distributed (see Chapter 7). Typically there are insufficient data available to estimate each of the $n \times J$ probabilities p_{ij} with any precision and so it is usual to make the following proportionality assumption

$$p_{ij} = q_j \times \theta_i. \tag{9.1}$$

Here, $q_j, j = 1, \ldots, J$, denote a set of *reference* disease probabilities and θ_i the *relative risk* of area i. Hence, the strong assumption has been made that the effect of being in area i is to change the disease probabilities across all strata by the common (multiplicative) factor θ_i. The assessment of this assumption is discussed in Section 9.5. The values q_j may be calculated either from the data in question or from a much larger region (e.g. the county or district containing A), thus leading to an *internally* or *externally* standardised set of rates, respectively (see Chapter 7). From the Poisson assumption it now follows that

$$Y_i = \sum_{j=1}^{J} Y_{ij} \sim \text{Po}(E_i\theta_i),$$

where the expected numbers

$$E_i = \sum_j N_{ij}q_j.$$

The quantity $\hat{\theta}_i = Y_i/E_i$ is referred to as the standardised mortality/morbidity ratio (SMR), and corresponds to the maximum likelihood estimator (MLE) of the relative risk in area i. Note that the standard error of $\hat{\theta}_i$ is proportional to $E_i^{-1/2}$ and so for very rare diseases and/or small areas (and hence small populations) the SMR may be very unstable. In a disease mapping framework it is conventional to stabilise the relative risks using a hierarchical model (Chapter 7); we return to this point shortly.

The null hypothesis that proximity to source does not influence risk may be represented by

$$H_0 : \theta_i = \rho \quad \text{for } i = 1, \ldots, n, \tag{9.2}$$

though this assumes that all other sources of variability in risk have been accounted for. In fact we could replace Equation (9.2) by $H_0 : \theta_i$ for $i = 1, \ldots, n$; however, typically not all risk factors will have been accounted for in the standardisation. If external standardisation is used the reference region may have elevated or lowered risk compared to the study region.

Let x_0 denote the (two-dimensional) geographical location of the point source, x_i the centroid of area i and d_i the distance from the source to the centroid of the area i (i.e. $d_i = |x_i - x_0|$). In the absence of an exposure measure that may be attached to each area, a natural additive distance/risk model is

$$\theta_i = \rho\{1 + g(d_i)\},$$

where ρ is the background relative risk in A and $g(\cdot)$ is a function of distance, with $g(d) \to 0$ as $d \to \infty$ (or in practice as d tends to the extent of the study region). Note that, by using distance as a surrogate for exposure, orientation information is lost (i.e. we have assumed an isotropic relationship). More generally, we may have a function that is not monotonic and is anisotropic (e.g. Lawson 1993). In Section 9.4 we describe methods that are non-specific about the form of $g(\cdot)$ while those described in Section 9.5 specify the form exactly up to a (finite) set of parameters.

Let z_i denote a $q \times 1$ vector of area-level risk factors. These may be incorporated either in the expected numbers (via a suitable discretisation), or via a regression model. In this latter case a natural form is given by

$$\theta_i = \rho\{1 + g(d_i)\} \exp(z_i^T \gamma).$$

The manner of adjustment, either through internal or external standardisation in the expected numbers, or via regression, is important (see Breslow *et al.* 1983). For example, if a measure of deprivation is available, then the use of internal standardisation is dangerous since some of the pollution effect may be lost since we are removing the deprivation effect *before* we model the pollution effect. If external standardisation is used, the choice of the reference area is important since the deprivation effect (say) should be specific to the area under consideration. A regression approach will correctly adjust standard errors of estimated relative risks but may be inefficient due to sparsity of data.

Even after accounting for the possibility of a distance/risk effect and known covariates, it is frequently the case that the data exhibit greater variability than that expected from a Poisson distribution. There are two possible ways of accommodating this extra-Poisson variability (overdispersion): a *quasi-likelihood* approach (McCullagh and Nelder 1989) simply specifies $E[Y_i|\theta_i] = E_i\theta_i$ and $\text{var}(Y_i|\theta_i) = \kappa \times E[Y_i|\theta_i]$ and estimates κ, while a hierarchical modelling approach assumes that the θ_i are random variables that arise from a probability distribution. This latter approach induces overdispersion (Chapter 7). Note that the assumption of (conditional) independence of the Y_i given the θ_i, may not be true due, for example, to unmeasured risk factors (e.g. genetic predisposition or environmental factors) that are smoothly varying across space. The common method of dealing with this is to follow a hierarchical modelling approach and to model the spatial dependence between the θ_i (Chapters 6, 7, 11, and 22). Great care must be used when such an approach is taken since the effect that one is aiming to detect may be 'smoothed' away. For this reason, disease mapping studies of the disease of interest, preferably at the same geographical scale as the point-source study, are vital to provide an indication of the 'baseline' spatial risk surface.

9.2.3   Bernoulli model for case-control data

When locations of cases and controls are available, the finer spatial information is preserved by adopting a Bernoulli model for the case-control label and modelling the probability of observing a case rather than a control at a particular location as a function of the exposure at that location (e.g. distance from x_0). Suppose that in A there are n_1 cases of the disease at locations $x_1, \ldots, x_{n_1}$ and n_0 controls at locations $x_{n_1+1}, \ldots, x_{n_1+n_0}$. Now define random variables Y_i using the status of the observation at the location x_i such that

$$Y_i = \begin{cases} 0 & \text{if the event is a control,} \\ 1 & \text{if the event is a case.} \end{cases} \tag{9.3}$$

As before, let d_i denote the distance from location x_i to the source location x_0. Then, conditional on the observed locations, the labels Y_i are independent Bernoulli random variables with probability of 'success' given by

$$\pi_i = \mathrm{Pr}(\text{case at } x_i \mid \text{case or control at } x_i). \tag{9.4}$$

In the absence of other risk factors, the null hypothesis that proximity to x_0 has no effect upon risk may be written as

$$H_0 : \pi_i = \pi_0 \quad \text{for } i = 1, \ldots, n_1 + n_0,$$

that is, the probability of disease is independent of location. Conceptually, we may think of the probability of there being a case at a location x as a smooth function of location, $\pi(x)$. Note that, as usual with case-control studies, this quantity does not represent absolute risk unless *all* cases and controls are selected.

By analogy with the aggregated data case we may assume the following general risk/distance model:

$$\frac{\pi_i}{1 - \pi_i} = \rho\{1 + g(d_i)\},$$

and individual level covariates z_i may be accommodated via the logistic model:

$$\frac{\pi_i}{1 - \pi_i} = \rho\{1 + g(d_i)\} \times \exp(z_i^T \gamma).$$

In Sections 9.4 and 9.5 we discuss various choices of $g(\cdot)$. Another method of adjusting for individual risk factors is via matching, see for example Breslow and Day (1980).

9.3 Conventional epidemiological methods

In this section we review methods that are applicable in general to cohort and case-control studies, and describe how they may be used in the context considered here. The methods are characterised by the use of a simple exposure measure that takes one of a small number of values (e.g. near to, or far from, the putative source). The data are then aggregated into groups defined by this measure and therefore methods for count data are the most appropriate (though the binomial formulation will typically be used for case-control data).

9.3.1 'Near versus reference' comparisons

The most straightforward approach to assessing the risk in relation to a point source is to compare the risk in the 'exposed' population (e.g. lying within a certain distance of the point source) with that in a reference population. For example, in the case of Sellafield, Craft and Birch (1983) and Gardner and Winter (1984) looked at registration and death rates for malignant disease in the surrounding area and compared these with national rates. This simple approach has two serious drawbacks: (a) the choice of the exposed population is not obvious (and is likely to be crucial); (b) a significant difference in risk will not necessarily be due to exposure since the reference population may be different in respects other than exposure. The method does, however, provide a simple first look at the data.

9.3.2 'Near versus far' comparisons

To address problem (b), the study region may be divided into 'near' and 'far' regions corresponding to exposed and unexposed areas, respectively. This approach is characterised by a 1/0 exposure variable and standard methods of analysis may be utilised (see Breslow and Day 1980, 1987; Clayton and Hills 1993).

We consider first a rare condition. Let Y_{1j} and N_{1j} denote the number of cases and population at risk in stratum j in the near region and Y_{2j} and N_{2j} the corresponding numbers in the far region. Further let Z_j and M_j denote the number of cases and population at risk in stratum j in a standard population. Summaries of the overall risk in region i ($i=1$ and 2 denoting near and far) are provided by directly and indirectly standardised rates that are given, respectively, by

$$\sum_{j=1}^{J} M_j \hat{p}_{ij}/M, \tag{9.5}$$

and

$$\frac{Y_i}{\sum_{j=1}^{J} N_{ij}\hat{q}_j} \times \frac{Z}{M}, \tag{9.6}$$

where $\hat{p}_{ij} = Y_{ij}/N_{ij}$, $\hat{q}_j = Z_j/M_j$, $Y_i = \Sigma_j Y_{ij}$, $Z = \Sigma_j Z_j$ and $M = \Sigma_j M_j$. The directly standardised rate corresponds to a 'counter-factual' argument in which the estimated rates within the area of interest are applied to the standard population. The indirectly standardised rate applies the estimated relative risk to the rate in the standard population. The directly standardised rate may be highly unstable since it is a function of the stratum-specific rate estimates $\hat{p}_{ij}$ and these may be based on small numbers, N_{ij}. Simple summaries of the rate ratios in the near or far regions compared to the standard population are obtained by taking the ratios of (9.5) or (9.6) to Z/M to give the comparative mortality figure (CMF) or the standardised mortality/morbidity ratio (SMR), respectively:

$$\text{CMF}_i = \frac{\sum_{j=1}^{J} M_j \hat{p}_{ij}/M}{Z/M},$$

and

$$\text{SMR}_i = \frac{Y_i}{\sum_{j=1}^{J} N_{ij}\hat{q}_j},$$

for $i = 1, 2$. A comparison of the near and far regions is provided by the ratios $\text{CMF}_1/\text{CMF}_2$ or $\text{SMR}_1/\text{SMR}_2$, but these suffer from a number of difficulties (Breslow and Day 1987, section 2). If the ratios of stratum-specific risks in the near and far regions are constant across strata (i.e. $p_{1j} = \psi \times p_{2j}, j = 1, \ldots, J$), then the ratio of directly standardised rates provides an estimate of $\psi = p_{1j}/p_{2j}$, the relative risk for the near area with respect to the far area. Note, however, that the variance of this estimator will depend on the standard population that is selected. If we have $p_{1j} = \psi \times p_{2j} = \phi \times q_j, j = 1, \ldots, J$ (which is equivalent to (9.1) with $\theta_1 = \phi$ and $\theta_2 = \phi/\psi$), then $\text{SMR}_1/\text{SMR}_2$ is equivalent to the MLE of ψ under the Poisson model of Section 9.2.2 (with $n = 2$). It is clear therefore that, before these summaries are calculated, the proportionality assumptions must be assessed. If proportionality is not found then a single summary of risk will be deceptive. Another disadvantage of the use of these summaries in anything but a descriptive role is that the conventional formulae for the variances of the CMFs and SMRs (Breslow and Day 1987, section 2.3) do not adjust for the overdispersion that typically arises in spatial epidemiology. The assessment of proportionality, and adjustment for overdispersion are discussed in Section 9.5.

Assuming for now that the assumption of proportionality is appropriate we consider 'exact' methods for obtaining an estimate of the relative risk ψ and a test of $\psi = 1$. We assume that $Y_i \sim \text{Po}(E_i\theta_i)$ with $\psi = \theta_1/\theta_2$. Following Cox and Hinkley (1974) we may then consider the conditional distribution of Y_1 given $Y = Y_1 + Y_2$. This distribution is binomial and only depends on ψ. Letting $\pi = \psi E_1/(E_2 + \psi E_1)$, we have

$$\Pr(y_1 | \pi, y) = \begin{cases} \binom{y}{y_1} \pi^{y_1}(1 - \pi)^{y - y_1}, & y_1 = 0, 1, \ldots, y \\ 0 & \text{otherwise,} \end{cases}$$

and so the conditioning has eliminated one of the parameters. The conditional MLE is given by $\hat{\pi} = Y_1/y$ and so $\hat{\psi} = (Y_1/E_1)/(Y_2/E_2)$ which is identical to the unconditional estimate (i.e. the ratio of SMRs). The null hypothesis $H_0 : \psi = 1$ (which is equivalent to $\pi = \pi_0 = E_1/(E_1 + E_2)$), versus $H_1 : \psi > 1$ is rejected for large values of y_1 and the observed significance level of the test is

$$\sum_{y=y_1}^{y} \binom{y}{y_1} \pi_0^{y_1} (1 - \pi_0)^{y - y_1}.$$

We now turn our attention to case-control data. Suppose first that we have a single stratum. Table 9.1 displays how the data may be summarised in the form of a 2×2 table with rows corresponding to cases and controls and columns exposed and non-exposed (i.e. near and far).

As with aggregated data, exact methods are available by conditioning on both table margins. The distribution of the number of exposed cases, Z_{11}, then follows a non-central

Table 9.1 2×2 table summarising near/far data

	Exposed	Non-exposed	Total
Cases	Z_{11}		n_1
Controls			n_0
	m_1	m_0	

hypergeometric distribution:

$$\Pr(Z_{11} = z | \psi, n_0, n_1, m_0, m_1) = \frac{\binom{n_1}{z_{11}} \binom{n_0}{m_1 - z_{11}} \psi^{z_{11}}}{\sum_{u=u_{\min}}^{u_{\max}} \binom{n_1}{u} \binom{n_0}{m_1 - u} \psi^{u}}, \tag{9.7}$$

for $z_{11} = u_{\min}, \ldots, u_{\max}$ where $u_{\min} = \max(0, m_1 - n_0)$ and $u_{\max} = \min(n_1, m_1)$ and ψ denotes the odds ratio for disease in the exposed versus non-exposed group. As before we may evaluate the conditional MLE though it is not available in closed form and does not correspond to the familiar unconditional MLE (cross-product ratio) that is given by

$$\frac{Z_{11} \times (n_0 - m_1 + Z_{11})}{(m_1 - Z_{11}) \times (n_1 - Z_{11})}.$$

Similarly, an exact test of $H_0 : \psi = 1$ may be carried out. The latter is particularly simple since for $\psi = 1$, (9.7) becomes a (central) hypergeometric distribution.

When, as is almost always the case, the data are stratified, we obtain a 2×2 table for each stratum. In this case the first question is whether the odds ratios are constant across strata, which may be assessed using a number of methods (Breslow and Day 1980). If this is established then the conditional MLE may be evaluated, though again it is not available analytically. Note that unlike the Poisson case, in which the conditional and unconditional MLEs both equal the ratio of SMRs, here the two estimators do not correspond though in large samples the difference is likely to be small. Alternatively, one may use the Mantel–Haenszel estimator. Breslow (1996) provides an interesting discussion of this and other estimators. Exact and Mantel–Haenszel tests of unity of the common odds ratio are also available. Severini (1999) discusses how the presence of overdispersion alters the properties of tests.

There are a number of examples of case-control analyses involving point or line sources of putative pollution. For example, Livingstone *et al.* (1996) investigated asthma incidence in Tower Hamlets, London and defined 'near' as being residence lying within 150 metres of a main road. Dolk *et al.* (1998, 1999) investigated the association between congenital anomalies and landfill sites across Europe using a case-control study. As part of the statistical analysis, odds ratios such as those described here were utilised.

For case-control data we have so far supposed that the data were selected without reference to the stratification variables. A more efficient analysis may result if the ratio of controls to cases is kept constant across confounding variables. In the above example, for instance, one might have wished to examine asthma risk with proximity to roads, matched on smoking status. In this case the selection procedure must be acknowledged in the analysis via the introduction of a (nuisance) parameter for each matching variable (e.g. smoking); regression methods (Section 9.5) may then be used. In the case of individually 1:1 matched data it is essential that a conditional likelihood is considered since the number of nuisance parameters increases with the number of case-control pairs, rendering standard likelihood methods inapplicable.

9.4 Semi-parametric tests

In this section we consider methods in which no specific form is chosen for the location/ risk function.

9.4.1 Besag and Newell's method

A number of authors (see Chapter 8) have proposed methods for surveillance (cluster detection) with count data that consist of multiple Poisson tests with each test considering the number of cases contained within circles centred on either pre-specified points or area centroids. Cluster detection is an inherently difficult problem due to the need for a definition of a 'cluster' (see Chapters 6 and 8). Depending on this definition the circles may be constructed to have constant radius (Openshaw *et al.* 1987), constant population at risk (Turnbull *et al.* 1990) or a constant number of cases (Besag and Newell 1991). We consider the last of these in a pre-specified point context. In this context the other two methods would simply correspond to near versus reference methods with the near area defined in terms of constant distance or population. Neither method are recommended for this context though Openshaw's method with different sized circles would give information on the size of any excess (though the multiple testing is not acknowledged). Similarly Besag and Newell's method gives information on the 'cluster' size.

Besag and Newell (1991) (see also Newell and Besag 1996) proposed an improved version of the geographical analysis machine (Openshaw *et al.* 1987, 1988) for the detection of clusters in routinely collected databases. Besag and Newell (1991) argue that proposed methods should acknowledge that, from a purely statistical perspective, the inaccuracies within such data are indistinguishable from aetiological effects. The key input to their method is a cluster size k. Here we describe the version that is appropriate for cluster investigation in relation to a pre-specified point source. The method could be used with point data but it is likely that a more specific exposure hypothesis would be available, in which case, a more refined approach would be taken.

The null hypothesis is that the cases are distributed at random over the population at risk in A. As in the basic Poisson model, assume that the region is divided into n disjoint areas. Label the area containing x_0 as A_1 and all other areas $A_2, \ldots, A_n$ by increasing distance from A_1 based on the area centroid. We first consider the case in which there are no strata. Define

$$D_i = \sum_{l=1}^{i} y_l \quad i = 1, \ldots, n$$

and

$$u_i = \sum_{l=1}^{i} N_l \quad i = 1, \ldots, n,$$

as the number of cases and population within the nearest i areas, respectively. The test statistic is $I = \min\{i : D_i \geq k\}$, the number of areas required to accrue at least k cases. A small observed value of I indicates that there is clustering around x_0. The observed significance level is calculated via

$$p\text{-value} = \Pr(I \leq i | k)$$

$$= 1 - \sum_{s=0}^{k-1} \frac{\exp(-E_i) E_i^s}{s!}, \tag{9.8}$$

where $E_i = u_i q$ and q is an estimate of risk obtained via, for example, internal or external standardisation. We note that a small p-value may result if the risk in the study region overall is high relative to the reference region from which q is derived. One may overcome this by using internal standardisation or by replacing E_i by $E_i^* = E_i \times Y/N$, where Y and N represent the total number of cases and the population at risk in the study region, respectively.

Adjustment for known risk factors is made by considering $u_{ij} = \sum_{l=1}^{i} N_{lj}$, the cumulative number at risk in stratum j within the nearest i areas. Then $E_i = u_i q$ in (9.8) should be replaced by $E_i = \sum_j u_{ij} q_j$ where q_j are a set of stratum-specific reference probabilities. Again, we may replace E_i by E_i^* where

$$E_i^* = E_i \times Y/E, \tag{9.9}$$

where $Y = \sum_i Y_i$ and $E = \sum_i E_i$, so that the overall difference between the risks in the study and the reference areas have been removed. If ranking the areas based on distance is not appropriate they can be ranked using some other measure. For example, if wind directions are thought to be important in determining the exposure of a region, this information can be used instead. The same procedure may be used for most rank-based methods.

The method of Besag and Newell is relatively simple to apply and is not unduly computer-intensive. In practice it is difficult to choose a value for the crucial cluster size k, however, and a range of values is typically chosen. The size of k should reflect both the level of aggregation of the data (see Waller and Lawson 1995) and the rarity of the disease since with large populations/non-rare diseases the expected number of cases in areas close to the focus (say) will be greater than a certain value under the null hypothesis. In this latter case it will be impossible to reject H_0 for small values of k (and so no information is contained in non-rejection). The method suffers from problems of multiple testing when different cluster sizes are considered, and the tests are not independent. These deficiencies could, however, be fixed via a Monte Carlo test. A drawback of the method is that, due to its genesis as a surveillance device, it does not provide an estimate of the risk around the putative source, only the presence of a cluster. When the method was developed it was explicitly designed for detecting discrepancies between numerator and denominator due to differences in risk *or* data inaccuracies, and hence is likely to provide many false positives by construction. The approach may be used with line sources if a measure of exposure can be used to rank areas.

9.4.2   Stone's test

Original version

The semi-parametric test developed by Stone (1988) was specifically designed to assess increased risk associated with a pre-specified source using area level data. The test takes the Poisson framework of Section 9.2.2 but only assumes that risk is a non-increasing function of increasing distance, or more precisely, a non-increasing function of the rank of the distance between x_0 and the sub-region centroid. In fact, although the method is commonly used with distance it may also be used with ranks based on exposure scores.

The standard Poisson model $Y_i \sim \text{Po}(\theta_i E_i)$ is assumed and areas are ordered with increasing distance from the source, so that $i = 1$ corresponds to the area closest to the source. In the *unconditional* test the null hypothesis $H_0 : \theta_1 = \cdots = \theta_n = 1$ is tested against the alternative hypothesis $H_1 : \theta_1 \geq \theta_2 \geq \cdots \geq \theta_n$ with at least one inequality holding. The estimates of θ_i under the alternative hypothesis can be found analytically using the theory of isotonic regression and implemented using the min-max formulae given in Stone (1988) or using the pooled adjacent violators (Barlow *et al.* 1972: 13–18; Robertson *et al.* 1988: 8–11). The hypothesis is tested using a generalised likelihood ratio test statistic and the observed significance level of the test is calculated via Monte Carlo simulation.

The unconditional test may reject H_0 simply because the study region has elevated or lowered risk. Bithell and Stone (1989) note this and suggest replacing E_i by the adjusted versions given by (9.9). Alternatively, a *conditional* test with $H_0 : \theta_1 = \cdots = \theta_n = \rho$ may be carried out (Shaddick and Elliott 1996). The significance level for this test can again be found by simulation but with a modification to allow for the unknown constant ρ.

In order to avoid the Monte Carlo test, Stone originally developed a *Poisson maximum* test, in which the test statistic was the maximum over $i = 1, \ldots, n$ of the observed SMRs. Clearly, the significance level of this SMR in isolation is not appropriate since we have selected the maximum. However, the test statistic has a tractable sampling distribution (and so avoids simulation), and has the attractive interpretation of relating to the circle centred at x_0 within which the observed risk is maximised (note that this corrects for the multiple testing problem that would be inherent if Openshaw's method was used in this context). Power calculations given in Stone (1988) showed that the two tests compared well. Later work (Bithell 1992), however, showed that for a range of situations of interest the Poisson maximum test has inferior power when compared to the likelihood ratio test. The cost of computing time is now so cheap that performing a Monte Carlo test is not an obstacle and hence the likelihood ratio test is more widely used.

The advantage of Stone's test is that it avoids the need to assume a fully specified distance/risk relationship and can be used when there is little information on the scale of the effect.

There are many applications of Stone's test in the epidemiological literature, particularly those studies conducted by the UK Small Area Health Statistics Unit (SAHSU) (Elliott *et al.* 1992a). The SAHSU studies routinely used Stone's test on a set of concentric bands radiating from the source, rather than on the original areas at which data were collected. The computational requirements of a large-scale study are thereby reduced but a somewhat arbitrary set of bands has been introduced. SAHSU has used Stone's test for a number of types of putative source: all incinerators of waste solvents and oils in Great Britain (Elliott *et al.* 1992*b*), a single petrochemical works at Baglan Bay, Wales (Sans *et al.* 1995), all municipal incinerators in Great Britain (Elliott *et al.* 1996), radio and TV transmitters (Dolk *et al.* 1997*a,b*), and cokeworks (Wilkinson *et al.* 1997). Viel *et al.* (1995) use the Poisson maximum test in an analysis of leukaemia in young people in the vicinity of the La Hague nuclear reprocessing plant. They compare this test with a near-intermediate-far exposure variable with different reference rates and also a kernel smoothing method (see Section 9.5.3). A number of additional comparisons between Stone's test and other methods have been carried out (see Sections 9.4.3 and 9.4.4).

Extensions

We now consider a number of extensions to the original method.

Case-control data

Stone (1988) proposed an extension to case-control data but did not implement the idea. Bithell (1992) noted that the 'Bernoulli maximum' test was ineffective but applied the likelihood ratio test to case-control data concerning childhood leukaemia and lymphoma around Sellafield. The idea is developed fully in Diggle *et al.* (1999), using the Bernoulli model that was described in Section 9.2.3. The null hypothesis $H_0 : \pi_i = \pi_0$, $i = 1, \ldots,$ $n_1 + n_0$ is tested against the isotonic alternative $H_1 : \pi_1 \geq \pi_2 \geq \cdots \geq \pi_{n_1+n_0}$, where the events (i.e. cases and controls) are ordered with increasing distance from the source as in the original test. Note that one difference between the two formulations is that, in the case-control version, a parameter for each case and each control is estimated rather than just each sub-region as in the Poisson model; since $n_1 + n_0$ is likely to be much larger than the number of areas the computation time can be much greater.

Multiple sites

Shaddick and Elliott (1996) discuss how Stone's test may be applied to multiple sites. As mentioned in Section 9.2.1, if an area falls within the exposure (distance) band of more than one site a simple solution is to take the exposure corresponding to the nearest source. Waller *et al.* (1992, 1994) used distance to the nearest site in the analysis of leukaemia in upstate New York.

In the case of S distinct sites, we first note that a single overall summary should only be considered if the sites are believed to be comparable in terms of their exposure. Under H_0 the *p*-value associated with site s, p_s, $s = 1, \ldots, S$, is uniformly distributed on $(0, 1)$ and so $-2 \log p_s$ follows a χ_2^2 distribution. Hence, for S independent sites, the combined statistic $-2 \sum_{s=1}^{S} \log p_s$ follows a χ_{2S}^2 distribution. Alternatively, the individual log likelihood ratio statistics may be summed and the significance assessed via simulation.

Covariate adjustment

In the original method it was only possible to adjust for known risk factors within the expected numbers. However, Morton-Jones *et al.* (1999) have developed a method for covariate adjustment in Stone's test using a generalised additive model (Hastie and Tibshirani 1990) which specifies a log-linear model for the risk factors and estimates the θ_i under the monotonicity constraint as above. The null hypothesis can still be tested using simulation, but only an approximate Monte Carlo test is available as the covariate parameters make the hypothesis composite. The adjustment for covariates in the case-control version of Stone's test follows similarly (Diggle *et al.* 1999).

Interval estimation

One drawback of Stone's test is that it only provides a point estimate of the distance/risk relationship. Diggle *et al.* (1999) suggest obtaining interval estimates of the fitted risk estimates using a Monte Carlo approach and simulating from the fitted model. Similarly, tolerance limits, estimated by simulating from the null hypothesis, can be a useful addition to a plot of the risk estimates against distance.

Another disadvantage of Stone's method is that no adjustment for overdispersion is made.

9.4.3   Score tests

Following from Section 9.3 there are a number of 'traditional' methods available for testing for a trend in a set of Poisson means as a function of a set of exposures. For example, suppose w_i denotes an 'exposure' associated with area i and E_i^* is defined as in (9.9). Then the statistic

$$\frac{\left\{\sum_{i=1}^{n} w_i (Y_i - E_i^*)\right\}^2}{\sum_{i=1}^{n} w_i^2 E_i^* - \left(\sum_{i=1}^{n} w_i E_i^*\right)^2 / Y} \tag{9.10}$$

may be used to compare the null hypothesis of constant risk in all areas, versus the general monotonic alternative. Under H_0 this statistic has an (asymptotic) chi-squared distribution with a single degree of freedom. If there is no specific quantitative exposure then we may take $w_i = i$ (where the areas are ranked according to distance x_0). This procedure may be justified as a score test (Tarone 1982; see also Breslow *et al.* 1983). Under certain regularity conditions score tests provide asymptotic *locally* most powerful tests (e.g. Gart and Tarone 1983).

Lawson (1993) and Waller *et al.* (1992, 1994) have advocated the use of score tests closely related to the above. Lawson (1993) considered bronchitis mortality around a reprocessing plant in Bonnybridge, Scotland. Waller *et al.* (1994) compare a score test with the Poisson maximum test of Stone (1988) and the method of Besag and Newell (1991) using leukaemia data from upstate New York in relation to hazardous waste sites containing trichloroethylene (TCE). Waller and Lawson (1995) compare these same tests on simulated data via examination of the power, although unfortunately such comparisons depend critically on the range of alternatives considered. In terms of power, however, the score test performed well for the alternatives considered. A fairer comparison would consider the likelihood ratio version of Stone's test. The asymptotic distribution of the score test statistic has been reported to be accurate in most situations (Waller *et al.* 1994) though Waller and Lawson (1995) give an algorithm for the numerical evaluation of the exact distribution using inversion of the characteristic function. Tango (1995) also contains a discussion of score tests for point sources.

Waller (1996) compares the performance of focused tests with respect to the varying amounts of data aggregation or sub-region size. He also illustrates how to use power functions to calculate the sample size required to detect a fixed effect. Waller and Poquette (1999) also advocate the use of '*post hoc*' power calculations in order to determine what effect sizes one could have expected to detect for the given population distribution across the area of interest.

9.4.4 Linear risk scores

Bithell (1995) considers likelihood ratio tests that result in statistics based on

$$\sum_{i=1}^{n} Y_i \log\{\theta_i(w_i)\},$$

where the $\theta_i(w_i)$ are risk 'scores' that are assigned by considering specific alternatives. For alternative hypotheses of the form

$$\rho \exp\left(-\frac{\beta}{w_i}\right),$$

the test takes the form $\Sigma_i Y_i \times w_i$. This class of tests are referred to as linear risk score (LRS) tests. Note that the 'score' here has nothing to do with the score test. In both this and the score test the 'exposures', w_i, may be used with such distance surrogates as $1/d_i$, $1/d_i^2$, $1/\text{rank}$ or $1/\text{rank}^{1/2}$. Bithell (1995) gives examples of situations under which each might be suitable and recommends the use of $1/\text{rank}$. This was subsequently used by Bithell *et al.* (1994) to examine the distribution of childhood leukaemia around nuclear installations in England and Wales (though other tests were also considered). An overall significance level across all sites was also reported, based on the distribution of the minimum of the collection of *p*-values.

Bithell (1992) implemented Stone's likelihood ratio and Poisson maximum tests and two LRS tests, based on inverse distance and inverse distance rank. These tests were illustrated using data from Sellafield and on simulated data. For the alternatives considered, the Poisson maximum test was the least powerful and the two LRS tests were superior to the likelihood ratio test.

In common with most of the test-based approaches of this section, a major disadvantage of both the score and LRS tests is that no estimated risk surface with interval estimates is produced.

9.4.5 Cuzick and Edwards' method

A method that was originally suggested for the detection of clustering in case-control data is that of Cuzick and Edwards (1990). Strictly, this method may be termed non-parametric but it is natural to include it here. We first describe two statistics that may be used in a point-source context with case-control data. The first, T_k, counts the number of cases within the k nearest cases or controls (or 'neighbours') of the source x_0. The second, T_k^{inv}, is defined as the number of cases that are closer to x_0 than the k nearest controls. This latter is referred to as the inverse sampling statistic (hence the superscript). For T_k the moments may be evaluated analytically under the null hypothesis of random allocation of cases and controls, and asymptotic normality appealed to in order to assess the significance of a given configuration. The choice of k is crucial and Cuzick and Edwards (1990) describe a combined T_k statistic (though the assumptions underlying its use are questioned by Stone 1990). Under H_0 the expectation of the T_k^{inv} statistic is simply available, but the variance is more unwieldy and asymptotic normality has not been established. Consequently, simulation is suggested to determine the significance level. Matching may be carried out to account for confounders, though the mean and variance are adjusted and simulation may be the easiest way to evaluate the significance level. No estimated risk surface is produced by the method.

We now describe the so-called *one-sample method* that may be used with small-area population counts. This approach is outlined in Cuzick and Edwards (1990) and described in more detail in Cuzick and Edwards (1996). The one-sample analogue of T_k^{inv} is to rank areas according to proximity to x_0 and then calculate expected numbers $E_1^*, E_2^*, \ldots$ for these areas (using 9.9). Areas are then combined until a distance is reached within which the expected numbers sum to as close to k as possible, call this value k'. The number of cases that occur within these areas is then compared with a Poisson distribution with expectation k'. This statistic is closely related to that of Turnbull *et al.* (1990), see Chapter 8 for further discussion. To the best of our knowledge the Cuzick and Edwards statistics have not been used in a pre-specified point-source context.

9.5 Regression methods

In this section we describe approaches in which an explicit parametric form is assumed for the relationship between risk and proximity to source.

9.5.1 Poisson regression models

For a rare disease and aggregated data the natural modelling framework is Poisson regression. For $Y_i \sim \text{Po}(E_i\theta_i)$, $i = 1, \ldots, n$, we may assume the generalised linear model (McCullagh and Nelder 1989)

$$\log \theta_i = \alpha + \beta w_i + z_i^T \gamma \tag{9.11}$$

where z_i represents a $q \times 1$ vector of area-level risk factors, w_i a measure of exposure and we write $\phi = (\alpha, \beta)$. The parameters (ϕ, γ) of this model may then be estimated via likelihood or Bayesian approaches. The near versus far exposure variable fits into this framework with $w_i = 1$ for those areas, i, the centroids of which lie near to x_0, and $w_i = 0$ otherwise. When there are no area-level risk factors, the MLE of $\exp(\beta)$ corresponds to the ratio of SMRs described in Section 9.3.2. There are many possible choices of w_i, for example d_i or d_i^{-1}. The choice of $w_i = d_i$ has been criticised by Diggle and Elliott (1995) since, with $\beta < 0$, $d_i \to \infty$ implies that $\theta_i \to 0$ and not to a background level of risk. The choice $w_i = d_i^{-1}$ has the desired behaviour as $d \to \infty$. This gives infinite risk at source (when $\beta > 0$), however, but this is not a problem for fitting unless the centroid of the closest area lies at x_0. The results may be very sensitive to the closeness of this area's centroid to x_0, however, and in terms of interpretation there is no estimate of the risk at source.

Lawson (1993) considers (9.11) with a multivariate w_i (see also Lawson and Williams 1994). Such a class allows for a non-monotonic distance/risk relationship and also for directional effects. For example the model

$$\log \theta_i = \alpha + \beta_1 \log d_i + \beta_2 d_i + z_i \gamma,$$

allows for a radial peak followed by a decline.

Diggle *et al.* (1997) assumes an *additive* exposure/risk model as an alternative to the multiplicative model (9.11) to give:

$$\theta_i = \rho\{1 + g(d_i, \boldsymbol{\phi})\} \exp(z_i^T \boldsymbol{\gamma}), \qquad (9.12)$$

with a variety of choices for $g(\cdot, \cdot)$ but with the property that $g(d, \cdot) \to 0$ as $d \to \infty$. The 'step' model

$$g(d, \boldsymbol{\phi}) = \begin{cases} \alpha, & d \leq \delta, \\ 0, & d > \delta, \end{cases} \qquad (9.13)$$

where $\boldsymbol{\phi} = (\alpha, \delta)$, corresponds to the near versus far approach but with the extent of the near region (δ) estimated from the data. The parameter α reflects the increased incidence at source. A more complex model that allows the risk to decrease smoothly to source is given by

$$g(d, \boldsymbol{\phi}) = \begin{cases} \alpha, & d \leq \delta, \\ \alpha \exp\left[-\dfrac{(d - \delta)^2}{\beta^2}\right], & d > \delta, \end{cases} \qquad (9.14)$$

where $\boldsymbol{\phi} = (\alpha, \beta, \delta)$. In (9.14), α has the same interpretation as in the step model, β is the rate of decline, and δ gives the width of the plateau. The decline from the plateau to baseline is given by a functional form equivalent to a half-normal density. Hence, β is seen to be similar to a standard deviation, with small β implying a swift decline and $\beta \to 0$ giving the step model. Unfortunately, the models (9.13) and (9.14) lead to a likelihood function that is not differentiable [since $g(d, \boldsymbol{\phi})$ is not differentiable with respect to δ] and so does not satisfy the usual regularity conditions. Consequently, the asymptotic properties of estimators and test statistics cannot be relied upon and Monte Carlo simulation must be used for standard errors and significance levels.

Extra-Poisson variation can be allowed for in these models using the quasi-likelihood approach described in Section 9.2.2. The linear model (9.11) with overdispersion was used by Cook-Mozaffari *et al.* (1989a,b) in the analysis of the spatial distribution of cancers and leukaemia around nuclear installations.

The models of this section all depend on the proportionality assumption (9.1). Wakefield and Morris (1999) suggest plotting $\hat{p}_{ij}$ versus q_j for selected areas in which there are abundant data (a plot of $\log \hat{p}_{ij}$ versus $\log q_j$ may be clearer). Alternatively, the model $Y_{ij} \sim \text{Po}(N_{ij}p_{ij})$ with $\log p_{ij} = \alpha + \gamma_{ij}$ (i.e. the saturated model), may be fitted and compared (via the deviance for example) with the model without stratum or area interactions (i.e. $\log p_{ij} = \alpha + \beta_j$). Comparison of $\hat{p}_{ij} = \exp(\hat{\alpha} + \hat{\gamma}_{ij})$ with $\hat{p}'_{ij} = \exp(\hat{\alpha} + \hat{\beta}_j)$ and q_j, allows the proportionality assumption to be assessed and strata with departures to be identified. If proportionality is not found to be appropriate then a more complex analysis must be performed, either by analysing sub-groups within which proportionality is reasonable separately, or via the inclusion of interaction terms.

For the case of S sites within the same study area one may take $w_i = \max_{s \in \{1,2,\ldots,S\}} w_{is}$, where w_{is} is the exposure in area i due to source s. This approach has been used with Stone's method (recall Section 9.4.2). Alternatively one may assume that each site contributes independently to the risk and the sum of exposures may then be taken (e.g. Diggle and Elliott 1995). So, for example, in this case, Equation (9.11) with inverse distance as exposure would become

$$\theta_i = \exp\left(\alpha + \sum_{s=1}^{S} \beta_s d_{is}^{-1} + z_i^T \gamma\right), \tag{9.15}$$

where d_{is} is the distance from centroid i to source s, whilst (9.12) becomes

$$\theta_i = \rho \prod_{s=1}^{S} \{1 + g(d_{is}, \phi_s)\} \times \exp(z_i^T \gamma). \tag{9.16}$$

In both (9.15) and (9.16) the parameters for each source have been taken as distinct (i.e. interactions between site and exposure have been included). An alternative is to assume constant effects across sites (i.e. $\beta_s = \beta$ and $\phi_s = \phi$ for $s = 1, \ldots, S$). An intermediate model that has been suggested by Wakefield and Morris (2000) for S distinct study areas, but which may be used in this situation, is to assume that β_s and ϕ_s are random effects. For example, in (9.15) we would have $\beta_s \sim N(\mu, \Sigma)$ where μ is the common effect and Σ describes the between-site variability in effect. If site-specific covariates Z_s exist (e.g. characteristics of the emitting source) then the model may be extended to

$$\beta_s \sim N\left(\mu_0 + Z_s^T \mu_1, \Sigma\right).$$

Dolk *et al.* (1998, 1999) describe a related meta-analysis approach in which a single summary relative risk parameter was obtained for each site (landfills) and combined using a random effects model; a test for homogeneity of the relative risk parameters was also carried out.

9.5.2 Logistic regression

By analogy with the Poisson regression models for aggregated data, case-control data may be analysed using logistic regression models:

$$\log \frac{\pi_i}{1 - \pi_i} = \alpha + \beta w_i + z_i^T \gamma.$$

For individual-level confounders z_i, a matched study may be carried out to improve efficiency. Matched case-control data should be analysed with a nuisance parameter for each matching variable, and using a conditional logistic regression approach if the number of matching variables is large (see Breslow and Day 1980). For frequency-based matching the difference between conditional and unconditional analyses is likely to be small whereas for $1:m$ matching a conditional approach is essential. Gardner *et al.* (1990*a,b*) used the latter method to estimate odds ratios from matched cases and controls in a study on leukaemia and lymphoma in under 25-year-olds near Sellafield.

Diggle and Rowlingson (1994) suggest the model

$$\frac{\pi_i}{1 - \pi_i} = \rho\{1 + g(d_i, \boldsymbol{\phi})\} \exp(z_i^T \boldsymbol{\gamma}),$$

with, for example,

$$g(d_i, \boldsymbol{\phi}) = \alpha \exp(-\beta d_i^2), \tag{9.17}$$

with $\boldsymbol{\phi} = (\alpha, \beta)$ The parameters ρ, $\boldsymbol{\gamma}$, and $\boldsymbol{\phi}$ are estimated using a Bernoulli likelihood function and numerical maximisation. This forms the basis for model (9.14), which was developed from aggregated data.

Biggeri *et al.* (1996), following Lawson (1993), give an example of an application of the Diggle and Rowlingson model with additional directional effects using

$$g(d, \boldsymbol{\phi}) = \alpha \exp\left\{\alpha + \sum_{k=1}^{3} w_k \beta_k\right\}$$

with $w_1 = d$, $w_2 = \sin \omega$, $w_3 = \cos \omega$ (where ω is the angle between the event location and the source location) and $\boldsymbol{\phi} = (\alpha, \beta_1, \beta_2, \beta_3)$. Unfortunately, they apply the model to matched case-control data, for which the model is not strictly appropriate. Diggle *et al.* (2000) illustrate conditional likelihood and Bayesian approaches to overcoming this problem. Multiple sites may be handled in an analogous fashion to the aggregated case.

Non-rare aggregated data may also be analysed using the above logistic regression framework.

9.5.3 Point process methods

The above approaches may be motivated from a point process perspective (Diggle 1990; Diggle and Rowlingson 1994; Diggle *et al.* 1997; Wakefield and Elliott 1999). Diggle (1990) proposes an inhomogeneous Poisson point process model for the distribution of a disease around a single point source as follows. Consider an inhomogeneous Poisson point process with intensity $\lambda_0(\boldsymbol{x})$ to model the distribution of the population at risk. Let the distribution of the cases be modelled by an inhomogeneous Poisson point process with intensity $\lambda_1(\boldsymbol{x})$, which is modelled as a function of the background intensity;

$$\lambda_1(\boldsymbol{x}) = \rho\lambda_0(\boldsymbol{x})\{1 + g(d, \boldsymbol{\phi})\}. \tag{9.18}$$

In (9.18), ρ represents a scaling factor and $g(\cdot, \cdot)$ is a parametric function of distance to the source describing the elevation in risk. Diggle (1990) estimates $\lambda_0(\boldsymbol{x})$ from a set of controls using a Gaussian kernel estimator and uses this estimate in a parametric maximum likelihood based estimation approach. There are a number of drawbacks of this model: uncertainty concerning the number of degrees of freedom to use in the likelihood ratio test; lack of flexibility in choices for $g(\cdot, \cdot)$; and sensitivity to the choice of smoothing parameter used to estimate the intensity $\lambda_0(x)$.

Bithell (1990, 1992) and Lawson (1993) have used kernel density estimation in the context of assessing risk in the vicinity of a pre-specified source. As noted above, however, the choice of smoothing parameter is vital, but these methods may be viewed as useful exploratory tools. When kernel surfaces are examined it is also important to consider the variance of this surface. Kelsall and Diggle (1995*a,b*) describe how tolerance intervals may be calculated.

9.5.4 Bayesian methods

Inference for the models described in Sections 9.5.1 and 9.5.2 may be carried out in a Bayesian framework by specifying a prior distribution for the unknown parameters. Wakefield and Morris (2000) consider the Poisson models of Section 9.5.1, induce overdispersion via the introduction of random effects (see Chapter 7) in the spirit of disease mapping and introduce a class of prior distributions. We refer the reader to Wakefield and Morris (2000) for further details. It should be noted, however, that the priors for γ and ρ may be taken to be relatively flat but those on the elements of ϕ are far more important, reflecting the lack of information in the likelihood function (see Section 9.6). The random effects may also be used for model assessment, in particular to assess the adequacy of the assumed distance/risk model. Diggle *et al.* (2000) consider matched data from a Bayesian perspective and combine the conditional likelihood with a prior distribution.

For the Bayesian approach, closed-form solutions are not available. Wakefield and Morris (2000) and Diggle *et al.* (2000) use a Markov chain Monte Carlo (MCMC) approach to generate samples from the posterior distribution (Gilks *et al.* 1996). This is more computationally expensive than likelihood-based approaches but does allow straightforward inference for functions of interest such as the distance/risk relationship. All of the models in this section may be analysed within a Bayesian framework using MCMC; in particular the BUGS software (Spiegelhalter *et al.* 1996) may be used.

9.6   Illustrative example

In a recent study, the incidence of specific cancers in relation to proximity to municipal solid waste incinerators in Great Britain was examined (Elliott *et al.* 1996). Here, we consider stomach cancer incidence data from a single site in order to illustrate a number of the techniques that we have described. In this example we only have the total disease counts and the expected numbers, by census enumeration district (ED), which contain on average approximately 400 people. In particular, we do not have the constituent cases and populations broken down by age and sex and so a number of approaches (e.g. direct standardisation) cannot be illustrated. Hence, our analysis should not be viewed as definitive. We have two sets of expected numbers; one adjusted for age and sex and the other for age, sex, and the Carstairs deprivation score (Carstairs and Morris 1991). This score is continuous and is a function of the four census variables overcrowding, access to a car, social class of head of household, and unemployment, available at the ED level. In what follows we adjust for deprivation within the regression in the parametric approaches, and within the expected numbers (using quintiles) for all other approaches (reference rates were taken from the health region within which the incinerator was situated). The study period was 1974–86; in the full study a ten-year lag was used from when the site became operable. Population data were obtained from the 1981 census.

Figure 9.1 shows some preliminary plots of the data. Figure 9.1(a) shows the locations of the 44 ED centroids with the smaller circles at each ED centroid indicating the relative size of the expected numbers in that ED. The location of the source is the origin. The two concentric circles have radius 3 km and 7.5 km. Figure 9.1(b) shows the SMRs plotted against distance. The solid line denotes a local (lowess) smoother with span 0.67 (and similarly for Fig. 9.1(c) and (d)), and the broken line denotes a relative risk of one. Figure 9.1(c) shows the deprivation score plotted against distance. The solid line denotes a lowess smooth with span 2/3. Figure 9.1(d) shows the relationship between raw risk and the deprivation score. Solid and broken lines are as in panel (b). We see that with the obvious interpretation of the distance/risk/deprivation relationship, deprivation is a true confounder. We now describe a number of analyses of these data.

Near versus reference
We chose the near region to consist of the 31 EDs with centroids within 3 km of the incinerator; this region contained 66 observed and 49.8 expected counts giving an SMR

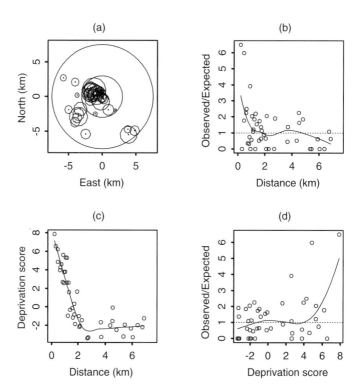

Fig. 9.1 Preliminary plots for the stomach cancer incidence data (see text for details).

of 1.33. The choice of 3 km is somewhat arbitrary but was thought a priori to correspond to a region within which the effect of emissions would be observed. The asymptotic standard error of this SMR is 0.16 indicating moderate evidence of an elevated risk, relative to the reference region, in the near region.

Near versus far

The far region was chosen to be 7.5 km as this would produce a region that was large enough for comparative purposes and did not contain other putative hazards. This region contained 19 observed and 21.4 expected cases in 13 EDs. The SMR of the far region was 0.89 with asymptotic standard error 0.20, providing no evidence that risk differs from that in the reference region. The exact Poisson test in Section 9.3.2 has a significance level of 0.0739. The sensitivity of the near versus far comparisons is illustrated by reanalysis using a near/far threshold of 0.5 km. Now the inner region consists of 4 EDs giving 21 observed cases and 5.4 expected cases, and the outer of 40 EDs, 64 observed cases and 65.7 expected cases. The exact test now rejects the null with $p < 0.001$.

Besag and Newell method

We implemented this method with $k = 4, 6, 8, 10$. Table 9.2 gives the results; the expected numbers E_i^* have been adjusted, via (9.9), so that the sum of the observed is equal to the sum of the expected. There are 10 cases in the first ED, giving $I = 1$ for each value of k used. We see highly significant results for $k \geq 6$. We note that for these data the majority of the data are never used since there is a concentration of cases close to the source.

Stone's test

We have implemented Stone's test in two ways, using either EDs or a small set of concentric bands. In the case of the band-based analysis we have used the band limits suggested by Shaddick and Elliott (1996). Table 9.3 shows the observed and expected numbers in each band as well as the crude risk ratios and the estimated risks $\hat{\theta}_i$ under the monotonicity constraint. The table shows a marked drop in risk between the first band and the rest. Both unconditional and conditional tests imply that there is a significant decline in risk as distance to the source increases; all tests (both at ED level and band level) give a *p*-value of 0.001 based on 999 simulations from the appropriate null hypothesis.

Figures 9.2(a) and (b) show the Monte Carlo-based confidence intervals on the estimated relative risk function calculated from data at ED and band level, respectively.

Table 9.2 Number of cases of k and resulting *p*-values for the method of Besag and Newell for the stomach cancer data

k	*p*-value using E_i	*p*-value using E_i^*
4	0.0939	0.150
6	0.00811	0.0179
8	0.000395	0.00123
10	1.23×10^{-5}	5.41×10^{-5}

Table 9.3 Stone's (unconditional) test on eight bands around the source

y_i	E_i	Band (km)	y_i/E_i	$\hat{\theta}_i$
21	5.41	0.5	3.881	3.881
11	14.77	1.0	0.745	1.061
28	22.25	2.0	1.258	1.061
6	7.33	3.0	0.818	1.061
11	8.42	4.6	1.307	1.061
3	5.20	5.7	0.577	0.618
1	4.23	6.7	0.236	0.618
4	3.51	7.5	1.138	0.618

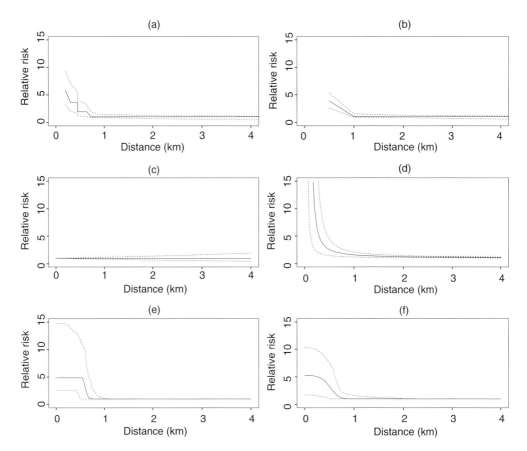

Fig. 9.2 Estimated relative risk function with interval estimates based on six different approaches: (a) Stone's test on 44 EDs, (b) Stone's test on eight bands, (c) Poisson regression linear in d_i, (d) Poisson regression linear in d_i^{-1}, (e) non-linear Poisson regression (full model), and (f) non-linear Bayesian Poisson regression. In panels (a) and (b) adjustment for deprivation is carried out within the expected numbers, in (c)–(f) via regression. See text for further details.

Dotted lines are the pointwise 2.5% and 97.5% points of 1000 simulations from the fitted model, given by the solid line. Plots are truncated at a distance of 4 km for clarity.

Score test

The observed value of the test statistic given by (9.10), with $w_i = d_i$, is 6.43. Using the chi-squared approximation gives a significance level of 0.011. We also used $w_i = 1/\text{rank}_i$ which gave a value of 35.9 for the test statistic and $p < 0.001$.

Linear risk score test

We have used scores based on $1/d_i$, $1/d_i^2$, $1/\text{rank}_i$ and the reciprocal of the square root of the rank. The unconditional tests based on 999 simulations from the Poisson distribution all gave simulated values of the test statistic less than the observed value, giving $p = 0.001$. We then applied the conditional test, simulating from the multinomial distribution. The same p-values were obtained, indicating that the increase in risk is a genuine trend, not just an overall decrease or increase in risk.

Poisson regression

Table 9.4 displays the result of fitting five models for the log relative risk $\log \theta_i$ in terms of a constant α, a deprivation score z_i, and the distance d_i. Deviance differences are with respect to model 1, the baseline model adjusting for deprivation. As expected, deprivation appears to significantly improve the fit. Of the distance-based models, $w_i = d_i^{-1}$ provides the greatest improvement. The large values of the residual deviance compared with the number of degrees of freedom in the model indicate extra-Poisson variation. The confidence intervals for β in models 3 and 4 do not include zero, providing evidence of increased risk.

To accommodate extra-Poisson variation we use the quasi-likelihood approach described in Section 9.2.2; for model 3 the estimate of the overdispersion parameter κ is 1.23. Note that no estimate of precision is available on this. Acknowledgement of the overdispersion can be made by multiplying the standard errors in Table 9.4 by $\kappa^{1/2}$; similarly deviance differences may be divided by κ. Figures 9.2(c) and 9.2(d) show the fitted relative risk/distance relationship, i.e. $\exp(\beta d_i)$. The broken lines represent asymptotic 95% confidence intervals (without adjustment for overdispersion). We see that using $w_i = d_i$ provides a very unrealistic assessment and the $w_i = d_i^{-1}$ model gives exceedingly wide confidence intervals close to source. Figure 9.3(a) shows standardised residuals from model 3 plotted against distance; no obvious trend is apparent.

Non-linear Poisson regression

Deviance differences and parameter values from fitting the null, step and full models are given in Diggle *et al.* (1997) along with Monte Carlo standard errors. Chi-squared tests comparing the deviances with that of the null model conclude that the full model provides the better fit. Figure 9.2(e) shows the fitted function $g(\cdot, \cdot)$ on the relative risk scale. The major difference between Fig. 9.2(d) and 9.2(e) is the estimated point and interval estimates close to source. A Monte Carlo 95% interval is denoted by the broken lines. Figure 9.3(b) shows the standardised residuals plotted against distance for the full model. Compared with Fig. 9.3(a) they indicate that the non-linear model provides a slightly improved fit. Diggle *et al.* (1997) estimated the overdispersion parameter κ to be

Table 9.4 Results from the log-linear model. First row of each section gives parameter estimates, second row gives estimated standard errors in parentheses. Deviance differences are with respect to model 1

Model	$\log \theta_i$	Parameters α	γ	β	Residual deviance	Df	Deviance difference w.r.t. model 1
0	α	0.169 (0.108)			80.86	43	-14.42
1	$\alpha + \gamma z_i$	0.012 (0.125)	0.132 (0.034)		66.44	42	$-$
2	$\alpha + \gamma z_i + \beta d_i$	0.064 (0.276)	0.124 (0.051)	-0.019 (0.0911)	66.40	41	0.04
3	$\alpha + \gamma z_i + \beta / d_i$	-0.294 (0.157)	-0.020 (0.0589)	0.472 (0.139)	55.52	41	10.92
4	$\alpha + \gamma z_i + \beta / \mathrm{rank}_i$	-0.102 (0.129)	0.030 (0.048)	1.784 (0.548)	56.72	41	9.72

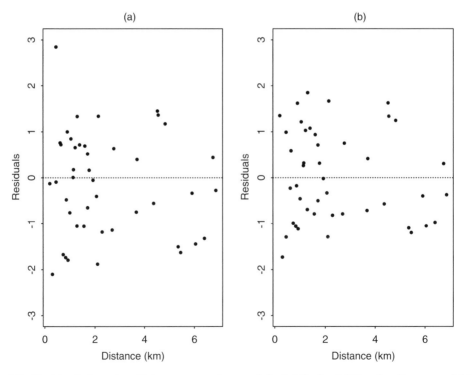

Fig. 9.3 Residuals from two Poisson regression models: (a) the best-fitting log-linear model in $1/d_i$ and (b) the full non-linear model.

approximately unity for the full model. Parameter estimates and standard errors (given in parentheses) for α, β, and δ are given by: 3.851 (3.707), 0.089 (0.113), and 0.531 (0.137), respectively.

Bayesian Poisson regression

Finally, we consider a Bayesian approach, implemented via MCMC. The Markov chain was given a 'burn-in' of 1000 iterations and then 30 000 samples were collected for inference. We consider the model (9.14) of Diggle *et al.* (1997). For α and δ the priors were uniform on the ranges $(-1, 10)$ and $(0, 3)$, respectively; the prior for β is more complicated being constructed to induce negative dependence between β and δ, see Wakefield and Morris (2000) for details. Figure 9.2(f) shows the fitted function $g(\cdot, \cdot)$ along with a 95% credible interval. When one compares the risk at source with the prior $\alpha \sim U(-1, 10)$ it is clear that there is very little information in the likelihood about the form of the distance/risk relationship close to source. Wakefield and Morris (1999) also consider a predictive distribution of the number of cases that would occur over a specified period of time, given a particular population size and age-sex distribution, at different distances from source.

Conclusion

We first note that this dataset was selected to provide an interesting example (there being an increased relative risk near the source). Each of the methods suggests a statistically significant increase in risk at source. Using inverse distance as exposure and the additive full model (with inference from a likelihood or Bayesian perspective) suggests that the increased risk extends approximately 1 km from source. There are clearly insufficient data (and no biological hypothesis) to predict accurately the form of the distance/risk relationship close to source. The Bayesian approach allows a subjective upper bound to be placed on the excess at source α, though care must be taken in its choice.

9.7 Concluding remarks

A major weakness of the majority of point-source studies is the lack of an adequate exposure measure. The ultimate gold standard would be to obtain for each individual the lifelong dose from a putative source but this is unachievable in practice. The best that one could hope for is perhaps the monitoring of personal exposure (Chapter 20) for individuals in a case-control study although this would only reflect current exposures, and some sort of modelling procedure (either explicit or assumed) would be needed to deal with historical exposures. For a routine enquiry it is feasible to obtain an exposure surface via the use of, for example, dispersion modelling (Chapter 21) or by the modelling of a complete surface from a network of monitors (Chapter 10). Area- or individual-level exposures may then be assigned on the basis of this surface, perhaps accounting for the non-exactness of these measures using errors-in-variables models (Fuller 1987; Carroll *et al.* 1995; Chapter 5). In this case, other data limitations such as inaccuracies in the health and population data should not be forgotten; the need for high quality data cannot be overstressed.

It is clear that an estimation approach to investigation is preferable to a simple hypothesis test; the contentious issue is whether the data are of sufficient quality and abundance to allow such an approach to be successfully carried out, given the small increases in risk often encountered and the localised effect. Data from multiple sites obviously leads to greater information on the location/risk surface. It is more likely that the data will be amenable to explicit modelling when a more rigorous epidemiological study (as opposed to a public or media motivated study) is carried out. In this case, the data are likely to be of higher quality and a better exposure variable may be available. When a parametric form is assumed for the risk surface, it is vital to consider the appropriateness of this surface via diagnostics.

Whether a testing or an estimation approach is taken, the reason for the selection of the sites is vital for interpretation. Simulating the statistical procedure under this selection mechanism and under a model of constant risk to all study individuals would allow the observed statistical analysis to be placed in proper context, but it is rare that the mechanism will ever be known in a particular case.

At this time, it would not be appropriate to recommend a single method for point-source studies, although estimation methods clearly give the most information. The methods of Section 9.3, and that of Besag and Newell, are straightforward to implement and provide a first look at the data. One of the test methods (Stone's score and LRS) may then be used to assess the null hypothesis of no association between risk and proximity to source, though more work is required to determine the power of these tests under specific alternatives. The interpretation of the resultant p-value is also not straightforward. In general, the size of a p-value has to be judged with reference to 'sample size' (here, the expected number of cases). One approach that has been advocated is to carry out an estimation procedure only when the null hypothesis of a constant location/risk relationship has been rejected. This two-stage approach is pragmatic but the pre-selection test mechanism leads to the optimal properties of estimators (e.g. unbiasedness) no longer being valid. It is straightforward to carry out estimation for all studies with a generalised linear model (with 1/distance or 1/rank), as long as care is taken when reporting the conclusions. In our experience, care should be taken when the non-regular models (9.13) and (9.14) are utilised; the likelihood surface of the alternative (9.17) is more straightforward to report. At this point there is a shortage of real studies and more experience is therefore required. There is, however, a clear need for continued methodological developments in order to extract the maximum information from the available data. Ultimately, interpretation and possible public health 'action' will not be determined by the statistical analysis alone, but it is important that they are informed by the best possible information that the data will allow.

Acknowledgement

This work was supported, in part, by an equipment grant from the Wellcome Trust (0455051/Z/95/Z).

References

Barlow, R. E., Bartholomew, D. J., Bremner, J. M., and Brunk, H. D. (1972). *Statistical inference under order restrictions: the theory and application of isotonic regression.* Wiley, New York.
Berger, J. O. and Sellke, T. (1987). Testing a point null hypothesis: the irreconcilibility of p-values and evidence (with discussion). *Journal of the American Statistical Association*, **82**, 112–39.

Besag, J. and Newell, J. (1991). The detection of clusters in rare diseases. *Journal of the Royal Statistical Society, Series A*, **154**, 143–55.

Best, N. and Wakefield, J. C. (1999). Accounting for inaccuracies in population counts and case registration in cancer mapping studies. *Journal of the Royal Statistical Society, Series A*, **162**, 363–82.

Biggeri, A., Barbone, F., Lagazio, C., Bovenzi, M., and Stanta, G. (1996). Air pollution and lung cancer in Trieste, Italy: spatial analysis of risk as a function of distance from source. *Environmental Health Perspectives*, **104**, 750–4.

Bithell, J. F. (1990). An application of density estimation to geographical epidemiology. *Statistics in Medicine*, **9**, 691–701.

Bithell, J. F. (1992). Statistical methods for analysing point-source exposures. In *Geographical and environmental epidemiology: methods for small area studies* (P. Elliott, J. Cuzick, D. English, and R. Stern, ed.), 221–30. Oxford University Press.

Bithell, J. F. (1995). The choice of test for detecting raised disease risk near a point source. *Statistics in Medicine*, **14**, 2309–22.

Bithell, J. F., and Stone, R. A. (1989). On statistical methods for analysing the geographical distribution of cancer cases near nuclear installations. *Journal of Epidemiology and Community Health*, **43**, 79–85.

Bithell, J. F., Dutton, S. J., Draper, G. J., and Neary, N. M. (1994). Distribution of childhood leukaemias and non-Hodgkin's lymphomas near nuclear installations in England and Wales. *British Medical Journal*, **309**, 501–5.

Breslow, N. E. (1996). Statistics in epidemiology: The case-control study. In *Advances in biometry* (P. Armitage and H. A. David, ed.). Wiley, New York.

Breslow, N. E. and Day, N. E. (1980). *Statistical methods in cancer research*. Vol. I: *The analysis of case-control studies*, IARC Scientific Publications. 32. International Agency for Research on Cancer, Lyon.

Breslow, N. E. and Day, N. E. (1987). *Statistical methods in cancer research*. Vol. II: *The analysis of cohort studies*, IARC Scientific Publications. 82. International Agency for Research on Cancer, Lyon.

Breslow, N. E., Lubis, J. H., Marek, P., and Langholz, B. (1983). Multiplicative models and cohort analysis. *Journal of the American Statistical Association*, **78**, 1–12.

Carroll, R. J., Ruppert, D., and Stefanski, L. A. (1995). *Measurement error in nonlinear models*. Chapman and Hall, London.

Carstairs, V. and Morris, R. (1991). *Deprivation and health in Scotland*. Aberdeen, Aberdeen University Press.

Clayton, D. and Hills, M. (1993). *Statistical models in epidemiology*. Oxford University Press.

Cook-Mozaffari, P., Darby, S., and Doll, R. (1989*a*). Cancer near potential sites of nuclear installations. *Lancet*, 1145–7.

Cook-Mozaffari, P., Darby, S., Doll, R., Forman, D., Hermon, C., Pike, M. C. *et al.* (1989*b*). Geographical variation in mortality from leukaemia and other cancers in England and Wales in relation to proximity to nuclear installations, 1969–78. *British Journal of Cancer*, **59**, 476–85.

Cox, D. R. and Hinkley, D. V. (1974). *Theoretical statistics*. Chapman and Hall, London.

Craft, A. W. and Birch, J. M. (1983). Childhood cancer in Cumbria. *Lancet*, **2**, 1299.

Cuzick, J. and Edwards, R. (1990). Spatial clustering for inhomogeneous populations (with discussion). *Journal of the Royal Statistical Society, Series B*, **52**, 73–104.

Cuzick, J. and Edwards, R. (1996). Cuzick-Edwards one-sample and inverse two-sampling statistics. In *Methods for investigating localized clustering of disease* (F. E. Alexander and P. Boyle, ed.), 200–2, IARC Scientific Publications 135. International Agency for Research on Cancer, Lyon.

Diggle, P. J. (1990). A point process modelling approach to raised incidence of a rare phenomenon in the vicinity of a pre-specified point. *Journal of the Royal Statistical Society, Series A*, **153**, 349–62.

Diggle, P. J. and Elliott, P. (1995). Statistical issues in the analysis of disease risk near point sources using individual or spatially aggregated data. *Journal of Epidemiology and Community Health*, **49**, S20–S27.

Diggle, P. J. and Rowlingson, B. S. (1994). A conditional approach to point process modelling of raised incidence. *Journal of the Royal Statistical Society, Series A*, **157**, 433–40.

Diggle, P. J., Morris, S. E., Elliott, P., and Shaddick, G. (1997). Regression modelling of disease risk in relation to point sources. *Journal of the Royal Statistical Society, Series A*, **160**, 491–505.

Diggle, P. J., Morris, S. E., and Wakefield, J. C. (2000). Point source modelling using matched case-control data. *Biostatistics*, **1**, 89–105.

Diggle, P. J., Morris, S. E., and Morton-Jones, A. (1999). Case-control isotonic regression for investigation of elevation in risk around a point source. *Statistics in Medicine*, **18**, 1605–13.

Dolk, H., Elliott, P., Shaddick, G., Walls, P., and Thakrar, B. (1997a). Cancer incidence near radio and television transmitters in Great Britain: All high power transmitters. *American Journal of Epidemiology*, **145**, 10–17.

Dolk, H., Shaddick, G., Walls, P., Grundy, C., Thakrar, B., Kleinschmidt, I. *et al.* (1997b). Cancer incidence near radio and television transmitters in Great Britain: Sutton Coldfield transmitter. *American Journal of Epidemiology*, **145**, 1–9.

Dolk, H., Vrijheid, M., Armstrong, B., Abramsky, L., Bianche, F., Garne, E. *et al.* (1998). Risk of congenital anomalies near hazardous-waste landfill sites in Europe: The EUROHAZCON study. *Lancet*, **352**, 423–7.

Dolk, H., Vrijheid, M., Armstrong, B. and the EUROHAZCON Collaborative Group (1999). Congenital anomalies near hazardous waste landfill sites in Europe. In *Disease mapping and risk assessment* (A. B. Lawson, ed.). Wiley, New York.

Elliott, P., Cuzick, J., English, D., and Stern, R. (1992a). *Geographical and environmental epidemiology: methods for small-area studies*. Oxford University Press.

Elliott, P., Hills, M., Beresford, J., Kleinschmidt, I., Jolley, D., Pattenden *et al.* (1992b). Incidence of cancer of the larynx and lung near incinerators of waste solvents and oils in Great Britain. *Lancet*, **339**, 854–8.

Elliott, P., Martuzzi, M. and Shaddick, G. (1995). Spatial statistical methods in environmental epidemiology: a critique. *Statistical Methods in Medical Research*, **4**, 139–61.

Elliott, P., Shaddick, G., Kleinschmidt, I., Jolley, D., Walls, P., Beresford, J. *et al.* (1996). Cancer incidence near municipal solid waste incinerators in Great Britain. *British Journal of Cancer*, **73**, 702–10.

Fuller, W. A. (1987). *Measurement error models*. Wiley, New York.

Gardner, M. J. (1992). Childhood leukaemia around the Sellafield nuclear plant. In *Geographical and environmental epidemiology: methods for small-area studies* (P. Elliott, J. Cuzick, D. English, and R. Stern, ed.), 209–309, Oxford University Press.

Gardner, M. J. and Winter, P. D. (1984). Mortality in Cumberland during 1959–78 with reference to cancer in young people around Windscale. *Lancet*, **1**, 216–17.

Gardner, M. J., Snee, M. P., Hall, A. J., Powell, C. A., Downes, S., and Terrell, J. D. (1990a). Results of case-control study of leukaemia and lymphoma among young people near Sellafield nuclear plant in West Cumbria. *British Medical Journal*, **300**, 423–39.

Gardner, M. J., Snee, M. P., Hall, A. J., Powell, C. A., Downes, S., and Terrell, J. D. (1990b). Methods and basic data of case-control study of leukaemia and lymphoma among young people near Sellafield nuclear plant in West Cumbria. *British Medical Journal*, **300**, 433–9.

Gart, J. J. and Tarone, R. E. (1983). The relation between score tests and approximate tests in exponential models common in biometry. *Biometrics*, **39**, 781–6.

Gilks, W. R., Richardson, S., and Spiegelhalter, D. J. (1996). *Markov chain Monte Carlo in practice*. Chapman and Hall, London.

Greenland, S. and Morgenstern, H. (1989). Ecological bias, confounding, and effect modification. *International Journal of Epidemiology*, **18**, 269–74.

Hastie, T. J. and Tibshirani, R. J. (1990). *Generalized additive models*. Chapman and Hall, London.

Hills, M. and Alexander, F. (1989). Statistical methods used in assessing the risk of disease near a point source of possible environmental pollution: a review. *Journal of the Royal Statistical Society, Series A*, **152**, 353–63.

Jolley, D., Jarman, B., and Elliott, P. (1992). Socio-economic confounding. In *Geographical and environmental epidemiology: methods for small-area studies* (P. Elliott, J. Cuzick, D. English, and R. Stern, ed.), 115–24. Oxford University Press.

Kelsall, J. E. and Diggle, P. J. (1995a). Kernel estimation of relative risk. *Bernoulli*, **1**, 3–16.

Kelsall, J. E. and Diggle, P. J. (1995b). Nonparametric estimation of spatial variation in relative risk. *Statistics in Medicine*, **14**, 2335–42.

Lawson, A. B. (1993). On the analysis of mortality events associated with a prespecified fixed point. *Journal of the Royal Statistical Society, Series A*, **156**, 363–77.

Lawson, A. B. and Williams, F. L. R. (1994). Armadale: a case study in environmental epidemiology. *Journal of the Royal Statistical Society, Series A*, **157**, 285–98.

Li, C.-Y., Thériault, G., and Lin, R. S. (1996). Epidemiological appraisal of studies of residential exposure to power frequency magnetic fields and adult cancers. *Occupational and Environmental Medicine*, **53**, 505–10.

Livingstone, A. E., Shaddick, G., Grundy, C., and Elliott, P. (1996). Do people living near inner city main roads have more asthma needing treatment? Case-control study. *British Medical Journal*, **312**, 676–77.

Marshall, R. J. (1991). A review of methods for the statistical analysis of spatial patterns of disease. *Journal of the Royal Statistical Society, Series A*, **154**, 421–41.

McCullagh, P. and Nelder, J. A. (1989). *Generalised linear models* (2nd edn). Chapman and Hall, London.

Morton-Jones, T., Diggle, P., and Elliott, P. (1999). Investigation of excess environmental risk around putative sources: Stone's test with covariate adjustment. *Statistics in Medicine*, **18**, 189–97.

Newell, J. N. and Besag, J. E. (1996). The detection of small-area database anomalies. In *Methods for investigating localized clustering of disease* (F. E. Alexander and P. Boyle, ed.), 88–100, IARC Scientific Publications. 135. International Agency for Research on Cancer, Lyon.

Openshaw, S., Charlton, M., Wymer, C., and Craft, A. W. (1987). A mark I geographical analysis machine for the automated analysis of point data sets. *International Journal of Geographical Information Systems*, **1**, 335–58.

Openshaw, S., Charlton, M., Craft, A. W. and Birch, J. M. (1988). Investigation of leukaemia clusters by the use of a geographical analysis machine. *Lancet*, 272–3.

Robertson, T., Wright, F. T., and Dykstra, R. L. (1988). *Order restricted statistical inference*. Wiley, New York.

Sans, S., Elliott, P., Kleinschmidt, I., Shaddick, G., Pattenden, S., Walls, P. *et al.* (1995). Cancer incidence and mortality near the Baglan Bay petrochemical works, South Wales. *Occupational and Environmental Medicine*, **52**, 217–24.

Severini, T. A. (1999). On the effect of overdispersion on exact conditional tests. *Journal of the Royal Statistical Society, Series B*, **61**, 115–26.

Shaddick, G. and Elliott, P. (1996). Use of Stone's method in studies of disease risk around point sources of environmental pollution. *Statistics in Medicine*, **15**, 1927–34.

Spiegelhalter, D. J., Thomas, A., Best, N. and Gilks, W. R. (1996). *BUGS: Bayesian inference using Gibbs sampling, Version 5.0*. Medical Research Council Biostatistics Unit, Cambridge.

Stone, R. A. (1988). Investigations of excess environmental risks around putative sources: Statistical problems and a proposed test. *Statistics in Medicine*, **7**, 649–60.

Stone, R. A. (1990). Spatial clustering for inhomogeneous populations (discussion of the paper by Cuzick and Edwards). *Journal of the Royal Statistical Society, Series B*, **52**, 101–2.

Tango, T. (1995). A class of tests for detecting 'general' and 'focused' clustering of rare diseases. *Statistics in Medicine*, **14**, 2323–34.

Tarone, R. E. (1982). The use of historical control information in testing for a trend in Poisson means. *Biometrics*, **38**, 457–62.

Turnbull, B. W., Iwano, E. J., Burnett, W. S., Howe, H. L., and Clark, L. C. (1990). Monitoring for clustering of disease: application to leukaemia incidence in upstate New York. *American Journal of Epidemiology*, **132**(Suppl.), S136–43.

Viel, J. F., Pobel, D., and Carré, A. (1995). Incidence of leukaemia in young people around the La Hague nuclear waste reprocessing plant: A sensitivity analysis. *Statistics in Medicine*, **14**, 2459–72.

Wakefield, J. C. and Elliott, P. (1999). Issues in the statistical analysis of small-area health data. *Statistics in Medicine*, **18**, 2377–99.

Wakefield, J. C. and Morris, S. E. (1999). Spatial dependence and errors-in-variables in environmental epidemiology. In *Bayesian statistics 6*. (J. M. Bernardo, J. O. Berger, A. P. David, and A. F. M. Smith, eds.), 657–84, Oxford University Press.

Wakefield, J. C. and Morris, S. E. (2000). The Bayesian modelling of disease risk in relation to a point source. Under review for *The Journal of the American Statistical Association*.

Waller, L. A. (1996). Statistical power and design of focussed clustering studies. *Statistics in Medicine*, **15**, 765–82.

Waller, L. A. and Lawson, A. B. (1995). The power of focussed tests to detect disease clustering. *Statistics in Medicine*, **14**, 2291–2308.

Waller, L. A. and Poquette, C. (1999). The power of focused score tests under mis-specified cluster models. In *Disease mapping and risk assessment* (A. B. Lawson, ed.). Wiley, New York.

Waller, L. A., Turnbull, B. W., Clark, L. C., and Nasca, P. (1992). Chronic disease surveillance and testing of clustering of disease and exposure: application to leukaemia incidence and TCE-contaminated dumpsites in upstate New York. *Environmetrics*, **3**, 281–300.

Waller, L. A., Turnbull, B. W., Clark, L. C., and Nasca, P. (1994). Spatial pattern analyses to detect rare disease clusters. In *Case studies in biometry* (N. Lange and L. Ryan, ed.), 3–23, Wiley, New York.

Wilkinson, P., Thakrar, B., Shaddick, G., Stevenson, S., Pattenden, S., Landon, M. *et al.* (1997). Cancer incidence around the Pan Britannica Industries pesticide factory, Waltham Abbey. *Occupational and Environmental Medicine*, **54**, 101–7.

10. Geostatistical methods for mapping environmental exposures

N. Cressie

10.1 Introduction

The agricultural and manufacturing sectors have traditionally dealt with waste by sending it downstream or into the air, in the hope that it will become diluted in the environment. However, it has become apparent that long-term exposure to even quite small doses of toxic substances (e.g. lead, mercury, PCBs) can have enormously harmful effects on flora and fauna, in particular on health effects. Industrial and urban development have produced growth and prosperity, but at a cost.

Harmful by-products disposed of indiscriminately can threaten neighbourhoods (e.g. the Love Canal residential area in upstate New York, built on a toxic chemical disposal site in the 1960s), communities (e.g. the Three Mile Island nuclear reactor leak in the 1970s), or whole regions (e.g. the Chernobyl nuclear reactor meltdown in the former Soviet Union in the 1980s). Obviously, there is increasing development and a growing population on a planet of fixed size and finite resources. The discovery, characterisation, and remediation of environmental damage require detailed spatial understanding and, in the characterisation phase, maps of exposures are an important component.

The aim of this chapter is to introduce the reader to some spatial statistical methods for mapping environmental exposures. The resultant map may be of interest in its own right, or it may provide the relevant information for a study on the health effects of the exposure. Geostatistical methods are particularly well suited to problems where monitoring data, possibly from different instruments, are distributed throughout a region of interest and the goal is to obtain the best map of the environmental exposure over the whole region. Parts of Chapter 6 also discuss this methodology with regard to disease mapping. Geostatistics' origins are in mining (France), meteorology (former Soviet Union), and time series analysis (UK), although it has been the French terminology due to Matheron (1963) that has persisted; see Cressie (1990) for an historical account.

The outline of this chapter is as follows. In Section 10.2, we motivate environmental-exposure mapping with a problem of great current interest in the USA and Europe, namely exposure to *particulate matter*. Section 10.3 discusses a number of approaches for obtaining exposure estimates at specific locations based on what we term 'naive' and smoothing methods, while in Section 10.4 geostatistical approaches are described. A detailed account of a particularly useful method, *ordinary kriging*, is presented in this section. In Section 10.5 we return to the particulate matter example in order to illustrate ordinary kriging.

Section 10.6 describes a fully parametric *hierarchical modelling* approach that has recently been developed in a geostatistical context and a discussion of related issues, including aggregation and disaggregation, is given in Section 10.5.

10.2   Illustrative example

In this chapter, we shall use the study of particulate matter (PM) to motivate the need for mapping of environmental exposures. *Particulate matter* is a generic term for a broad class of chemically and physically diverse substances that exist as either solids or liquid droplets; PM_{10} is defined by the United States Environmental Protection Agency (EPA) to be, 'particulate matter with an aerodynamic diameter less than or equal to a nominal 10 micrometers'. The EPA is involved with setting *particulate matter* regulations to ensure that its presence in ambient air is not dangerous to human health.

Numerous studies have been conducted to investigate the acute effects of air pollution on health; see Dockery and Pope (1997) for a review. Typical studies are described, for example, in Schwartz (1994), Pope *et al.* (1995), Seaton *et al.* (1995), and Styer *et al.* (1995). Health data that have been used in these studies include daily mortality counts and measures of morbidity in a variety of towns and cities across Europe and the US (with a variety of meteorological conditions and levels of different pollutants). In a typical study, non-accidental deaths in the over 65-year-olds are health endpoints of interest, and as many as twelve meteorological variables (e.g. pressure, temperature, humidity) have been included in some of the studies. Monitoring stations distributed around the study area deliver irregularly-spaced spatial data and daily temporal data on PM_{10}. Based on regression analyses and on health considerations, the US daily regulatory PM_{10} level has been set by the EPA at $150\,\mu g/m^3$.

A common feature of these epidemiological studies is that the spatial component has been removed by aggregation over the region of interest (often, the pollution level is taken to be a simple average over a number of monitors), leaving the possibility that conclusions are subject to ecological bias (see Chapter 11). Moreover, there is a need to know if certain sub-regions are in more danger of *particulate matter* contamination than others. Thus, a spatial analysis is needed to ensure 'environmental justice' for those who live in neighbourhoods whose spatial locations put them at risk of higher environmental exposures (e.g. downwind from a coal-burning power plant).

We now introduce briefly the data that will be used to motivate our discussion. Figure 10.1 shows a map of 26 air quality monitoring locations in the Pittsburgh area. The map is centred on downtown Pittsburgh and extends about 32 km in each of the compass directions. At the scale of the problem, the Earth's surface can be approximated to be flat and the units on each axis are given in miles. Site identifiers are written beside the locations; it is not known why there are site identifiers ranging from 2 to 9002 for only 26 sites. For illustrative purposes, we have chosen a particular day (day 226) in 1996 upon which to do a spatial analysis. On this day, there were 22 of the 26 monitoring locations reporting; these are marked by a ($\times$) on Fig. 10.1. The analysis we give should be viewed as illustrative, given the small number of data. One could attempt to validate the analysis using spatial data from other nearby days.

Geostatistical approaches to the modelling of air pollution surfaces have been considered by, for example, Brown *et al.* (1994) and Lajaunie (1984).

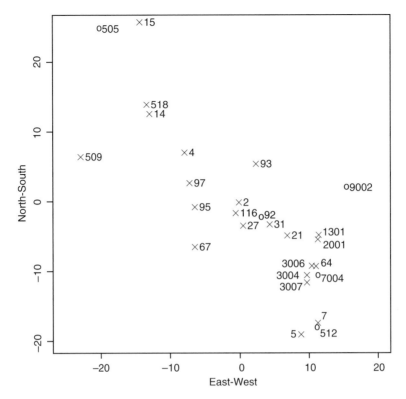

Fig. 10.1 Map of particulate matter monitoring stations ($\times$ and $\circ$) in a region around Pittsburgh, PA, USA ($\times$ denotes sites that recorded an observation on 13 August 1996). Units on both axes are miles.

In the next two sections we will describe a number of techniques for predicting the value of an unknown random variable (the exposure, in the context considered here) at specific locations. In general, we are not interested in a point estimate alone; a measure of the uncertainty attached to this estimate is also important. This is particularly true if one wants to link a health outcome to the prediction; unless the exposure is measured or predicted without error (which is never the case), we need to formulate the outcome/exposure model via an errors-in-variables approach, which requires information concerning the accuracy of the explanatory exposure variable (see Chapter 5).

10.3   Naive and smoothing methods

10.3.1   Basics

The structure of this section is as follows. We first introduce some basic notation and then, in Section 10.3.2, we discuss prediction methods that are essentially *ad hoc* techniques, while in 10.3.3 we concentrate on spline methods. In Section 10.4 we will describe a number of geostatistical methods, in particular concentrating on a technique known as *kriging*, a prediction method that has had a long and successful history in geostatistics.

A fundamental idea in this chapter is that we wish to make assumptions about the *random process* that gave rise to the exposure data. A random process is a collection of random variables that are indexed by another variable that may be discrete or continuous. A simple example of a random process is PM_{10} indexed by time; consideration of the daily maximum (say) is an example of a discrete indexing variable (time in days) while the consideration of pollutant continously over a day would lead to an indexing variable of continuous time. In the context described in Section 10.2 the indexing variable is the (continous) two-dimensional spatial location and the random variable is the PM_{10} concentration. The random process may then be thought of as generating the exposure across the region of interest. In the next section we present a number of naive approaches that, in general, do not acknowledge the stochastic nature of the mechanism. This approach is in contrast to that described in Section 10.6 in which methods that are optimal for a completely specified process are described. Between these two extremes we may wish to make assumptions only about features of the process such as the mean or variance-covariance structure. There are minimal assumptions that must be made and this leads to the important concept of *stationarity* that is discussed in Sections 10.4.2 and 10.4.3.

We finish this section by introducing some basic notation. We suppose that the exposure has been measured at n distinct sites, $s_1, \ldots, s_n$, and that the data are represented as

$$\mathbf{Z} = (Z(s_1), \ldots, Z(s_n))^T, \tag{10.1}$$

where $Z(s)$ denotes an observation (or a potential observation, such as the exposure at a location of interest) at location s in a region D of Euclidean space $\mathbb{R}^d$. Usually $d = 2$ or 3 and, if time is also included in the analysis, one could also have $d = 4$. In the example of Section 10.2 we have $d = 2$ since the elevation of the monitors is not available and we are not considering the time aspect. The locations $\{s_1, \ldots, s_n\}$ (in equation 10.1) are treated as known. We assume the data $\mathbf{Z}$ are a realisation from the random process

$$\{Z(s) : s \in D\},$$

where the index set D is a region. In the geostatistical literature $Z(s)$ is known as a *regionalised variable*.

Our goal is to predict the unobserved values at known spatial locations, using the observed data $\mathbf{Z}$. A generic location at which we wish to obtain a prediction will be denoted s_0. We note that, in general, we wish to predict the value of the *noise-free* exposure; that is, we wish to remove any measurement error component of $Z(s_0)$. We may also wish to estimate the exposure within a subregion B that is contained within D. For example, in a spatial epidemiological context the health and population data may be available as aggregated counts over sub-regions and we may wish to examine, at the ecological area level, the effect of the exposure health. However, such an analysis is subject to ecological bias (Chapter 11). In Chapter 22 an approach is described that combines the exposure and health data in such an analysis, and we also comment on this aspect in Section 10.6.

10.3.2   Naive methods

We start with a brief survey of a number of naive methods; further details may be found in Section 5.9.2 in Cressie (1993). Those we describe are mostly *ad hoc* with the only source of randomness in the model being measurement error; each approach has its own way of attempting to filter out this noise. A very simple approach is to predict $Z(s_0)$ to be the average of those points in a neighbourhood of s_0; this neighbourhood may be defined in terms of a constant radius or a constant number of neighbours. This naive method has a number of disadvantages, in particular the choice of the neighbourhood is likely to be crucial. One simple way of overcoming this difficulty is to include all of the points but to weight according to their 'proximity' to s_0. For example, the *inverse-distance-squared weighted average* predictor of $Z(s_0)$ is given by

$$\sum_{i=1}^{n} d_i^{-2} Z(s_i) \Big/ \sum_{i=1}^{n} d_i^{-2} = \sum_{i=1}^{n} q_i Z(s_i),$$

where d_i is the Euclidean distance, $|s_0 - s_i|$, between s_0 and s_i, and we have weights $q_i = d_i^{-2} / \sum_j d_j^{-2}$ and $\sum_i q_i = 1$. We see that locations s_i close to s_0 have large weights and the observed value of the exposure at these points contribute most to the prediction. If the true exposure surface is non-constant, this predictor reduces the variance of the prediction at the expense of increasing its bias. One could also choose weights inversely proportional to distance or, for that matter, any other increasing function of distance, which reveals the arbitrariness of this method. We would prefer a justification that is based on properties of the underlying process; in Section 10.4.4 we describe linear predictors that have such a justification.

10.3.3   Smoothing methods

A number of other 'non-parametric' smoothers are also available. For example, the locally weighted regression (lowess) method is a local weighted moving average procedure that has been adapted to two and more dimensions by Cleveland and Devlin (1988). The number of points that are used for prediction for a particular location may depend (for example) on the local density of points. Methods for determining an approximate measure of the variability of the prediction are described, for example, in Bowman and Azzalini (1997). Other possibilities for prediction include the Delauney triangulation, natural neighbour interpolation, multi-quadric biharmonic interpolation, and splines.

In general, we may write

$$Z(s) = \mu(s) + \epsilon(s); \qquad s \in D,$$

where $\mu(s)$ represents the expected value of the process and $\epsilon(s)$ a zero mean error term. Two fundamentally different approaches are then possible (though as we shall see they may result in similar predictions). The approaches of this section take the error terms $\epsilon(s)$ to be uncorrelated, and model the mean function $\mu(s)$ non-parametrically. In the next section we describe more traditional geostatistical approaches that take $\mu(s) = \mu$ and model the spatial dependence between $\epsilon(s)$ and $\epsilon(s')$ for $s \neq s'$. We note that the kriging approach may also include a non-constant mean in what is known as *universal kriging*. Proposed methods may also be compared by the number of assumptions that they make. In this and the following section, unless otherwise stated, no distributional assumptions are made concerning the error process $\epsilon(s)$; in Section 10.6 methods that assume a Gaussian process are described.

A spline function is basically a series of piece-wise polynomials over the region of interest (e.g. a cubic spline uses cubic polynomials). To prevent the function merely interpolating through the data, a *roughness penalty* term (e.g. penalising non-smoothness through consideration of the second derivative) is specified. There is now a large literature on spline fitting (e.g. see Green and Silverman 1994) with different methods having varying degrees of arbitrariness associated with the choice of roughness penalty. Further details of the use of splines in geostatistics may be found in Dubrule (1984), Wahba (1990), Cressie (1993), and Hutchinson and Gessler (1994).

More recently, Bayesian approaches to smoothing have become more widespread, for example, Denison *et al.* (1998) consider the use of piece-wise polynomials in which both the number and the position of the 'knots' (the locations of the changes in polynomial) are treated as random variables and assigned prior distributions. This flexibility is achieved at the expense of an increase in computational costs.

10.4   Geostatistical methods

In this section a brief description will be given of what we term *geostatistical methods* for prediction; further details may be found, for example, in Journel and Huijbregts (1978), Isaaks and Srivastava (1989), Cressie (1993, part I), and Wackernagel (1998).

10.4.1   Preliminaries

Typically, geostatistical methods only require assumptions about the first two moments of the Z-process, in contrast to the more sophisticated methods described in Section 10.6. By assuming that $\mathrm{var}\{Z(s)\} < \infty$, for all locations $s \in D$, we guarantee that the first two moments exist. We begin by discussing the important concept of stationarity. Intuitively, a process that is stationary across a region has a constant mean and the covariance between random variables at two locations depends only on the *relative locations* (i.e. the distance and angular direction between locations). The importance of stationarity stems from the fact that, if we have a stationary process, then realisations from the process from different parts of the region are comparable and so can be used for inference about the underlying *common* structure.

10.4.2   Second-order stationarity and the covariance function

Assume

$$E[Z(s)] = \mu; \qquad s \in D \tag{10.2}$$

$$\mathrm{cov}\{Z(s), Z(u)\} = C(s - u); \qquad s, u \in D, \tag{10.3}$$

where $C(\cdot)$ is a covariance function. Given (10.2),

$$\mathrm{cov}\{Z(s), Z(u)\} = E[\{Z(s) - \mu\}\{Z(u) - \mu\}].$$

Processes that satisfy (10.2) and (10.3) are said to be *second-order stationary*. In words, the mean is constant (with no trend, for example) and the covariance is merely a function of the vector difference between any two points. Thus, we have repeatability and so a basis for inference. If we let $h = s - u$ denote the vector difference between the locations s and u, then with the specification (10.3) the covariance between the process at the two locations may depend on both the magnitude *and* the direction of h. If $C(s - u)$ is a function only of $|h|$ then the covariance function is said to be *isotropic*.

In general, (10.2) and (10.3) say nothing about univariate distributions $[Z(s)]$, bivariate distributions $[Z(s), Z(u)]$, and so forth. (Notice our convention here, to write the distribution of the random vector Y as $[Y]$.) However, there is one situation where the assumptions (10.2) and (10.3) completely specify the Z-process. The process $\{Z(s) : s \in D\}$ is said to be a Gaussian process if any vector $(Z(u_1), \ldots, Z(u_m))^T$ has a multivariate normal distribution. Hence, if a Gaussian process has first two moments satisfying (10.2) and (10.3), then it is completely specified. We note that a Gaussian process in general may have a non-constant mean and can be simply transformed to stationarity by subtracting this mean.

There is another type of stationarity that again only involves the first two moments and is more general than second-order stationarity.

10.4.3 Intrinsic stationarity and the variogram

Assume (10.2) and,

$$\mathrm{var}\{Z(s) - Z(u)\} = 2\gamma(s - u); \quad s, u \in D, \tag{10.4}$$

where $2\gamma(\cdot)$ is known as the *variogram* ($\gamma(\cdot)$ is called the semi-variogram). Processes that satisfy (10.2) and (10.4) are said to be *intrinsically stationary*.

If the Z-process is second-order stationary, then

$$\gamma(h) = C(0) - C(h),$$

for $h \in \mathbb{R}^d$, but there are processes for which $\gamma(\cdot)$ is well-defined and $C(\cdot)$ is not. For example, standardized d-dimensional Brownian motion has

$$\mathrm{var}\{Z(s) - Z(u)\} = 2\gamma_b(s - u) = |s - u|, \tag{10.5}$$

but $\mathrm{cov}\{Z(s), Z(u)\}$ is not a function of the difference, $s - u$.

Clearly $\gamma(h) = \gamma(-h)$ and $\gamma(0) = 0$. If $\gamma(h) \to \theta_0 > 0$, as $h \to 0$, then θ_0 is termed the *nugget effect*. Mathematically speaking this phenomenon cannot occur for continuous processes (which require $\gamma(h) \to 0$, as $h \to 0$). One may hypothesise that the nugget effect θ_0 is actually made up of two components:

$$\theta_0 = c_{ms} + c_{me},$$

the microscale variance c_{ms} and the measurement-error variance c_{me}. Repeat measurements at specific locations allow c_{me} to be estimated; if no such data are available then we have no way of separating c_{me} from c_{ms}. We may think of the process as having the form

$$Z(s) = S(s) + \epsilon(s), \tag{10.6}$$

where $S(s)$ and $\epsilon(s)$ represent processes with and without spatial structure, respectively, and $\mathrm{var}\{\epsilon(s)\} = c_{me}$. Modelling the behaviour of the semi-variogram for small distances is difficult because the data cannot tell us anything about the variogram at distances smaller than $\min\{|s_i - s_j| : 1 \le i < j \le n\}$. However, by extrapolating this behaviour back to $h = 0$, we obtain an estimate of θ_0.

Suppose we have a process that is second-order stationary and that $C(h) \to 0$ as $|h| \to \infty$. Then $\gamma(h) \to C(0)$ as $|h| \to \infty$, and the quantity $C(0)$ is known as the *sill* of the semi-variogram. The *partial sill* is defined as $C(0) - \theta_0$. The *range* of the variogram in a particular direction is the distance at which the correlations are zero (or effectively zero). If $\gamma(\cdot)$ is a positive constant for all values of h, then $Z(s_1)$ and $Z(s_2)$ are uncorrelated for all s_1 and s_2 and there is no spatial structure.

To begin to make inference about the process, we first need to detrend the data to establish mean-stationarity, and then model the covariance function or the semi-variogram. In practice, covariance or semi-variogram models are chosen so that they are stationary and depend on only a finite number of parameters $\theta = (\theta_0, \ldots, \theta_k)^T$. Since the semi-variogram is more general than the covariance function, we will concentrate on this quantity. We will denote the semi-variogram as a function of the vector difference $h = s - u$ and θ, namely, as $\gamma(h; \theta)$. There are many families of semi-variogram models, for example, the *exponential* model is given by

$$\gamma(h; \theta) = \begin{cases} 0, & h = 0, \\ \theta_0 + \theta_1\{1 - \exp(-|h|/\theta_2)\}, & h \ne 0, \end{cases}$$

where $\theta = (\theta_0, \theta_1, \theta_2)^T$ and $\theta_j \ge 0$, $j = 1, 2, 3$. Cressie (1993, section 2.3) describes a number of other possibilities including spherical, power, wave, and rational quadratic models. The Matérn class (Matérn 1960) has recently been used successfully by Handcock and Wallis (1994) in a Bayesian approach to geostatistical analysis. See also the discussion of Diggle *et al.* (1998).

The model that will be used in the application of Section 10.5 is given by

$$\gamma(h; \theta) = \begin{cases} 0, & h = 0, \\ \theta_0 + \theta_1|h|, & h \ne 0, \end{cases} \tag{10.7}$$

where $\theta = (\theta_0, \theta_1)^T$ and $\theta_0, \theta_1 > 0$. The form (10.7) is a valid semi-variogram model and is obtained by taking a positive-coefficient linear combination of two valid semi-variogram models (which always produces a valid semi-variogram). The first is the standardized semi-variogram model with no spatial dependence, namely,

$$\gamma_0(h) = I(h \ne 0),$$

where $I(\cdot)$ is the indicator function that takes the value one if its argument is true and zero otherwise; the second is $\gamma_b(h)$ given by (10.5). Note that this model does not produce a well-defined covariance matrix for the underlying process because the variance function $\mathrm{var}\{Z(s)\}$ has not been specified.

Under the mean stationarity assumption (10.2),

$$2\gamma(s - u) = E[\{Z(s) - Z(u)\}^2],$$

which suggests that a natural way to estimate $\gamma(\cdot)$ is to replace $E(\cdot)^2$ by $ave(\cdot)^2$ in the expression above; that is, use a non-parametric method-of-moments estimator to obtain

$$\hat{\gamma}(\boldsymbol{h}) = (1/2)ave\{(Z(\boldsymbol{s}_i) - Z(\boldsymbol{s}_j))^2 : \boldsymbol{s}_i - \boldsymbol{s}_j = \boldsymbol{h}\}, \tag{10.8}$$

where $\boldsymbol{h}$ takes one of the values $\boldsymbol{h}_1, \ldots, \boldsymbol{h}_L$. In practice, the condition, $\boldsymbol{s}_i - \boldsymbol{s}_j = \boldsymbol{h}$, in (10.8) is modified to

$$\boldsymbol{s}_i - \boldsymbol{s}_j \in T(\boldsymbol{h}),$$

where $T(\boldsymbol{h})$ is a tolerance region around the spatial lag $\boldsymbol{h}$ that allows enough averaging in (10.8) so that $\hat{\gamma}(\cdot)$ has an acceptably small variance. The estimator (10.8) yields the so-called *semi-variogram estimator*. Further discussion of both parametric and non-parametric estimation of the variogram can be found in Cressie (1993, section 2.4). In an initial analysis, a non-parametric variogram estimator like (10.8) is preferred because we do not want to (or we are unable to) make assumptions about the joint distribution $[\boldsymbol{Z}]$.

Now, the non-parametric estimator $\hat{\gamma}(\cdot)$ is not generally itself a valid semi-variogram. The next step then is to fit a valid parametric model $\gamma(\cdot; \boldsymbol{\theta})$ to the estimates:

$$\{\hat{\gamma}(\boldsymbol{h}_l) : l = 1, \ldots, L\}.$$

One method of estimating the parameters of the variogram model that we shall use in Section 10.5 is a weighted least-squares criterion, proposed by Cressie (1985). In this approach we choose to minimise

$$\sum_{l=1}^{L} N(\boldsymbol{h}_l) \left\{ \frac{\hat{\gamma}(\boldsymbol{h}_l)}{\gamma(\boldsymbol{h}_l; \boldsymbol{\theta})} - 1 \right\}^2 \tag{10.9}$$

with respect to $\boldsymbol{\theta}$, where $N(\boldsymbol{h}_l)$ is the number of $(\boldsymbol{s}_i, \boldsymbol{s}_j)$ such that $\boldsymbol{s}_i - \boldsymbol{s}_j \in T(\boldsymbol{h}_l)$. Other ways of fitting the variogram (i.e. estimating $\hat{\boldsymbol{\theta}}$) include maximum likelihood and restricted maximum likelihood estimation of $\boldsymbol{\theta}$ (Cressie 1993; section 2.6). Ecker and Gelfand (1999) describe a Bayesian approach to estimation. For each of these other approaches a full specification of the underlying process is required. The geostatistical methodology described above, of estimating and fitting a variogram, is sometimes called *variography*.

10.4.4 Ordinary kriging

Based on the semi-variogram, we can draw an optimal map of the exposure surface $\{S(\boldsymbol{s}_0) : \boldsymbol{s}_0 \in D\}$ using a geostatistical technique known as ordinary kriging. The aim is to produce a linear predictor

$$\hat{p}(\boldsymbol{s}_0) = \boldsymbol{\lambda}^T \boldsymbol{Z}, \qquad \boldsymbol{s}_0 \in D, \tag{10.10}$$

that is *optimal* in the sense that it minimises the mean squared prediction error,

$$E\left[\{S(\boldsymbol{s}_0) - \boldsymbol{\lambda}^T \boldsymbol{Z}\}^2\right],$$

with respect to λ, subject to the unbiasedness constraint,

$$E[\lambda^T Z] = E[S(s_0)].$$

Assuming intrinsic stationarity and assuming that the parameter θ_0 in (10.7) has a component of measurement error, Cressie (1988) showed that the optimal choice of λ in (10.10) is given by

$$\Gamma\lambda + 1_n m = \gamma^*$$
$$1_n^T \lambda = 1. \tag{10.11}$$

Here m is a Lagrange multiplier that ensures that the sum of the elements in λ is one, Γ is an $n \times n$ matrix whose (i,j)th element is $\gamma(s_i - s_j)$, 1_n is an $n \times 1$ vector of 1s, γ^* is an $n \times 1$ vector whose ith component $\gamma^*(s_0 - s_i)$,

$$\gamma^*(h) = \begin{cases} c_{me}, & h = 0 \\ \gamma(h), & h \neq 0, \end{cases}$$

and c_{me} is the measurement error variance ($\leq \theta_0$).

Solving (10.11), we obtain,

$$\lambda + \Gamma^{-1}1 m = \Gamma^{-1}\gamma^*,$$

which implies that

$$m = -(1_n^T \Gamma^{-1} 1_n)^{-1}(1 - 1_n^T \Gamma^{-1} \gamma^*)$$
$$\lambda = \Gamma^{-1}(\gamma^* - 1_n m). \tag{10.12}$$

Furthermore, the minimised mean squared prediction error, known as the (ordinary) *kriging variance*, is given by,

$$\sigma_k^2(s_0) = \lambda^T \gamma^* + m - c_{me}. \tag{10.13}$$

Together, (10.12) and (10.13) are known as the (ordinary) kriging equations.

So far we have only considered isotropic processes. In general, exploratory analyses will he carried out in order to assess this assumption (see Section 10.5). Diggle and Verbyla (1998) describe a technique (in a non-spatial context) of examining a variogram simultaneously in two dimensions. If isotropy is not found to hold then one possibility is to consider a rotation and scaling of the coordinate system in order to obtain isotropy. This leads to the following semi-variogram function

$$\gamma(h) = \gamma^0(|Ah|), \tag{10.14}$$

where $\gamma^0(\cdot)$ is an isotropic semi-variogram. A semi-variogram γ that is represented as in (10.14) is said to possess *geometric anisotropy*. From Journel and Huijbregts

(1978: 179–81), we see that

$$A = \begin{bmatrix} \cos^2 \phi + \psi \sin^2 \phi & (1 - \psi) \sin \phi \cdot \cos \phi \\ (1 - \psi) \sin \phi \cdot \cos \phi & \sin^2 \phi + \psi \cos^2 \phi \end{bmatrix}.$$

This approach will be illustrated in Section 10.5.

Interestingly, there is a direct correspondence between splines and the geostatistical approach known as kriging; in kriging, the basis functions are actually (generalised) covariance functions (e.g. Cressie 1993, section 3.4.5). However, the geostatistical approach adapts to the quantity and quality of spatial dependence by incorporating an *estimation* step to precede the spatial prediction step. Here, the variogram (equivalently, the covariance function) is estimated from the data, Z, observed at known spatial locations $\{s_1, \ldots, s_n\}$. Moreover, once the variogram is estimated, one is able to produce kriging predictors, such as those given in this section, that minimise mean squared prediction errors. Thus, a geostatistical approach produces two maps, one being the predictor itself and the other being the kriging standard error (i.e. root mean squared prediction error). The spline approach also yields standard errors via cross-validation, and Wahba (1990) shows how standard errors may be obtained by defining splines within a Bayesian framework. An advantage of the spline approach is that they do not require the variography step but then they are not adaptive to spatial dependence in the data. Less importantly, kriging's prediction errors do not acknowledge the uncertainty in estimating the variogram parameters $\boldsymbol{\theta}$, ϕ, and ψ.

Apart from the advantages already mentioned, does kriging actually give better predictors in real problems? Laslett *et al.* (1987) and Laslett (1994) performed experiments where they held some spatial data back for validation of kriging-versus-spline prediction. When the data were regularly spaced, the two approaches were hard to distinguish, but when the data locations exhibited considerable irregularity, kriging showed improvement over splines. In the next section we present the classical geostatistical approach to spatial prediction, which we then use to analyse *particulate matter* data from a region centred on Pittsburgh, Pennsylvania.

We note in passing that there are a variety of other kriging procedures that may be used in certain situations. For example, *universal* kriging allows a more general form for the mean structure, *trans-Gaussian* kriging is relevant when the original data are transformed, *disjunctive* kriging considers generalised additive predictors, *block* kriging is concerned with prediction for the integrated exposure over an area, and *co-kriging* is used when there are multiple exposures; see Cressie (1993) for further details.

There are a number of examples in the literature of the kriging of various environmental exposures, including radon gas (Vincent and Gatrell 1991), ozone pollution (Lefohn *et al.* 1988), nitrogen dioxide (Campbell *et al.* 1994), and cyanide and cadmium pollution (Stein *et al.* 1995).

10.5   Illustrative example revisited

We begin by presenting the variography for PM_{10} exposure in the Pittsburgh region of the USA. Some basic exploratory data analysis indicated that the PM_{10} data should be logged in order to obtain a process whose distributions are approximately symmetric and whose variance does not depend on the mean. The advantage of symmetry is that the mean squared prediction error is then a very natural quantity to consider. That is, define

$$Z(s) = \log PM_{10}(s),$$

for $s \in D$, and where $PM_{10}(s)$ is the particulate matter reading (either observed or potential) at location s. In log units, the regulatory limit is $\log 150 = 5.0106$. Based on duplicate observations that were available at some sites, we obtained $c_{me} = 0.00706$ for $\log PM_{10}$ in the Pittsburgh region.

After some experimentation, we decided to rotate the usual axes counterclockwise by an angle of $22.5°$, where the directions ENE-WSW and NNW-SSE are now thought of as principal axes for representing the spatial variation. This was based on looking at plots of the variogram clouds in various directions, and it coincides with the prevailing wind direction on that particular day. For a given direction ϕ (defined clockwise from the N direction), the variogram cloud is defined to be a plot of $(Z(s_i) - Z(s_j))^2$ versus $\|s_i - s_j\|$, for all ordered location pairs belonging to $\{(s_i, s_j): \text{angle}(s_i - s_j) \in (\phi - 22.5°, \phi + 22.5°)\}$. Figure 10.2 shows variogram clouds for $\phi = -22.5°$ and $67.5°$.

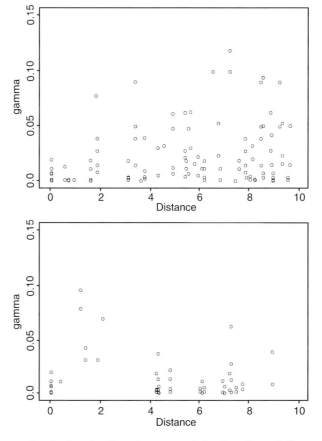

Fig. 10.2 Variogram cloud plots in directions $-22.5°$ (top) and $67.5°$ (bottom). Units on the horizontal axes are miles.

It is clear from Fig. 10.2 that there are spatial outliers near the origin in the second variogram cloud and there appears to be more spatial structure in the NNW direction ($-22.5°$) than in the ENE direction ($67.5°$). Upon closer inspection, the unusually high values, or spatial outliers, in the variogram cloud are mostly due to one monitoring site, namely 3004. Therefore, for the purpose of fitting a variogram, which is a measure of the 'global' spatial dependence, site 3004 was deleted. (However, for the purpose of spatial prediction, which uses 'local' information, site 3004 was included.)

Using the semi-variogram estimates defined by (10.8) and the weighted least-squares criterion given by (10.9), we fit individual semi-variograms in the directions $\phi = -22.5°$ and $\phi = 67.5°$. Model (10.7) was used and weighted least-squares parameter estimates of $\hat{\theta}_0 = 0.00851$ and $\hat{\theta}_1 = 0.00294$ were obtained. The resulting non-parametric semi-variogram estimates from (10.8), and resulting fits from (10.7) are shown in Fig. 10.3. We estimated $\hat{\phi} = -22.5°$ and $\hat{\psi} = 0.41353$.

Based on all the *particulate matter* data at the 22 sites on day 226 (site 3004 was included and also some duplicate *particulate matter* readings were available) and the

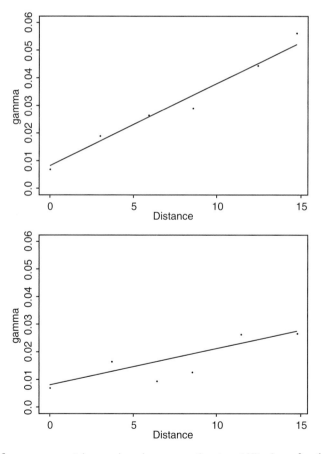

Fig. 10.3 Plot of non-parametric semi-variogram estimates $\hat{\gamma}(\boldsymbol{h})$ given by (10.8) and fitted semi-variogram $\gamma(\boldsymbol{h}; \boldsymbol{\theta})$ given by (10.7), in directions $-22.5°$ (top) and $67.5°$ (bottom). Units on the horizontal axes are miles.

estimated semi-variogram of the form of (10.14), spatial predictions were made at 500 locations where no data were observed. Then a standard contouring package was used to map the kriging predictors,

$$\{\hat{p}(s_0) : s_0 \in D\}, \tag{10.15}$$

and the kriging standard errors,

$$\{\sigma_k(s_0) : s_0 \in D\}, \tag{10.16}$$

where D is a convex region surrounding Pittsburgh and containing all the PM_{10} monitoring sites. Figure 10.4 shows a map with the prediction contours superimposed on the 22 monitoring-site locations and the 500 prediction locations. Figure 10.5 shows a map of the kriging standard errors, indicating how reliable various parts of the map shown in Fig. 10.4 are. We see, as expected, that prediction errors tend to be greatest at points furthest from the monitoring sites.

Finally, we would like to mention a recent development in predicting non-linear functions of the Z-process. For example, to determine whether a neighbourhood B in the Pittsburgh region is in compliance with the PM_{10} regulation, we may need to predict something like,

$$I(Z(B) < \log 150),$$

where $Z(B) = \int_B Z(\mathbf{u}) d\mathbf{u}/|B|$, $|B|$ is the area of B, and recall that $I(A)$ is an indicator function that equals 1 if A is true and equals 0 if A is not true. This is a problem of change of spatial support since the data are observed at point support but prediction is for the sub-region B.

The ordinary kriging predictor,

$$I\left(\int_B \hat{p}(\mathbf{u}) d\mathbf{u}/|B| < \log 150 \right),$$

is a very poor predictor because it is highly biased. This is due to the presence of both change of scale (log transformation) and change of support (point support to sub-region support). Either one can lead to non-linearities that result in ordinary kriging being no longer appropriate. Basically, for any non-linear functional $g(\cdot)$,

$$E[g\{Z(s)\}] \neq E[g\{\hat{p}(s)\}],$$

Aldworth and Cressie (2000) have developed a form of kriging that not only matches the first moment, $E[Z(s)] = E[\hat{p}(s)]$, but also variances and covariances, namely, $\text{cov}\{Z(s), Z(\mathbf{u})\} = \text{cov}\{\hat{p}(s), \hat{p}(\mathbf{u})\}$, for certain s and $\mathbf{u}$. This is called *covariance-matching constrained kriging* (CMCK) and it offers approximate unbiasedness and optimality within various classes of nonlinear predictors. Its advantage is that no matter what question one wants to ask, the CMCK map gives an (approximately) accurate and precise answer; the ordinary kriging map is only appropriate for 'linear' questions, although it is more precise than CMCK for those questions.

In the next section, a methodology is given that can, in principle, answer any question without compromising accuracy or precision. The price one pays for all this power is the need to specify fully (up to a finite number of parameters) all joint distributions, and the need to be patient as one waits for iteration-/simulation-based inferences to converge.

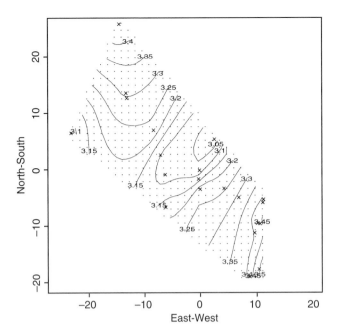

Fig. 10.4 Ordinary kriging prediction contours given by (10.10), superimposed on prediction sites (·) and monitoring sites.

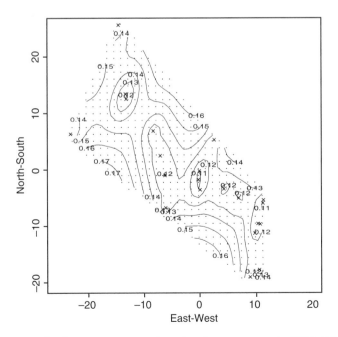

Fig. 10.5 Kriging standard error contours given by the square root of (10.13), superimposed on prediction sites (·) and monitoring sites.

10.6 Hierarchical modelling of spatial dependence

When the data are binary or are counts, linear predictors may not perform very well. If we drop the first- and second-moment assumptions, inherent in much of geostatistics, and replace it with a parametric specification that implies the full joint distribution of all random quantities, we should be able to find better spatial predictors than kriging predictors. We have also indicated previously that some uncertainties in parameters are not reflected in prediction variances; this problem can be overcome using the approach described by Diggle *et al.* (1998).

One approach that is proving very powerful is that of hierarchical modelling, which involves specification of various conditional distributions in a specific order defined by the hierarchical structure. Each specification is relatively simple. However, in combination, the joint distribution can be a complex (but realistic) model of the data and the underlying processes that generated them. Moreover, simulation-based inference using *conditional distributions* is well suited to hierarchical modelling of spatial dependence.

Recall that $[X]$ denotes the density of the random variable X, and we extend the notation so that $[X|Y]$ represents the conditional density of X given Y. In the geostatistical context, a hierarchical model might specify the first level of the hierarchy as $[Z(s)|S(s)]$; $s \in D$, and assume independence between any two of these conditional distributions whenever $s_1 \neq s_2$. The second level of the hierarchy might specify that some transformation of the underlying S-process, namely

$$\{h(S(s)) : s \in D\},$$

is a Gaussian process with mean function $\mu(s)$ and covariance function $C(s, u)$. These two moment functions would typically depend on a finite number of unknown parameters.

Now, one has a choice of whether to create a third level of the hierarchy by putting a (prior) distribution on the parameters or to estimate them from the data. Diggle *et al.* (1998) choose the former, while in the rest of this section we shall follow the usual geostatistical paradigm of separating out spatial prediction from parameter estimation.

Our goal is inference on $S(s_0)$; $s_0 \in D$, and hence we want to obtain the posterior distribution, $[S(s_0)|Z]$. For the purpose of presentation, assume $s_0 \notin \{s_1, \dots, s_n\}$. Then,

$$[S(s_0)|Z] \propto [Z, S(s_0)] = \int \cdots \int [Z, S, S(s_0)] \mathrm{d}S$$

$$= \int \cdots \int \left\{ \prod_{i=1}^{n} [Z(s_i)|S(s_i)] \right\} [S, S(s_0)] \mathrm{d}S.$$

Notice that each component in the integrand is available from the hierarchical model, however the posterior distribution is almost never available in closed form. An exception occurs when $[Z(s)|S(s)]$ is Gaussian with mean $Z(s)$, and $[\{S(s) : s \in D\}]$ is a Gaussian process, in which case the posterior distribution is also Gaussian (if all variances are known). Nevertheless, we can simulate from the posterior distribution in an iterative manner.

The Gibbs sampler (e.g. Smith and Roberts 1993) is a Markov chain Monte Carlo (MCMC) method that generates realisations successively from

$$[S(s_0)|\mathbf{S}, \mathbf{Z}] \propto [S(s_0)|\mathbf{S}], \qquad (10.17)$$

$$[S(s_i)|\mathbf{S}_{-i}, S(s_0), \mathbf{Z}] \propto [Z(s_i)|S(s_i)][S(s_i)|\mathbf{S}_{-i}, S(s_0)], \quad i = 1, \ldots, n, \qquad (10.18)$$

where $\mathbf{S}_{-i}$ is the $(n-1)$-dimensional vector of S-values with $S(s_i)$ removed. Once the $(n+1)$ simulations are carried out, one starts again with (10.17) followed by (10.18), and so forth; at each stage, one holds all conditioning variables fixed and equal to the previous values generated. For example, in both (10.17) and (10.18) one simply needs to know how to generate a univariate conditional distribution of one of $(n+1)$ S-values, given the remaining n S-values. Now, there is a large class of models for which such conditional distributions are readily available, namely Markov random fields (MRF) models. This class includes various non-Gaussian processes that are described in, for example, Besag (1974) and Cressie (1993). The models considered in Diggle *et al.* (1998) are not given directly through conditional distributions although they are still amenable to posterior generation using MCMC techniques. In non-Gaussian spatial applications, the Metropolis–Hastings algorithm (Smith and Roberts 1993) is often preferred to Gibbs sampling.

From (10.17) and (10.18), after a 'burn-in' period, we obtain simulations,

$$\{\mathbf{S}^{(t)}, S(s_0)^{(t)} : t = 1, \ldots, T\},$$

from the posterior distribution,

$$[\mathbf{S}, S(s_0)|\mathbf{Z}],$$

which can then be used to give empirical estimates of any summary of $[S(s_0)|\mathbf{Z}]$. For example, the spatial predictor that minimises the mean squared prediction error is

$$\mathrm{E}[S(s_0)|\mathbf{Z}] \simeq \frac{1}{T} \sum_{t=1}^{T} S(s_0)^{(t)}.$$

Furthermore, if one wishes to predict a non-linear function $g\{S(s_0)\}$ of $S(s_0)$, then the optimal predictor is

$$\mathrm{E}[g\{\mathbf{Z}(s_0)\}|\mathbf{Z}] \simeq \frac{1}{T} \sum_{t=1}^{T} g\{S(s_0)^{(t)}\}.$$

That is, all questions can in principle be answered accurately and precisely, provided parametric models can be specified and provided the iterations eventually yield realisations from the posterior distribution. There has been considerable research devoted to the latter problem of diagnosing convergence of the Gibbs sampler (e.g. Gelman *et al.* 1995), however, much remains to be done in this area. This is also true of model-diagnostics in the realm of hierarchical models; the assessment of assumptions is intrinsically more difficult because we are assessing quantities that are often not directly observed.

We note that although the hierarchical modelling framework is potentially very powerful and allows, for example, the joint modelling of health and exposure data, the implementation is not always easy. MCMC methods may not be straightforward to code, they are computationally expensive, and convergence remains a difficult issue.

10.7 Discussion

To keep the presentation in Section 10.4 simple, it was assumed in (10.2) that the exposure variable $Z(\cdot)$ had constant mean; the variogram is available to absorb small mis-specifications in the mean. However, it is known that meteorology can have an important effect on PM and hence the next stage in spatial modelling would be to replace (10.2) with

$$E[Z(s)] = x(s)^T \beta, \tag{10.19}$$

where $x(s)$ is a $p \times 1$ vector of explanatory variables (e.g. humidity, wind speed, wind direction, and so forth) and β is an unknown parameter vector. The assumption of (10.19) and (10.4) leads to a spatial-prediction approach that is briefly mentioned in Section 10.4.4 and is known as universal kriging. A more precise method of spatial prediction, also mentioned in that section, is known as co-kriging and takes the *joint* spatial variability of the exposure and the explanatory variables into account. We would only prefer the extra complication of co-kriging if $Z(s)$ and one of the variables $x_1(u)$ say, were correlated for $s \neq u$.

Notice the difference between exposure mapping and disease mapping. Disease counts are typically ascribed to disjoint administrative sub-regions $B_1, \ldots, B_r$ whose union is D. They are heteroskedastic and hence careful normalization is needed before a geostatistical approach can be taken. On the other hand, the exposure variable is referred to a point-level of aggregation and it can be aggregated up to the sub-regional level. As mentioned earlier, the more variables are aggregated, the greater the risk of falling foul of the ecological fallacy. Brillinger (1990) and Muller *et al.* (1997) take the opposite tack, of attempting to disaggregate the count or rate data from a choropleth map of sub-regions to a contour map of rates at all locations $s_0 \in D$. It may then be possible to relate these estimated rates with the exposure variable and hence to establish something like a regression relationship between disease rate and exposure.

Acknowledgements

The author would like to thank Jeremy Aldworth for his assistance with preparation of the figures and Jon Wakefield for his careful editorial work. This research was supported by the US Environmental Protection Agency under Co-operative Agreement CR 822919–01–0 between the EPA and Iowa State University.

References

Aldworth, J. and Cressie, N. (2000). *Prediction of nonlinear spatial functions*. Technical Report No. 649, Department of Statistics, Chio State University, Columbus, OH, USA.

Besag, J. E. (1974). Spatial interaction and the statistical analysis of lattice systems. *Journal of the Royal Statistical Society B*, **36**, 192–225.

Bowman, A. W. and Azzalini, A. (1997). *Applied smoothing techniques for data analysis*. Oxford Science Publications, Oxford.

Brillinger, D. R. (1990). Spatial-temporal modeling of spatially aggregate birth data. *Survey Methodology Journal*, **16**, 255–69.

Brown, P. J., Le, N. D., and Zidek, J. V. (1994). Multivariate spatial interpolation and exposure to air pollutants. *Canadian Journal of Statistics*, **22**, 489–509.

Campbell, G. W., Stedman, J. R., and Stevenson, K. (1994). A survey of nitrogen dioxide concentrations in the United Kingdom using diffusion tubes, July–December 1991. *Atmospheric Environment*, **28**, 477–87.

Cleveland, W. S. and Devlin, S. J. (1988). Locally weighted regression: an approach to regression analysis by local fitting. *Journal of the American Statistical Association*, **79**, 531–54.

Cressie, N. (1985). Fitting variogram models by weighted least squares. *Journal of the International Association for Mathematical Geology*, **17**, 563–86.

Cressie, N. (1988). Spatial prediction and ordinary kriging. *Mathematical Geology*, **20**, 405–21. [Erratum, *Mathematical Geology*, **21**, 493–4 (1989).]

Cressie, N. (1990). The origins of kriging. *Mathematical Geology*, **22**, 239–52.

Cressie, N. (1993). *Statistics for spatial data* (rev. edn). Wiley, New York.

Denison, D. G. T., Mallick, B. K., and Smith, A. F. M. (1998). Automatic Bayesian curve fitting. *Journal of the Royal Statistical Society, Series B*, **60**, 333–50.

Diggle, P. J. and Verbyla, A. P. (1998). Nonparametric estimation of covariance structure in longitudinal data. *Biometrics*, **54**, 401–5.

Diggle, P. J., Tawn, J. A., and Moyeed, R. A. (1998). Model-based geostatistics. *Applied Statistics*, **47**, 299–326.

Dockery, D. W. and Pope, C. A. (1997). Outdoor air. I: Particulates. In *Topics in environmental epidemiology* (K. Steenland and D. A. Savitz, ed.), 119–66. Oxford University Press, Oxford.

Dubrule, O. (1984). Comparing splines and kriging. *Computers and Geosciences*, **10**, 327–38.

Ecker, M. D. and Gelfand, A. E. (1999) Bayesian modelling and inference for geometrically anisotropic spatial data. *Mathematical Geology*, **31**, 67–83.

Gelman, A., Carlin, J., Rubin, D., and Stern, H. (1995). *Bayesian data analysis*. Chapman and Hall, London.

Green, P. J. and Silverman, B. W. (1994). *Nonparametric regression and generalized linear models: a roughness penalty approach*. Chapman and Hall, London.

Handcock, M. S. and Wallis, J. R. (1994). An approach to statistical spatio-temporal modeling of meteorological fields. *Journal of the American Statistical Association*, **89**, 368–78.

Hutchinson, M. F. and Gessler, P. E. (1994). Splines—more than just a smooth interpolator. *Geoderma*, **62**, 45–67.

Isaaks, E. H. and Srivastava, R. M. (1989). *An introduction to applied geostatistics*. Oxford University Press.

Journel, A. G. and Huijbregts, C. J. (1978). *Mining geostatistics*. Academic Press, London.

Lajaunie, C. (1984). A geostatistical approach to air pollution modelling. In *Geostatistics for natural resources characterisation* (G. Verly *et al.*, ed.), 877–91. NATO ASI Series C-122, Reidel, Dordrecht.

Laslett, G. M. (1994). Kriging and splines: An empirical comparison of their predictive performance in some applications (with discussion). *Journal of the American Statistical Association*, **89**, 391–409.

Laslett, G. M., McBratney, A. B., Pahl, P. J., and Hutchinson, M. F. (1987). Comparison of several prediction methods for soil pH. *Journal of Soil Science*, **38**, 325–41.

Lefohn, A. S., Knudsen, H. P., and McEvoy, L. R. (1988). The use of kriging to estimate monthly ozone exposure parameters for the southeastern United States. *Environmental Pollution*, **53**, 27–42.

Matérn, B. (1960). Spatial Variation. *Meddelanden fran Statens Skogsforskningsinstitute*, **49**, No. 5.

Matheron, G. (1963). Principles of geostatistics. *Economic Geology*, **58**, 1246–66.

Muller, H., Stadtmuller, U., and Tabrak, F. (1997). Spatial smoothing of geographically aggregated data, with application to the construction of incidence maps. *Journal of the American Statistical Association*, **92**, 61–71.

Pope, C. A., Thun, M. J., Namboodiri, M. M., Dockery, D. W., Evans, J. S., Speizer, F. E. *et al.* (1995). Particulate air pollution as a predictor of mortality in a prospective study of U.S. adults. *American Journal of Respiratory and Critical Care Medicine*, **151**, 669–74.

Schwartz, J. (1994). Air pollution and hospital admissions for the elderly in Birmingham, Alabama. *American Journal of Epidemiology*, **139**, 589–98.

Seaton, A., MacNee, W., Donaldson, K., and Godden, D. (1995). Particulate air pollution and acute health effects. *Lancet*, **345**, 176–8.

Smith, A. F. M. and Roberts, G. O. (1993). Bayesian computation via the Gibbs sampler and related Markov chain Monte Carlo methods. *Journal of the Royal Statistical Society, Series B*, **55**, 3–23.

Stein, A., Staritsky, I., Bouma, J., and van Groenigen, J. W. (1995). Interactive GIS for environmental risk assessment. *International Journal of Geographical Information Systems*, **9**, 509–25.

Styer, P., McMillan, N., Gao, F., Davis, J., and Sacks, J. (1995). The effect of outdoor airborne particulate matter on daily death counts. *Environmental Health Perspectives*, **103**, 490–7.

Vincent, P. and Gatrell, A. (1991). The spatial distribution of radon gas in Lancashire (UK): a kriging study. In *Proceedings of the Second European Conference on Geographical Information Systems*, 1179–86. EGIS Foundation, Utrecht.

Wackernagel, H. (1998). *Multivariate geostatistics* (2nd rev. edn). Springer, Berlin.

Wahba, G. (1990). *Spline models for observational data*. Society for Industrial and Applied Mathematics, Philadelphia, PA.

11. Ecological correlation studies

S. Richardson and C. Monfort

11.1 Introduction

In this chapter, our aim is to review some of the current issues relating to studies commonly known as 'ecological studies', with particular reference to the context of geographical epidemiology.

The existence of large contrasts in chronic disease incidence or mortality rates has long been noted. Some early references relating to geographical studies in the context of cancer epidemiology include those used to formulate aetiological hypotheses relating to diet (Armstrong and Doll 1975; Rose *et al.* 1986) and industrial factors (Blot and Fraumeni 1977). Recently, the focus of geographical studies in epidemiology has partially shifted from broad-scale studies carried out at an international or national level, to local studies of health-related outcomes (Alexander *et al.* 1990; Hatch and Susser 1990). A number of factors are responsible for this shift:

- the awareness that the interpretation of broad-scale studies is limited due to the problem of ecological bias, and in particular the existence of multiple confounding factors which may follow the same broad-scale geographical variations,
- the development of accurate databases and information systems at a small geographical scale, exemplified by the establishment of the Small Area Health Statistics Unit (Elliott *et al.* 1992),
- the statistical development of hierarchical models, in particular within the Bayesian framework, which allow the realistic modelling of small-scale variability and measurement error, and
- the necessity to examine localised environmental pollution effects at the small-area scale.

The aims of geographical studies range between:

- assessing heterogeneity and spatial structure of health outcomes in an exploratory manner,
- searching for clues to aetiology by examining the relationship between health outcomes and (for example) socio-economic, environmental, and genetic risk factors, this enterprise is sometimes known as 'hypothesis generation', and
- carrying out full ecological correlation studies, that is, studies of the association between sets of variables defined on *groups*, corresponding here to geographical areas; typically, the risk factors investigated via an ecological design have been connected to exposures related to industrial or agricultural employment, environmental pollutants (e.g. air, soil, water, background radiation), or to lifestyle factors such as dietary habits.

The level of inference of a geographical study depends on the aim of the study. For *exploratory studies* of spatial patterns, inference remains at the *aggregated level*. In such studies a statistical challenge is to account both for potential errors in the numerator and/or denominator of the rates (see Chapters 2 and 3), and for unequal population sizes inducing differential variability of the disease rates between areas, and to explore flexible classes of models for spatially correlated data. These last two issues are also discussed in Chapter 7. On the other hand, most *ecological analyses* are interested in inference at a level other than that of the group, and are typically trying to transfer inference on exposure effects from the group level down to the *individual-level*. However, ecological studies are 'incomplete' as they do not assess directly the link between exposure and effect. This creates the possibility of a difference between risk estimates at the individual and the aggregated level, a difference which is often referred to as *cross-level* or *ecological* bias.

The usefulness of geographical studies has thus been questioned in epidemiology (Greenland and Morgenstern 1989; Greenland and Robins 1994). That they are used reflects four considerations: geographical data are often straightforward to obtain (but the quality of such data needs to be checked, Chapter 2); the range of exposure is potentially much larger than that of (within-population) individual studies leading to an increase of power; the effect of measurement error on exposure is dampened by averaging; and they correspond to 'natural experiments' when the exposure has a physical geographical basis (e.g. soil, water) which can be usefully exploited. For these reasons, geographical studies are currently widely used. Nevertheless, in order to interpret ecological regression studies meaningfully, the following require consideration:

- how to relate individual-level and aggregated level dose-response relationships;
- the importance of considering confounders, including the use of appropriate summaries of confounder information at the aggregated level;
- the influence of unmeasured confounders, some of which potentially vary spatially, and which are implicitly modelled as spatially varying random effects.

In Section 11.2 we discuss the problem of model specification and inference between individual and aggregated level. In Section 11.3 we investigate issues relating to the sensitivity of aggregated level regression coefficients and to the specification of the spatial structure for the unmeasured confounders and present an illustrative study concerning childhood leukaemia. Section 11.4 contains a concluding discussion.

11.2   Ecological bias

11.2.1   General framework

We consider the following situation. At the *individual-level*, let $P(D|X=x)=f(x)$ denote the probability of contracting disease D for an individual exposed to a $p \times 1$ vector of risk factors X taking the values x. Within a group (area) G, we assume that the exposures of the individuals X has distribution $H(X)$ with mean μ_G.

At the *group level*, the disease rate for the whole group is given by

$$\lambda_G = E_G[P(D|X)] = \int_{x \in G} f(x)H(x)\,\mathrm{d}x, \tag{11.1}$$

so that the expectation is over the distribution of X in G. Implicitly this assumes that the dose-response $f(\cdot)$ is *the same* for all individuals in the group: this will be referred to as the 'common risk assumption'.

(a) For a linear dose-response relationship (i.e. an additive risk model), we have

$$f(x) = \alpha + x^T\beta \tag{11.2}$$

which integrates to

$$\lambda_G = \alpha + \mu_G^T\beta = f(\mu_G), \tag{11.3}$$

where β is a $p \times 1$ vector of parameters. Hence, in this simple case, the individual-level and the aggregated level relationships have the same shape with the same coefficients α and β.

(b) For an exponential dose-response relationship (i.e. a multiplicative risk model), we have

$$f(x) = \exp(\alpha + x^T\beta), \tag{11.4}$$

and integration involves higher order moments of the within-group exposure distribution $H(X)$ (Richardson *et al.* 1987). For example, if $H(X) = N(\mu_G, \Omega_G)$, then

$$\lambda_G = \exp(\alpha + \mu_G^T\beta + 0.5\beta^T\Omega_G\beta). \tag{11.5}$$

In this case, the aggregated level dose-response involves not only the mean μ_G of the exposure in each area, but a term which is a quadratic function of Ω_G, the within-area covariance of all the risk factors. We note that within-group normality may be obtained after transformation of the exposures.

Similarly, for any non-linear function f, $\lambda_G \neq f(\mu_G)$ and the convexity or concavity of f will determine the direction of the inequality. In what follows, we restrict our discussion to exponential f; one would proceed along similar lines for other non-linear forms for f.

Typically, ecological studies aim at estimating the coefficients α and β *on the basis of* n *groups*. Essentially ecological bias can occur due to confounding, and/or it may occur because of a non-linear f. We discuss these two possibilities in turn.

First, we suppose that the appropriate group summaries involved in Equations (11.3) or (11.5), (i.e. μ_G and Ω_G) are available. Using the aggregated relationships (11.3) or (11.5) for estimating α and β then requires a strong extension of the 'common risk assumption' to suppose that the coefficients α and β are *the same for all of the groups*. If this is not the case, for example if the baseline risk α and/or the slope β varies between the groups due to unmeasured confounders, then the ecological risk estimate will differ from the individual risk estimate and will suffer from 'ecological bias'. This has been extensively discussed and illustrated in the epidemiological literature (Richardson *et al.* 1987; Piantadosi *et al.* 1988; Greenland and Morgenstern 1989; Richardson 1992; Greenland and Robins 1994; Susser 1994*a, b*). In particular, sizeable ecological bias is produced if the baseline risk α varies between groups and is correlated with μ_G. This type of confounding occurs in some of the examples presented in Greenland and Robins (1994). It is thus of paramount importance to consider all the relevant confounders and to include them or to try to account for them statistically, for example by modelling them as random effects varying with the groups. Otherwise, the extension of the 'common risk assumption', which underlies many interpretations of ecological studies, is not tenable.

Second, we discuss the group summaries that are required in order to use (11.3) or (11.5). For the linear case (a), all that is needed are the values of λ_G and $\boldsymbol{\mu}_G$ for each of the groups and these are commonly available. However, this risk model has little appeal in epidemiology. When faced with the widely entertained multiplicative risk exponential model of Equation (11.4), we encounter further difficulties in carrying out ecological regressions based directly on (11.5). Indeed, it is uncommon that the exposure database would contain enough information to compute an estimate of $\boldsymbol{\Omega}_G$ in each area. Simplification of (11.5) by neglecting the quadratic term has been suggested by Plummer and Clayton (1996), so that (11.5) becomes

$$\lambda_G \approx \exp(\alpha + \boldsymbol{\mu}_G^T \boldsymbol{\beta}). \tag{11.6}$$

The attractiveness of (11.6) is that, as in the linear case, one seems to obtain a similar dose-effect relationship at the aggregated level as the individual one (11.4). Nevertheless, this simplification supposes that: (a) $\boldsymbol{\beta}$ is small, which is an uninteresting case; or (b) the elements of $\boldsymbol{\Omega}_G$ are small, corresponding to *homogeneous* exposure within the group; or (c) that $\boldsymbol{\Omega}_G$ does not vary across groups (in which case the $0.5\boldsymbol{\beta}^T \boldsymbol{\Omega} \boldsymbol{\beta}$ term is absorbed into the intercept), which is an unlikely assumption if there is enough contrast in exposure between the groups, but which could hold approximately after suitable transformation of the data. In order to control ecological bias due to the non-linearity of $f(\boldsymbol{x})$, in many cases one must thus include an assessment of the within-area distribution of the risk factors.

11.2.2   Dichotomous risk factors

We now discuss in some detail ecological analyses that involve dichotomous risk factors. For the sake of simplicity, we present our argument when there are only two dichotomous risk factors which we denote X_1 and X_2. We consider the exponential risk model given by (11.4), with β_1 associated with exposure to X_1 alone, and β_2 similarly defined. Thus $\exp(\beta_1)$ represents the risk ratio corresponding to exposure to X_1. To carry out the integration in (11.4), the *marginal* proportions p_1 (respectively p_2) of subjects in the group exposed to X_1 (respectively X_2), and the proportion p_{12} of subjects exposed to *both* X_1 and X_2, are required. Hence p_1, p_2, and p_{12} constitute $H(\cdot)$ here and the integration in (11.1) simplifies to a summation. We have suppressed some of the indexing by G to simplify the notation. This leads to the group rate

$$\lambda_G(p_1, p_2, p_{12}) = e^\alpha [1 + p_1(e^{\beta_1} - 1) + p_2(e^{\beta_2} - 1) + p_{12}(e^{\beta_1} - 1)(e^{\beta_2} - 1)]. \tag{11.7}$$

Neglecting the quadratic term gives

$$\lambda_G(p_1, p_2) \approx e^\alpha [1 + p_1(e^{\beta_1} - 1) + p_2(e^{\beta_2} - 1)]. \tag{11.8}$$

In a simple ecological study it is unlikely that p_{12} will be known, but it can simply be approximated by the product $p_1 p_2$, leading to

$$\lambda_G(p_1, p_2) \approx e^\alpha [1 + p_1(e^{\beta_1} - 1)][1 + p_2(e^{\beta_2} - 1)]. \tag{11.9}$$

This approximation is exact if exposure to X_1 and X_2 is independent within each group. More realistically, these exposures are assumed to be linked by an odds ratio ψ with $\psi = 1$ corresponding to independence. Hence, expressions (11.8) and (11.9) correspond respectively to different mis-specifications of the ecological regression (11.7), namely discarding the joint exposure or assuming $p_{12} = p_1 p_2$.

We summarise the results of an extensive comparative simulation study of the performance of (11.8) and (11.9) that was carried out by Lasserre *et al.* (2000). Typically, it was found that (11.9) was superior to (11.8), (i.e. approximating p_{12} by $p_1 p_2$ was better than ignoring this term altogether). Using (11.9) gave estimates of the risk ratios $\exp(\beta_1)$ and $\exp(\beta_2)$ centred on the 'true' values on average, with good coverage properties in terms of interval estimates. This was the case even when the within-group correlation between the two risk factors, characterised by ψ, was as large as 4. On the other hand, estimates using (11.8) were biased. A numerical illustration of these remarks can be found in table 1 in Richardson (1996).

To summarise: in the case of dichotomous risk factors, an improvement in estimation of the $\boldsymbol{\beta}$ coefficients of regression model (11.4) is gained by *approximating* the quadratic term, rather than *neglecting* it. This approximation is straightforward to implement since it only requires the marginal proportions. This is an advantageous case which should be fully exploited in designing ecological studies.

11.2.3 Continuous risk factors

For continuous risk factors, one should carefully consider whether there is any information available on within-group variability. Following the same lines of reasoning as for dichotomous risk factors, it may be hypothesised that knowledge of the full covariance matrix $\boldsymbol{\Omega}_G$ will not be required to provide a reasonably accurate approximation. For example, some progress may be made by assuming within-group independence of the risk factors (i.e. diagonal $\boldsymbol{\Omega}_G$).

A simple comparison of the performance of different approximations in the case of a linear-exponential dose-response relation of the form

$$f(x_1, x_2) = \alpha(1 + \beta_1 x_1) \exp(\beta_2 x_2) \tag{11.10}$$

was carried out in a geographical scenario suggested by Greenland and Robins (1994). The risk corresponding to β_1 was weaker than that corresponding to β_2. It was shown (Richardson *et al.* 1996) that the crude first order approximation

$$\lambda_G(\mu_{X_1}, \mu_{X_2}) \approx \alpha(1 + \beta_1 \mu_{X_1}) \exp(\beta_2 \mu_{X_2}) \tag{11.11}$$

produced biased estimates of β_1 and β_2, while the relation

$$\lambda_G(\mu_{X_1}, \mu_{X_2}) \approx \alpha(1 + \beta_1 \mu_{X_1}) \exp(\beta_2 \mu_{X_2} + 0.5 \beta_2^2 \sigma_{X_2}^2) \tag{11.12}$$

led to reasonably good estimates of β_1 and β_2. The difference between (11.11) and (11.12) is the inclusion of a quadratic term in β_2 involving $\sigma_{X_2}^2$ (the within-group variance of X_2). Further work along these lines needs to be carried out to study a variety of situations involving continuous risk factors and assessing different approximations.

In conclusion, we stress that, in all cases, it is important to first go back to the epidemiological dose-response relationship at the individual-level $P(D|X)$, and second to derive suitable approximations to its integrated form, $E_G[P(D|X)]$. In the simple case of dichotomous risk factors, cross-product terms involving the marginal proportions of the population exposed to the dichotomous factors in each area should be included in the ecological regressions. For continuous risk factors, inclusion of an estimate of the within-group variance-covariance matrix of the exposures should improve the situation.

11.3 Spatial structure in ecological regressions

In the preceding Section, we discussed the *functional specification* of ecological relationships. We are now concerned with the *estimation* of this relationship and the necessity of taking into account the residual spatial structure.

11.3.1 Why a spatial structure?

The statistical framework for estimating ecological regression depends on the scale of the geographical variations to be analysed. When within-area variability of the disease is negligible in comparison with between-area variability, ecological analyses are performed in a classical (non-hierarchical) regression framework. This is the case for studies concerning large areas and/or common diseases where it can be supposed that the usual epidemiological measures of disease rates (standardised mortality/morbidity ratios or directly standardised rates) are stable. This approach has been used to investigate the influence of water hardness on cardiovascular diseases in Great Britain (Cook and Pocock 1983), and of antioxidant status on cancer mortality in China (Chen *et al.* 1992). When the geographical scale is small and/or the disease is rare, inherent Poisson variability should be explicitly modelled at the first stage of a hierarchical model. Ecological relationships are specified at the second stage of the hierarchical model.

For studies at both the small and broad geographical scale, it is clear that in most cases there will be unidentified or unmeasured confounders, some of them potentially varying smoothly over space. There are many examples of such confounders, including genetic characteristics, sun exposure, and dietary habits. Spatial structure is therefore introduced to account indirectly for the *aggregated effect of these unobserved risk factors*.

Note that we are restricting our discussion to a chronic disease framework in which there is no direct dependence between the cases (as opposed to considering infectious diseases; see Chapter 14). For chronic diseases, there is no basis for the spatial structure in terms of contact processes; it is a parsimonious statistical device that is introduced to capture the effects of unobserved confounders. Using different spatial structures for the regression residuals or the random effects in a hierarchical model is analogous to carrying out different confounder adjustments in regression analyses. Hence, sensitivity of the results of ecological regressions to the choice of spatial structure must be investigated.

11.3.2 Broad-scale studies

For large-scale studies, the most straightforward statistical framework is that of multiple regression between rates Y_i and a set of covariates X_i, for $i = 1, \ldots, n$ areas:

$$Y_i = X_i \boldsymbol{\beta}^T + \epsilon_i,$$

where the zero-mean residual terms ϵ_i are assumed, approximately, to be normal with constant variance. Within this framework some normalisation of the rates (e.g. the logarithm), may be carried out in order to produce a set of 'responses' that are approximately normal with constant variance. As discussed above, the assumption that the residuals ϵ_i of such a regression are independent is not tenable for small-area studies and would lead to erroneous conclusions on the regression coefficients $\boldsymbol{\beta}$. In particular, the standard error of estimated coefficients will be too narrow. Thus, in spatial regression, it is supposed that the variance-covariance matrix of $\epsilon_1, \ldots, \epsilon_n$ is of the form $\sigma^2 \boldsymbol{\Sigma}_\epsilon$, where $\boldsymbol{\Sigma}_\epsilon$ models the spatial dependence and is usually parameterised in terms of a small number of parameters $\boldsymbol{\phi}$, i.e. $\boldsymbol{\Sigma}_\epsilon = \boldsymbol{\Sigma}_\epsilon(\boldsymbol{\phi})$. Generally, the spatial dependence between two areas is characterised by the distance between the area centroids.

The simultaneous estimation of the regression parameters $\boldsymbol{\beta}$ and those modelling the spatial dependence, ϕ, has been reviewed in Richardson (1992); here we will only give a brief outline of the issues. In a classical framework, this estimation usually involves first, the numerical maximisation of the profile likelihood for ϕ (i.e. a likelihood which is only a function of $\boldsymbol{\phi}$), to obtain $\hat{\boldsymbol{\phi}}$, and second, the computation of the usual generalised least square estimator for $\boldsymbol{\beta}$ using the covariance $\boldsymbol{\Sigma}_\epsilon(\hat{\boldsymbol{\phi}})$.

Two approaches have been taken for modelling $\boldsymbol{\Sigma}_\epsilon(\phi)$: either a *conditional* spatial autocorrelated model is specified for $\epsilon_i | \epsilon_j, j \neq i$, or a *joint* model is directly specified using classes of spatial covariance functions for which $\boldsymbol{\Sigma}_\epsilon(\boldsymbol{\phi})$ is positive definite. The choice of spatial model for the residuals is a delicate problem (Richardson *et al.* 1992). For any spatial analysis, the choice between the conditions of modelling $\epsilon_i | \epsilon_j, j \neq i$ or direct modelling through $\boldsymbol{\Sigma}_\epsilon(\boldsymbol{\phi})$ is mostly a matter of convenience, unless the data supports specific constraints which can be better expressed by using one or the other structure. For example, local independence can be expressed via conditional models for ϵ_i, whereas heteroscedasticity is more suited to specifying $\boldsymbol{\Sigma}_\epsilon(\boldsymbol{\phi})$. Empirically, a combination of residual plots, predictive fit, and other model choice criteria have been used. For a discussion of residuals in models with correlated errors see Haslett and Hayes (1998). It is thus important to use flexible classes of spatial models, in which complexity can be progressively increased. For example, in the conditional model, a zero-one neighbourhood structure can be extended to a parameterised distance-based neighbourhood structure. This implies different structures for $\boldsymbol{\Sigma}_\epsilon$ and allows the sensitivity of the spatial regression to be tested. An illustrative sensitivity analysis on geographical data relating to lung cancer and industrial factors in France can be found in Richardson *et al.* (1992).

11.3.3 Spatial structure in hierarchical models

The use of a hierarchical Bayesian approach to account for spatially structured extra-Poisson variability in small-area studies was first introduced by Clayton and Kaldor (1987) and was further developed by Besag *et al.* (1991) and Clayton and co-workers (1992, 1993). A review of hierarchical models in a spatial context may be found in Chapter 7. Basically, area-level relative risks are estimated by integrating: (a) local information consisting of the observed (Y_i) and expected (E_i) number of cases in each area, (b) prior information on the over-all variability and/or spatial structure of the relative risks, and (c) the potential effect of geographically defined covariates. These expected numbers are based on the age and sex (say) distribution of the area and a reference set of disease probabilities. In contrast to large-scale studies that use 'marginal' models, the hierarchical formulation explicitly decomposes the sources of variability. The random effect structure introduced at the second level of the model accounts for the extra-Poisson variability due to the aggregated effect of unknown confounders via a spatial 'clustering' component and an unstructured 'heterogeneity' component. In general, we are interested in investigating the sensitivity of the ecological regression to the prior specification of the sizes of these two components.

Let us first briefly recall the two-level formulation of the hierarchical model:

- First level—local variability (within area):

$$Y_i \sim \text{Poisson}(E_i\theta_i)$$

- Second level—structure between areas: log linear mixed model:

$$\log\theta_i = \alpha + X_i^T\boldsymbol{\beta} + U_i + V_i, \tag{11.13}$$

where X_i are area level covariates and U_i and V_i are random effects representing spatial clustering and unstructured heterogeneity, respectively. Note that U_i and V_i can be included separately.

Hence, the ecological regression is included at the second level and the previous discussion (Section 11.2) on the 'shape' of this regression is relevant here.

The following distributional forms are commonly adopted for the two random effects at the second level:

- Heterogeneity:

$$V_i \sim N(0, \sigma_v^2)$$

- Clustering:

$$U_i | U_j = u_j, j \neq i \sim N(\bar{u}_i, \omega_u^2/m_i)$$

where $\bar{u}_i = \sum_{j\neq i} W_{ij}u_j/m_i$, m_i is the number of neighbours of area i and $\{W_{ij}: i,j=1,\ldots,n\}$ is a 0–1 contiguity matrix in which $W_{ij}=1$ for neighbours and $W_{ij}=0$ otherwise, with $W_{ii}=0$ also. The constraint $\Sigma_i U_i=0$ is imposed for identifiability.

The variance parameters σ_v^2 and ω_u^2 control the amount of variability in V_i and U_i respectively and consequently the variability of the relative risks. Hence, the specification of their prior distribution has to be assessed carefully. Note that these parameters are not comparable since σ_v^2 characterises a marginal variability whilst ω_u^2 measures the local variability *conditional* on neighbouring random effects. As discussed above a joint model may also be specified for $U_1,\ldots,U_n$.

For a Bayesian approach, prior distributions are required for α, $\boldsymbol{\beta}$, σ_v^2, and ω_u^2. It is not possible to use uniform improper hyperpriors for the logarithms of σ_v^2 and ω_u^2 since this results in improper posteriors with an infinite spike at 0. Lower bounds on the variances need to be specified when using flat priors. Even with some proper priors such as gamma or χ^2 distributions, in the case of sparse data, lower bounds on the variances might also have to be set in order to avoid 'trapping' near zero. As suggested in Clayton

(1994) and Bernardinelli *et al.* (1995), we have chosen to specify proper chi-square distributions for the inverse variances (precisions). In particular

$$\omega_u^{-1} \sim \chi_{d_u}^2 / s_u,$$

and

$$\sigma_v^{-1} \sim \chi_{d_v}^2 / s_v,$$

where s_u, s_v denote scale parameters and d_u, d_v degrees of freedom, all of which are specified a priori. In Section 11.3.4 these will be varied in order to study sensitivity. For a generic inverse variance with distance χ_d^2 / s this leads to a mean and variance of d/s and $2d/s^2$, respectively. For α and β, uniform vague priors may be used.

The estimation of the parameters of this hierarchical model calls upon stochastic simulation techniques which belong to the family of Markov Chain Monte Carlo (MCMC) methods: see Gilks *et al.* (1996), for a general account and Mollié, (1996), for a review of their application in Bayesian disease mapping. The sample of values of U_i, V_i, σ_v^2, ω_u^2, α, and β produced may be considered (after an initial warm-up period) as values from the joint posterior distribution of the parameters conditional on the data. In the example that follows the BEAM (Bayesian Ecological Analysis Method) software (Clayton, 1994) was used to obtain samples from the posterior distribution. The WinBUGS software (Spiegelhalter *et al.* 1996) can also be used to obtain such samples. A summary of the variability of the random effects, allowing the assessment of their relative contribution to the overall variability of θ_i, given by

$$SD_u = \left(\frac{\Sigma U_i^2}{n-1} \right)^{1/2}$$

and similarly for SD_v. Note that $SD_v \approx \sigma_v$.

11.3.4 Sensitivity to the random effects prior variance: a case-study

There is considerable epidemiological interest in studying the role of environmental exposures in the aetiology of childhood leukaemia (Ross *et al.* 1994), and the role of radon exposure has been questioned recently.

We have therefore chosen to discuss the influence of the hyperprior specification of the random effects variances in the context of an ecological regression study concerned with the influence of background radiations, in particular radon levels and socio-economic factors on childhood leukaemia. The ecological regression term $X^T \beta$ at the second level of the model (11.13) thus contains two covariates, the socio-economic score and the (log) radon concentration. This study was carried out in England, Wales, and Scotland and has been reported in Richardson *et al.* (1995), where further details may be found. In the published analysis, flat priors for ω_u^{-2} and σ_v^{-2} with lower bounds were used. Here, we complement this analysis by contrasting different scaled chi-squared prior distributions for these parameters.

The data

The present study concerns 6691 cases of leukaemia diagnosed between 1969 and 1983, with 80.2% sub-classified as lymphocytic and unspecified leukaemias (LL). The geographical level is that of the 459 district level local authorities. The study period spans two national censuses in 1971 and 1981 and annual estimates of district populations are available. The study period was sub-divided into the three five years intervals: 1969–73, 1974–8, 1979–83. Expected number of cases per district were computed for each period.

Using census information, a socio-economic score was calculated for each district by averaging three (standardised) socio-economic characteristics: the proportion of economically active males who are working, the proportion of households with a car and the proportion of households that are owner-occupied.

The National Radiological Protection Board (NRPB) had undertaken a national survey of the concentration of radon, with a number of measurements per area. These measurements were combined using a geometric mean as indoor radon concentration has a skewed and approximately lognormal distribution.

A nearest neighbour structure for each district was created which can be summarised by a 459×459 contiguity matrix with the (i,j)th element W_{ij} being equal to 1 if districts i and j have a common border, and 0 otherwise.

Prior specification

The priors that we contrast are described in Table 11.1. The different scalings for the heterogeneity (s_u) and the clustering (s_v) component arise from the different interpretations (marginal versus conditional) of ω_u^2 and σ_v^2. Prior A has a larger coefficient of variation than prior B and a mass peaked near zero, thus favouring small values of the variances. When implementing the model, due to very sparse data, it became necessary to place lower bounds on the variances. For prior A, these were chosen to be 0.03, 0.02, and 0.01 and for prior B the value 0.01 was chosen. These lower bounds were selected for illustration only.

Table 11.1 Description of priors that were utilised for the precision parameters (inverse variance) of the heterogeneity and clustering models

Component	Degrees of freedom	Scale	Mean	Variance	Coefficient of variation
Prior A					
Heterogeneity V	$d_v = 0.5$	$s_v = 0.0005$	1000	4×10^6	2
Clustering U	$d_u = 0.5$	$s_u = 0.001$	500	1×10^6	2
Prior B					
Heterogeneity V	$d_v = 2$	$s_v = 0.02$	100	1×10^4	1
Clustering U	$d_u = 2$	$s_u = 0.04$	50	2.5×10^3	1

Results

(a) Overall variability due to the random effects

We first consider the quantification of the overall variability SD_v and SD_u of the heterogeneity and clustering components for models without covariates. Posterior densities corresponding to models including the heterogeneity and clustering components, alone or together, are presented in Fig. 11.1 for the period 1969–73. One can see that the prior exerts a strong influence, with a notable shift towards larger values of SD_u and SD_v for prior B. The overall density of the clustering component does not seem much influenced by the inclusion of the heterogeneity component while the heterogeneity component is less spread out when the clustering component is included. The heterogeneity component is also clearly sensitive to the lower bound used in prior A, whether estimated separately or together with the clustering component. This may indicate that there is a problem of identifiability of this component for these data. The clustering component is not affected by the choice of lower bound.

Table 11.2 summarises the estimation of SD_v for models that do not include the clustering term and Table 11.3 the estimation of SD_u for models not including the heterogeneity term. Both tables consider prior A with the lower bounds set to 0.01, models with or without covariate terms, and over three time periods. Again, one can see a consistent influence of the prior, with the mean variability under prior B, roughly double that of prior A. The inclusion of covariates, however, has only a small impact on the overall variability. The clustering component SD_u is consistently decreased, while for SD_v there

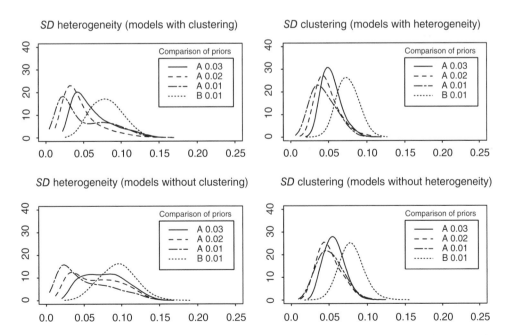

Fig. 11.1 Posterior distributions of SD_u and SD_v under different prior specifications (see Table 11.1) for the leukaemia data in the period 1969–73. The lower bound on the priors is indicated in the figure.

Table 11.2 Estimation of the heterogeneity component under different priors

SD_v (posterior s.d.)	Prior A		Prior B	
	No covariates	With covariates	No covariates	With covariates
1969–73	0.039 (0.026)	0.038 (0.024)	0.092 (0.031)	0.080 (0.027)
1974–8	0.052 (0.044)	0.048 (0.042)	0.111 (0.040)	0.115 (0.040)
1979–83	0.032 (0.022)	0.038 (0.026)	0.082 (0.027)	0.085 (0.028)

Table 11.3 Estimation of the clustering component under different priors

SD_v (posterior s.d.)	Prior A		Prior B	
	No covariates	With covariates	No covariates	With covariates
1969–73	0.048 (0.021)	0.042 (0.018)	0.092 (0.020)	0.082 (0.018)
1974–8	0.085 (0.042)	0.068 (0.036)	0.122 (0.031)	0.117 (0.031)
1979–83	0.055 (0.024)	0.043 (0.025)	0.099 (0.023)	0.096 (0.023)

is little change. There is a slight increase of SD_v in the 1979–83 period when covariates are included, which could be related to the weaker effect of the covariates for this period, adjustment creating some extra noise. It is also interesting to note that the size of the two components with and without covariates are comparable under prior B, but that the heterogeneity component becomes smaller for some time periods under prior A.

The influence of hyperpriors on the estimation of the relative risks is illustrated in Fig. 11.2 where the posterior density of the ratio of the 95% to 5% percentiles: $\theta_{0.95}/\theta_{0.05}$ of the distribution of the θ_i, $i = 1, \ldots, n$ is plotted for the 1969–73 period, for models estimated: (a) with or without covariates, (b) under hyperpriors A or B, and (c) including U_i, V_i or both. Note that prior A clearly produces more shrinkage than prior B (i.e. the relative risk ratio is narrower under prior A). As expected, there is less shrinkage when the covariates are included. The sensitivity of the ratio exhibited in Fig. 11.2 does not agree with the findings reported in Bernardinelli *et al.* (1995).

(b) Ecological regressions

In contrast to the marked sensitivity to the prior in the estimation of U_i and V_i demonstrated above, we found that the inference on the regression coefficients was quite robust to the different hyperprior specifications. This is demonstrated in Tables 11.4 and 11.5. There is an indication of a link, which becomes weaker over time, between leukaemia and the socio-economic score. The associated ecological regression coefficient stays stable under the different hyperpriors for the models including the heterogeneity term only. When clustering only is included, a small variation in the regression coefficient between priors A and B is notable for the last two time periods for the socio-economic score. Moreover, the posterior standard deviations of the regression coefficients are slightly

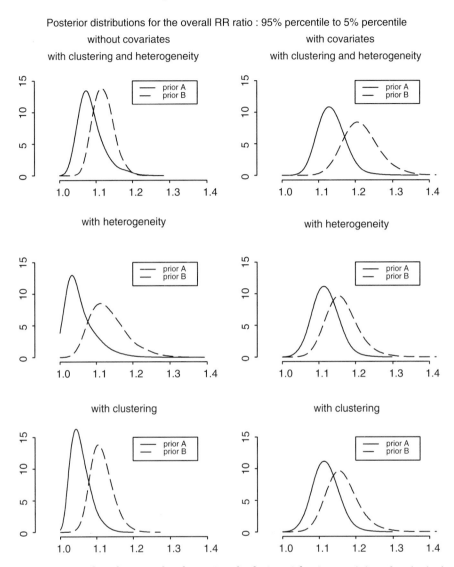

Posterior distributions for the overall RR ratio : 95% percentile to 5% percentile

Fig. 11.2 Posterior distributions for the ratio of relative risks $\theta_{0.95}$ and $\theta_{0.05}$ for the leukaemia data in the period 1969–73.

increased: (a) under Prior B, and (b) when the clustering component is included (rather than the heterogeneity term). There is no link with radon exposure; the sign of the coefficient is noticeably variable between the time periods. Note that these regression coefficients are comparable to those obtained previously by Richardson *et al.* (1995), in a model which included *both* U_i and V_i.

Hence, in this case-study, we have noted a small influence of the hyperprior specification on the ecological regression coefficient of the socio-economic score in the case of models including a clustering component. It is thus advisable to include such

Table 11.4 Estimation of the ecological regression corresponding to radon level and socio-economic score with heterogeneity component only and two different priors. The lower bound for the priors is 0.01

All leukaemia	Prior A		Prior B	
	Radon ($\times 10^2$)	SE score ($\times 10^2$)	Radon ($\times 10^2$)	SE score ($\times 10^2$)
1969–73				
Posterior mean	−0.27	3.03	−0.26	3.02
Posterior s.d.	(0.18)	(0.81)	(0.19)	(0.79)
1974–8				
Posterior mean	0.20	1.17	0.19	1.22
Posterior s.d.	(0.14)	(0.80)	(0.15)	(0.81)
1979–83				
Posterior mean	0.00	1.49	0.01	1.47
Posterior s.d.	(0.17)	(0.87)	(0.17)	(0.90)

Table 11.5 Estimation of the ecological regression corresponding to radon level and socio-economic score with clustering component only and two different priors. The lower bound for the priors is 0.01

All leukaemia	Prior A		Prior B	
	Radon ($\times 10^2$)	SE score ($\times 10^2$)	Radon ($\times 10^2$)	SE score ($\times 10^2$)
1969–73				
Posterior mean	−0.25	2.90	−0.24	2.93
Posterior s.d.	(0.20)	(0.87)	(0.20)	(0.93)
1974–8				
Posterior mean	0.17	1.22	0.14	1.11
Posterior s.d.	(0.14)	(0.87)	(0.17)	(0.93)
1979–83				
Posterior mean	−0.01	1.22	−0.03	0.78
Posterior s.d.	(0.17)	(0.93)	(0.20)	(0.99)

sensitivity analyses in any case study, as was done in Wakefield and Morris (1999) and Bernardinelli *et al.* (Chapter 16). Nevertheless the substantive conclusions regarding the link with the socio-economic score are not markedly affected by the change of hyperpriors.

11.4   Conclusions

From the previous discussion, it is clear that ecological correlation studies are open to misinterpretation. Despite this, there is an increasing call for such studies to assess the health effects of environmental exposures. Indeed, the latter are commonly difficult to assess at the individual-level, but can exhibit exploitable geographical contrasts. One must take care to consider specific design issues, however, as listed below.

(a) Are there known major risk factors for the pathology investigated and, if so, are there available summary measures at the ecological or within-area level that can be included? For example, studies of the influence of radon on lung cancer without correct assessment of tobacco and industrial factors are unlikely to yield interesting results, while studies of the influence of environmental exposure on childhood leukaemia do not suffer from the existence of major confounders. In this context, restricting the study to particular age groups might be beneficial because it is more straightforward to take latency effects into account by using a lagged summary exposure measure for one age class.

(b) What are the relative sizes of the within- and between-area variations of the exposure? Are there repeated measures available which can be exploited to assess the within-area variability and be incorporated into the geographical model? If the between-area variation is not larger than the within-area one, then the study should be reconsidered.

(c) Is there the possibility of investigating the constancy of the association between different time periods and/or of studying several pathologies which are a priori linked to the same environmental risk factors? The availability of several time periods allows the estimation of area-level random effects, independently of the introduction of a spatial structure. Consequently, in the space-time context, there is the possibility for a better control of confounding and less sensitivity to the choice of spatial models. Of course, the hypothesis here is that the area-level random effects take into account unmeasured risk factors *that are fairly stable over time*. Risk factors linked to socio-cultural habits are, on the other hand, likely to vary over time and should be incorporated for each time period.

References

Alexander, E.F., Cartwright R. A., McKinney, P. A., and Ricketts, T. J. (1990). Leukaemia incidence, social class and estuaries: an ecological analysis. *Journal of Public Health Medicine*, **12**, 109–17.

Armstrong, B. and Doll, R. (1975). Environmental factors and cancer incidence and mortality in different countries, with special reference to dietary practices. *International Journal of Cancer*, **15**, 617–31.

Bernardinelli, L., Clayton, D., and Montomoli, C. (1995). Bayesian estimates of disease map: how important are priors? *Statistics in Medicine*, **14**, 2411–31.

Besag, J., York, J., and Mollié, A. (1991). Bayesian image restoration with applications in spatial statistics (with discussion). *Annals of the Institute of Mathematical Statistics*, **43**, 1–59.

Blot, W. J. and Fraumeni, J. F. (1977). Geographical patterns of oral cancer in the United States: etiological implications. *Journal of Chronic Diseases*, **30**, 745–757.

Chen, J., Geissler, C., Parpia, B., and Campbell, T. C. (1992). Antioxydant status and cancer mortality in China. *International Journal of Epidemiology*, **21**, 625–35.

Clayton, D. (1994). BEAM: A program for Bayesian Ecological Analysis and Mapping. Technical Report. MRC Biostatistics Unit, Cambridge.

Clayton, D. and Bernardinelli, L. (1992). Bayesian methods for mapping disease risk. In *Geographical and environment epidemiology: methods for small area studies* (P. Elliott, J. Cuzick, D. English, and R. Stern ed.), 205–20. Oxford University Press.

Clayton, D. and Kaldor, J. (1987). Empirical Bayes estimates of age-standardised relative risks for use disease mapping. *Biometrics*, **43**, 671–81.

Clayton, D., Bernardinelli, L., and Montomoli, C. (1993). Spatial correlation in ecological analysis. *International Journal of Epidemiology*, **22**, 1193–202.

Cook, D. G. and Pocock, S. J. (1983). Multiple regression in geographical mortality studies, with allowance for spatially correlated errors. *Biometrics*, **39**, 361–71.

Elliott, P., Kleinschmidt, I., and Westlake, A. J. (1992). Use of routine data in studies of point sources of environmental pollution. In *Geographical and environment epidemiology: methods for small area studies* (P. Elliott, J. Cuzick, D. English, and R. Stern ed.), 106–14. Oxford University Press.

Gilks, W. R., Richardson, S., and Spiegelhalter, D. J. (ed.) (1996). *Markov chain Monte Carlo in practice*. Chapman and Hall, London.

Greenland, S. and Morgenstern, H. (1989). Ecological bias, confounding and effect modification. *International Journal of Epidemiology*, **18**, 269–74.

Greenland, S. and Robins, J. (1994). Ecological studies-biases, misconceptions and counter-examples. *American Journal Epidemiology*, **139**, 747–60.

Haslett, J. and Hayes, K. (1998). Residuals for the linear model with general covariance structure. *Journal of the Royal Statistical Society, Series B*, **60**, 201–15.

Hatch, M. and Susser, M. (1990). Background gamma radiation and childhood cancers within ten miles of a US nuclear plant. *International Journal of Epidemiology*, **19**, 546–52.

Lasserre, V., Guihenneuc-Jouyaux, C., and Richardson, S. (2000). Biases in ecological studies: utility of including within-area distribution of confounders. *Statistics in Medicine*, **19**, 45–59.

Mollié, A. (1996). Bayesian mapping of disease. In *Markov Chain Monte Carlo in Practice* (W. R. Gilks, S. Richardson, and D. J. Spiegelhalter ed.), 359–79. Chapman and Hall, London.

Piantadosi, S., Byar, D. P., and Green, S. B. (1988). The ecological fallacy. *American Journal of Epidemiology*, **127**, 893–904.

Plummer, M. and Clayton, D. (1996). Estimation of population exposure in ecological studies (with discussion). *Journal of the Royal Statistical Society, Series B*, **58**, 113–26.

Richardson, S. (1992). Statistical methods for geographical correlation studies. In *Geographical and environment epidemiology: methods for small area studies* (P. Elliott, J. Cuzick, D. English, and R. Stern ed.), 181–204. Oxford University Press.

Richardson, S. (1996). Discussion of paper by Plummer and Clayton. *Journal of the Royal Statistical Society, Series B*, **58**, 141–3.

Richardson, S., Montfort, C., Green, M., Draper, G., and Muirhead, C. (1995). Spatial variation of natural radiation and childhood leukaemia incidence in Great Britain. *Statistics in Medicine*, **14**, 2487–501.

Richardson, S., Stucker, I., and Hemon, D. (1987). Comparison of relative risks obtained in ecological and individual studies: some methodological considerations. *International Journal of Epidemiology*, **16**, 111–120.

Richardson, S., Guihenneuc, C., and Lasserre, V. (1992). Spatial linear models with autocorrelated error structure. *The Statistician*, **41**, 539–57.

Richardson, S., Guihenneuc-Jouhaux, C. and Lasserre, V. (1996). Ecological studies-biases, misconceptions, and counterexamples (Letter). *American Journal of Epidemiology*, **143**, 522–3.

Rose, D. P., Boyar, A. P., and Wynder, E. L., (1986). International comparisons of mortality rates for cancer of the breast, ovary, prostate, and colon, and per capita food consumption. *Cancer*, **58**, 2363–71.

Ross, J. A., Davies, S. D., Potter, J. D., and Robinson, L. L. (1994). Epidemiology of childhood leukaemia, with a focus on infants. *Epidemiologic Reviews*, **16**, 243–72.

Spiegelhalter, D. J., Thomas, A., Best, N. G., and Gilks, W. R. (1996). *BUGS: Bayesian inference using Gibbs sampling, Version 5.0*. Medical Research Council Biostatistics Unit, Cambridge.

Susser, M. (1994*a*). The logic in ecological? I: The logic of analysis. *American Journal of Public Health*, **84**, 825–9.

Susser, M. (1994*b*). The logic in ecological? II: The logic of design. *American Journal of Public Health*, **84**, 830–5.

Wakefield, J. and Morris, S. (1999). Spatial dependence and errors-in-variables. *Bayesian Statistics 6* (J. M. Bernardo, J. O. Berger, A. P. Dawid, and A. F. M. Smith ed.), 657–84. Oxford University Press.

III Disease mapping and clustering

Map 3: Stomach, women
1986–1990, all ages

Carte 3: Estomac, femmes
1986–1990, tous les âges

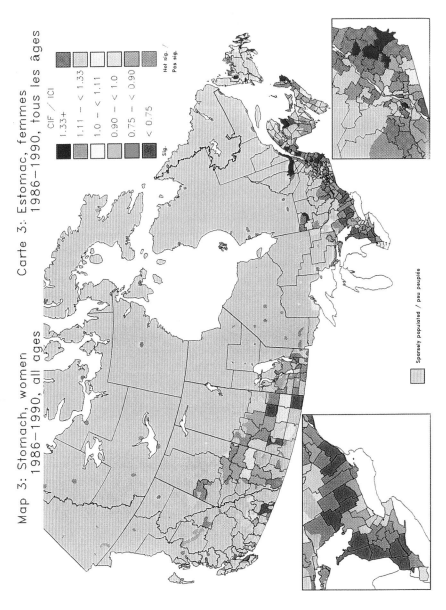

CIF / ICI

1.33+
1.11 — < 1.33
1.0 — < 1.11
0.90 — < 1.0
0.75 — < 0.90
< 0.75

Sig.   Not sig. /
                                              Pas sig.

Sparsely populated / peu peuplée

Plate 1   Stomach cancer incidence map. Canada 1986–90, females (from Le *et al.* 1996). Mapped function is the comparative incidence figure. Note map projection (Lambert conformal conic) to reflect large areas with sparse population, and incorporation of statistical significance into choropleth category definitions.

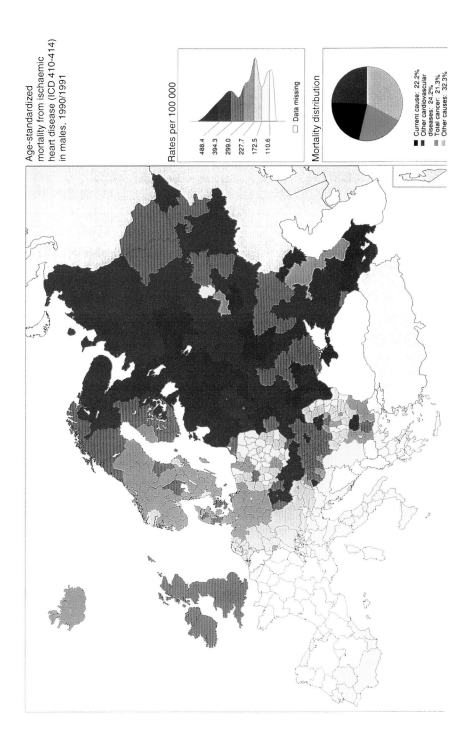

Age-standardized
mortality from ischaemic
heart disease (ICD 410-414)
in males, 1990/1991

Rates per 100 000

488.4
394.3
299.0
227.7
172.5
110.6

☐ Data missing

Mortality distribution

■ Current cause: 22.2%
■ Other cardiovascular diseases: 24.2%
▨ Total cancer: 21.3%
▨ Other causes: 32.3%

Plate 2 Ischaemic heart disease mortality in males, Europe 1990–1 (from WHO 1997). Note changes in risk at some international boundaries.

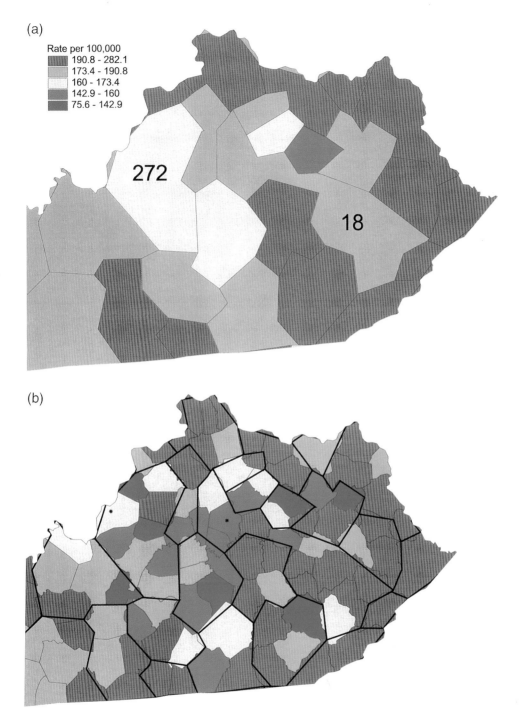

Plate 3   Age-adjusted death rates for coronary heart disease in Kentucky. (a) by health service areas, and (b) by counties. Asterisks (*) indicate cities with populations over 50 000.

HEART DISEASE
WHITE MALE

AGE-ADJUSTED DEATH RATES BY HSA, 1988–92

(a)

Age-adjusted

(U.S. rate = 205.0)

Rate per 100,000 population	Comparative mortality ratio (HSA to U.S.)
253.8 – 328.6	1.24 – 1.60
236.8 – 253.7	1.16 – 1.24
215.2 – 236.7	1.05 – 1.16
199.9 – 215.1	0.98 – 1.05
179.5 – 199.8	0.88 – 0.98
166.7 – 179.4	0.81 – 0.88
112.4 – 166.6	0.55 – 0.81

Distribution of HSA rates per 100,000 population

Proportion

ICD–9 Categories 390–398, 402, 404–429

SOURCE: CDC/NCHS

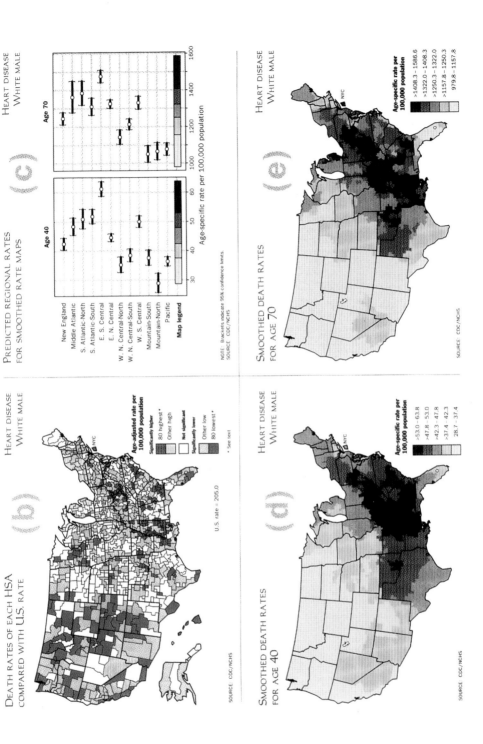

DEATH RATES OF EACH HSA COMPARED WITH U.S. RATE

HEART DISEASE
WHITE MALE

(b)

Age-adjusted rate per 100,000 population

Significantly higher
80 highest *
Other high

Not significant

Significantly lower
Other low
80 lowest *

* See text

U.S. rate = 205.0

SOURCE: CDC/NCHS

PREDICTED REGIONAL RATES FOR SMOOTHED RATE MAPS

HEART DISEASE
WHITE MALE

(c)

Age 40

Age 70

New England
Middle Atlantic
S. Atlantic-North
S. Atlantic-South
E. S. Central
E. N. Central
W. N. Central-North
W. N. Central-South
W. S. Central
Mountain-South
Mountain-North
Pacific

Map legend

Age-specific rate per 100,000 population

NOTE: Brackets indicate 95% confidence limits.
SOURCE: CDC/NCHS

SMOOTHED DEATH RATES FOR AGE 40

HEART DISEASE
WHITE MALE

(d)

Age-specific rate per 100,000 population
>53.0 – 63.8
>47.8 – 53.0
>42.3 – 47.8
>37.4 – 42.3
28.7 – 37.4

SOURCE: CDC/NCHS

SMOOTHED DEATH RATES FOR AGE 70

HEART DISEASE
WHITE MALE

(e)

Age-specific rate per 100,000 population
>1408.3 – 1586.6
>1322.0 – 1408.3
>1250.3 – 1322.0
>1157.8 – 1250.3
979.8 – 1157.8

SOURCE: CDC/NCHS

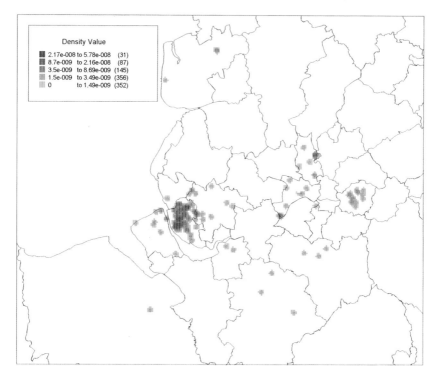

Plate 5 Two-dimensional density estimation map based on individual cases of 'Disease B'.

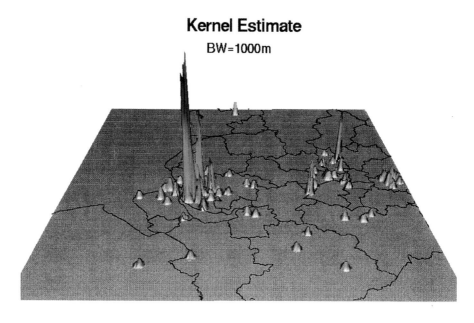

Plate 6 Three-dimensional density estimation map based on individual cases of 'Disease B'.

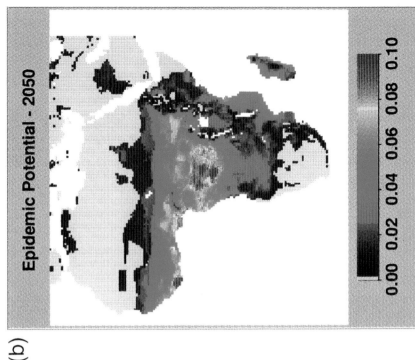

Plate 7 Calculation of epidemic potential for malaria in Africa, 1970–2050.

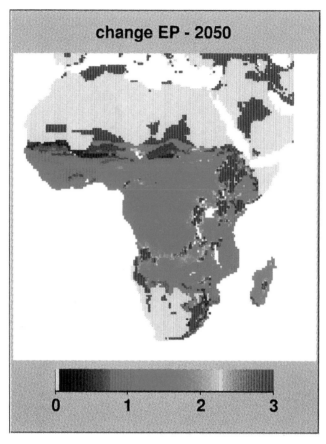

Plate 8 Calculation of change in epidemic potential for malaria in Africa, 2050.

12. Disease mapping: a historical perspective

S. D. Walter

12.1 Introduction

This chapter reviews the history of disease mapping over the past two hundred years. Medical geography is by now a substantial discipline, and space will permit only a sampling of the relevant literature; only selected examples of disease maps will be discussed, particularly those that illustrate points of methodology. There will be some emphasis on developments over the past ten years, and how they might suggest future directions in this field.

12.2 Early development of cartography

The creation of maps is an activity almost as old as recorded history. The earliest examples of maps from ancient civilisations in Mesopotamia and Egypt are as much as 5000 years old, and typically show important features of physical geography (such as mountains and bodies of water). Aspects of human activity were also mapped, for example to re-establish property lines after the annual floods of the Nile (Robinson *et al.* 1978).

In contrast to so-called *general* maps, which simultaneously represent several geographical phenomena, *thematic* maps display the spatial pattern of a single phenomenon, or sometimes the spatial relationships between several phenomena. Thematic cartography began around 1800, and was often stimulated by available data on the environment or society, for example on the weather or crime rates. Disease mapping began at about this time, motivated by a desire to evaluate geographical patterns in disease, and to identify risk factors that might explain those patterns.

12.3 Disease maps in the nineteenth century

Early disease maps often concerned infectious diseases, particularly yellow fever in the United States and cholera in Europe. Stevenson (1965) reports examples by Seaman just before 1800, spot maps that show the street locations of individual cases of yellow fever in New York. Similar maps in the early nineteenth century were used in the miasma-contagion debate. Areas with a suitable environment (warm temperatures and poor drainage) were supposed to suffer from a 'pathogenic mist' causing the disease, rather than the disease being spread by person-to-person transmission.

The cholera maps in Europe followed the same approach, sometimes showing mortality on a national scale, such as in Britain (Peterman 1852, cited by Howe 1989). A more recent example shows risks in parts of the Ganges Delta (Fig. 12.1); note that in addition to the case locations, it indicates areas of slow water flow below a certain height contour, a possible risk factor for the disease. At a local street level, the spot map approach was used most famously by John Snow (1855) in London, to demonstrate the spread of cholera through contaminated water.

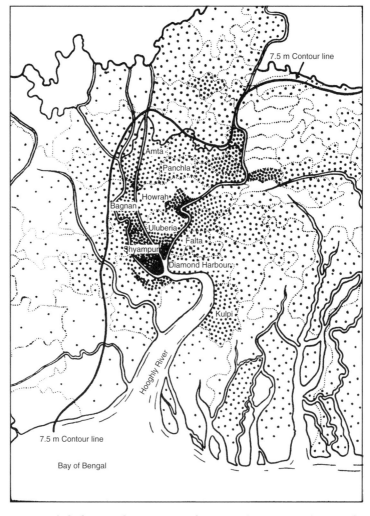

Fig. 12.1 Spot map of cholera in the Ganges Delta, 1936 (Jusatz 1977). Note that data reflect the case numerators only.

It should be noted that spot maps show only the case numerators, and do not take underlying population denominators into account. They therefore fail to provide disease rates, as would be expected by the contemporary epidemiologist. Interpretation of a spot map has to be supplemented by knowledge of the population residential density; or the distribution of potential risk factors. In examples, such as the Ganges cholera map, one cannot infer much about geographical differences in risk without also knowing about the population distribution in the area. In Snow's investigation interpretation was aided by information on the water distribution system.

Since the nineteenth century, interest in mapping infectious disease has continued, including the use of 'diffusion' maps to examine the spread of disease on a wider scale. Examples include the spread of cholera (see Fig. 12.2), influenza (Hunter and Young 1971), measles (Cliff *et al.* 1981), and a reconstruction of the spread of plague in the fourteenth century (Carpentier 1962). Other examples are considered in Chapter 14.

In a notable exception to the preoccupation at the time with the threat of infectious diseases, Haviland (1875) pioneered mapping of chronic disease, including heart disease and cancer in England and Wales. Haviland used mortality data from 1851–60: centralised, vital registration had been in existence since 1839. Combining mortality numerators

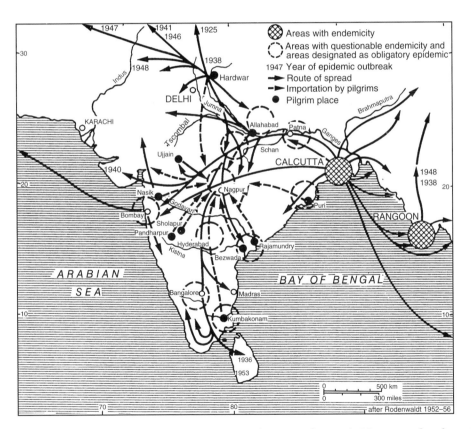

Fig. 12.2 Diffusion of cholera in Asia, 1931–55 (Learmonth 1972). Note postulated routes of transmission between endemic areas, dates of diffusion and postulated high risk groups (pilgrims).

with populations from the census, he computed crude death rates, thus becoming one of the first epidemiologists systematically to take denominators into account in a geographical analysis. Haviland recognised a problem that persists in disease maps even today, that of possible instability in the rates. He stated;

... the numbers ... that I use are proportional, not absolute: and being so, it is all the more necessary that the gross sum from which they are deduced should be as large as possible.

Haviland claimed to detect distinct regional patterns in mortality throughout the country; areas of high risk were coloured in blue (possibly by analogy with cyantotic blood) and low risk in red (healthy, oxygenated blood)—the opposite of the common modern convention to show *high* risk in red.

12.4   Disease maps 1900–90

Disease mapping in this century has been dominated by the production of numerous national and regional atlases of chronic diseases, particularly cancer. The United Kingdom and the United States were prominent early participants, and atlases published in those countries demonstrate some evolution in methodology.

12.4.1   The United Kingdom

In the 1920s and 1930s, Stocks produced a series of cancer mortality maps for England and Wales (Stocks 1928, 1936, 1937, 1939). An important methodological advance was an adjustment for regional differences in age and sex, thus avoiding possibly biased comparisons of crude rates, as in Haviland's work more than fifty years earlier. These maps also stimulated a formal statistical assessment of the spatial pattern in the data (Cruickshank 1947).

Stocks' work was updated by Howe (1963) in a national atlas for 13 major causes of death in 1954–8. A typical map is shown in Fig. 12.3; the standardised mortality ratio (SMR) is the function plotted, using the choropleth method in which each geographical area of analysis is shaded according to its data value. In a later revision (Howe 1970), a plotting symbol was used for each area, with size representing the base population. Modifications to the plotting symbols also indicated urban versus rural areas and statistical significance. Further updates in the 1980s (Gardner *et al.* 1983, 1984; Howe 1989) have followed essentially the same methods, with the addition of colour.

Use of plotting symbols was prompted in part by a desire to reduce the visual impact of large areas with small populations; these areas may dominate choropleth maps. Another option is the cartogram (Dorling 1995). This distorts the area (and shape) of the spatial units to make them proportional to the denominator variable. One example is the iso-demographic map, which distorts the base geographical map to have approximately equal population density. Figure 12.4 shows an iso-demographic map for influenza in England and Wales.

In Scotland, data from five regional registries were combined to show national maps of cancer incidence (Kemp *et al.* 1985). Geographical clustering of high risk areas was also examined using a rank adjacency statistic.

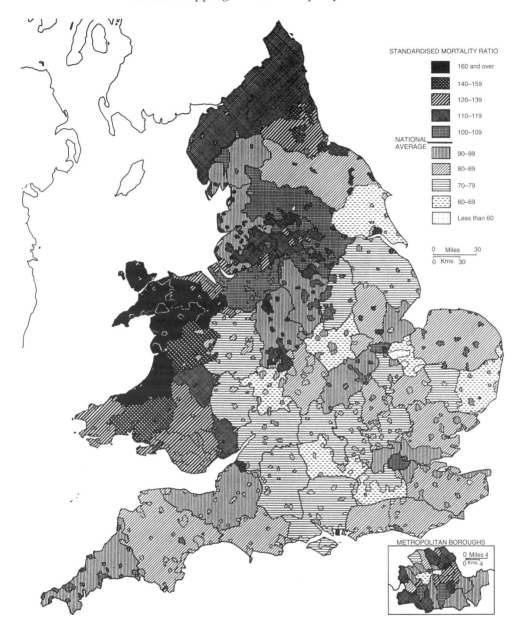

STANDARDISED MORTALITY RATIO

160 and over

140–159

120–139

110–119

100–109

NATIONAL
AVERAGE

90–99

80–89

70–79

60–69

Less than 60

0   Miles   30

0   Kms.   30

METROPOLITAN BOROUGHS

0 Miles 4

0 Kms. 4

Fig. 12.3 Choropleth map showing cancer mortality of the stomach (males) in England and Wales (from Howe 1963: 33). Note the use of classed choropleths, and the inset for densely populated area. Mapped function is the standardised mortality ratio.

12.4.2 The United States

Disease mapping at the national level in the US began somewhat later than in Britain. Early work (Burbank 1971) had suggested some geographical variation in mortality rates,

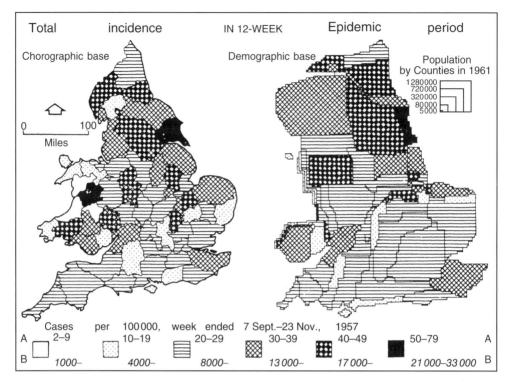

Fig. 12.4 Influenza in England and Wales, 1957, showing choropleth and iso-demographic maps (from Learmonth 1978). The left panel represents notified cases of acute pneumonia; the right panel represents estimated cases of influenza based on pneumonia rates. Note the increased impact of densely populated southeastern areas and reduced impact of areas such as North Wales in the iso-demographic projection.

although not as great as international differences. National atlases were produced showing approximately 3000 area-specific cancer mortality rates in whites (Mason *et al.* 1975) and non-whites (Mason *et al.* 1976), plus non-cancer mortality (Mason *et al.* 1981). Later updates showed trends in risk during 1950–80 (Pickle *et al.* 1987, 1990).

The American atlases used choropleths, with areas such as counties. The plotted data function has usually been the age-adjusted rate; areas in the highest decile of risk relative to the national rate are shown, together with an indication of statistical significance. Values significantly lower than the national rate are also differentiated, but without regard to their decile group. Some of the trend analyses (Pickle *et al.* 1987, 1990) have plotted only those areas in which mortality was increasing or decreasing at a statistically significant rate.

12.4.3 Other countries

Many other countries have initiated disease mapping over the last forty years. A survey of disease atlases and their methods in 1991 (Walter and Birnie 1991) showed that most concerned cancer in developed countries. The majority involved mortality data from the

1960s and later, although a few were able to use incidence figures, or data from earlier years (e.g. Finland accessed cancer incidence starting in 1953, Pukkala *et al.* 1987). Only a few examples existed of international collaboration, from the European Community and the Nordic countries. The 1991 survey revealed the following points:

1. ***Data selection*** There was considerable variation in the diseases selected, and in the diagnostic categories used. For example, cancer was variously grouped into as few as 4 or as many as 36 categories by different countries.

2. ***Numerators and denominators*** Information was often lacking on case numerators or population denominators, making it impossible to assess the precision of the mapped values of disease risk.

3. ***Units of analysis*** The regional units of analysis also varied considerably in size. Many regions had such small expected frequencies that random variation would dominate the data. Interestingly, the smaller regions tended to occur in atlases that covered larger total populations.

4. ***Criteria for mapping*** Criteria for selecting a diagnostic group for mapping, or for plotting regional values on a map, were frequently not stated. A few atlases offered criteria based on minimum case frequencies, population sizes, or population density.

5. ***Data function to be mapped*** The most commonly plotted data function was the relative risk (or equivalent), possibly in conjunction with statistical significance. Other functions included case frequencies or statistical significance alone. The choice of function makes an enormous difference to the appearance of the map, but the rationale for the choice adopted was rarely discussed.

6. ***Mapping method*** Most atlases used choropleth shading, but a few used plotting symbol to indicate the levels of other variables. Data smoothing was used only rarely.

7. ***Age-standardisation*** Age-standardisation was used by almost all atlases, most often with the indirect method. Contrary to expectation, atlases using the direct method tended to have smaller regional populations and case frequencies than those using the indirect method. Age groups used in the standardisation were often not reported.

8. ***Colour*** About half the atlases used colour. Red usually indicated high risk, but there were many exceptions. Colour schemes to represent average risk, low risk, and missing values were highly variable.

9. ***Trend and spatial analysis*** Time trend analysis was included in about half of the atlases, but only a few statistically assessed the spatial pattern. Some atlases provided informal verbal summaries of the patterns, but few attempted any substantive aetiologic interpretation. Few provided supplemental data or maps on important covariates (e.g. socio-economic status, smoking, occupation, climate).

In summary, the position in the early 1990s was that the methodology of disease mapping varied considerably between countries. Many atlases failed to provide the basic information needed for a rigorous appraisal of the geographical disease patterns they displayed. Comparisons between atlases, especially internationally, was made difficult by numerous differences in their methods, particularly concerning disease definitions, data summarisation and mapping techniques. The Walter and Birnie (1991) survey concluded with a set of proposed guidelines to alleviate these problems in the future.

A few maps published before 1990 illustrate specific points of interest. The Finnish cancer atlas (Pukkala *et al.* 1987) was one of the earliest to use data smoothing, with a geometric centroid approach. Although this alleviates the difficulty of unstable rates, it has the disadvantage of 'smearing out' the rates in regions with sparse populations. The impact of excess risks in isolated towns can then be magnified as the rates are smoothed out into surrounding rural areas. Finland also provides a rare example of mapping *prevalence* by region (Hakulinen *et al.* 1989). This work is also unique in offering projections of incidence and prevalence into the future, by modelling the incidence rates by region, age, period, and cohort.

Vershasselt and Timmermans (1987) have proposed a three-dimensional plot for cancer mortality, but this idea has not been widely adopted. The study by Martinez *et al.* (1998) of heat-related deaths is an example of mapping acute events in small geographical areas, using dot and choropleth methods. Some maps have used risk contours instead of choro-pleths, for example in Australia (Fig. 12.5), but this idea has not been adopted often.

In addition to the proliferation of disease atlases, the 1970s and 1980s saw the publication of a number of texts in the growing discipline of medical geography. They dealt with various diseases, often on a global scale, and associated methods (Howe 1977; McGlashen 1972; Learmonth 1978; McGlashen and Blunden 1983; Hutt and Burkitt 1986; Cliff and Haggett 1988; Boyle *et al.* 1989). Learmonth (1972) provided more details of mapping in the period 1950–70.

The existence of disease maps had the effect of stimulating epidemiologic studies to investigate areas of high risk. In the USA, for example, several studies of potential hazards from occupational exposures, lifestyle factors, or the environment were initiated (National Cancer Institute 1987).

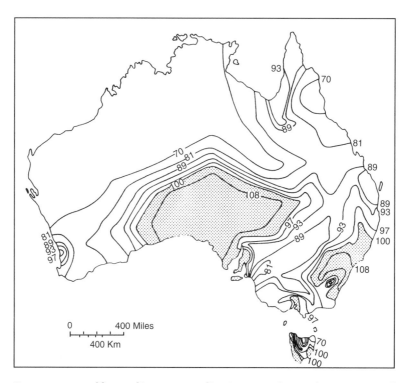

Fig. 12.5 Contour map of heart disease mortality in Australia, males, 1965–66 (from Howe *et al.* 1977). Map function if the standardised mortality ratio. Note use of inter-contour shading for areas of excess risk.

12.5   Developments since 1990

The 1990s have seen a widening of scope of disease maps. Many countries have expanded or updated their national atlases, while others have published them for the first time. Some local authorities have begun to map health data in smaller administrative areas. Several major international atlases have appeared, showing disease patterns on a wide scale. Some new causes of morbidity and mortality have been examined. Selected examples of these new publications will now be given.

The Canadian federal government has extended its series of atlases, to examine general mortality and time trends. Particular interest in the spatial pattern is evinced by the fact that causes of death were selected for mapping in part because of their 'quality and/or uniqueness of the spatial distribution'. In other words, regional differences themselves were used as a data selection criterion (Health and Welfare Canada 1991).

More recently, a Canadian atlas of cancer incidence has appeared (Le *et al.* 1996; see Plate 1). Cancer is registered provincially, so considerable attention was paid to the quality and comparability of the data from contributing registries. Geographical patterns may arise artefactually from differences in nosology, data completeness, and accuracy. Further points to note include: the stated criteria for the selection of cancer sites; a stated rationale for the choice of cut-points on the map's colour scale; and an assessment of the spatial pattern through Moran's I-statistic (see Chapter 8), with a new bootstrap estimate of its confidence interval. Relative to the large area of the country, Canada's population is highly concentrated; the base map projection is intended to reduce the impact of sparsely populated areas, and a neutral colour is used to indicate the substantial areas of the country with essentially no data.

In the Ontario cancer incidence atlas (Marrett *et al.* 1995; see Fig. 12.6), an unclassed choropleth method is used; this avoids subjective bias associated with the arbitrary choice of the number and width of class intervals. The atlas also allows for discrepancies between perceived and actual intensity of shading. Statistical significance in census districts is indicated by '+' and '−' overlays, and Moran's I-statistic is used to assess the spatial pattern. The base map uses an inset to show the sparsely populated northern areas on a larger scale.

Much smaller geographical areas (census sub-divisions) were examined in the Great Lakes Health Effects Program, which produced atlases of cancer, birth defects, and hospital morbidity in Ontario (Mills and Semenciw 1992; Johnson *et al.* 1992; Health Canada 1993).

The 1996 US mortality atlas (Pickle *et al.* 1996) shows age-adjusted rates by sex and race. As in previous US publications, the data are also shown as risks relative to the national average, with categories defined by a combination of percentiles and statistical significance. Smoothed regional rates are computed. Data on a given cause of death are presented in five different forms, with different colours for each. The style of presentation was guided by associated research on cognition; this indicated a preference for classed choropleths, and that plotting symbols were not feasible for the US map because of its large number of areas (see Chapter 13 and Plate 3).

An earlier US publication (Devine *et al.* 1991) investigated injury mortality, covering deaths such as homicide, falls, and drowning. Empirical Bayes smoothing (Chapters 7 and 15) was used on age-specific rates by county, which were subsequently

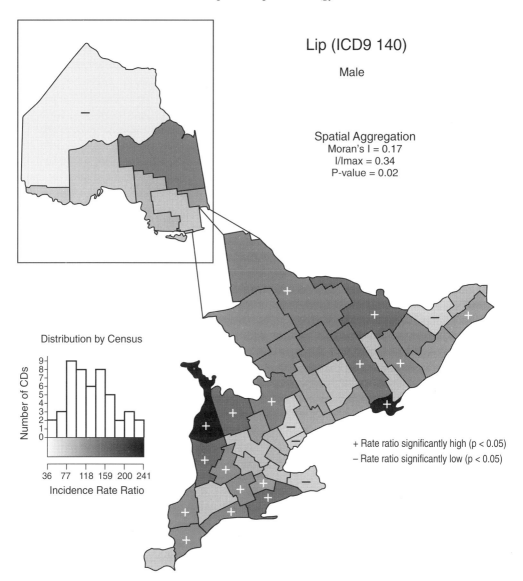

Fig. 12.6 Lip cancer incidence, Ontario 1980–91 (from Marrett *et al.* 1995). Note the use of unclassed choropleths, inset for sparsely populated areas, map overlays to indicate statistical significance, rate histogram, and summary index of spatial aggregation.

age-standardised. National and state maps include an estimate of the excess deaths, relative to the national mean.

Several European countries have recently published disease maps, and some present new methodological points. The cancer mortality atlas of Poland (Zatoñski *et al.* 1993) used a geographical centroid smoothing method, with weights inversely proportional to the distance from the point being smoothed, and directly proportional to the population denominator. Special plotting symbols show the rates in large cities.

Special plotting symbols are also used in the mortality atlas for Estonia (Baburin *et al.* 1997), which discussed the difficulty of converting the several Russian versions of the ICD that had been in use during the data collection period (1968–92). Some jurisdictions, for example, Norway (Cancer Registry 1998) and Sweden (Regional Oncologic Centres 1996), have continued to exploit their high quality disease registration systems to issue atlases of cancer incidence, thus also avoiding interpretational problems associated with mortality data (Boyle 1989).

An atlas of cancer mortality in Switzerland (Schüler and Bopp 1997) stabilises the mapped rates with a new method based on mean ranks over time. Continuous shading with overlays to indicate statistical significance is used, similar to the Ontario cancer incidence atlas. Other features include the display of data by language regions of the country and by size of community; and the detailed attempt at aetiological explanation of the geographical patterns observed.

In its mortality atlas, Spain (Ortega *et al.* 1996) joins the small group that have included a statistical examination of the spatial pattern, using the rank adjacency statistic pioneered in atlases in Scotland (Kemp *et al.* 1985) and Italy (Cislaghi *et al.* 1986). Maps of southern Sweden (Southern Swedish Regional Tumour Registry 1994) use plotting symbol overlays to show the number of cancer cases in each region.

The Europeans have also made considerable progress in the field of international disease mapping, with the recent publication of three major atlases. The European Community (EC) atlas of cancer mortality (Smans *et al.* 1992) assembled data from nine countries, with 355 regions. International mortality comparisons involve additional questions of data comparability and accuracy. Although previous literature suggests substantial international differences in how deaths are coded (Percy *et al.* 1981; Boyle 1989), no study of this question had been carried out in all the countries contributing to the EC atlas. Some indirect markers of data quality were available, such as the proportion of deaths occurring in hospital, but the potential for systematic between-country bias is strong. Indeed, several maps in this atlas show evidence of changes in risk at international boundaries. It is not clear if these effects are related to true differences in risk, or to cultural differences in how deaths are classified.

The EC authors discuss some other issues of methodology that arise when considering such a large and diverse geographical area. The role of chance in labelling particular regions as having extreme risk is prominent. They also consider potential biases associated with inaccurate denominators and migration effects, especially with respect to the surprisingly low risk seen in Southern Italy for many causes of death.

The atlas of cancer mortality in Central Europe (Zatoñski *et al.* 1996) used mortality and trend data from nine other countries. Major issues of data quality and comparability arose here also. The authors discussed the process of death coding in the various countries, and considered measures of quality such as the proportion of autopsies, ill-defined causes of death, and 'vague site' classifications. Substantial international variation existed in these indices, with the implication that some of the geographical patterns found could be artefactual. While these potential problems in the mortality data should be recognised, the preferred incidence data are not yet available in these countries.

Lastly, the atlas of mortality in Europe (WHO 1997) is perhaps the most ambitious collaborative project of this type to date. It covers 50 countries in the European Region of the WHO, with a total population of approximately 850 million people. Mortality data are shown as rates and histograms for 1980/91 and 1990/91. Numerous discrepancies and idiosyncracies occurred in the assembly of data. Compilation required elimination of non-comparable data groupings, and 'plausibility checking' to eliminate clerical and programming errors. Despite these attempts to improve data quality, apparent risk differences are still observed at national boundaries, as occurred in the EC atlas. For example (Plate 2), international boundaries can be discerned quite easily in the map of mortality from ischaemic heart disease. The European atlas has the progressive feature of allowing Internet access via its website (http://www.euromort.rivm.nl). Users can access maps of their own choosing, with control over data time period, cause of death, and sex. Some details of contributing nations and local area data are also available.

The worldwide distribution of AIDS has been examined recently (Smallman-Raynor *et al.* 1992). This atlas uses conventional mapping techniques, but also includes maps of the disease diffusion based on stochastic modelling. A considerable amount of data at the national and regional levels is also provided. This atlas represents an interesting return to mapping infectious diseases, but with modern techniques.

As in earlier years, the existence of disease maps has stimulated the execution of targeted epidemiological studies, and the development of new mapping methods. There has been some interest in trend surface analysis, to identify local deviations in risk after adjustment for regional effects or relevant covariates (e.g. Cislaghi *et al.* 1990; Jones *et al.* 1992; Sturgeon *et al.* 1995; Sinha and Benedict 1996). Smoothing, in conjunction with covariate adjustment, has also been proposed (Kafadar 1997). Some studies attempt to use geographical patterns to demonstrate the effect of preventive interventions, such as cervical cancer screening (Lazcano-Ponce *et al.* 1996).

A small amount of work has taken place concerning the perceptual psychology of maps. Experimental evidence has shown that the impact of a map can be substantially affected by 'incidental' features such as the type of shading used, and that there may be differences between the statistical and visual impressions of the data. Perception may also depend on the inherent complexity of the base map (Walter 1993). Map features, such as plotting symbols, have been used very successfully in some circumstances, but they may not be feasible for maps with large numbers of areas (Pickle *et al.* 1996). Use of colour, while having aesthetic appeal, may nevertheless be confusing to the map reader (Wainer and Francolini 1980); and makes accurate photo-reproduction more difficult. The choices of data collection periods and mapping categories can also be debated (Hole and Lamont 1992; Cromley and Cromley 1996).

Interpretation of the spatial relationships of diseases to risk factors are complicated by the so-called ecological fallacy (Walter 1991; Greenland and Robins 1994; Chapter 11). Even greater analytic complexity occurs when risk factors are measured at several levels of geographical scale (e.g. Duncan *et al.* 1993; Langford *et al.* 1998).

12.6   Mapping in the twenty-first century

Recent years have seen a rapid growth in the availability of data suitable for geographical analysis, and in the methods for producing disease maps. The 1991 survey (Walter and Birnie 1991) highlighted the diversity in approaches used in various countries, and this diversification has continued in the past decade. Accordingly, it seems dangerous to make detailed prognostication about future directions. There are, however, a few broad trends, which might be conjectured to persist.

1. ***International cooperation***   As noted earlier, international comparisons between national disease atlases have previously been hampered by their substantial differences in methodology. Continued collaboration between the European countries is therefore an encouraging sign. With the new European atlases, one can make broad-scale geographical comparisons, based on methods that are nominally consistent. There remain concerns about data quality, and some of the apparent regional trends may be due in part to methodological artefacts, rather than true environmental effects. The same may also be true within countries, such as between the provinces of Canada. *We may anticipate further efforts at inter-jurisdictional cooperation in the future.*

2. ***Use of incidence data***   There have been an increasing number of cancer atlases based on incidence data. As noted earlier, incidence data are much preferable, avoiding many biases associated with mortality data. Many countries, however, still do not possess population-based cancer registries to estimate incidence. *One may hope for an expansion of cancer incidence registration to the many places that currently have to rely on mortality data.*

3. ***Maps of non-cancer diseases***   Incidence data for non-cancer disorders is at a primitive stage, and only isolated examples of maps for problems, such as birth defects exist currently. *There may be greater emphasis in future disease maps on causes of morbidity such as injuries, mental disease, and non-cancer chronic disease, which have received little attention to date.*

4. ***Adoption of statistical methods***   *As shown elsewhere in this book, there has been a dramatic increase in the scope and complexity of statistical techniques for the analysis of geographical health data, but so far this has had relatively little impact on how disease maps are produced in practice.* For example, while a few atlases show smoothed rates (using geographical smoothers or empirical Bayes methods), the vast majority continue to show only unsmoothed data. It seems that this is partly because of some distrust of statistical manipulation of any kind by local heath authorities; administrators and medical officers of health want to see their rates, uncontaminated (as they see it) by statistical adjustments of any kind.
    A case in point arose during the production of the Ontario cancer atlas (Marrett *et al.* 1995). It was discovered that Bayesian smoothed rates in many smaller regions were substantially affected by the dominant effects of one or two locations that had much larger populations. Future users of the atlas had a strong preference to see the data in 'raw' form in the first place; showing smoothed data as well would have meant approximately doubling the size of the atlas, which then became infeasible. It may be assumed that this experience is not an isolated one. Smoothing was employed, however, in the most recent US mortality atlas (Pickle *et al.* 1996); smoothing may be more feasible here, given the relatively large number of units of analysis.
    A similar picture emerges with respect to the analysis of spatial pattern. Despite the wide range of statistical techniques available, to date only a few atlases have included statistical measures of geographical clustering in the data. Most present merely a subjective verbal description of the data patterns.

5. ***Trend analysis***   *There have been an increasing number of atlases that consider changes in the pattern of risk over time.* This may reflect the increasing data collection periods provided by centralised disease and death registration systems. Analysis of space-time interaction is an appealing way to obtain greater insight into disease aetiology, but as the time-span of the analysis increases, one must be cautious about possible artefactual changes in the data. These would include issues, such as changes in disease coding, and completeness and accuracy over time, especially if such changes might have a geographical component.

6. ***Choice of data function to be mapped***   The earlier survey (Walter and Birnie 1991) revealed substantial inconsistencies between countries in the methods used, including the choice of function to be mapped. *Inconsistency persists in more recent atlases, with a mixture of rate values and statistical significance being plotted simultaneously or separately.* Recently, there has perhaps

been greater recognition of the potential misinterpretation of statistical *p*-values, in particular that significant deviations in risk are more likely to occur in large populations, even if the actual deviations are small. Nevertheless, one continues to see maps where this problem is not acknowledged. The reluctance of map publishers to used smoothed data probably reflects lack of familiarity on the part of users and a continuing desire by consumers to inspect their basic data at the local level.

7. ***Increasing access to mapping technology*** The development of powerful computers has been a major force in the potential for disease mapping. It is likely that this trend will continue, so that larger databases and more rigorous analytical methods will become accessible to a wide circle of consumers. The availability of the European mortality atlas on the Internet is probably only the first such venture. *In the future we will likely see capability for on-line manipulation of data to create maps to the user's specifications, and an interface with other databases containing information on relevant covariables.*

8. ***Reduction of publication times*** To date the interval between data collection and map publication has typically been measured in years. *We may expect the greater availability of rapid computing to reduce publication times, and make disease maps more useful as a tool for ongoing health surveillance.*

9. ***Integration of risk factor information*** Atlases to date have focused primarily on the disease data, with little attention to possible risk factors. *It is likely that we will see improved integration of disease and risk factor databases, enhanced capability to map such data simultaneously, and to understand their relationships.*

    Multi-level analysis is emerging as an important statistical technique for risk factor analysis in epidemiology, but limited methodology exists for effectively mapping this type of data. *A particular challenge will be to develop suitable cartographic methods to display covariates measured at several levels of scale.*

10. ***Geographical scope of future maps*** In the early development of disease maps, there was much concern with the worldwide spread of infectious diseases, including the interplay between the developed and the developing world. *Most of the activity in this century has nonetheless been dominated by work in the developed countries.* Large parts of the world's population live in territory still uncharted by the medical geographer. *One may hope that this situation will improve with increasing globalisation of science, the growing importance of the developing countries, and the recognition that disease does not respect political boundaries.*

Acknowledgements

This work was supported in part through a National Health Scientist award from Health Canada

References

Baburin, A., Gornoi, K., Leinsalu, M., and Rahu, M. (1997). *Atlas of mortality in Estonia*. Institute of Experimental and Clinical Medicine, Tallinn.
Boyle, P. (1989). Relative value of incidence and mortality data in cancer research. In *Cancer mapping* (P. Boyle, C. S. Muir, and E. Grundmann ed.). Springer, Berlin.
Boyle, P., Muir, C., and Grundmann, E. (ed.) (1989). *Cancer mapping*. Springer, Berlin.
Burbank, F. (1971) Patterns in cancer mortality in the United States: 1950–70. *National Cancer Institute Monograph*, **33**, 1–594.

Cancer Registry (1998). *Cancer in Norway 1995.* Cancer Registry of Norway, Oslo.

Carpentier, E. (1962). Autour de la peste noire: famines et epidemies dans l'histoire du xiv eme siécle. *Annals of Economic and Social Civilisations*, **17**, 1062–92.

Cislaghi, C., DeCarli, A., LaVecchia, C., Laverda, N., Mezzanotte, G., and Smans, M. (1986). *Data, statistics and maps on cancer mortality, Italy 1975/77.* Pitagora Editrice, Bologna.

Cislaghi, C., DeCarli, A., LaVecchia, C., Mezzanotte, G., and Vigotti, M.A. (1990). Trend surface models applied to the analysis of geographical variations in cancer mortality. *Revue d'Epidemiologie et de Santé Publique*, **38**, 57–69.

Cliff, A. D. and Haggett, P. (1988). *Atlas of disease distributions: analytic approaches to epidemiologic data.* Blackwell, Oxford.

Cliff, A. D., Haggett, P, Ord, J. K., and Versey, G. R. (1981). *Spatial diffusion.* Cambridge University Press.

Cromley, E. K. and Cromley, R. G. (1996). An analysis of alternative classification schemes for medical atlas mapping. *European Journal of Cancer*, **32A**, 1551–9.

Cruickshank, D. B. (1947). Regional influences in cancer. *British Journal of Cancer*, **1**, 109–28.

Devine, O. J., Annest, J. L., Kirk, M. L., Holmgreen, P., Emrich, S. S., Rosenberg, M. L. *et al.* (1991). *Injury mortality atlas of the United States, 1979–87.* US Department of Health and Human Services, Atlanta.

Dorling, D. (1995). *A new social atlas of Britain.* Wiley, Chichester.

Duncan, C., Jones, K., and Moon, G. (1993). Do places matter? A multi-level analysis of regional variations in health-related behaviour in Britain. *Social Science and Medicine*, **37**, 725–33.

Gardner, M. J., Winter, P. D., Taylor, C. P., and Acheson, E. D. (1983). *Atlas of cancer mortality in England and Wales 1968–78.* Wiley, Chichester.

Gardner, M. J., Winter, P. D., and Barker, D. J. P. (1984). *Atlas of mortality from selected diseases in England and Wales 1968–78.* Wiley, Chichester.

Greenland, S. and Robins, J. (1994). Ecologic studies—biases, misconceptions and counter-examples. *American Journal of Epidemiology*, **139**, 747–60.

Hakulinen, T., Kenward, M., Luostarinen, T., Oskanen, H., Pukkala, E, Söderman, B. *et al.* (1989). *Cancer in Finland in 1954–2008.* Finnish Cancer Registry, Helsinki.

Haviland, A. (1875). *The geographical distribution of diseases in Great Britain.* Smith Elder, London.

Health and Welfare Canada (1991). *Mortality atlas of Canada.* Vol. 4: *General mortality patterns and recent trends.* Government of Canada, Ottawa.

Health Canada (1993). *Hospital morbidity atlas, Ontario: 1985–88.* Government of Canada, Ottawa.

Hole, D. J and Lamont, D. W. (1992). Problems in the interpretation of small area analysis of epidemiologic data. *Journal of Epidemiology and Community Health*, **46**, 305–10.

Howe, G. M. (1963). *National atlas of disease mortality in the United Kingdom.* Nelson, London.

Howe, G. M. (1970). *National atlas of disease mortality in the United Kingdom*, (2nd edn). Nelson, London.

Howe, G. M. (ed) (1977). *A world geography of human diseases.* Academic Press, London.

Howe, G. M. (1989). Historical evolution of disease mapping in general and specifically of cancer mapping. In *Cancer mapping* (P. Boyle, C. S. Muir, and E. Grundmann ed.), 1–21. Springer, Berlin.

Howe, G. M., Burgess, L., and Gatenby, P. (1977). Cardiovascular disease. In *A world geography of human diseases* (G. M. Howe, ed.). Academic Press, London.

Hunter, J. M. and Young, J. C. (1971). Diffusion of influenza in England and Wales. *Annals of the Association of American Geographers*, **61**, 627–31.

Hutt, M. S. R. and Burkitt, D. P. (1986). *The geography of non-infectious diseases.* Oxford University Press.

Johnson, K., Rouleau, J., and Stweart, C. (1992). *Birth defects atlas of Ontario 1978–88.* Health Canada, Ottawa.

Jones, M. E., Shugg, D., Dwyer, T., Young, B., and Bonett, A. (1992). Interstate differences in incidence and mortality from melanoma. *Medical Journal of Australia*, **157**, 373–8.

Jusatz, H. (1977). Cholera. In *A world geography of human diseases* (G. M. Howe ed.). Academic Press, London.

Kafadar, K. (1997). Geographical trends in prostate cancer mortality: an application of spatial smoothers and the need for adjustment. *Annals of Epidemiology*, **7**, 35–45.

Kemp, I., Boyle, P., Smans, M., and Muir, C. (1985). *Atlas of cancer in Scotland, 1975–80*. International Agency for Research on Cancer, Scientific Publication 72. IARC, Lyon.

Langford, I. H, Bentham, G., and McDonald, A. (1998). Multi-level modelling of geographically aggregated data. *Statistics in Medicine*, **17**, 41–57.

Lazcano-Ponce, E. C., Rascon-Pacheco, R. A., Lozano-Ascencio, R., and Velasco-Mondragon, H. E. (1996). Mortality from cervical carcinoma in Mexico: impact of screening, 1980–90. *Acta Cytologica*, **40**, 506–12.

Le, N. D., Marrett, L. D., Robson, D. L., Semenciw, R. M., Turner, D., and Walter, S.D. (1996). *Canadian cancer incidence atlas*. Government of Canada, Ottawa.

Learmonth, A. (1972). Atlases in medical geography 1950–70: a review. In *Medical geography: techniques and field studies* (N. D. McGlashen ed.). Methuen, London.

Learmonth, A. (1978). *Patterns of disease and hunger*. David & Charles, London.

Marrett, L. D., Nishri, E. D., Swift, M. B., Walter, S. D., and Holowaty, E. J. (1995). *Geographical distribution of cancer in Ontario*. Vol. II: *Atlas of cancer incidence 1980–91*. Ontario Cancer Treatment and Research Foundation, Toronto.

Martinez, B F., Annest, J. L, Kilbourne, E. M., Kirk, M. L., Lui, K-J., and Smith, S. M. (1989). Geographical distribution of heat-related deaths among elderly persons. *Journal of American Medical Association*, **262**, 2246–50.

Mason, T. J., McKay, F. W., Hoover, R., Blot, W. J., and Fraumeni, J. F. (1975). *Atlas of cancer mortality for U.S. counties: 1950–69*. US Government Printing Office, Washington, DC.

Mason, T. J., McKay, F. W., Hoover, R., Blot, W. J., and Fraumeni, J. F. (1976). *Atlas of cancer mortality among U.S. nonwhites: 1950–69*. US Government Printing Office, Washington, DC.

Mason, T. J., Fraumeni, J. F., Hoover, R., and Blot, W. J. (1981). *An atlas of mortality from selected diseases*. US Government Printing Office, Washington, DC.

McGlashen, N. D. (ed.) (1972). *Medical geography: techniques and field studies*. Methuen, London.

McGlashen N. D. and Blunden, J. R. (ed.) (1983). *Geographical aspects of health*. Academic Press, London.

Mills, C. and Semenciw, R. (1992). *Cancer incidence in the Great Lakes region, Ontario: 1984–88*. Health Canada, Ottawa.

National Cancer Institute (1987). *Backgrounder: research contributions made possible by the NCI cancer atlases published in the 1970s*. Office of Cancer Communications. NCI, Bethesda, MD.

Ortega, G. L-A., Santamaría, M. P., Pujolar, A. E., Saizar, M. E., and Santos, V. A. (1996). *Atlas of cancer mortality and other causes of death in Spain 1978–92*. Fundación Científica de la Asociación Española contra el Cáncer, Madrid.

Percy, C., Stanek, E., and Gloeckler, L. (1981). Accuracy of death certificates and its effect on cancer mortality statistics. *American Journal of Public Health*, **71**, 242–50.

Petermann, A. H. (1852). *Cholera map of the British Isles showing the districts attacked in 1831, 1832 and 1833. Constructed from official documents*. Betts, London.

Pickle, L. W., Mason, T. J., Howard, N., Hoover, R., and Fraumeni, J. F. (1987). *Atlas of U.S. mortality among whites: 1950–80*. US Government Printing Office, Washington, DC.

Pickle, L. W., Mason, T. J., Howard, N., Hoover, R., and Fraumeni, J. F. (1990). *Atlas of US mortality among nonwhites: 1950–80*. US Government Printing Office, Washington, DC.

Pickle, L. W., Mungiole, M., Jones, G. K., and White, A. A. (1996). *Atlas of United States mortality*. National Centre for Health Statistics, Hyattsville, MD.

Pukkala, E., Gustavsson, N., and Teppo, L. (1987). *Atlas of cancer incidence in Finland 1953–82*, publication 37. Cancer Society of Finland, Helsinki.

Regional Oncologic Centres (1996). *Atlas of cancer incidence in Sweden*. Karolinska Hospital, Stockholm.

Robinson, A., Sale, R., and Morrison, J. (1978). *Elements of cartography* (4th edn). Wiley, New York.

Schüler, G. and Bopp, M. (1997). *Atlas der Krebsmortalität in der Schweiz 1970–90*. Birkhäuser, Basel.

Sinha, T. and Benedict, R. (1996). Relationship between latitude and melanoma incidence: international evidence. *Cancer Letters*, **99**, 225–31.

Smallman-Raynor, M., Cliff, A. D., and Haggett, P. (1992). *International atlas of AIDS*. Blackwell, Oxford.

Smans, M., Muir, C. S., and Boyle, P. (1992). *Atlas of cancer mortality in the European Economic Community.* International Agency for Research on Cancer, Scientific Publication 107. IARC, Lyon.

Snow, J. (1855). *On the mode of communication of cholera* (2nd edn). Churchill, London.

Southern Swedish Regional Tumour Registry (1994). *Cancer incidence in southern Sweden 1988–92.* Lund.

Stevenson, L. G. (1965). Putting disease on the map: the early use of spot maps in the study of yellow fever. *Journal of History of Medicine and Allied Sciences,* **20,** 226–61.

Stocks, P. (1928). On the evidence for a regional distribution of cancer prevalence in England and Wales. *Report of the International Conference on Cancer,* 508–19. British Empire Cancer Campaign, London.

Stocks, P. (1936). *Distribution in England and Wales of cancer of various organs,* 239–80. Annual Report. British Empire Cancer Campaign, London.

Stocks, P. (1937). *Distribution in England and Wales of cancer of various organs,* 198–223. Annual Report. British Empire Cancer Campaign, London.

Stocks, P. (1939). *Distribution in England and Wales of cancer of various organs,* 308–43. Annual Report. British Empire Cancer Campaign, London.

Sturgeon, R., Schairer, C., Gail, M., McAdams, M., Brinton, L. A., and Hoover, R. N. (1995). Geographical variation in mortality from breast cancer among white women in the United States. *Journal of the National Cancer Institute,* **87,** 1846–53.

Verhasselt, Y. and Timmermans, A. (1987). *World maps of cancer mortality.* Geografisch Instituut VUB, Brussels.

Wainer, H. and Francolini, C. M. (1980). An empirical inquiry concerning human understanding of two-variable colour maps. *American Statistician,* **34,** 81–93.

Walter, S. D. (1991). The ecologic method in the study of environmental health. *Environmental Health Perspectives,* **94,** 61–65.

Walter, S. D. (1993). Visual and statistical assessment of spatial clustering in mapped data. *Statistics in Medicine,* **12,** 1275–91.

Walter, S. D. and Birnie, S. E. (1991). Mapping mortality and morbidity patterns: an international comparison. *International of Journal of Epidemiology,* **20,** 678–89.

WHO (World Health Organisation) (1997). *Atlas of mortality in Europe.* WHO Regional Publications, European series. 75. WHO, Copenhagen.

Zatoñski, W., Pukkala, E., Didkowska, J., Tyczyñski, J., and Gustavsson, N. (1993). *Atlas of cancer mortality in Poland, 1986–90.* Cancer Center, Warsaw.

Zatoñski, W., Smans, M., Tyczyñski, J., and Boyle, P. (ed.) (1996). *Atlas of cancer mortality in central Europe.* International Agency for Research on Cancer, Scientific Publication 134. IARC, Lyon.

13. Mapping mortality data in the United States

L. W. Pickle

13.1 Introduction

Mapping incident cases of disease has been a tool by which epidemic patterns have been studied for at least two hundred years (Howe 1989). Most notable of these was the map of cholera cases around London water pumps in the mid 1800s which clearly pointed to the source of the epidemic (Snow 1855). With rapid improvements in computing power and mapping software over the past thirty years, map-making has become automated and, most recently, available to everyone on their desktop computers. These advances launched the field of medical geography and led to the production of disease atlases around the world, over 50 at last count (Walter and Birnie 1991). Nearly all of these atlases mapped mortality rather than incidence data. These atlases generated field studies that have made important discoveries about the causes of these diseases (Anderson 1987; Blot *et al.* 1979). In this chapter, we will discuss the advantages and disadvantages of mapping mortality data, methods used in producing a mortality atlas, and recent research suggesting improvements in map design that can enhance the accurate communication of the underlying data patterns to the reader. Experiences in mapping mortality data for the *Atlas of United States Mortality* (Pickle *et al.* 1996) will be used to illustrate the general methods.

13.2 Incidence versus mortality

Epidemiologists generally prefer to examine patterns of incidence rather than mortality because their primary interest is in uncovering factors that contribute to the occurrence of disease and in measuring the disease burden in a population. However, other public health researchers may also be interested in finding reasons for high case fatality rates or in explaining high mortality rates for a disease which is easily detectable and treated. For example, after elevated cervical cancer death rates during the 1970s were noticed in West Virginia (Pickle *et al.* 1987), the state Medicaid programme was changed to cover Pap smears for poor women. Thus, mortality data may be preferred to incidence data when the focus is on providing better health care once the disease has occurred, rather than preventing its occurrence in the first place.

Regardless of the researcher's preference, adequate incidence data often do not exist. The time of progression from initiation of disease to clinically apparent symptoms, to either cure or death varies widely with the disease. For external causes of death, such as unintentional injuries, homicides, and suicides, the progression is too rapid for cases to be ascertained prior to death, making mortality data the only source of information. At the other extreme, death certificate data are nearly useless for diseases with a very low case fatality rate, such as for many common infectious diseases, as too few cases occur for analysis and mapping.

Even for diseases where there may be sufficient time for case identification, a mechanism must be in place for their ascertainment. Procedures for case ascertainment, data collection, and recording must be accurate and uniform across all reporting areas and must encompass all geographical units to be mapped (see Chapters 2 and 5). For example, US cancer incidence statistics are published by the National Cancer Institute (NCI) for eleven scattered geographical areas, covering about 14% of the US population (Ries *et al.* 1997). Although the data collected by the tumour registries in this programme are of high quality and can provide information on treatment choices, histology, and stage of cancer at diagnosis unavailable elsewhere, the geographical coverage is too limited to study the spatial variation of cancer and the sample is not necessarily representative of the entire population. Under Congressional mandate, the Centers for Disease Control (CDC) initiated a programme to implement tumour registries in each US state in 1992, setting standards of data quality and timeliness of reporting for each participating registry (CDC 1994). As of 1997, all but one US state is participating so that, in the near future, cancer incidence data will be available for the entire US, at least at the state level. In many smaller countries, nationwide cancer registries have been maintained for many years (Shanmugaratnam 1989).

Because of the limited availability of cancer incidence data, the NCI initiated a series of cancer mortality atlases in 1975 (Mason *et al.* 1975, 1976). These atlases uncovered a number of cancer 'hot spots', clusters of areas with high cancer death rates, which later led to important aetiological discoveries (Anderson 1987). For example, high rates of oral cancer were found in southeastern states among white women (Mason *et al.* 1975). At first thought to be due to occupational exposures to textile fibres, this pattern was found to be caused by snuff dipping, the use of smokeless tobacco common among women in this region (Winn *et al.* 1981). Later cancer atlases examined the changing geographical patterns over time revealing, for example, new clusters of high rates in the 1970s for lung cancer on the West Coast among white women and prostate cancer in the southeast among black men (Pickle *et al.* 1987, 1990). Although at first questioned as to their usefulness, these atlases proved the utility of mapping mortality data by leading to hundreds of correlation and field interview studies which confirmed the cancer excesses and offered plausible explanations for them.

13.3 Mortality data collection in the United States

The US government first established 'registration areas' for deaths in 1880. Although only a few states participated at first, participation expanded during the 1930s when public demand grew for birth and death certificates to meet eligibility requirements for new social programmes (Hetzel 1997). By 1933, all US states had passed laws requiring the certification and reporting of each death that occurred. The collection of death information has a longer history in Europe; the reader is referred to a discussion by

Lopez *et al.* (1996) for further details. Demand for improved quality of information on US certificates grew as state and local governments tried to define their needs and qualify for new federal welfare programs. What had begun as a listing of births and deaths for purposes of establishing property rights, following the British system, suddenly needed to be accurate enough to generate statistics in order to qualify for federal funding.

The standard US death certificate contains basic information about each death which occurs within the US, including demographic information about the decedent, the date and place of death, and the immediate, underlying, and contributing causes of death as certified by a physician. Each state is free to modify this standard certificate to include additional information. Selected data from each certificate are sent to the National Center for Health Statistics (NCHS), which processes and compiles the information into an annual nationwide mortality database.

The NCHS enters into contracts with each of the US states to purchase certain data fields from each death certificate. Data contained on the centralised NCHS files are limited to those that comply with confidentiality requirements and legal contractual restrictions. Because of these limitations, not all data from the certificate are available for mapping or analysis. For example, exact address of the decedent's residence is reported to the State Health Department, but the smallest geographical unit reported to NCHS is the county. There are 3141 counties in the US, containing, on average, around 87 000 people.

13.4   Quality of data

The issue of accuracy of cause-of-death statistics is fundamental to the interpretation of patterns shown on mortality maps. The quality of cause-of-death determination is affected by the accuracy and completeness of information, from medical diagnosis to final coding and processing of underlying cause of death. Beginning with mortality data for 1968, the underlying cause of death for US certificates has been determined by a computerised system at NCHS which consistently applies World Health Organisation coding and selection rules to each death certificate, using all conditions reported by the medical certifier (NCHS 1990). Automation of this task and cross-verification of medical condition coding is believed to have reduced errors in assigning underlying cause from death certificate information to less than 1% (Harris and French 1980). However, the completeness and accuracy of the information supplied on the certificate and the decedent's medical diagnosis remain as potential sources of error (Sirken *et al.* 1987).

There are indications that the quality of medical information on the death certificate has improved over time. In particular, there has been a steady reduction of deaths assigned to the residual category of 'Symptoms, signs, and ill-defined conditions' (ICD categories 780–799) from 1.5% prior to 1988 to 1.07% in 1992 (NCHS 1994), presumably because of improved specificity of information provided by the medical certifier. The increasing number of medical conditions reported on death certificates also supports an improvement in detailed diagnostic information and greater care in completing the medical certification of death (Israel *et al.* 1986). Validation studies suggest that, for most broad categories, the reported underlying cause of death agrees well with hospital records of the decedents (Gittlesohn and Senning 1979; Gittlesohn and Royston 1982; Percy *et al.* 1981; Kircher *et al.* 1985). However, for deaths which occur away from a medical setting, as for an unobserved sudden death, the medical certifier may not have sufficient information about the decedent's medical history to report correctly the underlying and contributing causes of death. For example, long-term diabetics are at high risk of heart disease and stroke as a consequence of their disease, but studies have shown substantial under-reporting of diabetes on their death certificates (Michael *et al.* 1991). Other errors may occur where the cause of death is classified to a related, but incorrect, disorder or to a non-specific disease category. These types of errors can be addressed by grouping the related causes which are often confused, or by not sub-setting the broadly specified disease for analysis.

It should not be assumed that incidence data, if they exist, are error-free. Indeed, they are subject to similar problems of inadequate detail on medical records (Boyle 1989), particularly when precise histological information is required for ICD (WHO 1977) coding. In fact, Doll and Peto (1981), in a landmark paper, argue strongly that mortality data are to be preferred to registry data for assessing cancer trends.

13.5 Diseases to map

The potential for errors in assigning underlying cause of death must be considered in defining the diseases to be mapped. For the NCHS *Atlas of United States Mortality*, we attempted to create cause groups that were broad enough to avoid these problems, yet specific enough to be meaningful for a etiological research. For example, cancers of the colon and rectum were combined because of the potential for misclassification between these diagnoses (Percy *et al.* 1981). All chronic obstructive pulmonary diseases (COPD, ICD categories 490–496, including chronic bronchitis, emphysema, and asthma) were combined for mapping because approximately 75% of all COPD deaths in 1988–92 were coded as 'other', with the majority of these 'not otherwise specified'. Use of the ICD category groups to define diseases to be mapped aids comparisons with other published data, but specific ICD category definitions of the mapped causes should always be provided so that the reader can judge comparability of code groupings. Even within the US, the few mortality atlases that have been produced have not used exactly the same definitions; for example, colon and rectal cancer were mapped separately in the NCI series but combined into colorectal cancer for the NCHS atlas.

The decision of what diseases to map must also consider the number of deaths which occur due to each cause. Mapping a rare cause of death will typically be uninformative, with no apparent spatial patterns. Sufficient numbers for these rare diseases can be obtained by aggregating data over several years or by combining smaller geographical units into larger ones. One approach is to map the leading causes of death according to broad ICD groupings which have a predetermined minimum number of deaths. For the NCHS atlas, we grouped over geographic unit and over time, then mapped the leading causes with approximately 10 or more deaths per 100 000 population per year, arguing that for rarer causes the coefficient of variation would be high for over a quarter of the geographical units.

13.6 Statistical methods

Some researchers have advocated mapping the exact residence of each decedent on a dot map. Aside from confidentiality concerns, this method would work for a relatively small number of deaths in a limited geographical area, but is impracticable for a nationwide map or even a regional map of a common cause of death. In the US, approximately two million deaths occur each year, so that even regional maps could not clearly show so many locations. In addition, a dot map does not take into account the underlying heterogeneity of population size across the geographical units from which the cases arose. Crude death rates for distinct geographic units may be mapped to account for these population differences, but further adjustment is usually necessary to remove the bias in crude rates due to different age distributions in different regions. Both direct and indirect age-adjustment procedures are available (Fleiss 1981); the direct method uses the same standard population to compute each geographical unit's adjusted rate (Pickle and White 1995), while the indirect method uses the same set of standard rates applied to the observed population in each geographical unit. Crucially, if two areas (units) are to be compared, both procedures rely on the assumption that the ratio of rates in the two areas are approximately constant across the strata (see Chapter 9). Occasionally, when the focus of the map is on a narrow age range, age-specific rather than age-adjusted rates are presented. Recently, there has been interest in mapping 'years of potential life lost' (McDonnell *et al.* 1998), a sum of the number of years lost by each death prior to that individual's expected lifespan. This measure can reflect the population burden due to a particular cause of death better than the age-adjusted rates because of its heavy weight given to deaths among younger persons.

Statistical models have been proposed for mortality data ranging from simple binomial models for count data (Brillinger 1986) to empirical Bayes methods (Manton *et al.* 1989; Clayton and Kaldor 1987) and, more recently, to fully Bayesian (e.g. Besag *et al.* 1991; see also Chapters 7, 15, and 16) and non-Bayesian (Pickle *et al.* 1997) methods based on generalised linear mixed effects models. Recent developments in non-parametric smoothing techniques (Kafadar 1994; Hansen 1991; Mungiole *et al.* 1999) offer a third choice of mapping non-parametrically smoothed (as opposed to Bayesian parametrically smoothed) observed or modelled rates. These techniques are outlined in the next section.

13.6.1 Non-parametric smoothing techniques for georeferenced data

We see the results of smoothing techniques for georeferenced (spatial) data daily in our weather maps—many observed points have been smoothed in some way to provide a map showing broad patterns of temperature or precipitation. For spatial data in general, we wish to remove background noise and bring into focus the patterns in the original data, but these patterns are often too complex to allow global surface modelling. Local smoothers provide a method of highlighting structure in the data without having to specify that structure parametrically. Both linear and non-linear (typically median-based) smoothers are available but few methods account for heteroscedasticity (i.e. where some values being smoothed are more reliable statistics than others). This is nearly always the situation with health data (e.g. mortality rates by county), where the standard errors are highly dependent on the varying population sizes across geographical units.

Although non-parametric statistical techniques for smoothing one-dimensional data, such as moving averages for time series data, have been available for many years, it has only been recently that these methods have been extended to two-dimensional data. A brief summary of these methods follows; the reader is referred to Isaaks and Srivastava (1989), Hansen (1991), and Kafadar (1994) for a more extensive review (see also Chapter 10).

Spatial smoothers were first developed for gridded data, such as geological samples taken at regular intervals; health data typically are collected at irregularly spaced points or for aggregated areas. Kriging was developed to interpolate values between collection sites; Chapter 10 provides a comprehensive discussion on this methodology. Later, robust thin-plate spline and local polynomial regression methods (loess) were applied to spatial data using a least squares estimation criterion. Methods such as thin-plate splines which include a smoothness penalty tend to blur edges which may be important features in the data. 'Head-banging', a two-dimensional median-based smoothing algorithm, was suggested by Tukey and Tukey (1981) for non-gridded spatial data and implemented by Hansen (1991). Simple two-dimensional moving averages with weights inversely proportional to inter-point distances can capture much of the pattern in spatial data, but Hansen (1991) and Kafadar (1994) have shown that head-banging performs well in the presence of wild outliers, edge effects, or ridges in the data.

Conceptually, head-banging lowers unusually high points and raises unusually low points so that their values are more in line with nearby points. This is accomplished by examining a collection of nearly collinear triples of neighbouring points around each point to be smoothed. For each collection of triples, the median of the lower end-points and the median of the higher end-points are determined. If the point to be smoothed is at a boundary, neighbours are extrapolated to provide triples. The median of the lower median, the centre point, and the higher median is taken to be the smoothed value for the centre point. This process is repeated for each point, then repeated a specified number of times over the entire dataset. The user can specify the number of iterations to be performed, the maximum number of nearest neighbours and triples considered, and the minimum angle which defines 'near collinearity' of the points in a triple. Specific details of the algorithm are provided in Hansen (1991).

A limitation of the original head-banging algorithm for health data is that only unweighted medians are calculated. As a consequence, reliable city values can be smoothed to resemble neighbouring small town values which are less reliable. Mungiole *et al.* (1999) modified the original algorithm to calculate weighted medians. Pickle *et al.* (1996) found that this modified algorithm worked well for maps of mortality rates, with weights proportional to the inverse variances of the rates. 'Spikes' in the data, such as high HIV mortality rates in core cities, and ridge effects, such as high heart disease mortality along the Mississippi and Ohio rivers, were retained when they were values based on large samples but were smoothed away when based on few deaths. This modified algorithm shows promise as a tool for highlighting complex patterns in health data. Note that these methods are similar in spirit to the Bayesian local smoothing models that are becoming popular in disease mapping (see Chapter 7).

Because these are new techniques for analysing and presenting mortality data, no guidelines exist for deciding when such smoothing is most appropriate. The NCHS atlas includes an observed age-adjusted rate map and age-specific maps of smoothed, modelled rates. The former may be appropriate to answer questions about rates in individual geographical units (although it should be remembered that observed rate maps may be unreliable if the data are sparse), whilst questions about general spatial patterns in the data are better answered by modelled or smoothed rates, both of which supposedly remove random background noise in the rates due to small numbers of deaths. Combining these methods reveals the broadest patterns in the data by applying the non-parametric smoothing algorithm to data already smoothed by the model.

The choice of which quantities to map depends on the aim of the mapping exercise. The earliest US atlases included choropleth maps with only those geographical units shaded which had rates significantly different from the US rate or were in the highest 10% of all rates. This 'blanking out' of many geographical units because of non-significance removes information about the spatial patterns in the data that can be gained by looking for trends or clusters of similar rates on the map (Lewandowsky *et al.* 1995). Therefore, if the significance of the small-area rates compared to an overall rate is of interest, this information should be presented in a separate map which is in addition to a map showing the estimated rates. Recently, several new statistical methods of identifying clusters of high or low rates on a map have been proposed that are an improvement over the significance method (Kulldorff and Nagarwalla 1995; Munasinghe and Morris 1996). The posterior probability of exceeding a threshold of interest (e.g. relative risk > 1) may also be mapped (Chapter 7).

13.7   Geographical units

The geographical unit used for a mortality map can range from exact location (dot map) to broad geographical region, depending on the availability of data and on confidentiality concerns. The geographical unit to be used must be uniquely defined across the entire area to be mapped. For example, metropolitan statistical areas are useful aggregations of core cities and surrounding counties but are defined, as the name implies, only in metropolitan areas of the US. In some cases, similar administrative entities exist that may be used as comparable units for mapping, such as parishes, boroughs, and counties in the US. Choosing the geographical unit to use from what is available is always a compromise between choosing units small enough to illustrate local patterns of interest but large enough to provide stable rates for mapping.

In addition to these considerations, the map designer must take publication details into account, such as the size of the printed map or the availability of zooming capability for an electronically published map. Choice of a geographical unit that is too small will make some patterns impossible to discern or boundary lines will overwhelm the interior shading. Health service areas (HSAs) in the NCHS atlas were aggregated to a minimum size of 250 square miles so that each unit's colour could be seen on a quarter-page map. In addition to minimum size, the range of sizes of the geographical units can bias the visual impression of the map, such as when a few areas are much larger than the others. These large areas will draw the reader's eye, even though it is often the smallest units that contain the majority of the country's population. For US data, the HSAs are of more uniform size than counties.

In the past, US counties have been aggregated to stabilise rates for mapping on the basis of socio-demographic (Mason *et al.* 1975) or economic (Levine *et al.* 1987) characteristics or population size. In contrast, grouping areas based on medical service utilisation for purposes of mortality mapping, such as by the recently defined HSAs (Makuc *et al.* 1991), may reduce the variation of diagnosis, treatment, and death certification practices within the aggregated units. In addition to stabilising the mortality statistics, small geographical units are sometimes aggregated to preserve the confidentiality of the data. For example, US mortality data at the county level is released by NCHS for public use only for counties with a minimum population size of 100 000 or the data must be aggregated to three or more years. Some have also suggested aggregating county data to achieve a minimum population size for rate stability (Munasinghe and Morris 1996) or to combine places with similar levels of urbanisation for homogeneity in ecological analyses (Goodall *et al.* 1998).

To illustrate the impact of the choice of geographical unit on the map patterns, we present two examples. The first US cancer atlas (Mason *et al.* 1975) showed two adjacent counties in Montana that had significantly high lung cancer death rates among white males, whereas the remainder of the state had low rates. This 'hot spot' was found to be the former site of a copper smelter plant which had polluted the community with arsenic, most likely the cause of the high lung cancer rates (Lee and Fraumeni 1969). In a subsequent atlas which mapped data for the same time period, data for these counties were absorbed into a larger unit (four state economic areas compared to 57 counties in Montana); mapped in this way, the 'hot spot' was no longer apparent (Pickle *et al.* 1987).

As a second example of pattern differences due to choice of geographical unit, Plate 3 shows coronary heart disease mortality rates among white males in eastern Kentucky stratified into quintile categories. HSAs 272 and 18 include Louisville and Lexington, Kentucky, respectively (shown by dots in Plate 3b). At the HSA level, these areas have average or slightly high mortality rates (Plate 3a). However, when mapped at the county level (Plate 3b), both of these HSAs contain counties in four or five of the five possible colour categories, indicating a wide range of rates. It is interesting to note that rates in and near the cities of Louisville and Lexington are average or low, whereas rates in more rural counties further from these cities, although still within the same HSA, are higher. However, because of greater population and numbers of deaths, the cities' rates dominate the aggregated HSA rates, hiding some very high county rates in eastern Kentucky.

13.8   Map design

Once the mortality data for selected causes of death are aggregated to the desired geographical units and the appropriate statistics are computed, presentation issues must be considered, particularly if the map is to be widely disseminated. Several basic map styles are available and for each of these specific design issues must be addressed. Unfortunately, experts differ in their preferred map type for disease rates (Tukey 1979; Tufte 1993; Monmonier 1993; Dent 1993; Cleveland and McGill 1984). Because of these conflicting opinions, NCHS started a research programme focused on the design of mortality rate maps. The research group was multidisciplinary, including statisticians, demographers, psychologists, geographers, and cartographers. Results of this research will be briefly summarised here; details are available elsewhere (Pickle and Herrmann 1995).

What factors affect map reading? Obviously, the characteristics of the map are important, but so are the characteristics of the reader, such as what experience and training they have had and whether they are colour blind. What is sometimes forgotten is that the best map design also depends on what questions will be asked of the map. Following Bertin's classification (Bertin 1983), a typical map reader wants to ask one or more of three basic questions. The first is a very specific rate readout task: what is the mortality rate in a certain place? The second is a more general pattern recognition task: are there geographical trends in the data or clusters of high or low rate areas? The last is the most general map comparison task: for example, are the mortality patterns similar for males and females, or for blacks and whites? When the expected audience is diverse, the map design and page layout should allow *all* of these questions to be answered by either a single map or a set of maps.

At the beginning of our research, we sketched out a cognitive model of map reading consisting of four specific stages: orienting to the map, legend comprehension, integration of map and legend, and data extraction (Herrmann and Pickle 1996). There are other possible models that describe how a person extracts information from a map, but this one helped us to focus our experiments on a single stage (e.g. legend comprehension), resulting in fewer confounding variables to be controlled.

Basic map styles tested included choropleth (area shaded) maps, isopleth maps (like a weather map, where each line follows a contour of equal rates), and dot maps (where a dot was placed on the population centroid of each geographical unit). The choropleth and dot maps were constructed either as unclassed (proportional) maps, where the intensity of colour or size of dot is proportional to the actual rate in each area, or classed maps, where rates are first categorised into ranges, then each range is assigned a colour or dot size.

Our first study showed that of all map styles examined, epidemiologists preferred the classed choropleth maps and used them most accurately (Pickle *et al.* 1994). People who had some training in cartography preferred the more complex map designs, but they were equally accurate on all types (White *et al.* 1995). Therefore, we decided to use classed choropleth maps for the NCHS atlas.

Consistent with the recommendations of cartographers, Hastie *et al.* (1996) found that very distinct colours (e.g. a rainbow palette) were best for reading a single rate off the map, but this was contrary to Lewandowsky's finding that a colour gradient was best for cluster recognition (Lewandowsky *et al.* 1993). We decided to use a double-ended colour scheme for our main atlas map—this is a combination of a colour gradient for each of two hues (one for high rates, one for low rates). We hoped to be able to select colours for this scheme that would allow both accurate rate readout and cluster identification/pattern recognition.

Carswell *et al.* (1995) tested various double-ended colour schemes and found that map readers performed better when the colour choices followed 'convention', such as the use of darker shades for high rates and lighter shades for low rates, or red for high and blue for low rates. Using these accepted cartographic conventions, Brewer conducted an experiment to compare colour schemes, using quarter-page five-category and full-page seven-category choropleth maps (Brewer *et al.* 1997). The colours used in the experiment included double-ended, sequential, and spectral colour schemes. These colours were carefully chosen so that lightness was balanced for both hues in the double-ended schemes, and increased evenly for the sequential schemes. The pairs of hues for the double-ended schemes were chosen to avoid pairs that would confuse colour blind readers. For the rate readout task, the sequential schemes were worse than the double-ended ones, although all could be used fairly accurately. This finding probably results from the greater similarity of colours in the sequential scheme (5 or 7 shades of the same hue) compared to the double-ended, where at most three shades must be distinguished. The choice of colour had little effect on cluster recognition, except that the number of clusters identified was greater for the grey scheme. The grey scheme was significantly worst for perceived pleasantness and ease of use.

In another study, a number of innovative legend designs were tested, including fixed box and proportional box legends, vertical and horizontal orientations, single and double labelling. The epidemiologists wanted to read a simple legend quickly and gain access to the more interesting map content. Therefore, they preferred the more traditional fixed box legend in vertical orientation (Pickle *et al.* 1995).

In the cancer atlases, most non-significant counties were grouped into a single colour category, regardless of their actual rate. In hindsight, it seemed that this masked important information about local patterns, but at the same time the reader must be warned that some rates are based on very small numbers, and therefore are unreliable. MacEachren *et al.* (1998) tested three methods for indicating unreliability on a map: (1) the rate and reliability information were shown in separate maps; (2) a bivariate colour scheme; and (3) a double hatching of both white and black lines to indicate unreliability overlaid on the rate colour. The study subjects had trouble answering reliability questions from the map pair and could not use the bivariate colour scheme very accurately to identify clusters and patterns on the map. The innovative double-hatching is visible over all colours and allows readers to separate the information about the level of the rate and its reliability. That is, they can ignore the hatching and find patches of similar colour for a clustering task, but are warned about unreliability during a rate readout task.

To illustrate the application of these research findings, Plate 4 shows the two-page layout for heart disease mortality rates from the *Atlas of United States Mortality* (Pickle *et al.* 1996). This integrated graphical presentation includes both observed age-adjusted rates (Plate 4a) and estimated age-place-specific rates (Plate 4c,d,e) predicted from a mixed effects model which includes a geographical hierarchy of age effects. The second page includes a map indicating the significance of each HSA's rate compared to the US rate (Plate 4b), and regional (Plate 4c) and HSA (Plate 4d,e) rates estimated from the model. Questions of the rate in a particular HSA are best answered by the observed rate map (Plate 4a); unreliable rates would be hatched on this map, but all rates are reliable for this example. Whether a rate is significantly higher or lower than the overall US rate is determined from the significance map (Plate 4b). Questions about the broad geographical patterns in the data and the effects of age on these patterns are best answered by the model results, shown in Plate 4c, d, and e. Map colours were chosen to avoid common colour vision deficiencies and to balance levels of darkness so that no single colour visually dominated a map. Colours for each type of map are unique within the atlas so that the reader can quickly memorise the page layout and map content.

13.9 Summary

Characteristics of the cause of death to be mapped, such as its case fatality rate, lag time between clinical onset and death, diagnostic accuracy and treatment availability, need to be considered in deciding which causes of death may be mapped confidently or which causes should be combined for mapping. Likewise, rate stability and confidentiality must be considered in choosing the geographical unit to map. Recent research in the area of map design has shown the impact of map elements and page layout on accurate reader extraction of statistical data from the map. Despite these concerns, with careful design, mapping mortality data can provide valuable insight into the aetiology and treatment patterns for many causes of death. As Tufte (1983) has observed, 'The most extensive data maps ... place millions of bits of information on a single page before our eyes. No other method for the display of statistical information is so powerful'.

References

Anderson, L. (1987). *Research contributions made possible by the NCI cancer atlases published in the 1970s.* Backgrounder. National Cancer Institute, Office of Cancer Communications, Bethesda, MD.

Bertin, J. (1983). *Semiology of graphics: diagrams, networks, maps.* University of Wisconsin, Madison, WI.

Besag, J., York, J., and Mollie, A. (1991). Bayesian image restoration, with two applications in spatial statistics. *Annals of the Institute of Statistical Mathematics*, **43**, 1–21.

Blot, W. J., Fraumeni, J. F., Jr., Mason, T. J., and Hoover, R. N. (1979). Developing clues to environmental cancer: A stepwise approach with the use of cancer mortality data. *Environmental Health Perspectives*, **32**, 53–8.

Boyle, P. (1989). Relative value of incidence and mortality data in cancer research. In *Cancer Mapping* (P. Boyle, C. S. Muir, and E. Grundmann ed.), 41–63. Springer, Berlin.

Brewer, C. A., MacEachren, A. M., Pickle, L. W., and Herrmann, D. (1997). Mapping mortality: Evaluating color schemes for choropleth maps. *Annals of the Association of American Geographers*, **87**, 411–38.

Brillinger, D. R. (1986) The natural variability of vital rates and associated statistics. *Biometrics*, **42**, 693–712.

Carswell, C. M., Kinslow, H. S., Pickle, L. W., and Herrmann, D. (1995). Using color to represent magnitude in statistical maps: The case for double-ended scales. In *Cognitive aspects of statistical mapping* (L. W. Pickle and D. J. Herrmann ed.), 201–28. Working Paper Series Report 18. National Center for Health Statistics. Hyattsville, MD.

Centers for Disease Control and Prevention (1994). Announcement 426. 1994 National Program of Cancer Registries. *http://www.cdc.gov/nccdphp/dcpc/npcr/npcrpdfs/pa426-94.pdf*, 7 Oct. (1998).

Clayton, D. and Kaldor, J. (1987). Empirical Bayes estimates of age-standardized relative risks for use in disease mapping. *Biometrics*, **43**, 671–81.

Cleveland, W. S. and McGill, R. (1984). Graphical perception: Theory, experimentation, and application to the development of graphical methods. *Journal of the American Statistical Association*, **79**, 531–4.

Dent, B. D. (1993). *Cartography: thematic map design.* Wm. C. Brown, Dubuque, IA.

Doll, R. and Peto, R. (1981). The causes of cancer: Quantitative estimates of avoidable risks of cancer in the United States today. *Journal of the National Cancer Institute*, **66**, 1192–1308.

Fleiss, J. L. (1981). *Statistical methods for rates and proportions* (2nd edn). Wiley, New York.

Gittelsohn, A. and Royston, P. N. (1982). Annotated bibliography of cause-of-death validation studies, 1958–80. *Vital Health Statistics*, **2**(89). National Center for Health Statistics, Hyattsville, MD.

Gittelsohn, A. and Senning, J. (1979). Studies on the reliability of vital and health records: I. Comparison of cause of death and hospital record diagnoses. *American Journal of Public Health*, **69**, 680–9.

Goodall, C. R., Kafadar, K., and Tukey, J. W. (1998). Computing and using rural versus urban measures in statistical applications. *The American Statistician*, **52**, 101–11.

Hansen, K. M. (1991). Headbanging: Robust smoothing in the plane. *IEEE Transactions on Geoscience and Remote Sensing*, **29**, 369–78.

Harris, K. W. and French, D. K. (1980). A methodological study of quality control procedures for mortality medical coding. *Vital Health Statistics*, **2**(81). DHEW Publication No. (PHS) 79-1355. National Center for Health Statistics, Hyattsville, MD.

Hastie, R., Hammerle, O., Kerwin, J., Croner, C. M., and Herrmann, D. J. (1996). Human performance reading statistical maps. *Journal of Experimental Psychology: Applied*, **2**, 3–16.

Herrmann, D. J. and Pickle, L. W. (1996). A cognitive subtask model of statistical map reading. *Visual Cognition*, **3**(2), 165–90.

Hetzel, A. M. (1997). *History and organization of the vital statistics system*. National Center for Health Statistics, Hyattsville, MD.

Howe, G. M. (1989). Historical evolution of disease mapping in general and specifically of cancer mapping. In *Cancer mapping* (P. Boyle, C. S. Muir, and E. Grundmann ed.), 1–21. Springer, Berlin.

Isaaks, E. H. and Srivastava, R. H. (1989). *Applied geostatistics*. Oxford University Press, New York.

Israel, R. A., Rosenberg, H. M., and Curtin, L. R. (1986). Analytical potential for multiple cause-of-death data. *American Journal of Epidemiology*, **124**, 161–79.

Kafadar, K. (1994). Choosing among two-dimensional smoothers in practice. *Journal of Computing Simulation*, **18**, 419–39.

Kircher, T., Nelson, J., and Burdo, H. (1985). The autopsy as a measure of accuracy of the death certificate. *New England Journal of Medicine*, **313**, 1263–9.

Kulldorff, M. and Nagarwalla, N. (1995). Spatial disease clusters: detection and inference. *Statistics in Medicine*, **14**, 799–810.

Lee, A. M. and Fraumeni, J. F., Jr. (1969). Arsenic and respiratory cancer in man: an occupational study. *Journal of the National Cancer Institute*, **42**, 1045–52.

Levine, P. H., McKay, F. W., and Connelly, R. R. (1987). Patterns of nasopharyngeal cancer mortality in the United States. *International Journal of Cancer*, **39**, 133–7.

Lewandowsky, S., Herrmann, D. J., Behrens J. T., Li, S. C., Pickle, L., and Jobe, J. B. (1993). Perception of clusters in statistical maps. *Applied Cognitive Psychology*, **7**, 533–51.

Lewandowsky, S., Behrens, J. T., Pickle, L. W., Herrman, D. J., and White, A. A. (1995), Perception of clusters in mortality maps: Representing magnitude and statistical reliability. In *Cognitive aspects of statistical mapping* (L. W. Pickle and D. J. Herrmann ed.), 107–32. Working Paper Series Report **18**. National Center for Health Statistics, Hyattsville, MD.

Lopez, A. D., (1996). Mortality data. In *Geographical and environmental epidemiology: methods for small-area studies* (P. Elliott, J. Cuzick, D. English, and R. Stern ed.), 37–50. Oxford University Press.

MacEachren, A. M., Brewer, C. A., and Pickle, L. W. (1998). Visualizing georeferenced data: Representing reliability of health statistics. *Environment and Planning A*, **30**, 1547–61.

Makuc, D. M., Haglund, B., Ingram, D. D., Kleinman, J. C., and Feldman, J. J. (1991). Health service areas for the United States. *Vital Health Statistics*, **2**(112), National Center for Health Statistics, Hyattsville, MD.

Manton, K. G., Woodbury, M. A., Stallard, E., Riggan, W. B., Creason, J. P., and Pellom, A. C. (1989). Empirical Bayes procedures for stabilizing maps of U.S. cancer mortality rates. *Journal of the American Statistical Association*, **84**, 637–50.

Mason, T. J., McKay, F. W., Hoover, R., Blot, W. J., and Fraumeni, J. F. (1975). *Atlas of cancer mortality for U.S. counties: 1950–1969*. USGPO, DHEW Publication No. (NIH) 75-780, Washington, DC.

Mason, T. J., McKay, F. W., Hoover, R., Blot, W. J., and Fraumeni, J. F. (1976). *Atlas of cancer mortality among U.S. nonwhites: 1950–1969*. USGPO, DHEW Publication No. (NIH) 76-1204, Washington, DC.

McDonnell, S., Vossberg, K., Hopkins, R. S., and Mittan, B. (1998). Using YPLL (years of potential life lost) in health planning. *Public Health Reports*, **113**, 55–61.

Michael, S., Gard, S., Schurman, E., and Kurth, D. (1991). Sensitivity of death certificate data for monitoring diabetes mortality. Diabetic eye disease follow-up study, 1985–1990. *Morbidity and Mortality Weekly Report*, **40**, 739–741.

Monmonier, M. (1993). *Mapping it out*. University of Chicago Press, Chicago, IL.

Munasinghe, R. L. and Morris, R. D. (1996). Localization of disease clusters using regional measures of spatial autocorrelation. *Statistics in Medicine*, **15**, 893–905.

Mungiole, M., Pickle, L. W., and Simonson, K. H. (1999). Application of a weighted head-banging algorithm to mortality data maps. *Statistics in Medicine*, **18**, 3201–9.

National Center for Health Statistics (1990). *Vital statistics, ICD-9 ACME decision tables for classifying underlying causes of death, 1990*. NCHS instruction manual: part 2c. Public Health Service, Hyattsville, MD. (Published annually).

National Center for Health Statistics (1994). *Vital statistics of the United States, 1990*. Vol II: *mortality*. Public Health Service, Washington, DC.

Percy, C., Stanek, E., and Gloeckler, L. (1981). Accuracy of cancer death certificates and its effect on cancer mortality statistics. *American Journal of Public Health*, **71**, 242–50.

Pickle, L. W. and Herrmann, D. J. (ed.) (1995). *Cognitive aspects of statistical mapping*, 201–8. Working Paper Series Report 18. National Center for Health Statistics, Hyattsville, MD.

Pickle, L. and White, A. A. (1995). Effects of the choice of age-adjustment method on maps of death rates. *Statistics in Medicine*, **14**, 615–27.

Pickle, L. W., Mason, T. J., Howard, N., Hoover, R., and Fraumeni, J. F., Jr. (1987). *Atlas of U.S. cancer mortality among whites: 1950–1980*. USGPO, DHHS Publication No. (NIH) 87-2900, Washington, DC.

Pickle, L. W., Mason, T. J., Howard, N., Hoover, R. and Fraumeni, J. F., Jr. (1990). *Atlas of U.S. cancer mortality among nonwhites: 1950–1980*. USGPO, DHHS Publication No. (NIH) 90-1582, Washington.

Pickle, L. W., Herrmann, D., Kerwin, J., Croner, C. M., and White, A. A. (1994). The impact of statistical graphic design on interpretation of disease rate maps. *Proceedings of the Statistical Graphics Section of the 1993 Annual Meeting of the American Statistical Association*, 111–16, San Francisco, CA.

Pickle, L. W., Mungiole, M., Jones, G. K., and White, A. A. (1996). *Atlas of United States mortality*. National Center for Health Statistics, Hyattsville, MD.

Pickle, L. W., Mungiole, M., Jones, G. K., and White, A. A. (1997). Analysis of mapped mortality data by mixed effects models. *Proceedings of the Biometrics Section, American Statistical Association 1996 Meeting, Chicago*, 227–32.

Pickle, L. W., Herrmann, D. J., and Wilson, B. F. (1995). A legendary study of statistical map reading: The cognitive effectiveness of statistical map legends. In *Cognitive aspects of statistical mapping* (L. W. Pickle and D. J. Herrman ed.), 233–48. Working Paper Series Report 18. National Center for Health Statistics, Hyattsville, MD.

Ries, L. A. G., Kosary, C. L., Hankey, B. F., Miller, B. A., Harras, A., and Edwards, B. K. (ed.) (1997). *SEER Cancer Statistics Review, 1973–1994*. NIH Publication No. 97-2789, National Cancer Institute, Bethesda, MD.

Shanmugaratnam, K. (1989). Availability and completeness of cancer registration worldwide. In *Cancer Mapping* (P. Boyle, C. S. Muir, and E. Grundman ed.), 28–33. Springer, Berlin.

Sirken, M. G., Rosenberg, H. M., Chevarley, F. M., and Curtin, L. R. (1987). The quality of cause-of-death statistics. *American Journal of Public Health*, **77**, 137–9.

Snow, J. (1855). *On the mode of communication of cholera* (2nd edn). The Commonwealth Fund, New York.

Tufte, E. R. (1983). *The visual display of quantitative information*, 26. Graphics Press, Cheshire, CT.

Tufte, E. R. (1993). *Design of a cancer atlas*. Contract report. National Center for Health Statistics, Hyattsville, MD.

Tukey, J. W. (1979). Statistical mapping: what should not be plotted. In *Proceedings of the 1976 Workshop on Automated Cartography and Epidemiology*. DHEW Publication No. (PHS) 79-1254, National Center for Health Statistics, Hyattsville, MD.

Tukey, P. A. and Tukey, J. W. (1981). Graphical display of data sets in 3 or more dimensions. In *Interpreting multivariate data* (V. Barnett ed.). Wiley, New York.

Walter, S. D. and Birnie, S. E. (1991). Mapping mortality and morbidity patterns: An international comparison. *International Journal of Epidemiology*, **20**, 678–89.

White, A. A., Pickle, L. W., Herrmann, D. J., Croner, C. M., and Wilson, B. F. (1995). Map design preferences associated with professional discipline. *Proceedings of the Statistical Graphics Section of the 1994 Annual Meeting of the American Statistical Association*, 54–9, Toronto, Canada.

Winn, D. M., Blot, W. J., Shy, C. M., Pickle, L. W., Toledo, A., and Fraumeni, J. F. (1981). Snuff dipping and oral cancer among women in the southern United States. *New England Journal of Medicine*, **304**, 745–9.

WHO (World Health Organisation) (1977). *Manual of the international statistical classification of diseases, injuries, and causes of death, based on the recommendations of the Ninth Revision Conference, 1975*. WHO, Geneva.

14. Geographical analysis of communicable disease data

P. Atkinson and A. Molesworth

14.1 Introduction

This chapter takes a *geographical* approach to the analysis of disease distribution across the population, with a focus on the communicable (infectious) diseases.

Communicable diseases are illnesses 'due to an infectious agent or its toxic products that arise through transmission of that agent or its products either directly or indirectly from an infected person, animal, or reservoir to a susceptible host' (Last 1988). Understanding the geographical variation in communicable disease has, in the past, greatly increased our knowledge of disease distribution and spread (Robinson 1982; Cliff *et al.* 1986; Smallman-Raynor *et al.* 1992) and our understanding of causal mechanisms and factors associated with the risk of becoming infected or of developing disease (Snow 1855; Bruce 1926; Burkitt and Wright 1970). Despite this, there is currently little appreciation amongst public health professionals of the value in mapping communicable diseases or associated risks. Some of the data used to inform them are collected, at local and national levels, through intensive research projects, but much is also collected through surveillance—the ongoing scrutiny of all aspects of occurrence and spread of disease that are pertinent to effective control (Last 1988). The need to collect, analyse and disseminate information in a timely manner means that communicable disease surveillance systems generally use methods distinguished by their practicality rather than their accuracy. Limited resources, large datasets, and concern for the maintenance of patient anonymity—combined with under-recognition of the benefits of conducting geographical analysis by those providing, analysing, and using data—mean that the spatial references required for disease mapping are frequently not made available. The situation is slowly improving. Further exploration is nevertheless needed of analytical methods capable of describing geographical variation in the distribution of communicable diseases which are comprehensible and amenable to those working in the public health environment.

From a public health perspective, this chapter presents methods used to map and analyse communicable disease data, discusses their limitations and raises possible solutions or alternative approaches to minimising some of these problems. The discussion is based primarily on experience of the surveillance of communicable diseases in England and Wales. In all examples, the relative geographical location of disease cases are based on real data, but for reasons of confidentiality they are withheld.

14.2   Mapping area-based communicable disease data

The geographical distribution of the majority of spatially referenced communicable disease data can only be described in terms of areal units. Area-based representations describe counts of data associated with, and delimited by, specific geographical zones or areas, commonly pre-defined for administrative purposes. Mapping area-based data over time also assumes that the zoning system used is stable or, if it changes, that the area distribution on one year's cases can be matched to the next. Unfortunately, many communicable disease data are mapped onto administrative areas which change frequently; hence problems common to the analysis of non-infectious diseases (see Chapter 5) are encountered. Most such changes involve mergers of pre-existing spatial units. If these new boundaries are used for disease mapping, some reduction in the spatial resolution of the data inevitably occurs, and information on spatial variation in disease distribution is lost. However, a number of changes involve sub-division of previous areas. In this case, unless more detailed information is available on the location of the cases which would enable them to be mapped on to the new zones, this extra information has to be ignored in analysis. Creating and interpreting maps based on area data at a particular instance in time cause problems, which are well documented elsewhere (Monmonier 1993; Bailey and Gatrell 1995). As we shall see, mapping area based data *over* time exacerbates these problems. Communicable disease data cause a number of further difficulties.

Among these, some of the most difficult problems arise directly from the fact that, because of their infectious nature, communicable diseases and associated risks tend to cluster. The most common representations of areal-based distributions are 'area-value' choropleth maps, which use shading to represent the variability in data constrained by the unit boundaries being mapped. Each unit is thus represented as self-contained, with change occurring independently of that unit and only at the boundaries; within each areal unit, the spatial distribution of data appears homogenous. In reality this is not the case. The distribution of disease within any unit may be markedly heterogeneous, and in the case of communicable diseases, clustering is likely to be especially marked. This can have serious implications, for example in directing resources for the care of patients, or targeting action to prevent further infection. Figure 14.1a shows a choropleth map of the count of a disease—referred to here as 'Disease A'—for a ward in a local government area in England. The actual location of the individual cases, shown by the dots, demonstrates how the choropleth map struggles to represent the true clustered pattern of the disease. For example, the group of cases in the top right of the map occupies a small geographical area, yet they are represented by high incidences in two large wards on the choropleth visualisation. The implication of homogeneity within wards is clearly false (see also Chapter 5).

These effects exacerbate what has been called the modifiable area unit problem (MAUP) (Openshaw 1984) in that the observed disease distribution will be more likely to change as a function of the zoning system used. Figure 14.1b shows a choropleth map based on a different set of boundaries, for the same disease data. As can be seen, the clustered disease cases make the choropleth extremely sensitive to the location of boundaries, resulting in a very different pattern.

One possible solution to the MAUP would be to re-aggregate data to another set of zones. Without the availability of alternative zoning systems or higher resolution data,

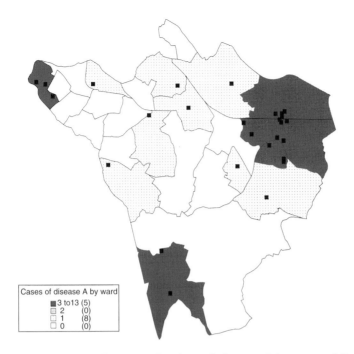

Fig. 14.1a Dot map of individual cases and a choropleth map of the count of disease by ward, for 'Disease A'.

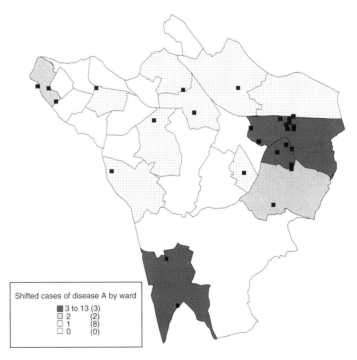

Fig. 14.1b Dot map of 'shifted' individual cases and a choropleth map of the count of 'shifted' disease by ward, for 'Disease A'.

however, this is almost always impossible. The limited availability of higher resolution data also means that the degree of ecological fallacy is extremely difficult to assess (Robinson 1950; Langbein and Lightman 1980). Simply stated, this refers to the fact that what holds at one level of spatial aggregation may not hold at another or for individual members of the population; its effects are endemic to areal-based data (see Section 11.2 of Chapter 11 for further discussion of the ecological fallacy). This is a particular issue in relation to disease mapping, since aggregated data are often used for research and the results applied to target prevention strategies at the individual level.

A second problem, again common to non-infectious disease, concerns the more indirect effects of clustering, seen when the observed disease distribution is adjusted for covariates such as population size. Health data areal units are commonly based on the administrative areas of health services, which are of relatively low spatial resolution, each covering a substantial surface area and population. A choropleth map of the distribution of cases alone would, of course, be misleading: areas with high caseloads may simply have large populations (i.e. a larger denominator). One solution to adjust for the number of people at risk of disease would be geometrically to transform each of the zones to make its area proportional to its attribute value, in this case population size. The resulting map is known as a density equalised map or a cartogram (Dorling 1996). However, cartograms can be difficult to create and interpret. Alternatively, a choropleth map showing disease rates can be constructed, giving the distribution of cases as rates in the usual way (i.e. adjusted for the size of the population). The rates observed will nevertheless still be a product of the zoning system used and just as prone to the MAUP as the areal distribution of the cases themselves.

Whichever approach is used, population data must be available for the same areal units as the disease data to allow for correction. Otherwise, the population characteristics need to be mapped to those of the health zone used (see Flowerdew and Green 1991). A problem arises in these cases when the population is large and no account is taken of the spatial clustering of the disease. The effect may be to mask locally high rates of disease, occurring as clusters within an area unit. Conversely, small population denominators, combined with the clustered nature of communicable diseases, produce 'unstable' values for some spatial units (see Chapter 7). Typically, areas with small populations tend to be rural and to be relatively large in spatial extent. They thereby dominate the map and draw the reader's attention to the very areas in which there is least confidence. Confounding factors, such as age, sex, or deprivation, can also affect the map. These need to be adjusted for before any associations can be inferred between risk factors and disease occurrence. Allowing for each of these confounders means that the number of maps which need to be produced may increase markedly. Possible solutions include mapping relative risk or odds (Clayton and Kaldor 1987), probability mapping (Choynowski 1959; Rhind 1983), and Bayes estimation (Bernardinelli and Montomoli 1992; Langford 1994; see also Chapter 7).

A third problem is one of visualisation. Disease clustering is likely to increase the range of data values across the zone system. Some zones will contain very few or no cases, whereas others will contain a large cluster, depending on the arrangement of zones. This may complicate presentation. Shading systems should avoid the problems of large zones or areas visually dominating the map. It is even more important than usual that the number of classes, their intervals (Tobler 1973; Evans 1977), and the type of shading (Bailey and Gatrell 1995) are chosen wisely to represent the full range of data.

14.3   Mapping point-based communicable disease data

Point-based disease maps either describe the point location of individual cases or 'summary' points describing the surrounding areas. In this section we concentrate on the former. Good examples of 'summary' point disease maps are general practitioner sentinel surveillance datasets, such as the Royal College of General Practitioners Weekly Returns Service in England and Wales (Fleming and Crombie 1985), and the Sentinel Network of General Practitioners in France (Chauvin 1994).

Point-based infectious disease data are, in practice, relatively rare, partly because of concerns about confidentiality. However, the added flexibility and spatial precision of such data mean that they are increasingly being collected to assist in determining who should pay for health care (Atkinson and Watson 1999). Maps describing the point location of individual cases certainly have a number of advantages. Manipulation and analysis of the data can be performed independently of any fixed set of areal units. The data can also be readily aggregated to different spatial levels, according to need. This allows the relationship between disease distribution and other covariates to be examined at a variety of resolutions, thus providing an indication of the severity of the ecological fallacy. Even so, there are problems in creating and manipulating point-based representations, common to all health data, as well as additional problems specific to communicable disease data.

First, there are problems encountered in georeferencing individual disease case data. A number of countries now produce datasets that provide a point georeference based on some part of the postal address: for example, the UK Office for National Statistics provides an Ordinance Survey National Grid reference describing the point location of each unit postcode in Great Britain in the Royal Mail Address Manager Postzon file (Post Office 1985). The georeferenced datasets vary in precision and accuracy (Raper *et al.* 1992). The outcome of this may be either to hide patterns in the data, or to produce patterns in the map that were not present in the original data. The accuracy of such datasets is gradually improving, so these problems are likely to be reduced. The UK Address Point dataset, for example, provides georeferenced data on each address to an accuracy of 1 metre. It is also possible manually to georeference each case from the postal address. Such approaches are, however, extremely costly, and are thus often not feasible for many research applications and most health organisations. Inaccuracies and imprecision thus remain important concerns in many studies, and may systematically bias the map (see Chapter 5). A number of strategies have been discussed for dealing with this problem (Gatrell 1989; Gatrell *et al.* 1991), many of which are applicable to international georeferenced postal datasets.

Second, problems occur in representing point distributions, related to multiple representation and high symbol density. Some georeferenced postal datasets use one point to describe the spatial location of a group of households; each group of households is thus represented by one symbol on the map. Consequently, the reader cannot distinguish between symbols describing one case and those referring to multiple cases. This problem may be exacerbated by the low accuracy of georeferenced postal datasets. If, for example, this provides spatial references to an accuracy of only 100 m, and two groups of

households are located close to one another, they may be allocated the same georeference. The distance between two or more symbols in high density areas can also be so
small to make them appear as one. As noted already, infectious diseases have a tendency
to cluster, making the problems of multiple representation and high symbol density particularly troublesome. It thus becomes extremely difficult to visualise the degree of
disease intensity in areas of high infection. One solution to these problems is to use
techniques of density estimation (Silverman 1986; Bithell 1990; Diggle 1990; Brunsden
1991). These attempt to measure the density of a point distribution at a series of sample
points across the area of interest. These sample points are located so that they describe a
two-dimensional density surface representing the spatial variation in the intensity of the
spatial process of interest. Surface 'height' varies according to the local disease
incidence, even if cases are located at the same geographical point. The density surface
thus provides a visualisation of the overall variation in true disease density, including the
detail inherent in areas of high density. Chapters 6 and 8 describe kernel density
estimation.

Figure 14.2 and Plates 5 and 6 show an example. Figure 14.2 presents the distribution
of cases of 'Disease B' in northwest England in 1990–1. In this form, it is not possible to
tell whether one dot signifies one or more cases. Higher densities of cases are seen in

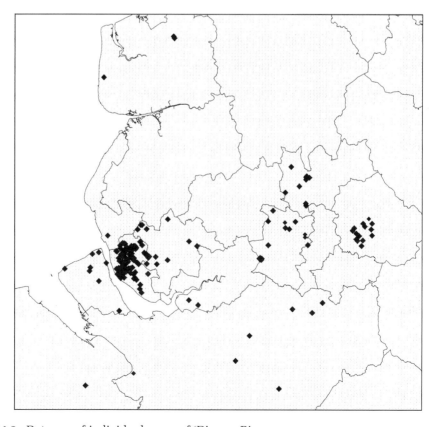

Fig. 14.2 Dot map of individual cases of 'Disease B'.

Merseyside, but it is difficult to identify variations of density within this area. Plate 5 shows a 'naive' two-dimensional density estimate of the same disease cases, using a grid of 375×375 metre squares and a bandwidth of 750 metres. This figure suffers from all the usual area-based mapping problems, and distinguishing high density variation remains difficult. Plate 6 shows the same density estimate in three dimensions (Atkinson and Unwin 1997). The surface counts each case at each location, even where they overlap, and enables the reader to detect both the overall and local variations in density. The distribution is also free from the constraints of confidentiality on individual-level data, and can be manipulated to reduce or accentuate clusters of cases in certain areas without loss of accuracy. This transfer of highly confidential point data to a density surface has proved an extremely useful method of 'anonymising' patient records.

A third problem is that of adjusting point data distributions for those of covariates, such as population. The geographical location of each individual in a population is not usually available. Most population datasets are aggregated to small administrative areas to maintain confidentiality. Two possible solutions to link disease and population data are to aggregate disease data to the smallest population administration areas, or to use continuous disease and population surfaces simultaneously. In the first, point referenced data can be aggregated to any combination of population administration areas using basic point-in-polygon techniques. Unfortunately, this approach reintroduces the MAUP described above. In the second, density estimation is used to create a continuous disease surface; the covarying population data are then interpolated to create a similar continuous surface. The area under the surface can then be used to calculate population for any arrangement of zones. The continuous population surface can be generated by redistributing census data based on population weighted enumeration district centroids (Bracken and Martin 1989; Martin 1988, 1989, 1991). Population data are redistributed to the surrounding areas assuming that the closer an area is to the centroid, the greater the contribution of the population data. Dividing the disease surface by the population surface produces a population corrected surface, or a rate surface. Kelsall and Diggle (1995) present methods for producing such a surface using samples of cases and controls.

Mapping covariate-corrected infectious disease data produces one particular problem: that of small population values on continuous surfaces. Detailed population surfaces created using the above method show substantial variability within small areas. Some have very high counts, whereas nearby there may be almost no counts. These variations in population produce 'unstable' rate estimates.

Finally, detailed infectious disease surfaces contain clusters of cases over small geographical areas. These produce extremely high localised density values. These variations in disease density, combined with unstable populations, produce 'spiky' rate surfaces which are difficult to visualise. They can be dealt with in two possible ways. One is to build the population surfaces using local data, as close as possible to the individual level. In England and Wales, this can be achieved approximately by distributing population data on to postcodes and forming density estimated surfaces on the population postcode centroids (Martin and Tate 1998). Alternatively, the covariate surface can be smoothed to provide a more robust denominator to the ratio surface. Unfortunately, this may result in local clusters of disease being missed in areas of population undersmoothing, while false clusters may be generated in areas of population oversmoothing.

14.4   Mapping mixed resolution data

A different problem is encountered when the resolution of the geographical reference linked to individual case records varies within the dataset. Although such 'mixed resolution' data occur in many health datasets, they are especially common in data from communicable disease surveillance, where spatial references are frequently incomplete and imprecise. In mapping such data, it is important to ensure that as much as possible of the variation in spatial resolution and type of geographical reference afforded by the data is accommodated, if the full value of the information is to be retained (Unwin *et al.* 1996).

An example of this is given here—the distribution of the 6200 cases of communicable 'Disease C' known to be living in London at the start of 1998. Surveillance of C requires that data supplied for each case includes a reference to the location of residence—the unit postcode. However, the spatial reference available for each case is often incomplete, and not always what was originally requested (Table 14.1). The aim is to portray the spatial variation in Disease C in map form. Three approaches are considered here.

14.4.1   Using the resolution for which all cases are available

Information on the health authority (HA) is available for all cases in the study (although an unknown number of additional cases will have been missed by the disease registration system); choropleth mapping at this level thus allows all the known cases to be included, and minimises risks of bias due to data omission (Fig. 14.3). It is also appropriate if the results are to be used at the HA level and will capture relationships to other factors, if these also vary at the HA level. However, such associations should not be assumed a priori; in England and Wales HA boundaries are defined by the National Health Service for internal administrative purposes, and there is no inherent reason why any disease should vary in accordance with these arbitrary units. A more precise description of the spatial variation in Disease C might confirm this, but this requires mapping its distribution at higher resolution.

Table 14.1   Spatial resolution of data collected in surveillance of 'Disease C'

Spatial reference type		No. in London (approx.)	Availability	
			n	%
Postcode unit	(PCU)	160 000	3300	53
Postcode sector	(PCS)	1000	3400	55
Postcode district	(PCD)	300	5100	82
Postcode area	(PCA)	20	5200	84
Local government district	(LA)	30	5100	82
Health authority	(HA)	15	6200	100

14.4.2   Comparing spatial distribution at different resolutions

The choice of map resolution should be balanced against the availability of data at each resolution. In this case, a similar number of cases (about 80% of the total) can be referenced by postcode districts, postcode areas, and local authorities (LAs); only about half the data can be referenced by unit postcode. The postcode districts, however, offer a resolution about 10 times greater than that of the LAs and 15 times that of postcode area, while the unit postcode essentially represents point data. It is therefore useful to compare distributions between HAs, postcode districts, and unit postcodes. Results are shown in Figs 14.3 and 14.4.

As can be seen, HAs and postcode districts give clearly different pictures; the density estimate produced by unit postcodes, although based on considerably less data, gives a similar picture (not shown here) to the postcode district. This approach may thus help determine the optimum resolution for mapping Disease C: in this case the postcode district or unit postcode. It may also help clarify the extent to which MAUP affects the results and provide an indication of the magnitude of the ecological fallacy when interpreting the results in relation to covariates. Nevertheless, each map may still be unrepresentative of the distribution of C, because of biases introduced by omitting cases for which the required spatial reference was unavailable. This is especially likely in the surveillance of communicable diseases, because of the clustering of cases. Cases occurring in a locality will tend to be reported by the same service; any bias in reporting is therefore likely to be spatially heterogeneous and may act to mask or exaggerate clustering in the data.

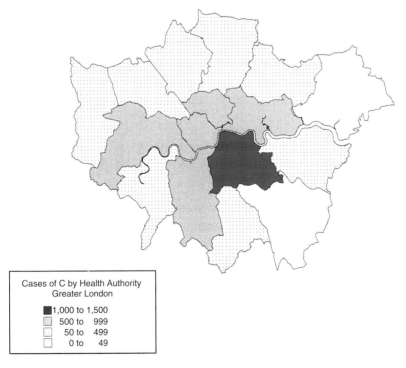

Cases of C by Health Authority
Greater London

■ 1,000 to 1,500
  500 to   999
   50 to   499
    0 to   49

Fig. 14.3 Choropleth map of the count of 'Disease C' by health authority.

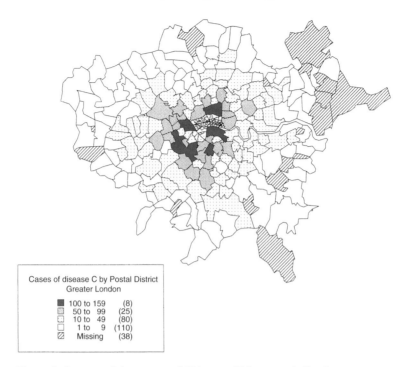

Fig. 14.4   Choropleth map of the count of 'Disease C' by postal district.

14.4.3   Mapping to an optimal resolution

Mapping the data at the optimal resolution is likely to be the most informative, but is also likely to suffer significantly due to gaps in georeferencing. To counteract this, it is necessary to impute locations for these missing cases. This can be based on the distribution of either the general population or the cases already referenced. Suppose in this case that the reference level of choice is the postcode district. Data on postcode district is available for 82% of the reported cases of Disease C. The remaining 18% need to be allocated to a postcode district.

One approach is to distribute these according to the underlying population. If 5% of the general population is in a specific postcode district, then 5% of the remaining unassigned cases can be allocated to that postcode district. The postcode district distribution of the general population can be derived from known population distributions, such as that of residential postal delivery points within each postcode district (using, for estimates in the UK, the Royal Mail Address Manager). Alternatively, the postcode district of unassigned cases can be derived from that already observed in the 82% of cases for which postcode district is available. If the incubation period is short, and the disease highly contagious, then the 'best estimate' location of each case may be assumed to relate to that of other cases, and may thus be derived from the previously established disease distribution. Conversely, if the latent period is very long, then the distribution of missing cases is more likely to reflect that of the general population distribution.

Unfortunately, the methods described above assume that the data are unbiased, and may force similarities in the spatial distribution of cases or the characteristics of the underlying population where none exist. The final representation may also not accurately reflect spatial variations in the certainty with which cases can be located, or with which they can be analysed. Another statistical inference carried out on the full (imputed) dataset will also be anti-conservative because the uncertainty in the location of the computed cases will not be acknowledged. Furthermore, allocating caseloads is simple, but subsequent consideration of other factors (attributes of the cases) that may explain spatial variation in disease distribution can still only be based on the 82% of cases for whom the spatial reference was already assigned. The alternative, selecting *n* cases at random and assigning them to a location on a case-by-case basis, will introduce a random element into what may be a non-random distribution and diffuse the strength of any such associations.

The choice of methods to map and explain spatial variation in disease and exposure distribution depends clearly on the nature of the disease data and the purpose of the analysis. Ultimately the end-user must also be able to interpret the maps. Some problems associated with this are described in the next section.

14.5 Interpreting the spatial distribution of communicable disease data

14.5.1 Bias

Maps of disease and exposure may often reflect the distribution only of a sample of the diseased population. In these cases, bias is a particular problem (Goodchild and Gopal 1989; see also Chapters 2 and 5). All health data suffer from reporting bias, but the geographical analysis of communicable disease data is especially affected because of their spatial clustering and because their detection is geographically sensitive. As noted earlier, cases are likely to be reported by services that provide care for the local population; differences in efficiency of detection and reporting between services will thus create spurious patterns in the data. It is also more likely that cases will be identified and reported when the disease is endemic to an area, where there are a large number of cases, or where there are clinicians specialised in diagnosing disease, than if the cases are few or apparently sporadic. In order to test for reporting biases of this type, it is necessary to compare the distribution of cases with the distribution of service areas. If much of the variation is between, rather than within, service areas, this may imply the presence of reporting bias.

14.5.2 Understanding the origin of georeferences

Frequently, public health specialists need to know where infection was acquired to implement a prevention strategy aimed at removing or reducing the risk of new infection. Geographical location of infection is often impossible to determine, especially if infection is transmitted through multiple exposure routes, if the source of infection is particularly common, or if the case may not wish to disclose such information because the nature of the exposure is sensitive (e.g. if the infection is sexually transmitted). Instead, the location of infection or cause may only be inferred from the spatial variation in the distribution of patients, according to a proxy georeference such as the location of diagnosis or location of death (Snow 1855).

In communicable disease datasets, the data items available for georeferencing are limited (see Section 14.1), and the outcome of mapping such references is consequently often to describe spatial variation in where cases live, have lived, or receive care. If cases are detected and georeferenced soon after infection was acquired, then mapping their distribution may provide an insight into the source or cause of infection. Infections are frequently detected when a patient actually develops disease—the symptomatic stage of infection. For diseases with a short incubation period, such as influenza or measles, where a patient was living at diagnosis may well be related directly or indirectly to where they were infected; this information can thus indicate how diseases spread (Cliff *et al.* 1986). For diseases with a long latent period, like TB or AIDS, however, this is less likely to be the case. A person may develop disease many years after infection, during which time they may have moved several times. Knowledge of migration prior to development of the disease may aid analysis, but such information is rarely readily available. Rates of migration in the general population can provide information about the likelihood that cases have changed residence, but their application is limited and will be unsuitable if the infected population is in some way characterised by its pattern of migration (e.g. if it comprises an itinerant population). An alternative approach is to map the distribution of asymptomatic cases that are diagnosed soon after infection. However, these data are, again, often not readily available and the interpretation of such maps is likely to be limited because the ascertainment of infection in otherwise 'healthy' individuals tends to be biased towards those who may perceive themselves at risk or to areas where specific diagnostic services are most readily available (e.g. for HIV).

Information on the source of infection is clearly of great importance in attempts to prevent the spread of infection, but in general is rarely available, especially for those diseases where the incubation period is long. In the absence of such information, prevention strategies can best be targeted at, or designed specifically to include, those groups classified as 'high risk', such as those who already have an infection or disease and can presumably transmit their infection. In these instances the use of maps describing the distribution of disease should not be under-rated. It may be more appropriate to base prevention strategies on the information which already exists, describing spatial variation in disease occurrence, than to use public health resources to identify an often hypothetical source of infection.

14.6   Conclusions

This chapter has discussed some of the problems of communicable disease surveillance data, the difficulties in mapping area, point, and mixed resolution data, and the need for care in the interpretation of communicable disease patterns.

The quality and availability of georeferenced information is slowly improving, but the nature of surveillance systems designed to provide timely data to inform intervention mean that complete data are unlikely to be achieved. For this reason, the geographical analysis of communicable disease data will require the ongoing development of robust spatial analytical techniques that can cope with clustered patterns, minimise the impact of missing data, and incorporate mixed resolution data. At the same time, there is a continuing need to find novel, appropriate, and profitable ways to use existing georeferenced data in order to demonstrate the value of geographical enquiry as part of health analysis. In this way, those working in communicable disease might begin to realise the potential of the analysis by 'place', in the same way as generations of epidemiologists before them.

References

Atkinson, P. and Unwin, D. (1997, September). The use of density estimation techniques in mapping the distribution of hepatitis A. *Proceedings of the International Workshop on Geomedical Systems*, Rostock, Germany.

Atkinson, P. and Watson, J. (1999). Communicable disease data sources in England and Wales. In *Official health statistics: an unofficial guide* (S. H. Kerrison and A. MacFarlane ed.) Edward Arnold, London.

Bailey, T. C. and Gatrell, A. C. (1995). *Interactive spatial data analysis*. Longman, Harlow.

Benardinelli, L. and Montomoli, C. (1992). Empirical Bayes versus fully Bayesian analysis of geographical variation in disease risk. *Statistics in Medicine*, **11**, 938–1007.

Bithell, J. F. (1990). An application of density estimation to geographical epidemiology. *Statistics in Medicine*, **9**, 691–701.

Bracken, I. and Martin, D. (1989). The generation of spatial population distributions from census centroid data. *Environment and Planning A*, **21**, 537–43.

Bruce, R. (1926). Trail of the Tsetse. In *Microbe Hunters* (P. de Kruif ed.), 246–70. Harvest Books, San Diego, CA.

Brunsden, C. (1991). Estimating probability surfaces in GIS: an adaptive technique. In *Proceedings of the First European Conference on Geographical Information Systems* (J. Harts, H. F. L. Ottens, and H. J. Scholten ed.), 155–64. EGIS Foundation, Amsterdam.

Burkitt, D. P. and Wright, H. D. (1970). *Burkitt's lymphoma*. Livingstone Press, Edinburgh.

Chauvin, P. (1994). Constitution and monitoring of an epidemiological surveillance network with sentinel general practitioners. *European Journal of Epidemiology*, **10**, 1–3.

Choynowski, M. (1959). Maps based on probabilities. *Journal of the American Statistical Association*, **54**, 385–8.

Clayton, D. and Kaldor, J. (1987). Empirical Bayes estimates of age-standardised relative risks for the use in disease mapping. *Biometrics*, **43**, 671–81.

Cliff, A. D., Haggett, P., and Ord, J. K. (1986). *Spatial aspects of influenza epidemics*. Pion, London.

Diggle, P. (1990). A point process modelling approach to raised incidence of a rare phenomenon in the vicinity of a prespecified point. *Journal of the Royal Statistical Society*, **153**, 349–62.

Dorling, D. (1996). *Area cartograms: their use and creation. CATMOG No. 59*. Geo Books, Norwich.

Evans, I. S. (1977). The selection of class intervals. *Transactions of the Institute of British Geographers*, **2**, 98–124.

Fleming, D. M. and Crombie, D. L. (1985). The incidence of common infectious diseases: The Weekly Returns Service of the Royal College of General Practitioners. *Health Trends*, **17**, 13–16.

Flowerdew, R. and Green, I. (1991). Data integration: methods for transferring data between zonal systems. In *Handling geographical information: methodology and potential applications* (I. Masser and M. Blakemore ed.), 38–54. Longman, Harlow.

Gatrell, A. C. (1989). On the spatial representation and accuracy of address-based data in the United Kingdom. *International Journal of Geographical Information Systems*, **3**, 335–48.

Gatrell, A. C., Dunn, C. E., and Boyle, P. J. (1991). The relative utility of the Central Postcode Directory and Pinpoint Address Code in applications of geographical information systems. *Environment and Planning A*, **23**, 1447–58.

Goodchild, M. and Gopal, S. (ed.) (1989). *The accuracy of spatial databases*. Taylor & Francis, London.

Kelsall, J. and Diggle, P. (1995). Non-parametric estimation of spatial variation in relative risk. *Statistics in Medicine*, **14**, 2335–42.

Langbein, L. I. and Lightman, A. J. (1980). *Ecological inference*. Sage, London.

Langford, I. (1994). Using empirical Bayes estimates in the geographical analysis of disease risk. *Area*, **26**, 142–90.

Last, J. M. (ed.) (1988). *A dictionary of epidemiology*. International Epidemiological Association, Oxford.

Martin, D. (1988). *An approach to surface generation from centroid-type data*. Technical Reports in Geo-Information Systems 5, Computing and Cartography. The Wales and South West Regional Research Laboratory.

Martin, D. (1989). Mapping population data from zone centroid locations. *Transactions of the Institute of British Geographers* (new series), **14**, 90–7.

Martin, D. (1991). Representing the socio-economic world. *Papers in Regional Science: The Journal of the RSAI*, **70**, 317–27.

Martin, D. and Tate, N. J. (1998). Small area population geography: a comparison of alternative models for Northern Ireland. *Proceedings of GIS Research UK Conference* (Extended Abstract), (B. M. Gittings and A. Lewis ed.), 4.12–4.14. Edinburgh.

Monmonier, M. (1993). *Mapping it out: expository cartography for the humanities and social sciences*. University of Chicago Press, Chicago and London.

Openshaw, S. (1984). *The modifiable areal unit problem. CATMOG No. 38*. Geo Books, Norwich.

Post Office (1985). *The postcode address file digest*. The Post Office, London.

Raper, J., Rhind, D. W., and Shepherd, J. (1992). *Postcodes: the new geography*. Longman, London.

Rhind, D. (1983). Creating new variables and new areas from the census data. In *A census users handbook*. (D. Rhind, ed.), 151–79. Methuen, Andover.

Robinson, A. H. (1950). Ecological correlation and the behaviour of individuals. *American Sociological Review*, **15**, 351–57.

Robinson, A. H. (1982). *Early thematic mapping in the History of cartography*. University of Chicago Press, Chicago.

Silverman, B. W. (1986). *Density estimation*. Chapman & Hall, London.

Smallman-Raynor, M., Cliff, A. D., and Haggett, P. (1992). *London international atlas of AIDS*. Blackwell, Oxford.

Snow, J. M. (1855). *On the mode of communication of cholera* (2nd edn). Churchill Livingstone, London.

Tobler, W. R. (1973). Choropleth maps without class intervals. *Geographical Analysis*, **5**, 26–8.

Unwin, A. R., Hawkins, G., Hofmann, H., and Siegl, B. (1996). Interactive graphics for datasets with missing values—MANET. *Journal of Computational and Graphical Statistics*, **5**, 113–22.

Unwin, D. (1981). *Introductory spatial analysis*. Methuen, London and New York.

15. Bayesian mapping of Hodgkin's disease in France

A. Mollié

15.1 Introduction

The aim of a map is to demonstrate the distribution of a phenomena in space. By illustrating patterns in disease distribution, disease maps stimulate the formulation of aetiological hypotheses. The conventional approach of mapping standardised disease rates based on Poisson inference gives a good illustration of the geographical distribution of the underlying rates when the disease is not rare. However, for rare diseases or small areas, these maps often produce a patchwork of colours which are difficult to interpret and on which the most highlighted geographical areas are often those based on the least reliable data. The numbers of disease cases observed in each small area are often more variable than that implied by the standard Poisson model. Bayesian models have been developed in disease mapping in order to take into account this extra-Poisson variation. One way is to shrink the most unreliable standardised rates towards the overall mean rate, thereby producing smoothed maps. This approach is part of the general theory of Bayesian analysis using generalised linear mixed models, developed and discussed, for example, in Breslow and Clayton (1993) and Clayton (1996).

Extensions to the above approach follow on recognition that some spatial pattern could be present in the disease rates (i.e. geographically close areas tend to have similar rates). This phenomenon may occur, for example, if the disease process depends on some unknown or unmeasured risk factor which itself is spatially distributed. In this case, prior information on the rates which allows for local geographical dependence is pertinent. With this prior information, a Bayesian estimate of the disease rate in an area is shrunk towards a local mean, according to the rates in the neighbouring areas. A parallel can be drawn with the image restoration problem (e.g. Besag 1986), our goal being to reconstruct the true image (disease rates) from noisy observed data (event counts).

Various methods are available for obtaining Bayesian shrinkage estimates. Empirical Bayes methods yield acceptable point estimates of the rates but underestimate their uncertainty. A direct fully Bayesian approach is not tractable with the non-conjugate distributions typically involved. However, a Monte Carlo technique called the Gibbs sampler has been used to simulate posterior distributions and produce satisfactory point and interval estimates for disease rates (see Chapter 7, Section 7.3).

In this chapter we present a case study of mapping mortality rates for Hodgkin's disease in French départements in which we illustrate and compare the various methods for estimation of rates for rare diseases. We also discuss some practical issues for implementing the fully Bayesian approach, in particular the choice of prior distributions.

15.2   Hodgkin's disease

Hodgkin's disease is a malignancy of the immune system which is distinguished from other lymphomas on histological criteria (Mueller 1996). Its aetiology remains unknown, although the clinical and histological features of the disease suggest a chronic infectious process. There is some support for the hypothesis that Hodgkin's disease may develop as a rare consequence of a common infection, particularly if the infection is delayed until early adulthood. However, the evidence is not strong. Linkage studies have demonstrated a genetic component to the disease, and there is some evidence from occupational studies of a link with exposure to various agricultural pesticides and other chemicals, although no specific compounds have been identified. Geographical and space-time clustering of the disease have been repeatedly sought, but not consistently found.

Unfortunately, cancer incidence data are not available in France, except for a few registers. Instead we consider two illustrations using cancer *mortality* data for Hodgkin's disease in the 94 mainland French départements during the period 1986–1993 (Rezvani *et al.* 1997). The first example consists of 1063 deaths among females (0.5 per 100 000), giving an average of 11.27 deaths per département over the eight-year period. The second example deals with 1693 deaths among males (0.8 per 100 000) giving an average of 17.91 deaths per département over the study period.

The prognosis for Hodgkin's disease has improved greatly due to better treatment over the last twenty years. Hence, mortality data do not reflect incidence and may be less useful for postulating potential risks factors. Nevertheless, the study described below identifies important differences in the geographical distribution of Hodgkin's disease mortality between males and females which may provide some clues as to the disease aetiology.

15.3   Maximum likelihood estimation of relative risks

We begin by discussing standard maximum likelihood methods for estimating the relative risk of Hodgkin's disease in small areas (départements). Separate studies were carried out for males and females as follows. Suppose the map is divided into n contiguous areas labelled $i = 1, \ldots, n$ and let $Y = (Y_1, \ldots, Y_n)$ denote the number of deaths from Hodgkin's disease for males (females) in each area during the study period. Expected numbers of deaths $E = (E_1, \ldots, E_n)$ are assumed to be known and constant during the study period. They are calculated via internal standardisation, that is, by applying the overall male (female) age-specific death rates p_j to the stratified population at risk in the area, N_{ij}. That is, $E_i = \Sigma_j p_j N_{ij}$ where j indexes age strata.

Independently in each area, the number of deaths Y_i is assumed to follow a Poisson distribution with mean $E_i \theta_i$ where $\theta = (\theta_1, \ldots, \theta_n)$ are the unknown area-specific relative risks of mortality from the disease. The data likelihood is thus:

$$Y_i \,|\, \theta_i \sim \mathrm{Po}(E_i \times \theta_i)$$

$$\text{i.e.} \quad f(Y_i \,|\, \theta_i) = \frac{e^{-E_i \theta_i} (E_i \theta_i)^{Y_i}}{Y_i!}. \tag{15.1}$$

It follows from (15.1) that the maximum likelihood estimate (MLE) of θ_i is $\hat{\theta}_i = Y_i/E_i$, termed the standardised mortality ratio (SMR) for the ith area; the estimated standard error of the SMR is $\sqrt{Y_i}/E_i$.

15.3.1 SMRs for Hodgkin's disease in France

Figure 15.1a presents a map of SMRs for Hodgkin's disease in females. The map shows very wide differences between départements: the five with the highest SMRs (départements 27, 47, 51, 53, 58) are shaded in black or dark grey and the five with the lowest SMRs (départements 05, 46, 48, 73, 87) are shown in white. The results for these 10 départements are also presented in Table 15.1. The SMRs vary around their overall mean of 0.96 with standard deviation 0.37, and range from 0 for départements 05 and 48 (which have the smallest populations and expected numbers of deaths) to 1.93 for département 51. The standard errors of the SMRs are 0 for départements 05 and 48 and range from 0.132 for département 69 (which has one of the largest populations) to 0.653 for département 04 (which has one of the smallest populations, i.e. twelve times less than département 69).

For each SMR we also computed a 95% confidence interval (CI) based on the Poisson standard errors. Those which exclude unity, and are therefore regarded as statistically significant, are presented in Table 15.1. However, there are a number of problems associated with the interpretation of variations shown in maps of SMRs and with the comparison of SMRs for different areas; these are emphasised in the present application since Hodgkin's disease mortality is very rare in France. In particular, the départements highlighted in Fig. 15.1a (i.e. with the most extreme point estimates of SMR) are not necessarily those for which the SMR is statistically significantly different from unity. For instance, among the five départements with lowest SMRs only two (73, 87) are statistically significant; among the five départements with the highest SMRs only one (51) is statistically significant. On the other hand, the SMRs for départements 22, 56, 59, 60, and 69, which are based on large populations, are all significantly different from unity despite having point estimates which are less extreme than for those départements highlighted in white or black/dark grey in Fig. 15.1a but which are non-significant. This is because SMRs based on only a few cases have large standard errors; thus although these SMRs are often extreme they tend not to achieve statistical significance. By contrast, départements with large populations will yield SMRs with small standard errors and therefore tend to achieve statistical significance even when the SMR is only moderately different from 1.0.

Similar problems are seen for the SMRs of Hodgkin's disease mortality for males. The SMRs (Fig. 15.2a) vary around their overall mean of 0.97 with standard deviation 0.29, and range from 0.27 for département 05 (which has the second smallest population size and expected number of deaths) to 1.88 for département 80. The four départements with the lowest SMRs and the four with the highest are presented in Table 15.2. Départements whose 95% confidence intervals exclude unity are also presented in Table 15.2. Again, we note that five of the eight most extreme SMRs shown in dark or light shading in Fig. 15.2a (départements 55, 72, 05, 48, and 87) are not statistically significantly different from unity due to the small populations in those départements.

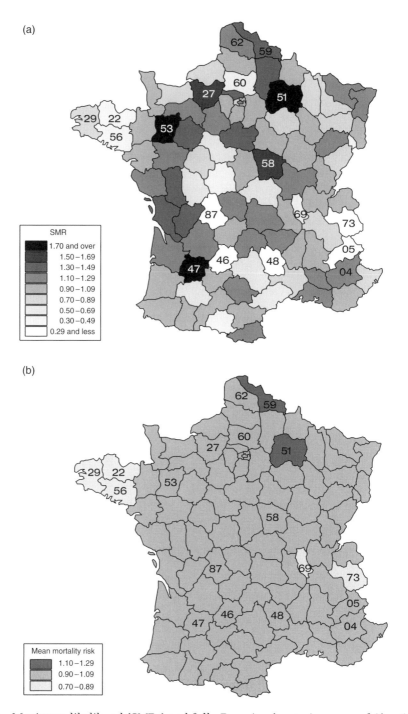

Fig. 15.1 Maximum likelihood (SMRs) and fully Bayesian (posterior mean of θ_i) estimates of the relative risk of mortality from Hodgkin's disease for females in France, 1986−93; numbered départements are those listed in Table 15.1.

Table 15.1 Maximum likelihood (SMR) and fully Bayesian estimates of the relative risk of mortality from Hodgkin's disease for females in France, 1986–93 for selected départements (shown ordered by decreasing SMR)

i	Département	Y_i	E_i	SMR	95% CI_{SMR}	θ_i^*	95% CI_{Bayes}
51	Marne	19	9.83	1.93	(1.16–3.01)	1.11	(0.89–1.50)
53	Mayenne	9	5.24	1.72	(0.79–3.26)	1.02	(0.81–1.35)
47	Lot-et-Garonne	11	6.43	1.71	(0.85–3.06)	1.03	(0.82–1.35)
27	Eure	14	8.75	1.60	(0.87–2.69)	1.05	(0.85–1.37)
58	Nièvre	8	5.19	1.54	(0.66–3.04)	1.01	(0.80–1.30)
59	Nord	61	43.48	1.40	(1.08–1.82)	1.17	(0.96–1.47)
62	Pas-de-Calais	31	25.26	1.23	(0.83–1.75)	1.09	(0.87–1.41)
04	Alpes-de-Haute-Provence	3	2.65	1.13	(0.23–3.30)	0.96	(0.73–1.24)
29	Finistère	12	16.84	0.71	(0.37–1.25)	0.87	(0.61–1.11)
69	Rhône	13	27.33	0.48	(0.25–0.81)	0.84	(0.61–1.04)
22	Côtes-d'Armor	4	11.17	0.36	(0.10–0.92)	0.85	(0.58–1.09)
56	Morbihan	4	11.80	0.34	(0.09–0.87)	0.85	(0.61–1.09)
60	Oise	4	11.76	0.34	(0.09–0.87)	0.92	(0.67–1.15)
46	Lot	1	3.52	0.28	(0.01–1.58)	0.94	(0.71–1.18)
87	Haute-Vienne	2	7.80	0.26	(0.03–0.93)	0.91	(0.67–1.14)
73	Savoie	1	6.38	0.16	(0.00–0.87)	0.88	(0.63–1.11)
05	Hautes-Alpes	0	2.19	0.00	(0.00–1.68)	0.92	(0.67–1.17)
48	Lozère	0	1.55	0.00	(0.00–2.38)	0.94	(0.69–1.19)

$*\theta_i$ is the posterior mean relative risk estimated using the fully Bayesian model with a convolution Gaussian prior on the log relative risks.

Table 15.2 Maximum likelihood (SMR) and fully Bayesian estimates of the relative risk of mortality from Hodgkin disease for males in France, 1986–93 for selected départements (shown ordered by decreasing SMR)

i	Département	Y_i	E_i	SMR	95% CI_{SMR}	θ_i^*	95% CI_{Bayes}
80	Somme	30	15.92	1.88	(1.27–2.70)	1.40	(1.10–1.80)
59	Nord	108	66.42	1.63	(1.33–1.98)	1.49	(1.25–1.78)
72	Sarthe	24	15.82	1.52	(0.97–2.25)	1.08	(0.87–1.38)
55	Meuse	9	5.97	1.51	(0.69–2.86)	1.08	(0.83–1.42)
76	Seine-Maritime	51	34.20	1.49	(1.11–1.97)	1.30	(1.04–1.62)
62	Pas-de-Calais	50	38.72	1.29	(0.96–1.70)	1.32	(1.05–1.63)
02	Aisne	17	15.60	1.09	(0.64–1.74)	1.16	(0.92–1.47)
90	Territoire-de-Belfort	4	3.85	1.04	(0.28–2.66)	0.99	(0.74–1.33)
60	Oise	20	19.67	1.02	(0.62–1.57)	1.10	(0.87–1.36)
42	Loire	21	22.47	0.93	(0.58–1.43)	0.89	(0.71–1.11)
44	Loire-Atlantique	25	29.25	0.85	(0.55–1.27)	0.89	(0.70–1.12)
57	Moselle	24	28.21	0.85	(0.55–1.26)	0.89	(0.68–1.17)
29	Finistère	15	25.93	0.58	(0.32–0.95)	0.74	(0.54–0.99)
69	Rhône	21	42.33	0.50	(0.31–0.76)	0.75	(0.58–0.94)
87	Haute-Vienne	6	12.28	0.49	(0.18–1.07)	0.89	(0.69–1.12)
48	Lozère	1	2.64	0.38	(0.01–2.11)	0.86	(0.64–1.13)
05	Hautes-Alpes	1	3.73	0.27	(0.01–1.49)	0.86	(0.63–1.14)

$*\theta_i$ is the posterior mean relative risk estimated using the fully Bayesian model with a convolution Gaussian prior on the log relative risks.

15.4   The Bayesian approach

Estimation of the relative risks by SMRs supposes that the disease rate is constant over each area so that all individuals of a given age in this area experience the same risk. However, for rare diseases, individual risk levels may often vary *within* the same area, producing variation in the observed number of events that exceeds that expected from standard Poisson inference upon which the SMR is based. That is, in a given area, variation in the observed number of events is due partly to Poisson sampling, but also to extra-Poisson variation. The latter results from heterogeneity in individual risk levels within the area, possibly due to clustering of cases in space or time (see Appendix I in Chapter 7 for further discussion of this phenomenon in the context of binomial data).

Extra-Poisson variation in the observed disease counts can be accommodated by allowing the area-specific relative risks to depend on a latent variable (random effect), the variance of which reflects the degree of extra-Poisson variation. Note that this latent variable may also be used to capture the effects of unknown or unmeasured area level covariates. This adjustment for excess variation in the data leads to area-specific relative risk estimates which are smoothed or shrunk towards each other compared to the crude SMR estimates. Estimation is most naturally carried out using Bayesian methods (Chapter 7).

Bayesian approaches in this context combine two types of information: (i) the information provided in each area by the observed deaths—this is described by the *Poisson likelihood* in Equation (15.1); (ii) information about the relative risks in each area and their variability across the map—this is summarised by the *prior* distribution. This prior distribution is parameterised by (a vector of) hyperparameters $\boldsymbol{\phi}$ which control the degree of variability in the relative risks across areas, and is denoted $f(\boldsymbol{\theta}|\boldsymbol{\phi})$. Under the fully Bayesian approach, a *hyperprior* distribution for $\boldsymbol{\phi}$, denoted $f(\boldsymbol{\phi})$, is also specified. We discuss suitable choices for $f(\boldsymbol{\theta}|\boldsymbol{\phi})$ and $f(\boldsymbol{\phi})$ in Sections 15.4.1 and 15.4.3, respectively.

Applying Bayes theorem gives the joint posterior distribution of the parameters $\boldsymbol{\theta}$ and $\boldsymbol{\phi}$ conditional on the data, namely

$$f(\boldsymbol{\theta}, \boldsymbol{\phi}|\boldsymbol{Y}) \propto f(\boldsymbol{Y}|\boldsymbol{\theta}) \times f(\boldsymbol{\theta}|\boldsymbol{\phi}) \times f(\boldsymbol{\phi}).$$

Bayesian inference about the unknown relative risk in a particular area i is based on the marginal posterior distribution for θ_i given the data Y_i which is obtained by integrating the joint posterior over the hyperparameters $\boldsymbol{\phi}$ and the remaining relative risk parameters $\theta_j, j \neq i$. That is

$$f(\theta_i \mid Y_i) = \int_{\boldsymbol{\phi}} \int_{\theta_1} \cdots \int_{\theta_{i-1}} \int_{\theta_{i+1}} \cdots \int_{\theta_n} f(\boldsymbol{\theta}, \boldsymbol{\phi}|\boldsymbol{Y}) \, \mathrm{d}\boldsymbol{\phi} \, \mathrm{d}\theta_1 \ldots \mathrm{d}\theta_{i-1} \mathrm{d}\theta_{i+1} \ldots \mathrm{d}\theta_n.$$

A point estimate of the relative risks is given by a summary measure of the location of this distribution, such as the posterior mean $E[\theta_i|Y_i]$ or the posterior median. However direct evaluation of these parameters through analytic or numerical integration is not generally possible. An alternative which, in certain situations, produces closed-form solutions, is to consider using a completely specified prior distribution $f(\boldsymbol{\theta}|\boldsymbol{\phi})$ with known hyperparameters $\boldsymbol{\phi}$, although this is seldom used in practice. The empirical Bayes (EB) approach assumes that the hyperparameters are unknown, but rather than specify the hyperprior distribution $f(\phi)$, replaces the unknown ϕ by a point estimate $\hat{\phi}$ based on the marginal likelihood of ϕ given the data Y. Alternatively, the fully Bayesian approach comprises a three-stage hierarchical model in which the hyperprior distribution $f(\phi)$ is specified (see Chapter 7).

15.4.1 Prior distributions for the area-specific relative risks

We now describe various prior models that may be assumed for the area-specific relative risk parameters (i.e. the second stage of the Bayesian hierarchical model). Further details of the models discussed here can be found in Section 7.2.2 in Chapter 7.

Independent priors

If prior beliefs suggest that there is no systematic pattern to the variability of the relative risks θ, then we consider each θ_i to be independent conditional on the hyperparameters ϕ. A mathematically convenient choice is the conjugate gamma prior (Manton *et al.* 1981, 1987, 1989; Tsutakawa 1988); see also Chapter 22 for discussion of a variation on the usual conjugate Poisson-gamma disease mapping model. Alternatively, a normal prior distribution on the logarithm of each relative risk is often used since this leads to the generalised linear mixed model formulation and allows for the inclusion of covariate information where available (Tsutakawa *et al.* 1985; Clayton and Kaldor 1987). Writing $\log \theta_i = V_i$, we typically specify:

$$V_i \sim N(0, \sigma_v^2) \tag{15.2}$$

where the variance σ_v^2 corresponds to the hyperparameter ϕ in the previous section.

Spatially structured priors

Prior knowledge may suggest that geographically close areas tend to have similar relative risks, (i.e. there exists local spatially structured variation in relative risks). This prior knowledge can be expressed using Gaussian autoregressive models (Besag, 1974) which originated in the image processing literature and were first applied in the context of disease mapping by Clayton and Kaldor (1987). In the most common case, the conditional distribution of the log relative risk in each area i, given all the other log relative risks in areas $j \neq i$ and the hyperparameter ω_u^2, is normal with mean given by the mean of the log relative risks in areas $j \in \partial i$ and variance proportional to ω_u^2/m_i. Here, ∂i defines the set of areas neighbouring area i and m_i is the number of areas belonging to this set. Writing $\log \theta_i = U_i$, we typically specify

$$U_i | U_j = u_j, j \neq i \sim N\left(\bar{u}_i, \frac{\omega_u^2}{m_i}\right) \tag{15.3}$$

where $\bar{u}_i = (1/m_i) \sum_{j \in \partial i} u_j$. Note that the joint prior distribution for $U = (U_1, \ldots, U_n)$ corresponding to model (15.3) is improper since the mean level for each U_i is not defined (see Section 7.2.2 in Chapter 7). However, the posterior distribution for the U_i is identifiable in the presence of any informative data (Y_i); alternatively, we may reparameterise the model to include a separate intercept term (representing the mean level) and impose the constraint $\sum_i u_i = 0$ to ensure that the model is identifiable. This is the approach taken in Chapter 7.

Convolution priors

In practice it is often unclear how to choose between an unstructured prior and a purely spatially structured prior. An intermediate distribution on the log relative risks that ranges from prior independence to prior local dependence, called a convolution Gaussian prior, has therefore been proposed (Besag 1989; Besag and Mollié 1989; Besag *et al.* 1991; Mollié 1996). In this prior model, the log relative risk in each area is defined to be the sum of two independent components:

$$\log \theta_i = U_i + V_i$$

where the prior distributions for V_i and U_i are defined as in (15.2) and (15.3), respectively, Thus, the V_i describe the unstructured heterogeneity of the relative risks, whilst the U_i represent local spatially structured variation. The conditional prior expectation of $\log \theta_i$ given all the other $\log \theta_j$s ($j \neq i$) and hyperparameters $\phi^T = (\sigma_v^2, \omega_u^2)$ is thus the sum of the expectations of the independent components U_i and V_i, i.e.

$$\mathrm{E}[\log \theta_i | u_j, v_j, j \neq i, \sigma_v^2, \omega_u^2] = \mathrm{E}[V_i | \sigma_v^2] + \mathrm{E}[U_i | U_j = u_j, j \in \partial i, \omega_u^2]$$

$$= 0 + \bar{u}_i = \bar{u}_i.$$

Likewise, the conditional prior variance is

$$\mathrm{var}[\log \theta_i | u_j, v_j, j \neq i, \sigma_v^2, \omega_u^2] = \mathrm{var}[V_i | \sigma_v^2] + \mathrm{var}[U_i | U_j = u_j, j \in \partial i, \omega_u^2]$$

$$= \sigma_v^2 + \frac{\omega_u^2}{m_i}. \tag{15.4}$$

The parameters σ_v^2 and ω_u^2 control the strength of each component. Setting $\omega_u^2 = 0$ leads to a total independence of the risks whereas $\sigma_v^2 = 0$ corresponds to purely local dependence modelled by the intrinsic Gaussian autoregression. A small value for the ratio ω_u^2 / σ_v^2 reflects mainly unstructured heterogeneity, whereas a large value indicates that spatially structured variation dominates. However, calibration of this ratio is complicated by the fact that ω_u^2 is only *proportional* to the *conditional* spatial variation of the log relative risks, with each area having a different constant of proportionality given by the inverse of its number of neighbours (15.4). Ideally, we would like to compare the ratio of *marginal* spatial and unstructured variances for a given model in order to determine which (if either) one dominates. The marginal variance may be found by considering the form of the joint distribution for the collection $\log \theta_i$, $i = 1, \ldots, n$ (see Section 7.2.2 and Appendix II in Chapter 7). This gives a theoretical marginal prior covariance of $\sigma_v^2 I + \omega_u^2 (I - W)^{-1} D$, where W is the weight matrix with elements $w_{ij} = m_i^{-1}$ if i and j are adjacent areas, and $w_{ij} = 0$ otherwise, and D is an $n \times n$ diagonal matrix with elements $D_{ii} = m_i^{-1}$ (see Section 7.2.2 in Chapter 7). However $(I - W)$ is a singular matrix and so the marginal covariance does not exist. Instead, we may approximate the marginal variability of the spatial random effects by calculating the *empirical* marginal variance

$s_u^2 = (1/(n-1)) \sum_i (U_i - \bar{U})^2$. The ratio s_u^2/s_v^2 (where $s_v^2 = (1/(n-1)) \sum_i (V_i - \bar{V})^2$, is the corresponding empirical variance for the unstructured random effects) may be used to estimate the relative importance of each component to the total random effects variation. (Note that $s_v^2 \approx \sigma_v^2$ but $s_u^2 \neq \omega_u^2$.)

The convolution prior model has been generalised to allow for covariate effects (Mollié 1990; Clayton and Bernardinelli 1992; Clayton *et al.* 1993; see also Chapter 16).

15.4.2 Empirical Bayes estimation of the relative risks

The empirical Bayes (EB) estimate of the vector of relative risks θ is the mean of the posterior distribution for θ evaluated at the MLE of the marginal likelihood of ϕ, i.e. $E[\theta|Y, \hat{\phi}]$. With the non-conjugate convolution Gaussian prior, a multivariate Normal approximation for the marginal posterior distribution of the collection $\log \theta_i$, $i = 1, \ldots, n$, is needed (Clayton and Kaldor 1987). In addition, since the marginal likelihood of ϕ is rarely tractable, its maximisation requires the EM algorithm (Dempster *et al.* 1977). This consists of an iterative process which maximises the conditional expectation of the prior log density given the data Y and the current values of the hyperparameters ϕ.

The main disadvantage of EB estimation is that the variability of the EB estimates is difficult to assess. In addition, we have found that in practice, EB estimation of the hyperparameters of the convolution Gaussian prior often produces either the heterogeneity component alone ($\omega_u^2 \to 0$) of the clustering component alone ($\sigma_v^2 \to 0$); mixing of both components is rarely found. This can be due to the fact that the function maximised is an approximation of the posterior log likelihood, which is flat around its maximum, and is therefore very difficult to distinguish from the likelihood at the boundary (i.e. at 0).

EB results for Hodgkin's disease mortality in France

EB estimates of the relative risks of Hodgkin's disease mortality were computed as described above, assuming the convolution Gaussian prior. For females, the estimated convolution prior reduces to the heterogeneity component V only, with $\sigma_v^2 = 0.011$ and $\omega_u^2 \approx 0$. This produces smoothing of the rates in each département towards the overall relative risk ($= 1$). For males, the model reduces to the clustering component U only, with $\omega_u^2 = 0.044$ and $\sigma_v^2 \approx 0$. The observed rates are thus smoothed towards a local mean given by the mean of the relative risks in the adjacent départements.

15.4.3 Fully Bayesian estimation of the relative risks

The fully Bayesian approach provides an alternative way to incorporate variability in the hyperparameters ϕ by specifying a hyperprior distribution $f(\phi)$ and basing inference about θ on the marginal posterior distribution $f(\theta|Y)$ integrated over ϕ.

Hyperpriors for ϕ

Classical choices for the hyperprior distribution $f(\phi) = f(\sigma_v^2, \omega_u^2)$ generally assume independence between the unstructured and spatial hyperparameters σ_v^2 and ω_u^2 of the convolution model. It is also tempting to assume the distributions to be non-informative, which, for the variance parameter of a normal distribution, corresponds to assuming an improper uniform distribution on $(-\infty, +\infty)$ for the logarithm of this parameter. However, when used as the hyperprior for σ_v^2 or ω_u^2 in the convolution Gaussian prior (or indeed, in any hierarchical Gaussian model) this results in an improper posterior with an infinite spike at $\sigma_v^2 = 0$ or $\omega_u^2 = 0$, respectively. A convenient alternative which allows the prior to be *proper* but diffuse, is to assume a conjugate gamma distribution with specified parameters for the *inverse* variance (precision) of the normal distribution. The choice of parameters for this distribution is important as Bayesian estimates may be relatively sensitive to this choice. The mean of the gamma distribution represents a prior guess at the value of the inverse of the variance parameter (i.e. σ_v^{-2} or ω_u^{-2}), and its variance reflects the uncertainty about this prior belief.

One way to specify these parameters is to assume that, on average, 95% of the log relative risks lie in a symmetric interval $(-a, +a)$. That is, to guess a value a so that the interval (e^{-a}, e^a) contains 95% of the relative risks a priori. In terms of the convolution prior we have seen that we cannot consider the marginal variance, and so instead, we must make a guess at the range of relative risks conditional on their neighbours. Then, under the assumption of normality, the prior conditional variance of the log relative risks may be approximated by

$$\mathrm{var}[\log \theta_i | u_j, v_j, j \neq i, \sigma_v^2, \omega_u^2] = \sigma_v^2 + \frac{\omega_u^2}{m_i} \approx (a/1.96)^2.$$

In the absence of information about the relative contributions of the unstructured (σ_v^2) and spatial (ω_u^2/m_i) components of this variance, it is reasonable to assume a priori that they have the same strength. This suggests that a priori $\sigma_v^2 = \omega_u^2/\bar{m} = 0.5 \times (a/1.96)^2$, where $\bar{m}$ is the average number of neighbours across the study region. We therefore choose gamma hyperpriors for the *inverses* of the unstructured and spatial (conditional) variance parameters with means

$$2 \times \left(\frac{1.96}{a}\right)^2 \qquad \text{for } \sigma_v^{-2}$$

$$\frac{2}{\bar{m}} \times \left(\frac{1.96}{a}\right)^2 \qquad \text{for } \omega_u^{-2}.$$

The variances of both gamma hyperpriors are taken to be large to reflect uncertainty about the values specified for the prior means.

As already noted, the difficulty with this method of choosing the hyperpriors is that our guess at the value of a should reflect the *conditional* variability of the relative risks across the map. This is a very non-intuitive quantity to specify, and in practice, our prior guess at a is likely to reflect our beliefs about the overall marginal variation in relative risks. Since we assume large variances for the hyperprior (reflecting high uncertainty about our prior guess at a), this is unlikely to matter very much; we investigate this issue via a sensitivity analysis reported in Section 15.4.4. A related approach to specifying the hyperprior distribution for the spatial variance parameter, this time based on a guess at the *marginal* variation in relative risks across the map, is given in the Appendix in Chapter 16.

The mean of the number of neighbours is $\bar{m} = 5$ for départements in France. For Hodgkin's disease in females, a reasonable guess (based on the observed SMRs) for the

95% plausible range of relative risks is 0.4–2.5, which gives a ≈ 0.9. That is, 95% of the relative risks for Hodgkin's disease in females lie within $\exp(2a) \approx 6:1$ range of variation under our prior guess. Gamma hyperpriors were therefore chosen to have a mean of 10 for σ_v^{-2} and 2 for ω_u^{-2}, the variance of each hyperprior distribution was set to 10^4. These prior guesses correspond to the following shape and inverse scale parameters for the gamma distribution: 10^{-2} and 10^{-3}, respectively for σ_v^{-2} and 4×10^{-4} and 2×10^{-4}, respectively for ω_u^{-2}.

For males, according to the observed SMRs, the range of variation of the relative risks is smaller than for females and a 95% plausible interval is $0.5 - 1.9$. Hence $a \approx 0.64$, which means that 95% of relative risks lie within $3.6:1$ range of variation a priori. Gamma hyperpriors on the inverse variances were thus chosen to have a mean of 19 for σ_v^{-2} and 3.8 for ω_u^{-2}, with both prior variances equal to 10^{-4}. These prior guesses correspond to the following shape and inverse scale parameters for the gamma distribution: 3.61×10^{-2} and 1.9×10^{-3}, respectively for σ_v^{-2}, and 1.44×10^{-3} and 3.8×10^{-4}, respectively, for ω_u^{-2}.

Fully Bayesian results for Hodgkin's disease mortality in France

We used Markov chain Monte Carlo (MCMC) methods to obtain fully Bayesian estimates of the relative risk of Hodgkin's disease mortality in the 94 French départements. This involves simulation of samples from the joint posterior distribution $f(\boldsymbol{\theta},\boldsymbol{\phi}|Y)$ which may then be used to obtain estimates of the marginal posterior distributions of interest that is, $f(\boldsymbol{\theta}|Y)$ and, $f(\boldsymbol{\phi}|Y)$. Details of the Gibbs sampling algorithm used to carry out the simulations are given elsewhere (e.g. Gilks *et al.* 1996). This algorithm is implemented in the WinBUGS statistical software (Spiegelhalter *et al.* 1998), which may be used to carry out fully Bayesian estimation of the models described in this chapter. We performed a single run of the Gibbs sampler with a burn-in (pre-convergence cycle) of 1000 iterations followed by 10 000 further iterations for each set of data (males and females).

Posterior estimates of the unstructured and spatial variance components are shown in the first (females) and second (males) rows of Table 15.3. Plots of the prior and posterior distributions of the inverse variance parameters σ_v^{-2} and ω_u^{-2} for males are also shown in Fig. 15.3. For females the ratio of the empirical marginal spatial to unstructured variances (s_u^2/s_v^2) is 0.49, indicating that unstructured heterogeneity dominates. For males, the spatially structured component dominates, with a ratio of 3.03 for the marginal spatial to unstructured variances. As expected, the posterior means of the empirical and theoretical variances of the unstructured components (s_v^2 and σ_v^2, respectively) are very similar in each analysis, since both reflect marginal variability. However the posterior mean of the empirical variance of the spatial component (s_u^2) is about half the value of the theoretical variance ω_u^2 for both males and females, reflecting the difference between the marginal and conditional variances respectively. Note that our prior guess at the scaling factor for the ratio of marginal to conditional spatial variances was $1/5$, somewhat smaller than the posterior distributions indicate.

The posterior distribution of the ratio of the 97.5th to 2.5th percentiles of the relative risks $\theta_{0.975}/\theta_{0.025}$ (i.e. the 95% relative risk ratio or range of variation) has mean 1.91, median 1.82, and 95% Bayesian credible interval (1.24–3.07) for females, but is somewhat larger for males (mean 2.37, median 2.33 and 95% Bayesian credible interval; 1.77–3.17).

The fully Bayesian estimates of relative risks shown in Fig. 15.1b (females) and Fig. 15.2b (males) show much less variation than the observed SMRs (Figs 15.1a and

Table 15.3 Posterior mean (95% CI) for the hyperparameters of the fully Bayesian convolution model for Hodgkin's disease in females (row 1) and males (rows 2–7); results for males are given for each of the six hyperprior choices considered in the sensitivity analysis

	Unstructured component		Spatial component		Ratio
	σ_v^2	s_v^2	ω_u^2	s_u^2	s_u^2/s_v^2
Females					
1	0.0115	0.0112	0.0123	0.0055	0.49
	(0.0007–0.0423)	(0.0007–0.0403)	(0.0002–0.0654)	(0.0001–0.0264)	
Males					
1	0.0072	0.0070	0.0432	0.0211	3.03
	(0.0008–0.0252)	(0.0008–0.0242)	(0.0102–0.1010)	(0.0059–0.0414)	
2	0.0097	0.0094	0.0386	0.0189	2.01
	(0.0018–0.0274)	(0.0018–0.0263)	(0.0059–0.0960)	(0.0034–0.0389)	
3	0.0090	0.0087	0.0407	0.0201	2.31
	(0.0022–0.0267)	(0.0021–0.0252)	(0.0102–0.0980)	(0.0061–0.0399)	
4	0.0048	0.0047	0.0452	0.0220	4.66
	(0.0001–0.0223)	(0.0001–0.0215)	(0.0092–0.1066)	(0.0059–0.0421)	
5	0.0093	0.0089	0.0390	0.0195	2.18
	(0.0017–0.0286)	(0.0016–0.0270)	(0.0097–0.0905)	(0.0055–0.0387)	
6	0.0098	0.0096	0.0310	0.0163	1.71
	(0.0024–0.0278)	(0.0022–0.0266)	(0.0068–0.0788)	(0.0040–0.0342)	

Fig. 15.2a, respectively). These are summarised for selected départements in the right-hand columns of Table 15.1 (females) and Table 15.2 (males). For females, the posterior mean relative risks vary from 0.84 for département 69 to 1.17 for département 59, with overall mean 0.98 (s.d. = 0.05). Extreme SMR estimates based on small populations, for instance for départements 05, 27, 46, 47, 48, 53, and 58, have disappeared and much of the map has been almost totally smoothed. On the other hand, extreme estimates based on very large populations for départements 59 and 69, or on moderate populations for départements 22, 51, and 56 are maintained. However, none of the 95% Bayesian credible intervals exclude unity (Table 15.1), indicating that the variations observed on the map (Fig. 15.1b) are statistically insignificant.

The posterior relative risks for males, although smoothed compared to the observed SMRs show more variation than for females, with means ranging from 0.74 for département 29 to 1.49 for département 59 (mean SMR across départements = 0.97; s.d. = 0.12). The relatively large posterior variance associated with the spatial component of risk for males leads to *local* smoothing of the relative risk estimates. Thus, extreme SMR estimates based on small populations for départements 55 and 72 have disappeared, having been smoothed towards their larger neighbours whose risk estimates are in the opposite direction. However, estimated relative risks for départements 05, 48 and 87, although having small populations, are less changed from their SMRs because their neighbours also have similar risk estimates (Table 15.2). Extreme relative risk estimates

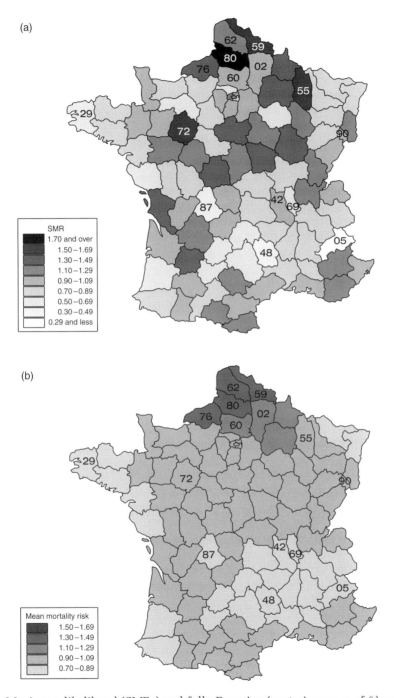

Fig. 15.2 Maximum likelihood (SMRs) and fully Bayesian (posterior mean of θ_i) estimates of the relative risk of mortality from Hodgkin's disease for males in France, 1986–93; numbered départements are those listed in Table 15.2.

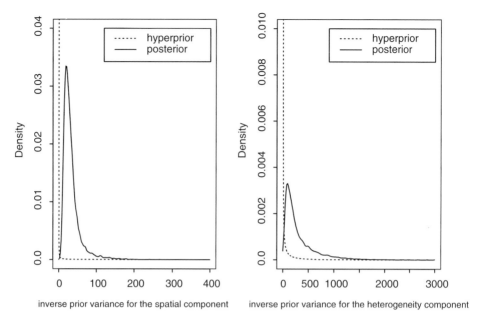

Fig. 15.3 Prior and posterior distributions of the inverse variance of each component of the convolution Gaussian prior for the log relative risks (using hyperprior 1) for males.

based on large populations for départements 59, 69, and 80 remain relatively unchanged from their SMRs. Moreover, risk estimates for départements 02, 60, 62, and 76, which have neighbours with high estimated risks, have been raised, while that of département 42 has been reduced. Bayesian 95% credible intervals for all the four départements coloured in dark grey (59, 62, 76, and 80) exclude unity, indicating significantly elevated risk of mortality from Hodgkin's disease for males living in these areas. The spatial structure of the relative risks is shown in Fig. 15.2b: risks are low in the south and the west but high in the north.

15.4.4 Sensitivity to the choice of hyperprior

To investigate the influence of the choice of hyperprior on estimates of Hodgkin's disease mortality among males, we carried out a sensitivity analysis to different choices of the prior mean for the inverse variance parameters σ_v^{-2} and ω_u^{-2}. We considered six combinations of priors for these two parameters, summarised in Table 15.4 in terms of the shape and inverse scale parameters of the gamma distribution and the corresponding range within which 95% of the département-specific relative risk parameters lie a priori, that is, (e^{-a}, e^a). The first choice is the one based on the data, as discussed in Section 15.4.3, which concentrates around small values of σ_v^{-2} and ω_u^{-2}; for the second and the third choices we increased the prior means for both σ_v^{-2} and ω_u^{-2}, keeping their ratio equal to 5 (i.e. $\bar{m}$); for the last three choices, this ratio was set to 1 (i.e. the prior means for σ_v^{-2} and ω_u^{-2} were taken to be equal). The variance of the hyperprior distribution was set to 10^4 in all cases. Thus, hyperpriors 2, 3, 5, and 6 correspond to relatively small ranges of relative risks a priori; hyperprior 1 to an intermediate range; and hyperprior 4 to a huge range of

Table 15.4 Mean, scale, and inverse shape parameters for the six combinations of gamma hyperpriors considered for the hyperparameters of the convolution model for males

	Unstructured component inverse variance (σ_v^{-2})			Spatial component inverse variance (ω_u^{-2})			Prior 95% range for θ (e^{-a}, e^{a})	Prior mean ratio*
	Mean	Shape	Inv. scale	Mean	Shape	Inv. scale		
1	19	0.0361	0.0019	3.8	0.00144	0.00038	(0.5, 1.9)	5
2	50	0.25	0.005	10	0.01	0.001	(0.7, 1.5)	5
3	100	1	0.01	20	0.04	0.002	(0.8, 1.3)	5
4	1	0.0001	0.0001	1	0.0001	0.0001	(0.1, 16.0)	1
5	50	0.25	0.005	50	0.25	0.005	(0.7, 1.5)	1
6	100	1	0.01	100	1	0.01	(0.8, 1.3)	1

*Ratio between prior mean for σ_v^{-2} and ω_u^{-2}.

relative risks that is very unlikely to occur in epidemiology (see penultimate column of Table 15.4).

Results based on the posterior distribution estimated from 10 000 iterations of the Gibbs sampler for each choice of hyperprior are given in Table 15.3 for the hyperparameters ω_u^2 and σ_v^2, and in Table 15.5 for the relative risks in selected départements. The posterior variance of the spatially structured component (ω_u^2) is fairly similar across all priors, whereas for the variance of the unstructured component (σ_v^2), the choice of hyperprior leads to much greater differences, particularly for hyperprior 4.

Concerning the relative importance of each component, the ratios of the posterior means of the empirical marginal spatial to unstructured variances (s_u^2/s_v^2) are all greater than unity, indicating that spatially structured variation dominates for each prior. Hyperprior 4 leads to the strongest dominance $(s_u^2/s_v^2 = 4.66)$ and hyperprior 6 to the weakest $(s_u^2/s_v^2 = 1.71)$. As found for the original analysis reported above, the posterior means of the empirical and theoretical unstructured variances $(s_v^2$ and σ_v^2, respectively) were very similar for each hyperprior, whilst the empirical marginal spatial variance was about half the theoretical conditional spatial variance in each case. Despite the sensitivity of the unstructured variance σ_v^2 to the prior specification, the posterior distribution of the 95% relative risk ratio $(\theta_{0.975}/\theta_{0.025})$ under each hyperprior is very similar for all six choices (Fig. 15.4).

Posterior estimates of the relative risks are similar for all six hyperpriors: over the 94 départements, the average of the posterior mean relative risks is 0.97 for each choice, with standard deviation 0.12 for all choices except for hyperprior 6, where the standard deviation was 0.11. The posterior mean estimate of relative risk for each département differs by 0.012 on average across the six hyperpriors, with a maximum difference of 0.03 for each of two départements (02 and 62). The maps obtained are also very similar under all hyperpriors: compared with the map for hyperprior 1 (Fig. 15.2b) there are only two départements that change category under hyperpriors 3 and 4, three départements that change under hyperprior 5 and four that change under hyperprior 2. These changes concerned mainly départements 57, 60, 62, and 76 and, for some

Spatial epidemiology

Table 15.5 Comparison of the posterior mean (95% CI) estimates of relative risk of mortality from Hodgkin's disease for males in France, 1986–93, using each of the six hyperpriors (selected départements shown ordered by decreasing SMR)

			Hyperprior			
i	1	2	3	4	5	6
80	1.40	1.39	1.40	1.39	1.40	1.37
	(1.10–1.80)	(1.09–1.78)	(1.09–1.80)	(1.11–1.76)	(1.09–1.80)	(1.08–1.76)
59	1.49	1.49	1.49	1.49	1.49	1.47
	(1.25–1.78)	(1.24–1.78)	(1.25–1.78)	(1.24–1.78)	(1.25–1.77)	(1.23–1.76)
72	1.08	1.09	1.09	1.07	1.08	1.08
	(0.87–1.38)	(0.86–1.40)	(0.86–1.40)	(0.86–1.35)	(0.86–1.40)	(0.86–1.38)
55	1.08	1.08	1.08	1.08	1.08	1.07
	(0.83–1.42)	(0.82–1.43)	(0.83–1.43)	(0.83–1.40)	(0.83–1.43)	(0.83–1.40)
76	1.30	1.29	1.30	1.29	1.30	1.28
	(1.04–1.62)	(1.04–1.61)	(1.04–1.62)	(1.05–1.62)	(1.05–1.62)	(1.03–1.59)
62	1.32	1.29	1.30	1.32	1.31	1.29
	(1.05–1.63)	(1.03–1.62)	(1.04–1.62)	(1.05–1.65)	(1.04–1.63)	(1.03–1.60)
02	1.16	1.14	1.15	1.17	1.15	1.14
	(0.92–1.47)	(0.90–1.45)	(0.91–1.46)	(0.94–1.45)	(0.90–1.46)	(0.89–1.43)
90	0.99	0.98	0.99	0.99	0.99	0.98
	(0.74–1.33)	(0.73–1.33)	(0.73–1.33)	(0.74–1.30)	(0.74–1.34)	(0.73–1.31)
60	1.10	1.08	1.09	1.10	1.09	1.08
	(0.87–1.36)	(0.86–1.35)	(0.86–1.37)	(0.89–1.35)	(0.86–1.36)	(0.86–1.35)
42	0.89	0.89	0.89	0.89	0.90	0.90
	(0.71–1.11)	(0.71–1.12)	(0.71–1.10)	(0.71–1.09)	(0.71–1.12)	(0.72–1.12)
44	0.89	0.89	0.89	0.90	0.89	0.89
	(0.70–1.12)	(0.70–1.12)	(0.70–1.11)	(0.70–1.13)	(0.69–1.12)	(0.70–1.13)
57	0.89	0.90	0.89	0.90	0.90	0.90
	(0.68–1.17)	(0.67–1.17)	(0.67–1.16)	(0.69–1.17)	(0.68–1.17)	(0.68–1.17)
29	0.74	0.75	0.74	0.74	0.74	0.76
	(0.54–0.99)	(0.53–1.01)	(0.54–1.00)	(0.53–1.00)	(0.54–1.00)	(0.56–1.01)
69	0.75	0.74	0.74	0.76	0.74	0.75
	(0.58–0.94)	(0.57–0.93)	(0.57–0.93)	(0.59–0.95)	(0.57–0.94)	(0.58–0.94)
87	0.89	0.88	0.88	0.90	0.89	0.89
	(0.69–1.12)	(0.67–1.13)	(0.67–1.12)	(0.70–1.12)	(0.68–1.13)	(0.68–1.12)
48	0.86	0.86	0.86	0.86	0.87	0.87
	(0.64–1.13)	(0.64–1.15)	(0.65–1.14)	(0.65–1.12)	(0.64–1.14)	(0.66–1.14)
05	0.86	0.86	0.85	0.86	0.86	0.86
	(0.63–1.14)	(0.63–1.15)	(0.63–1.13)	(0.64–1.13)	(0.62–1.14)	(0.64–1.14)

hyperpriors, départements 42, 44, and 87, since the original relative risk estimates for these départements were very close to a cut-point on the scale used to shade the maps (see Table 15.5 for details). The greatest differences occurred between the maps for hyperpriors 1 and 6, with six changes involving départements 60, 62, and 76 (shaded in lighter grey under hyperprior 6) and 42, 44, and 57 (shaded in darker grey under

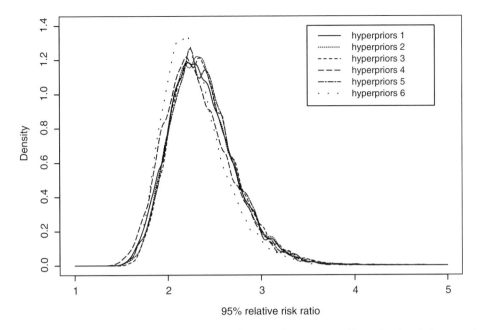

Fig. 15.4 Posterior distributions of the 95% relative risk ratio $\theta_{0.975}/\theta_{0.025}$ for the six hyperprior choices for males.

hyperprior 6). However, the overall visual impact given by the smoothed maps was similar for all hyperpriors. Moreover, five of the six départements (59, 62, 69, 76 and 80) whose 95% Bayesian credible interval excluded unity under hyperprior 1 have intervals which exclude unity under all the six hyperpriors; only the 95% credible interval for département 29 no longer excludes unity under hyperpriors 2–6 (see Table 15.5).

15.5 Discussion

This case study has illustrated some of the problems typically associated with standard Poisson maximum likelihood approaches to disease mapping for rare diseases and for small areas. The most extreme SMRs are usually based on only a few cases, whilst the most extreme *p*-values of hypothesis tests comparing SMRs to unity and confidence intervals which exclude unity may simply identify areas with large populations. Bayesian approaches may overcome the problem of overdispersion and unreliability of the classical SMRs. Indeed, they smooth SMRs based on sparse data but preserve those based on large populations, as shown in the examples. Bayesian estimates of the relative risks are then easier to interpret.

Both the empirical Bayes and fully Bayesian methods lead to similar conclusions concerning the pattern of variation in relative risk of Hodgkin's disease across French départements: for females, unstructured variation dominated, whilst for males, strong spatial correlation was found with départements in the far north being at greatest risk. This elevated risk in northern France deserves further investigation.

The fully Bayesian method, which consists of simulating the joint posterior distribution, has a number of advantages over the EB method: not only does it produce both point and interval estimates of the relative risks, but it also permits computations of appropriate statistics for a specific problem, such as the posterior distributions of the empirical marginal spatial variance, s_u^2, and of the 95% relative risk ratio, $\theta_{0.975}/\theta_{0.025}$.

The use of a fully Bayesian approach introduces the problem of choosing an appropriate prior for the relative risks. The convolution Gaussian model avoids us having to choose between prior independence and a purely local spatially structured dependence of the risks. However our example shows that the choice of hyperprior for the variance parameters of the convolution model may have a large influence on the posterior estimates of these variance components. Despite this, the relative risk estimates and maps seem robust to this choice. Thus, if the primary goal of the analysis is to obtain area-specific estimates of disease risk, such prior sensitivity may be of little consequence; however, if the primary objective is to quantify and explain the underlying pattern of variation in disease risks across a region, then careful interpretation may be required.

Acknowledgements

This work was partially supported by an EU BIOMED II Concerted Action grant number PL96 3488.

References

Besag J. (1974). Spatial interaction and the statistical analysis of lattice systems. *Journal of the Royal Statistical Society, Series B*, **36**, 192–236.

Besag J. (1986). On the statistical analysis of dirty pictures. *Journal of the Royal Statistical Society, Series B*, **48**, 259–302.

Besag J. (1989). Towards Bayesian image analysis. *Journal of Applied Statistics*, **16**, 395–407.

Besag J. and Mollié A. (1989). Bayesian mapping of mortality rates. *Bulletin of the International Statistical Institute*, **53**, 127–8.

Besag J., York J., and Mollié A. (1991). Bayesian image restoration, with two applications in spatial statistics. *Annals of the Institute of Statistical Mathematics*, **43**, 1–21.

Breslow N. and Clayton D. (1993). Approximate inference in generalized linear mixed models. *Journal of the American Statistical Association*, **88**, 9–25.

Clayton D. (1996). Generalized linear mixed models. In *Markov chain Monte Carlo in practice* (W. R. Gilks, S. Richardson, and D. J. Spiegelhalter ed.), 275–301. Chapman & Hall, London.

Clayton D. and Bernardinelli L. (1992). Bayesian methods for mapping disease risk. In *Small Area Studies in Geographical and Environmental Epidemiology* (P. Elliott, J. Cuzick, D. English, and R. Stern ed.), 205–20. Oxford University Press.

Clayton D. and Kaldor J. (1987). Empirical Bayes estimates of age-standardised relative risks for use in disease mapping. *Biometrics*, **43**, 671–81.

Clayton D., Bernardinelli L., and Montomoli C. (1993). Spatial correlation in ecological analysis. *International Journal of Epidemiology*, **22**, 1193–1202.

Dempster A. P., Laird N. M., and Rubin D. B. (1977). Maximum likelihood from incomplete data via the EM algorithm. *Journal of the Royal Statistical Society, Series B*, **39**, 1–38.

Gilks W. R., Richardson S., and Spiegelhalter D. J. (1996). Introducing Markov chain Monte Carlo. In *Markov chain Monte Carlo in practice* (W. R. Gilks, S. Richardson, and D. J. Spiegelhalter, ed.), 1–19. Chapman & Hall, London.

Manton K. G., Woodbury M. A., and Stallard E. (1981). A variance components approach to categorical data models with heterogeneous cell populations: analysis of spatial gradients in lung cancer mortality rates in North Carolina counties. *Biometrics*, **37**, 259–69.

Manton K. G., Stallard E., Woodbury M. A., Riggan W. B., Creason J. P., and Mason T. J. (1987). Statistically adjusted estimates of geographic mortality profiles. *Journal of the National Cancer Institute*, **78**, 805–15.

Manton K. G., Woodbury M. A., Stallard E., Riggan W. B., Creason J. P. and Pellom A. C. (1989). Empirical Bayes procedures for stabilizing maps of U. S. cancer mortality rates. *Journal of the American Statistical Association*, **84**, 637–50.

Mollié A. (1990). Représentation géographique des taux de mortalité: Modélisation spatiale et méthodes bayésiennes. Thèse de Doctorat, Université Paris VI.

Mollié A. (1996). Bayesian mapping of disease. In *Markov chain Monte Carlo in practice* (W. R. Gilks., S. Richardson, and D. J. Spiegelhalter ed.), 359–79. Chapman & Hall, London.

Mueller. N. E. (1996). Hodgkin's disease. In *Cancer epidemiology and prevention* (D. Schottenfeld and J. F. Fraumeni, Jr. ed.). Oxford University Press.

Rezvani A., Mollié A., Doyon F., and Sancho-Garnier H. (1997). *Atlas de la mortalité par cancer en France: 1986–1993.* INSERM, Paris.

Spiegelhalter D. J., Thomas A., and Best N. G. (1998). *WinBUGS user Manual, Version 1.1.1.* Medical Research Council Biostatistics Unit, Cambridge, UK. (Available from http://www.mrc-bsu.cam.ac.uk/bugs)

Tsutakawa R. K. (1988). Mixed model for analyzing geographic variability in mortality rates. *Journal of the American Statistical Association*, **83**, 37–42.

Tsutakawa R. K., Shoop G. L., and Marienfeld C. J. (1985). Empirical Bayes estimation of cancer mortality rates. *Statistics in Medicine*, **4**, 201–12.

16. Investigating the genetic association between diabetes and malaria: an application of Bayesian ecological regression models with errors in covariates

L. Bernardinelli, C. Pascutto, C. Montomoli, and W. Gilks

16.1 Introduction

There is scientific interest in studying the association between diabetes and malaria, because both diseases are associated with the human leukocyte antigen (HLA) system, which is responsible for most immune responses in humans. The underlying hypothesis is that endemic malaria may have genetically selected individuals less susceptible to insulin-dependent diabetes mellitus (IDDM), which is an autoimmune disease. This hypothesis may be investigated via an ecological correlation study. Such studies are concerned with geographical variation in disease occurrence and its association with ecological covariates (i.e. explanatory variables measured at an area level) (Walter 1991*a*,*b*; Morgenstern 1982; Chapter 11). In the present application, past malaria prevalence is treated as a proxy covariate for genetic selection operated by the disease in each area: the assumption is that the higher the prevalence of malaria, the stronger its selective pressure on the population.

The simplest approach to ecological analysis would be to fit a multiple regression model for disease occurrence allowing only for Poisson (or binomial) variation (Clayton and Hills 1993). However, in many situations, the residual variation not explained by the ecological variables might be substantially in excess of that expected from Poisson or binomial sampling theory, leading to overdispersion in the area-specific disease risks (prevalence). If the risk depends on unmeasured covariates which themselves have a spatial distribution, this may induce spatial correlation in the area level residuals. Furthermore, the use of area-specific malaria prevalence as a proxy for the true covariate of interest (i.e. genetic selection) introduces measurement error that may bias the estimated association with diabetes.

These issues can be properly accounted for by adopting a fully Bayesian modelling approach implemented using Markov chain Monte Carlo (MCMC) simulation methods (Besag *et al.* 1991; Bernardinelli and Montomoli 1992; Clayton and Bernardinelli 1992; Bernardinelli *et al.* 1995*a*,*b*). We have previously developed such a model for ecological regression with an imprecisely observed covariate and used it to investigate the hypothesised association between IDDM and malaria in Sardinia (Bernardinelli *et al.* 1997).

A significant negative association was found between IDDM incidence and past malaria prevalence in each commune. In this chapter, we describe a similar Bayesian hierarchical-spatial model and apply it to a new dataset on IDDM prevalence among 18-year-old males born in Sardinia between 1936 and 1973, using malaria prevalence in 1938–40 as the ecological covariate. We show how to deal with the potential bias associated with using such a proxy by extending our Bayesian model to allow for covariate measurement error. We also provide a method for choosing the hyperprior distributions for the spatial variation parameters of the model, and discuss the sensitivity of the results to different choices.

16.2   Scientific background

IDDM incidence in Sardinia is quite atypical of other Mediterranean countries (Muntoni and Songini 1992). Sardinia has the second highest incidence in Europe (33.2 per 100 000 person years; Songini *et al.* 1998) after Finland (40 per 100 000; Tuomileto *et al.* 1995). A study carried out on the cumulative prevalence of IDDM in 18 years-old military conscripts born in the period 1936–71 showed that the risk for IDDM began increasing with the male birth cohort of 1950 and that the increasing trend is much higher than the one observed in the rest of Europe (Songini *et al.* 1993).

The association between IDDM and the HLA system, which is known to be involved in controlling immunological responses, has long been established (Todd *et al.* 1988; Thomson 1988; Green 1990). In particular, many studies have demonstrated association between IDDM and the HLA loci A, B (class I), DR (class II) (Langholz *et al.* 1995; Thomas *et al.* 1995), and the tumour necrosis factor-α gene (TNF-α) localised in the HLA region (class III) (Davies *et al.* 1994; Tracey *et al.* 1989). In Sardinia, a particular HLA haplotype is associated with IDDM (Cucca *et al.* 1993).

Malaria has been recognised as an important parasitic disease of humans for centuries. The parasite responsible for malaria is Plasmodium, which is transmitted to the human host by the Anopheles mosquito. In infected individuals, Plasmodium can be found primarily inside of the red blood cells (RBC). The parasite reproduces asexually inside of the RBC, and following this the RBC breaks open releasing many new parasites. These parasites then infect more RBCs, and this ultimately leads to the destruction of massive numbers of RBCs. Despite the introduction of control programmes in many parts of the world over the past few decades, the impact of malaria on human populations continues to increase. For this reason, malaria is the most important natural selective factor on human populations that has been discovered to date (Jacob 1992).

A West African study showed that an allele of HLA class I and an unusual haplotype of HLA class II are associated with protection from malaria (Hill *et al.* 1991; Ebert and Lorenzi 1994). The association between susceptibility to cerebral malaria and the TNF2 allele, a variant located in the promoter region of the TNF-α associated with higher levels of TNF transcription, has also recently been established (McGuire *et al.* 1994). These elements support the hypothesis that in areas of high endemicity, malaria operates the genetic selection responsible for influencing susceptibility to autoimmune diseases (Greenwood 1968; Wilson and Duff 1995).

The Sardinian population has a long history of malaria. The disease spread gradually over the island after the Carthaginian conquest, became established after Roman occupation, and was a major cause of death in the island until the mid twentieth century, when it was completely eradicated (Fantini 1991). Population genetic studies carried out by Piazza *et al.* (1985) suggest that, in the plains of Sardinia where malaria had been endemic, some genetic traits were selected to provide greater resistance to the haemolysing action of Plasmodium. In the hilly and mountainous areas, where malaria was almost absent, this adaptation did not occur. The genetic traits that protect against malaria are also known to be responsible for some serious hereditary diseases in Sardinia such as β-thalassemia, Cooley's disease and favism, the latter caused by glucose-6-phospate dehydrogenase (G6PD) enzyme deficiency (Siniscalco *et al.* 1961; Meloni *et al.* 1992; Bernardinelli *et al.* 1994).

   Given this background, we have carried out a series of studies to investigate the aetiological hypothesis that the occurrence of IDDM in Sardinia may be linked to genetic selection factors operated by endemic malaria on the island. Using malaria prevalence in the years 1938–40 as a proxy to indicate areas of high endemicity (i.e. where the greatest genetic adaption is likely to have occurred), we found evidence of a significant negative correlation with incidence of IDDM in Sardinians aged under 29 years observed in the period 1989 and 1992 (Bernardinelli *et al.* 1997). This finding remained even after adjusting for potential confounding variables such as altitude (Bernardinelli *et al.* 1999*a*) and proportion of males affected by G6PD deficiency (Bernardinelli *et al.* 1999*b*). In this chapter, we consider a new and larger dataset on cumulative prevalence of IDDM in Sardinian military conscripts in order to establish further evidence of a genetic link between diabetes and malaria.

16.3   Data

The cumulative prevalence of IDDM was observed at the military medical examination of 18-year-old male conscripts born in Sardinia between 1936 and 1973 and resident in Sardinia at the time of the visit (Songini *et al.* 1993). We let Y_i denote the number of IDDM cases observed in commune i ($i = 1, 2, \ldots, n = 366$), and N_i, denote the number of conscripts examined in commune i.

   The number of individuals affected by malaria during the period 1938–40, Z_i, was reported for each Sardinian commune by Fermi (1938, 1940). This is the most accurate and complete data source on malaria available, and is based on Fermi's pioneering work to gather information on malaria morbidity in every Sardinian village and to estimate the prevalence of malaria in each commune of the island. The population M_i for each commune was taken from the 1936 census.

16.4   Statistical model

The Bayesian ecological regression model used here is similar to that applied in our previous analyses (Bernardinelli *et al.* 1997, 1999*a,b*). However, these studies were concerned with population-based counts of IDDM incidence in each commune, which were assumed to follow a Poisson distribution. The present data set concern cumulative prevalence of IDDM amongst a cohort of military conscripts, and hence a binomial sampling distribution is more appropriate.

16.4.1 A model for IDDM prevalence

Suppose we observe Y_i events (IDDM cases in our application) in a sample of N_i individuals in area i. We assume

$$Y_i \sim \text{Bin}(N_i, p_i), \tag{16.1}$$

where p_i is the true area-specific prevalence of IDDM. To investigate whether prevalence is geographically related and shows patterns similar to the pattern of malaria endemicity in Sardinia, we would ideally like to map the true prevalence p_i. Since it is unknown, the most obvious strategy is to calculate its maximum likelihood estimate, $\hat{p}_i = Y_i/N_i$. Mapping the set $\{\hat{p}_i\}$, however, can be misleading because sampling variability can dominate the map and disguise genuine trends (e.g. see Chapter 15). Furthermore if the disease risk is not constant *within* communes or depends on some unknown or unmeasured covariate, the observed data may display *extra-binomial variation* (overdispersion). That is, the data are more variable than the binomial model supposes (see Appendix I in Chapter 7 for further discussion of this issue).

Several strategies for dealing with sampling variability in maps have been proposed. The current state of the art is to adopt a fully Bayesian hierarchical-spatial model (see Chapter 7). An important feature of this type of model is that the prior distribution for the $\{p_i\}$ may incorporate spatial correlation, allowing the estimate of p_i to formally 'borrow strength' from neighbouring areas. In this way, the empirical map is smoothed, and geographical trends and inferences are made more reliable.

Mapping Bayesian estimates of disease occurrence may reveal geographical trends across the map, or may suggest links with area-specific covariates X_i. To incorporate these covariates into the model, a natural assumption, in conjunction with the binomial assumption (16.1), would be

$$\text{logit}(p_i) = \log \theta_i + X_i^T \beta, \tag{16.2}$$

where $\log \theta_i$ represents the covariate-adjusted log odds ratio (i.e. logistic-transformed prevalence) in commune i and β is the (possibly vector valued) unknown regression coefficient(s) associated with the ecological covariate(s) X. Minimally informative Bayesian prior distributions, such as independent normal distributions with zero mean with very large variance, are typically specified for each regression coefficient. Such a model is called an *ecological regression model* (see Chapter 11).

Spatial smoothing of the $\{p_i\}$ can be effected via a Markov random field prior on the $\{\log \theta_i\}$. This prior will tend to produce similar estimates for $\log \theta_i$ and $\log \theta_j$ if areas i and j are geographically close.

16.4.2 A Markov random field prior

In this section we describe a *Markov random field* (MRF) prior distribution for the $\{\log \theta_i\}$ parameters in (16.2). Following the development and notation in Section 7.2 of Chapter 7 we let

$$\log \theta_i = \alpha + U_i \tag{16.3}$$

and assume a minimally informative prior for the intercept α and a MRF prior for the vector $U = (U_1, \ldots, U_n)^T$ with the constraint $\sum_i U_i = 0$ to ensure identifiability.

The Gaussian MRF prior we employ is the intrinsic conditional autoregressive (CAR) model given in Equation (7.8) of Chapter 7, namely

$$U_i | U_j = u_j, j \neq i \sim N\left(\bar{u}, \frac{\omega_u^2}{m_i}\right). \tag{16.4}$$

This assumes that each U_i is normally distributed with mean $\bar{u}$ given by the average value of u_j among its set of neighbours, and variance proportional to the number of neighbours m_i. The amount of overall smoothing of the random effects $\{U_i\}$ is controlled by the variance parameter ω_u^2 in (16.4). A large value of ω_u^2 will induce little smoothing, whilst a zero-value would force all the $\{U_i\}$ to be equal. Since we do not wish to impose any fixed amount of smoothing on the random effects, but rather wish to let the data themselves determine how much smoothing should be induced, we treat ω_u^2 as a model parameter and assign it a prior distribution. Here we assume a χ^2 prior distribution for the *inverse* variance (i.e. the precision parameter)

$$\omega_u^{-2} = \tau_u \sim \frac{1}{\phi} \chi_\nu^2, \tag{16.5}$$

where ϕ and ν are fixed a priori and represent the scale factor and degrees of freedom of the χ^2 distribution, respectively. The mean and variance of the prior for τ_u are given by

$$\text{mean} = \frac{\nu}{\phi}; \quad \text{var} = \frac{2\nu}{\phi^2}.$$

16.4.3   Choosing the parameters of the prior distribution for τ_u

The choice of a suitable combination of scale factor ϕ and degrees of freedom ν for the prior for τ_u is an important issue, especially if there is little information in the data. Sometimes it can be difficult to make a reasonable guess for the precision parameter, which is not an intuitive quantity. It is generally easier to think in terms of geographical variability rather than precision of the area-specific estimates. For example, we may be willing to make a prior guess at the range of prevalences expected across the map, or the rate ratio between a commune with a high prevalence (say the 95th percentile) and one with a low prevalence (say the 5th percentile).

Unfortunately, such guesses intuitively reflect our prior belief about the *marginal* variability of the $\{U_i\}$ across the map, whereas the parameter for which we must specify a prior (τ_u) is the inverse of the *conditional* variance parameter. As noted in Chapters 7 and 15, the marginal variance of the vector $U = (U_1, \ldots, U_n)$ does not exist since the intrinsic CAR prior does not define a proper joint density for U. However, Bernardinelli *et al.* (1995a) carried out a simulation study to show that there is an approximate connection between the conditional precision parameter τ_u and the *empirical* marginal variability of the $\{U_i\}$ which depends on the pattern of adjacencies between areas. For Sardinia, the empirical standard deviation of the area-specific effects across communes turned out to be about $0.7/\sqrt{\tau_u}$. A description of how to estimate this relationship for a map with a different neighbourhood structure is provided in the Appendix. On the basis of this relationship, we may express the ratio of the 95th percentile to the 5th percentile of the area-specific prevalence rates as $e^{3.29 \times 0.7/\sqrt{\tau_u}}$ (see Appendix for details). We are thus able to translate our prior guess at an intuitive quantity (the 90% prevalence rate ratio) into a prior point estimate for the model parameter τ_u.

In order to move from a point guess to the specification of a complete prior distribution for τ_u, we must choose suitable values for ν and ϕ in (16.5) which reflect this point estimate and our uncertainty about it. As a 'rule of thumb', ν is a measure of the strength of belief in one's prior guess about the rate ratio: larger values of ν represent greater certainty in the guess. Having fixed a value for ν, ϕ can be chosen so that the mean of the distribution is close to the prior guess for τ_u. However, we recommend plotting a range of prior distributions obtained for different combinations of ϕ and ν on the scale of the rate ratio, and then selecting the distribution whose shape best fits one's prior belief about the amount of geographical variation in the map (see Fig. 16.3).

In this analysis, we chose $\nu = 20$ and $\phi = 2$, corresponding to a quite strong prior belief that 90% prevalence rate ratio for IDDM in Sardinia is approximately 2 and thus that the geographical variability is not very high.

16.4.4   Covariate measurement error

When dealing with ecological covariates, the available data Z_i may be either imperfect measurements of, or proxies for, the true covariate of interest X_i. The simplest approach to this problem would be to estimate X_i from Z_i for each area independently, and use this estimate $\hat{X}_i$ in place of the true unknown X_i in the ecological regression (16.2). When Z_i is an accurate measure of X_i, this approach may be reasonable. However, when there is a weaker correspondence between X_i and Z_i, this approach has several disadvantages. First of all, the estimate of the regression coefficient β would probably be underestimated (e.g. see Richardson and Gilks 1993; Chapter 5). Second, the precision of the parameter estimates would be overestimated, through failure to take account of uncertainty in the $\{\hat{X}_i\}$. Third, if it were reasonable a priori to expect spatial correlation in the true covariate, improved estimates of the $\{X_i\}$ and other unknowns could be obtained through a Bayesian procedure incorporating a spatial smoothing prior on the unknown $\{X_i\}$.

In our application, the true ecological covariate X_i (representing genetic selection factors) is related to underlying malaria prevalence, and Z_i is the observed number of malaria cases in commune i at one period in time. We will assume that

$$Z_i \sim \mathrm{Bin}(M_i, \psi_i) \tag{16.6}$$

where M_i is the population size of commune i taken from the 1936 Census. Initially, we take the covariate X_i in (16.2) to be the logistic-transformed expectation of Z_i, i.e.

$$\log\left(\frac{\psi_i}{1 - \psi_i}\right) = X_i. \tag{16.7}$$

Since the areal units (communes) in our analysis are small, and the covariate of interest is a measure of occurrence of a disease, it is reasonable a priori to expect the covariate to vary smoothly across areas. Hence, we should account for spatial correlation in the ecological covariate. To achieve this, we assumed the same MRF prior structure as described in Section 16.4.2 for the $\{X_i\}$

$$X_i|X_j = x_j, j \neq i \sim N\left(\bar{x}, \frac{\omega_x^2}{m_i}\right) \tag{16.8}$$

where $\bar{x}$ is the mean of the values $X_j = x_j$ in communes neighbouring area i, m_i is the number of neighbours as before, and $\omega_x^2 > 0$ controls the overall variability of the true covariate values across the map.

We chose $\nu = 20$ and $\phi = 3$ as the degrees of freedom and scale factor of the χ^2 prior distribution for the inverse variance $\omega_x^{-2} = \tau_x$. This choice allows for slightly higher geographical variability than for IDDM prevalence.

This part of the model accounts for sampling error in the covariate X_i, but there is a further source of measurement error we wish to account for in this application. The hypothesis of interest concerns how genetic adaptation in areas of endemic malaria affects susceptibility to IDDM. Thus the true covariate is the long-term malaria endemicity averaged over many centuries in each commune. In order to model the long-term malaria endemicity, we may replace the deterministic relationship in (16.7) by the following stochastic relationship

$$\log\left(\frac{\psi_i}{1 - \psi_i}\right) \sim N(X_i, \zeta) \tag{16.9}$$

We have thus introduced an extra layer of uncertainty into the model. This may be interpreted as follows: the true log odds of malaria prevalence in commune i (i.e. log $\psi_i/(1 - \psi_i)$) represents a single realisation from a latent Normal distribution with mean X_i (i.e. the long-term average endemicity of malaria in commune i) and unknown long-term variance, ζ. Since the data contain no information by which to estimate ζ, we must specify its value a priori. Exploratory analyses (see Bernardinelli *et al.* 1997) suggested that a suitable value might be $\zeta = 2.27$, which represents moderate variation in the odds of malaria in each commune over time.

Subjectively fixing a value for ζ is a potentially controversial aspect of our analysis. We therefore carried out a sensitivity analysis to investigate the influence of different values of ζ on β, the regression coefficient for the covariate.

16.5   Estimation

We estimated the models using Markov chain Monte Carlo (MCMC) methods as implemented in the WinBUGS software (Spiegelhalter *et al.* 1998). In each case, we ran the sampler for 10 000 iterations and discarded the first 5000 'burn-in' samples. Convergence of the model parameters was checked by examining the sample traces and using a variety of diagnostics implemented in the CODA software (Best *et al.* 1995). Computation took about 10 minutes for each model on a personal computer Pentium 200 Pro running Windows NT 4.0.

16.6 Results

Figures 16.1a and b show maps of the maximum likelihood estimates of IDDM prevalence (Y_i/N_i) and malaria prevalence (Z_i/M_i) by commune respectively. Unfortunately, any similarities between the pattern on risk for each disease tend to be obscured by the high geographical variability and imprecision of these raw estimates.

Table 16.1 presents posterior summaries of the regression coefficient β obtained by fitting the Bayesian smoothing model (16.1)–(16.5) with (i) the logistic transformed observed malaria prevalence ($Z_i/M_i)/(1 - Z_i/M_i$) as a *fixed* ecological covariate, and (ii) accounting for all sources of covariate measurement error using model (16.6)–(16.9).

As expected from our previous analyses on the association between malaria and IDDM, the point estimate of the regression coefficient indicates a negative association between the two diseases in both models. Even though the 95% credible intervals include zero, and hence the association is not highly significant, the posterior distribution of β is shifted towards negative values. However, accounting for covariate measurement errors in the second model resulted in a more negative regression coefficient, with a higher standard deviation than in the model with a fixed covariate.

Figure 16.1b shows the map of posterior mean IDDM prevalence obtained by fitting model (16.1)–(16.5) with the observed malaria covariate. The map shows a considerable

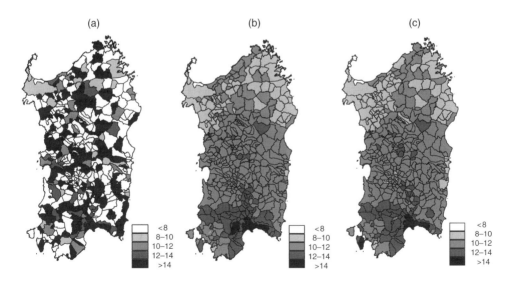

Fig. 16.1 IDDM: (a) observed prevalence, Y_i/N_i; (b) smoothed prevalence, p_i, obtained by fitting the ecological regression model (16.1)–(16.5) with the logistic transformed malaria prevalence as a fixed covariate; (c) smoothed prevalence, p_i, obtained by fitting the ecological regression model (16.1)–(16.9) accounting for all sources of covariate measurement error.

Table 16.1 Posterior mean, posterior standard deviation (s.d.), and 95% credible interval (95% CI) of the regression coefficient β in the model with the observed covariate (M1) and the model allowing for covariate measurement error (M2)

Model	Posterior mean	s.d.	95% CI
M1	−0.004	0.009	−0.021, 0.013
M2	−0.027	0.024	−0.075, 0.020

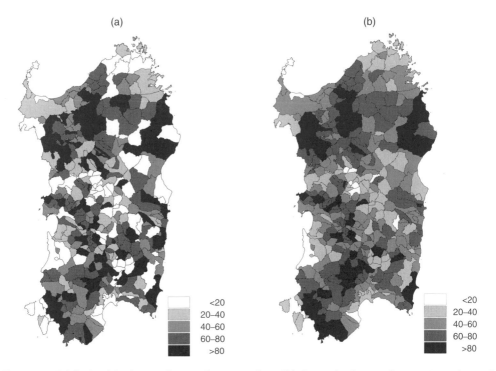

Fig. 16.2 Malaria: (a) observed prevalence, Z_i/M_i; (b) Smoothed prevalence, ψ, estimated using the final model (16.6)–(16.9).

amount of smoothing compared to observed prevalence (Fig. 16.1a), and a north-to-south gradient in risk is evident.

Figures 16.1c and b show, respectively, the posterior mean estimates of IDDM prevalence and of malaria prevalence obtained by fitting the final model (16.6)–(16.9). Careful comparison of these two maps suggests a negative association between IDDM and malaria: dark-coloured areas in Fig. 16.1c tend to be light-coloured in Fig. 16.2b, and vice versa.

In order to investigate the sensitivity of the results to the choice of ζ, we refitted the final model (16.1)–(16.9) using two extreme values for ζ: $\zeta = 0.1$ (which corresponds to minimal long-term variability in malaria endemicity within each commune) and $\zeta = 10$ (which corresponds to very high long-term variability). Posterior summaries of the

Table 16.2 Posterior mean, posterior standard deviation (s.d.), and 95% credible interval (95% CI) for the regression coefficient in the final model (16.1)–(16.9) for different choices of long-term variance ζ

ζ	Posterior Mean	s.d.	95% CI
0.1	−0.019	0.016	−0.051, 0.013
2.27	−0.027	0.024	−0.075, 0.020
10	−0.87	0.326	−1.542, 0.350

Table 16.3 Prior mean, 95% prior interval, posterior mean, and 95% credible interval (95% CI) for the 90% prevalence rate ratio (90% PRR) for IDDM, and posterior mean and 95% CI for the regression coefficient β in the final model (16.1)–(16.9) for different combinations of degrees of freedom (ν) and scale factor (ϕ) in hyperprior (16.5) for the spatial precision parameter τ_u

			Prior 90% PRR		Posterior 90% PRR		Regression coefficient, β	
Prior	ν	ϕ	Mean	(95% interval)	Mean	(95% CI)	Mean	(95% CI)
1	5	0.5	1.26	(1.11, 2.73)	2.18	(1.58, 3.21)	−0.025	(−0.077, 0.030)
2	5	2	2.50	(1.52, 55.76)	2.27	(1.59, 3.56)	−0.020	(−0.080, 0.030)
3	20	0.5	1.06	(1.04, 1.11)	2.22	(1.59, 3.45)	−0.030	(−0.079, 0.017)
4	20	2	1.24	(1.16, 1.53)	2.15	(1.57, 3.12)	−0.027	(−0.075, 0.024)

regression coefficient β are reported in Table 16.2 for each value of ζ considered. The results for $\zeta = 10$ seem unrealistic, and in fact lead to a map of true malaria prevalence which is unrealistically oversmoothed. On the contrary, our original choice of $\zeta = 2.27$ is rather conservative, because it leads to results which do not differ qualitatively from those obtained with lower values of $\zeta = 0.01$ and from those obtained without accounting for measurement errors in the covariate (see Table 16.1).

Finally, we analysed the sensitivity of the results to the choice of ν and ϕ for the prior distribution of the precision parameter τ_u. We considered four different combinations of ν and ϕ, as given in Table 16.3. The corresponding prior densities, plotted as a function of the ratio between the 95th and the 5th centile of the area-specific prevalence rates (i.e. the 90% prevalence rate ratio; see Section 16.4.3), are reported in Fig. 16.3. Priors 1 and 2 are weak priors: they are rather flat and hence do not particularly favour any values for the rate ratio. Priors 3 and 4 are stronger priors favouring a low geographical variability, because most of their mass is centred on low values for the rate ratio.

Table 16.3 shows the sensitivity of the posterior estimates of the 90% prevalence rate ratio and the regression coefficient β to each of the four hyperpriors: the results do not show appreciable differences. Similarly, the regression coefficient did not show sensitivity to different choices for the prior distribution for τ_x, the inverse of the spatial variance ω_x^2 in the covariate measurement error model (16.8).

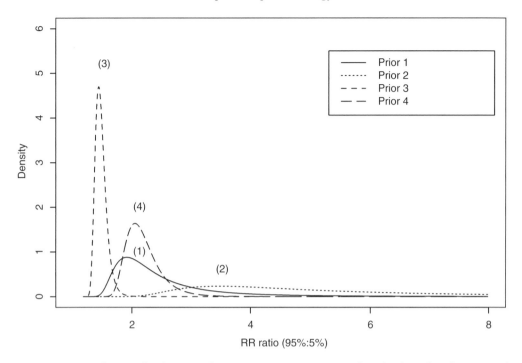

Fig. 16.3 Prior density for the spatial precision parameter τ_u in (16.5), plotted as function of the 90% prevalence rate ratio for IDDM in Sardinia, for four combinations of degrees of freedom ν and scale factor ϕ.

16.7 Discussion

16.7.1 Substantive conclusions

Sardinians are known to be susceptible to autoimmune diseases. A significant negative association between long-term malaria endemicity and diabetes relative risk emerged in previous analyses (Bernardinelli *et al.* 1997), even after accounting for potential confounders, such as altitude (Bernardinelli *et al.* 1999*a*) and the proportion of males in each commune affected by G6PD deficiency (Bernardinelli *et al.* 1999*b*). The results obtained in the present analysis, in which we used a different dataset on IDDM, are consistent with the previous findings, even though the negative association between malaria and IDDM is less strong. Note that the present analysis was based on a binomial model, and so the regression coefficient β refers to the *odds ratio* of IDDM as long-term malaria endemicity in the commune increases; our previous analyses considered Poisson regression models, and hence yielded estimates of the *relative risk* of IDDM associated with long-term malaria endemicity.

A possible interpretation of this finding is that, since malaria has been endemic in the plains of Sardinia for centuries, places with high prevalence of malaria in 1938 are those in which a stronger selection process took place, providing resistance to malaria and also preventing the onset of autoimmune conditions (Jacob 1992).

16.7.2 Methodological issues

In this chapter we have shown how it is possible to carry out an ecological regression analysis accounting for imprecisely measured covariates using a Bayesian hierarchical-spatial model allowing for errors-in-variables. Such a model can be implemented via MCMC techniques. This approach to ecological correlation studies involving covariate measurement error can be applied in many situations. As in the present study, the rate of another disease may be used as a surrogate for true exposure: for example, lung cancer rates could be used as a proxy for smoking. Many environmental covariates, such as air pollution, are also typically measured using imprecise instruments.

The use of spatial smoothing priors for both disease occurrence and the ecological covariate is of particular value when, as in our application, the covariates are themselves incidence or prevalence data for other diseases. In this case it is reasonable to expect spatial correlation in both the covariate and the disease rate. Malaria prevalence tends to be higher in low-lying and humid regions and lower in the mountains and hills. The spatial prior for the covariate allowed us to obtain a map of the geographical variation of malaria prevalence in which the random variation has been filtered out.

Specifying a spatial smoothing prior for the random effects U_i in Equation (16.2) is a way of controlling for residual confounding due to unmeasured spatially correlated risk factors. If the pattern of variation in these unknown covariates is similar to that of disease risk, location may act as a confounder representing a surrogate for these other factors (Clayton *et al.* 1994). In our application, the introduction of a spatial prior for the U_i allowed the model to adjust for other genetic or environmental factors which may be spatially correlated and which affect risk of IDDM but which are not captured by the malaria covariate.

We wish to stress that the results we obtained rely on the assumptions of our model. New data and/or different model assumptions could lead to different results. With models as complex as those considered here it is important to investigate the sensitivity of any conclusions to changes in model specification.

First, the choice of a fixed value for the long-term variance ζ is a fundamental step in the construction of the model. It greatly affects the amount of smoothing in the true covariate value and also influences the estimate of the regression coefficient β. Although smaller values of ζ than the one we originally specified did not change the results qualitatively, larger values of ζ lead to coefficient estimates that were larger in absolute value, with much wider credible intervals. Since no other data were available on malaria prevalence in Sardinia, we had to rely on our judgement about the amount of variation over time in malaria prevalence in order to chose a realistic value for ζ. However, our research on this issue is continuing: there is a possibility of obtaining new data on prevalence of malaria in Sardinia in different time periods which would enable us to obtain better informed estimates for the long-term variability ζ.

Second, the choice of the hyperpriors for the precision parameters in the MRF priors must be done subjectively. We illustrated our method for choosing a combination of degrees of freedom and scale factor parameters for this hyperprior on the basis of one's prior belief on the amount of geographical variability across the map. We also showed that the regression coefficient estimates are not heavily influenced by the chosen combination.

Appendix

Relationship between the conditional variance parameter and the
empirical marginal variance of the spatially structured random effects

As discussed in Section 16.4.3, using epidemiological knowledge to specify an informative prior for the precision hyperparameter, τ_u, of the MRF model is an important issue, but thinking in terms of the *precision* of the area-specific effects U_i is not straightforward. Instead, it is more appealing to construct a prior for τ_u starting from a prior guess about the geographical variability of the area-specific disease rates. Intuitively, this guess refers to the overall (marginal) variability of the $\{U_i\}$ across the map, whilst τ_u is proportional to the inverse of the *conditional* variance of each U_i given values for the U_j in all other areas $j \neq i$. The theoretical relationship between the marginal and conditional variances of the $\{U_i\}$ depends on the spatial neighbourhood structure (and hence varies for each different map). Furthermore, it cannot be calculated directly because the marginal covariance matrix is singular for the intrinsic CAR model used in this application (see Chapters 7 and 15). However, we may approximate this relationship for a given map using the *empirical* distribution of the spatial random effects, as described below.

Let $U_{.05}$ and $U_{.95}$ denote the 5th and 95th percentiles, respectively, of the empirical distribution of the spatial random effects across the map. In the absence of covariates, Equations (16.2) and (16.3) imply that $U_{.95} - U_{.05} = \log \theta_{.95} - \log \theta_{.05} \approx \log(p_{.95}/p_{.05})$ where $p_{.95}$ and $p_{.05}$ are the 95th and 5th percentiles of the distribution of area-specific IDDM prevalence rates across the map. If we assume that the empirical distribution of the random effects is approximately normal, then we would expect

$$\log \frac{p_{.95}}{p_{.05}} \approx 2 \times 1.645 \times s_u \tag{16.10}$$

where s_u is the square root of the empirical marginal variance of the random effects $\{U_i\}$ across the map (i.e. the quantity about which we are willing to express prior beliefs). Note that it would be more correct to consider the distribution of area-specific odds ratios rather than prevalences since a logistic transformation of prevalence appears in the ecological regression model (16.2). However, when prevalence is not very high the two quantities are approximately equal. In addition, if covariates are included in the model, then (16.10) refers approximately to the log ratio of the 95th and 5th percentiles of the *residual* area-specific prevalences across the map.

The relationship between s_u and the conditional precision parameter τ_u may be estimated by carrying out a series of simulations in which realisations of the vector of random effects U are generated from the intrinsic CAR model (16.4) (with sum-to-zero constraint imposed for identifiability) using different *pre-specified* values of the hyperparameter τ_u. For the present application, six different values between 2 and 30 were chosen, and a single realisation of U was generated in each case. The square root of the empirical variance of the elements of $U = (U_1, \ldots, U_n)$ for each simulation, i.e. $\sqrt{\sum_{i=1}^{n}(U_i - \bar{U})^2/(n-1)}$, provides an estimate of s_u under that CAR model. We then calculated the ratio

$$r = \frac{s_u}{\omega_u}.$$

This provides an estimate of the scaling factor between the empirical and conditional standard deviations for the CAR model and was found to be identical to two decimal places for all six simulations in the present application. We may then translate our prior guess at the 90% range of geographical variation in the disease rate, which gives us s_u via (16.10), into a point prior for the precision parameter of the CAR model using the relationship

$$\tau_u = \frac{r^2}{s_u^2},$$

hence giving a prior estimate of τ_u. Note that the value of τ depends on the choice of neighbourhood structure and weights for the model, and so must be re-estimated for different maps.

Acknowledgements

This work was partially supported by an EU Biomed II Concerted Action grant number PL96 3488.

References

Bernardinelli, L. and Montomoli, C. (1992). Empirical Bayes versus Fully Bayesian analysis of geographical variation in disease risk. *Statistics in Medicine*, **11**, 983–1007.

Bernardinelli, L., Clayton, D., and Montomoli, C. (1995a). Bayesian estimates of disease maps: how important are priors? *Statistics in Medicine*, **14**, 2411–31.

Bernardinelli, L., Clayton, D., Pascutto, C., Montomoli, C., Ghislandi, M., and Songini, M. (1995b). Bayesian analysis of space-time variation in disease risk. *Statistics in Medicine*, **14**, 2433–43.

Bernardinelli, L., Pascutto, C., Best, N. G., and Gilks, W. R. (1997). Disease mapping with errors in covariates. *Statistics in Medicine*, **16**, 741–52.

Bernardinelli, L., Pascutto, C., Montomoli, C., Komakec, J., Gilks, W. R., Songini, M. *et al.* (1999a). Bayesian analysis of ecological data for studying the association between insulin-dependent diabetes mellitus and malaria. In *Statistics for the environment*. Vol. 4. *Statistical aspects of health and environment* (V. Barnett, A. Stein, and K. F. Turkman ed.), Wiley, Chichester.

Bernardinelli, L., Pascutto, C., Montomoli, C., Komakec, J., and Gilks, W. R. (1999b). Ecological regression with errors in covariates: an application. In *Advanced methods of disease mapping and risk assessment for public health decision making* (A. B. Lawson, D. Boehning, E. Lessafre, A. Biggeri, J-F. Viel, R. Bertollini ed.), Wiley, Chichester.

Besag J., York J., and Mollié, A. (1991). Bayesian image restoration, with applications in spatial statistics (with discussion). *Annals of the Institute of Statistical Mathematics*, **43**, 1–59.

Best, N. G., Cowles, M. K., and Vines, S. K. (1995). *CODA: convergence diagnostics and output analysis for Gibbs sampling output, Version 0.30*. Medical Research Council Biostatistics Unit, Cambridge.

Clayton, D. G. and Bernardinelli, L. (1992). Bayesian methods for mapping disease risk. In *Small Area Studies in Geographical and Environmental Epidemiology* (P. Elliott, J. Cuzick, D. English, and R. Stern ed.), 205–20. Oxford University Press.

Clayton, D. and Hills, M. (1993). *Statistical models in epidemiology*. Oxford University Press.

Clayton, D. G., Bernardinelli, L., and Montomoli, C. (1994). Spatial correlation in ecological analysis. *International Journal of Epidemiology*, **22**, 1193–202.

Cucca, F., Muntoni, F., Lampis, R., Frau, F., Argiolas, L., Silvetti, M. *et al.* (1993) Combinations of specific DRB1, DQA1, DQB1 haplotypes are associated with insulin-dependent diabetes mellitus in Sardinia. *Human Immunology*, **37**, 859–94.

Davies, J. L., Kawaguchi, Y., Bennet, S. T., Copeman, J. B., Cordell, H. J., Pritchard, L. E. *et al.* (1994). A genome-wide search for human type 1 diabetes susceptibility genes. *Nature*, **371**, 130–6.

Ebert, D. and Lorenzi, R. (1994). Parasites and polymorphisms. *Nature*, **369**, 705–6.

Fantini, B. (1991). La lotta antimalarica in Italia fra controllo ed eradicazione: l'esperimento Sardegna. *Parassitologia*, **33**, 11–23.

Fermi, C. (1938). Provincia di Nuoro. Malaria, danni economici. Risanamento e proposte per il suo risorgimento. *Gallizzi*, **2**, 1–311.

Fermi, C. (1940). Provincia di Cagliari. Malaria, danni economici. Risanamento e proposte per il suo risorgimento. *Gallizzi*, **3**, 1–610.

Green, A. (1990). The role of genetic factors in the development of insulin-dependent diabetes mellitus. *Current Topics in Microbiology and Immunology*, **164**, 3–16.

Greenwood B. M. (1968). Autoimmune disease and parasitic infections in Nigerians. *Lancet*, **30**, 380–2.

Hill, A. V. S., Allsopp, C. E. M., Kwiatkowski, D., Anstey, N. M., Twumasi, P., Rowe, P. A. *et al.* (1991). Common West African HLA antigens are associated with protection from severe malaria. *Nature*, **352**, 595–600.

Jacob, C. O. (1992). Tumor necrosis factor α in autoimmunity: pretty girl or old witch? *Immunology Today*, **13**, 122–5.

Langholz, B., Tuomilehto-Wolf, E., Thomas, D., Pitkaniemi, J., Tuomilehto, J., and the DiMe Study Group (1995). Variation in HLA-associated risks of childhood insulin-dependent diabetes mellitus in the Finnish population. I: Allele effects at A, B, and DR loci. *Genetic Epidemiology*, **12**, 441–53.

McGuire, W., Hill, A. V., Allsopp, C. E., Greenwood, B. M., and Kwiatkowski, D. (1994). Variation in the TNF-alpha promoter region associated with susceptibility to cerebral malaria. *Nature*, **371**, 508–10.

Meloni, T., Pacifico, A., Forteleone, G., and Meloni, G. F. (1992). Association of G6PD Deficiency and diabetes mellitus in northern Sardinian subjects. *Haematology*, **77**, 94–100.

Morgenstern, H. (1982). Uses of ecologic analysis in epidemiologic research. *American Journal of Public Health*, **72**, 1336–44.

Muntoni, S. and Songini, M. (1992). High incidence rate of IDDM in Sardinia. *Diabetes Care*, **15**, 1317–22.

Piazza, A., Mayr, W. R., Contu, L., Amoroso, A., Borelli, I., Curtoni, E. S. *et al.* (1985). Genetic and population structure of four Sardinian villages. *Annals of Human Genetics*, **4**, 47–63.

Richardson, S. and Gilks, W. R. (1993). Conditional independence models for epidemiological studies with covariate measurement error. *Statistics in Medicine*, **12**, 1703–22.

Siniscalco, M., Bernini, L., Latte, B., and Motulsky, A. G. (1961). Favism and thalassaemia in Sardinia and their relationship to malaria. *Nature*, **190**, 1179–80.

Songini, M., Loche, M., and Muntoni, S. (1993). Increasing prevalence of juvenile onset Type 1 (insulin dependent) diabetes mellitus in Sardinia: the military service approach. *Diabetologia*, **36**, 457–552.

Songini, M., Bernardinelli, L., Clayton, D., Montomoli, C., Pascutto, C. *et al.* and the Sardinian IDDM Study Group (1998). The Sardinian IDDM Study 1. Epidemiology and geographical distribution of IDDM in Sardinia during 1989 to 1994. *Diabetologia*, **41**, 221–7.

Spiegelhalter, D. J., Thomas, A., and Best, N. G. (1998). *WinBUGS user manual, Version 1.1.1.* Medical Research Council Biostatistics Unit, Cambridge. (Available from http://www.mrc-bsu. cam.ac.uk/bugs)

Thomas, D., Pitkaniemi, J., Langholz, B., Tuomilehto-Wolf, E., Tuomilehto, J., and the DiMe Study Group (1995). Variation in HLA-associated risks of childhood insulin-dependent diabetes mellitus in the Finnish population. II: Haplotype effects. *Genetic Epidemiology*, **12**, 441–53.

Thomson, G. (1988). HLA disease associations: Models for insulin dependent diabetes mellitus and the study of complex human genetic disorders. *Annual Reviews of Genetics*, **22**, 31–50.

Todd, J. A., Bell, J. I., and McDevitt, H. O. (1988). A molecular basis for genetic susceptibility in insulin dependent diabetes mellitus. *Trends in Genetics*, **4**, 129–34.

Tracey, K. J., Vlassara H., and Cerami A. (1989). Cachetin/tumour necrosis factor. *Lancet*, **i**, 1122–6.

Tuomilehto, J., Virtala, E., Karvonen, M., Lounama, R., Pitkaniemi, J., Reunanen, A. *et al.* (1995). Increase in incidence in insulin-dependent diabetes mellitus among children in Finland. *International Journal of Epidemiology*, **24**, 984–92.

Walter, S. D. (1991*a*). The ecologic method in the study of environmental health. I: Overview of the method. *Environmental Health Perspective*, **94**, 61–5.

Walter, S. D. (1991*b*). The ecologic method in the study of environmental health. II: Methodologic issues and feasibility. *Environmental Health Perspective*, **94**, 67–73.

Wilson, A. G. and Duff, G. W. (1995). Genetic traits in common diseases support the adage that autoimmunity is the price paid for eradicating infectious diseases. *British Medical Journal*, **310**, 1482–3.

17. Do cancers cluster?

F. E. Alexander and P. Boyle

17.1 Clusters and clustering: definitions and interpretation

This chapter addresses the issue of cancer clustering with particular reference to childhood leukaemia. Clustering is a poorly defined concept in the medical literature. An important distinction must be made between the notion of an individual cluster—corresponding to an excess number of cases in one small area, around one infrequent point source or subject to one source of environmental pollution—and the concept of a general tendency to cluster. Here, a more heterogeneous or 'clumped' distribution of cases than can be attributed to variations in population density and the play of chance is then implied.

Following Alexander and Cuzick (1992), the appropriate null hypothesis (H_0) of 'no clustering' may be formulated in terms of a partition of the study area A into a large number of small areas $\{A_i\}$. Suppose that stratum-specific reference disease (incidence, mortality) rates $\{R_j\}$ and counts of the population-at-risk $\{n_{ij}\}$ are available. Then under H_0, the number of cases in A_i has Poisson distribution with mean equal to the 'expected number'

$$E_i = \theta \sum R_j n_{ij}$$

where θ is the relative risk for some large area containing A_i (taking account of regional trends, large-scale heterogeneity, variations in known risk factors, etc.). Spatial clustering may be defined as any departure from H_0 in which the variability of the observed cases in each A_i is increased over that expected under the Poisson distribution. If this occurs, then cases will tend to group together in some areas and these will be clusters. Some authors will focus specifically on departures in which rates of disease follow adjacencies in the A_is and these authors will often refer to other variability as 'heterogeneity' (e.g. Richardson *et al.* 1990). Other authors have reserved the term 'clustering' for variations within the small areas irrespective of their spatial relationships (e.g. Alexander *et al.* 1998a). In truth, both are important but they tend to focus on clustering acting at different scales. In this chapter we use the term mainly in the second sense.

If the time period under study is lengthy, then the above truly represents spatial clustering. If, on the other hand, the time period is short and the cases are localised in time as well as in space, then we have 'space-time' clustering. Historically, valid methodology (both for data collection and statistical analysis) was available first for space-time clustering. Space-time interaction methods, due initially to Knox (1964), adjust for *local* geographical variations (keeping time constant) and *global* temporal variations in reported disease risk. Valid statistical methodology for the analyses of spatial clustering of disease in human populations has been developed more recently (Lawson *et al.* 1995; Alexander and Boyle 1996; Statistics in Medicine 1996).

17.1.1 Philosophical approaches

There are four broad philosophies underlying investigations of spatial clustering or extra-Poisson variation (Alexander and Boyle 1996). Under the first, the prime interest is the analysis of putative geographically defined disease determinants; testing for and/or allowing for extra-Poisson variation is an essential first step, but is not in itself the main interest.

In the second approach, the focus is directly on the investigation of clusters and clustering. A positive result from a global test of whether there is an overall tendency to cluster in the total dataset is normally regarded as a prerequisite for further study (Cuzick and Edwards 1990; Alexander and Cuzick 1992). With this approach, a single localised excess will often be dismissed when it is part of the analysis of a large series. The result of such a global test applied to data containing just one striking excess will, of course, depend upon the size of the total dataset. This dependence on the size of the reference area is considered unacceptable by advocates of the third philosophy whose aim is to identify for further scrutiny localised 'anomalies' (or clusters) in the dataset without recourse to any global testing (Openshaw *et al.* 1988; Besag and Newell 1991).

In the absence of a predetermined putative risk, for example from a point source S, these three are the choices available. If, however, one (or one type) of putative risk has been identified then different questions became appropriate, for example:

- Is there an excess of cases in the vicinity of the source S? Does this decrease with distance from S?
- Is there an excess of cases in the vicinity of sources of type S? Does this decrease with distance from S and/or with estimated decline in environmental exposure?

Methods for investigating 'focused clustering' are then applicable (see Chapter 9).

Whatever the approach, it should be noted that the question of generalised clustering remains important: formally it is necessary to test for, and if necessary allow for, generalised clustering; informally we can conclude that an excess of observed to expected numbers in a specific area is more impressive if cases do not, in general, tend to occur in clusters.

17.1.2 Interpretation

Generalised clustering arises when one of two biological mechanisms is influencing the distribution: (i) cases are not independent of one another; or (ii) cases are independent but are influenced by local geographical heterogeneity of risk determinants. These have been described as 'true contagion' and 'apparent contagion', respectively (Cliff and Ord 1981).

The paradigms for the first are diseases caused by infectious agents and/or inherited factors transmitted between cases. The second includes both local geographical variation in relatively ubiquitous risk factors (such as smoking) and excess risk around one or a small number of point sources where an otherwise rare environmental exposure is present. Under reasonable assumptions these two have mathematical formulations as Poisson cluster processes and heterogeneous Poisson processes, respectively, and, crucially, the two are mathematically equivalent (Bartlett 1953; see also Appendix I in Chapter 7 for discussion of a related issue). The biological distinction also becomes blurred with chronic diseases because of the inclusion of healthy carriers, migration, and long or variable latent periods.

Under either of these models the clustering is 'real' in the sense that there is some aetiological factor which is shared by the cases in each cluster. Then, a generalised tendency to cluster will point to one of three things: an infectious agent as a cause of the disease, geographical variations in inherited genetic risk, or inequitable geographical distribution of environmental factors.

Interpretation of clusters and clustering, especially by the general public, is based on this assumption of causality. Thus, an individual cluster will usually be interpreted in terms of (substantial risk from) a local environmental hazard (e.g. point source) even when the association was identified '*post hoc*', invalidating formal statistical inference. It is often not appreciated, however, that clusters and clustering can also arise because of 'clusters of risk factors'; here, a number of cases occur close together but each can be attributed to a different causal pathway. In these circumstances the cluster is meaningless in that it has no implications for either public health surveillance or aetiological research: in other words it is a chance finding.

It is, of course, not possible for data analysis to determine for any individual cluster whether it is real in the sense defined above, or at least whether it is impossible, until all the causes of the relevant disease have been elucidated. Significant results for global tests of clustering can assist in assigning strength of belief here, but cannot provide definitive conclusions.

17.1.3 Estimation of magnitude

An important distinction is required between statistical significance and size of effect here as elsewhere in statistical analysis, but it is frequently forgotten (Boyle *et al.* 1996). As MacMahon (1968) has said: 'It is hard to think of any aetiological factor—from genes to lightning bolts—that would not show some degree of clustering if sufficient data were analysed by sufficiently sensitive means'. Statistical significance depends both on the magnitude of the effect and the quantity of data available; biological significance depends primarily on the magnitude of the effect. Thus, it is appropriate to define measures of the effect (these depend on the type of clustering under investigation) and then to provide estimates for these measures. Weak clustering will correspond to small estimates and strong clustering to large estimates.

17.1.4 Reports of cancer clusters

Investigation of generalised (geographical) clustering of cancer has largely been restricted to leukaemias, lymphomas, and childhood cancers. These diseases have also appeared prominently in analyses of clustering but, in addition, laryngeal cancer and other respiratory system cancers have been investigated quite frequently. Reports of individual geographical cancer clusters are commonly made: Caldwell (1990) identifies 108 studies in the USA in twenty years, all of which remain 'unexplained' in terms of any 'cause' and the majority (79%) of which involve childhood leukaemia.

In the next section we focus on clusters and clustering of childhood leukaemia both on account of the importance of these studies and also to provide concrete illustration of points relevant to other cancer cluster studies. A detailed account of studies of clustering of childhood leukaemia in the UK is given in Chapter 18.

17.2. Clusters of childhood leukaemia

17.2.1 Investigative phases

Three eras of research can be identified (Boyle *et al.* 1996) although the temporal distinction between them is limited. The first era relates to reports of individual clusters; the majority of these are anecdotal reports of which one of the earliest was in 1905 (Arnspreger 1905) and included cases of all ages. From that time until the end of the 1970s, the usual interpretation involved infectious organisms. Until now, reports of individual clusters have continued to emerge and their initial identification is a direct continuation of the early phases; methods of subsequent investigation are now, however, lengthy, costly, and sophisticated (e.g. COMARE 1996). The primary focus of concern regarding childhood leukaemia clusters in recent times has been the possibility of a causal association with an environmental pollutant.

The second era was one in which wide ranging searches were conducted and elementary statistical analyses applied. A large number of examples of these reports are listed by Boyle *et al.* (1996). The third era is the formal statistical analysis of population data; these include applications of space-time interaction methodologies (Gilman and Knox 1991), analyses of general spatial clustering (e.g. Alexander *et al.* 1998a), systematic searches for clusters (e.g. Openshaw *et al.* 1988; Kuldorff and Negawalla 1995), and analyses in the vicinity of all examples of a specified putative source of risk (e.g. Cook-Mozaffari *et al.* 1987).

During this period, two distinct aetiological paradigms have persisted with changes over time in the degree of belief attached to each. Historically, the first paradigm was that leukaemia arose as a consequence of exposure to an unknown infectious agent. This has persisted to the present, albeit with subtle modifications. Most early observers tended to the belief that there was one specific 'leukaemia' virus to which exposure was relatively uncommon. Recent focus has been driven largely by the work of Greaves and colleagues (1988, 1993, 1997) and Kinlen and colleagues (1990, 1995); these authors predict that leukaemia is a rare consequence of exposure to a common infectious agent and that risk is increased by certain *patterns* of exposure: specifically, delayed exposure (Greaves) and exposure in circumstances involving population mixing (Kinlen). Other current variants of the general paradigm include exposure *in utero* (Smith 1997). Since the majority of cases would be infected by 'healthy' carriers, clustering is not a necessary consequence of this hypothesis. There has never been strong evidence to implicate any specific agent; limited data suggest a role for varicella (reviewed in Alexander 1993), the Epstein–Barr virus (Schlehofer *et al.* 1996) and other herpes viruses, *Mycoplasma pneumoniae* (Alexander 1997), and the JC virus (Smith 1997). In the absence of an identifiable agent it is almost impossible to invoke this paradigm as the established cause of any individual cluster but there is strong evidence to support this explanation of the Niles cluster (see below).

The second paradigm involves exposure to an environmental leukaemogen; this was not favoured until the 1980s but, since that time, has probably been the first 'explanation' in the minds of lay people and public health specialists alike when a cluster of childhood leukaemia is observed. Ionising radiation has been the suspect identified most frequently but pesticides, solvents, and others have been considered. There is a 'popular perception that childhood leukaemia is a sentinel environmental disease' (Hoffman *et al.* 1997). No cluster has ever been satisfactorily explained as a consequence of any of these exposures.

With time there has also come greater appreciation that 'childhood leukaemia' is not one single disease and the different sub-types are unlikely to have a common aetiology. The dominant sub-type, acute lymphoblastic leukaemia (ALL), is itself frequently divided into immunophenotypic sub-groups of which common-ALL is the most frequent. Marked international variations in common-ALL incidence (Greaves *et al.* 1993) suggest a distinct aetiology.

17.2.2   Some individual clusters

The examples in the next section illustrate these issues; recent examples from several countries have been included together with Niles. With the exception of Niles, case-control studies and environmental assessments have been conducted or are in progress for all of these. Such studies are expensive and time-consuming yet because of the small numbers involved are unlikely to yield aetiological insights. Nonetheless, while clusters continue to be reported and the causes of childhood leukaemia are not understood, it is the responsibility of public health officials to investigate potential clusters and address the fears and concerns of the public. Note that for these and the majority of reported clusters it is location at diagnosis which is critical; after all, it is this which is likely to be observed, whereas the fact that a group of cases had been close together when born could remain unnoticed. We must emphasise, however, that we do not know the times of the critical exposures which may lead to childhood leukaemia; this should be borne in mind when reading the next section.

Niles, USA (Heath and Hasterlick 1963)

A cluster of eight cases of childhood leukaemia was identified in a suburb of Chicago following a special data search (looking for clusters at a time when it was believed that they could lead to identification of a 'leukaemia virus'). This cluster was associated with one single primary school; six children attended the school, the sibling of another case and the best friend of the final case were also pupils. The ratio of observed (O) to expected (E) is in the range 15–20, but not all boundaries were delineated in advance. The cluster was localised in two distinct time periods and was synchronous with 'rheumaticky' illness in the school and congenital abnormalities in the population (Heath *et al.* 1964). Unusual immune responses were also noted in the families of the cases (Schwartz *et al.* 1963). Crucially, there was very rapid population growth in the suburb together with overcrowding in the school (Kinlen *et al.* 1990). Although many scientists continue to interpret this cluster in terms of an infectious origin, as was the case initially, no specific 'culprit' agent has been identified and it will never now be possible to identify one.

Seascale, UK (Draper et al. 1993)

This is possibly the most extensively researched cluster of childhood leukaemia world-wide. It arose in a small village in the vicinity of a composite nuclear facility, now including the Sellafield reprocessing plant, and was initially identified by researchers for a television company in 1983. The cluster includes young adults (16–24 years) as well as children and non-Hodgkin's lymphoma in addition to leukaemia. Altogether, 10 cases arose in Seascale ward in the period 1953–90 (Draper *et al.* 1993) and, since the excess of O to E in the period 1990–4 remains statistically significant, the excess risk appears persistent in time. A further case was diagnosed in 1991 (COMARE 1996). Early concern focused on the possible effects of environmental exposure to ionising radiation (Black 1984). Subsequently, a case-control study identified a strong statistical association of cases with high paternal preconception occupational exposure to ionising radiation—the PPI hypothesis (Gardner *et al.* 1987*a*,*b*). Intense research has, however, failed to confirm the PPI hypothesis and current evaluations of the Seascale cluster conclude that, while it is unlikely to be due to chance, the cause remains unknown (Draper *et al.* 1993; COMARE 1996).

The most focused study to address the PPI hypothesis has recently been published (Draper *et al.* 1997). This applied record linkage techniques to identify children of registered radiation workers in the UK and cancers in these children. After excluding the cases in the study of Gardner *et al.* (1990), there were 40 'exposed' cases of leukaemia and non-Hodgkin's lymphoma (the fathers were radiation workers before their conception). When cases were compared with population controls there was evidence of excess risk in exposed cases (odds ratio = 1.77, 95% confidence interval: 1.05–3.03). However, risk was highest in children whose father's dose was too small to measure and, after adjusting for radiation worker status, the odds ratio for the high exposure category of Gardner *et al.* was 0.92 (95% CI: 0.28–2.98). These results therefore provide no support for the PPI hypothesis; the authors themselves attribute them to chance, or to another characteristic of the radiation workers, the 'most likely' being 'exposure to an oncogenic infective agent resulting from high levels of population mixing'. This is similar to the conclusions of the most recent UK government report on the Seascale cluster (COMARE 1996). Cohort studies (Gardner *et al.* 1987*a*,*b*; Kinlen 1993) demonstrate that there is no excess risk for school-aged children who moved to the area, although at pre-school ages there is an excess-both for children born in Seascale and for immigrants. Despite all this research, the cluster remains unexplained (see the next chapter).

Woburn, USA (Lagakos et al. 1986)

A chance discovery of toxic wastes and their leaching into the water supply in East Woburn led to health surveys which discovered 20 cases of leukaemia in 'children' (19 years and under) between 1964 and 1983. This is somewhat over twice the expected number and statistically highly significant. Statistical modelling of childhood leukaemia in the whole of Woburn found a significant association with proximity to the contaminated wells. However, while contaminants included trichlorethylene and other known leukaemogens, the dose was insufficient to 'explain' the excess according to accepted dose-response models. It has not been demonstrated that the association is not due to confounding by another unknown characteristic of the East Woburn population. The cluster has persisted in time and was accompanied by an excess of congenital abnormalities, including

Downs' syndrome. Later, immune abnormalities were identified in the population and families involved (Byers *et al.* 1988). More recently, the possibility that toxic leakage into the water supply from a metal waste site might have led to high exposure of parts of the Woburn population has been explored. Analyses of hair samples do not, however, show evidence to support this (Rogers *et al.* 1997).

Elbmarsh, Germany (Hoffman et al. *1997)*

In 1990–1, five cases of childhood leukaemia were diagnosed in a small community in northern Germany within 5 km of the Krummel nuclear facility. A further case was diagnosed in 1995. The overall ratio of O to E for the 5 km circle around the plant is 4.6. Measurements of air, soil, drinking water, milk, vegetables, and other garden products have failed to show any unusual contamination by known leukaemogens. This cluster has generated intense concern in the state involved (Lower Saxony). It is extremely unlikely that there is a causal link to the nuclear facility (Alexander and Greaves, 1998) but 'we cannot presently exclude the possibility that an underlying causal process might be ongoing' (Hoffman *et al.* 1997). These authors are correct—until the causes of childhood leukaemia are properly understood. The same applies to the other small recent clusters described below.

Barcelona, Spain (Gonzalez et al. *1997)*

Between 1991 and 1995, four cases of acute lymphoblastic leukaemia were diagnosed in children resident in a small town in Barcelona (O : E = 26). Three of the children attended the same school. Investigations have failed to uncover any unusual exposure of the cases to known risk factors or any unusual incidence in small towns nearby. The authors have suggested that infection(s) and/or pesticides may be the culprit.

Carbonia, Italy (Cocco et al. *1995)*

Between 1983 and 1985, seven cases of childhood leukaemia were diagnosed in children living in a town on the island of Sardinia (O : E = 8.1) and the local media generated considerable public concern by suggesting that environmental pollution from a nearby large industrial complex might be the cause. A further two cases were diagnosed between 1986 and 1988 (E = 0.63) but no cases occurred during 1989–94. This cluster is therefore relatively localised in time; it is interesting that all the cases were of one subtype (common-ALL). All the cases were born in the city and lived there until diagnosed. Marked associations of birth cohort with age-at-diagnosis suggest an exposure preceding diagnosis by a relatively small constant interval. Subsequent investigations demonstrated that 'no meaningful concentrations of industrial pollutants could have reached Carbonia at the time the cluster was forming' (Cocco *et al.* 1993). The authors investigated spatial clustering within Carbonia and found none, but their analysis is essentially restricted to location at birth (since control locations were known only at birth). The cluster remains unexplained.

17.2.3   What is the critical location and time?

It is generally agreed that childhood leukaemia, like other cancers, requires at least two 'hits' when critical DNA damage occurs; either or both of these hits could be associated with geographically varying risk capable of generating clustering in the location where they occurred, and, for space-time clustering, at the time when they occurred. If an infectious agent is involved, however, then clustering would relate to time and place of exposure and infection, although the time when this infection leads to clinically apparent cancer might be considerably later (e.g. for a persistent infection which is often established as a consequence of exposure *in utero*/neonatally). A related childhood condition, Burkitt's lymphoma (BL), often displays space-time clustering when occurring in tropical areas. BL is known to be caused by early exposure to the Epstein–Barr virus, with infection by malaria frequently acting as a co-factor (via its immune suppressive effect). BL provides a salutary reminder of the vagaries of clustering, since the space-time clustering of BL is believed to relate to the distribution of malaria infection rather than that of the causative (Epstein–Barr) agent.

Our knowledge of the timing of the genetic events underlying childhood leukaemia is slowly increasing but still very imperfect. It is now clear that infant leukaemia with MLL gene rearrangement (over 80% of cases of infant leukaemia) is fully established *in utero* (Gale *et al.* 1997; Greaves 1997). If clustering of these cases occurs then it can only be related to geographical variation in aetiological factors, if locations (and times) relevant to the *in utero* period are involved.

It is also clear that some cases of common-ALL (all those with TEL-AML1 rearrangements—around 30% of all cases) occurred in one genetic lesion *in utero* (Ford *et al.* 1998). This does not necessarily mean that clustering should relate to this period although some authors have hypothesised a causative role for exposure to a virus *in utero* (Smith 1997).

Usually, analyses of spatial clustering take location at residence at just one time—often birth or diagnosis—but sometimes death or onset of symptoms. Since many children diagnosed with leukaemia have moved at least once between birth and diagnosis—47% in a recent study of 1104 UK cases (Alexander, unpublished data)—there will be substantial dilution of an effect and loss of statistical power if the 'wrong' location is taken for analyses. For 'classical' analyses of space-time interaction, the critical time is taken as just one of the times above. If the latent periods (between exposure and leukaemia) were constant and no children changed residence, this would cause no problems; however, since neither of these is likely to apply, considerable loss of statistical power will result.

Although the time from the appearance of the first leukaemic cell to symptomatic leukaemia may be short (a few weeks or months) we know that the last critical exposure does not occur at the time of diagnosis; it need, therefore, not occur at the residence of diagnosis. The latter usually serves as a proxy for residence in a moderately short period before diagnosis. In the same way, residence at birth can be taken as a proxy for residence *in utero* and during the neonatal period. Neither are perfect and they do not cover all times at potential risk. Complete residential histories are much more difficult to obtain and require contact with individual families.

Only one published study has analysed these (Alexander *et al.* 1992) and this generated the hypothesis that the critical times (related to clustering and aetiology) differed by age-at-diagnosis; in particular: (i) the year preceding diagnosis appeared to be critical for the childhood peak of ALL (as hypothesised by Greaves); while (ii) the neonatal period appeared to be critical for older cases (diagnosed at 5 years of age and older). There was, in addition, evidence to suggest that (iii) the same agent was applicable to both.

Substantial (indirect) epidemiological evidence supports the first component of this hypothesis; this has been reviewed by Greaves and Alexander (1993) and Greaves (1997) and includes the observation that both space-time and spatial clustering by place of diagnosis are most clearly seen for young cases of ALL. More limited epidemiological support for the second and third components is now available, including recent reports of space-time and spatial clustering at place of birth for older cases (Alexander 1992; Alexander *et al.* 1998*a,b*; Gustaffson and Carstensen 1999; Dockerty *et al.* 1999); and proximity in space and/or space-time of young cases of ALL (at diagnosis) and older cases (at presumed place of birth). Two recent reports (Alexander *et al.* 1998*a,b*) also point to the possibility that infant cases have, at their time and presumed residence of birth, lived close to other cases at their critical times.

These results provide preliminary evidence that, when looking for aetiologically meaningful clusters of childhood leukaemia, we should focus on:

- cases of ALL in the childhood peak where they lived at/shortly before diagnosis,
- older children with leukaemia where they lived at/close to birth,
- infant cases where they lived at/before birth,
- aggregations involving combinations of these.

If this is true then inclusion of *all* cases of childhood leukaemia for analyses of space-time or spatial clustering related to residence at either birth or diagnosis will dilute the effect. Analyses may need to be restricted to appropriate sub-groups; the alternative—use of more complex and focused methodology—is not discussed further in the present volume, although present methods may be refined to incorporate the 'critical' period.

17.2.4   Space-time interaction clustering

Analyses of space-time clustering related to birth, onset of symptoms, report of disease, and death have been reviewed in Boyle *et al.* (1996) and earlier publications. Analyses by the Knox method (1964) and derivatives are the most frequently reported. Although this methodology has low statistical power for 'reasonable' models of chronic disease (Chen *et al.* 1984) analyses using this methodology continue to be reported. One reason is, undoubtedly, the difficulty that is often found in estimating valid denominators of person-years-at-risk for small areas for times overlapping two or more decennial censuses (see Chapter 3). The second main reason is likely to be the belief that, while extraneous factors may influence both spatial and temporal distributions, the interaction of these should be consistent (under H_0) with the assumption of independence.

More recent analyses include those for the UK (Gilman and Knox 1995), Greece (Petridou *et al.* 1996), and Sweden (Gustaffson and Carstensen 1999). The overall impression (Alexander 1993; Boyle *et al.* 1996) is that space-time clustering is strongest for cases of ALL at time/place of diagnosis and, particularly, for younger cases. The recent Swedish analysis reports significant space-time clustering by time/place of birth for *older* cases only. Gilman and Knox (1995) report significant space-time clustering for the UK related to *both* birth and diagnosis (involving different 'close' pairs for each) but do not separate their results by age group at diagnosis.

Space-time interaction clustering is usually interpreted in terms of infectious processes but this is not essential and an alternative involving localised environmental hazards with short latent periods is almost equally tenable.

17.2.5 Spatial clustering

Several analyses of large datasets of childhood leukaemia are now available, almost all related to location at diagnosis. One of the first was Draper (1991). Several independent analyses found statistically significant evidence of spatial clustering of childhood leukaemia and non-Hodgkin's lymphoma in the UK (1966–82). The magnitude of the effect was, however, such that it could be attributable to data artefacts (see Chapter 18).

Analyses of spatial clustering of childhood leukaemia are reviewed by Boyle *et al.* (1996). The most recent analysis of a large dataset, EUROCLUS, includes data from 12 countries and 4 regions within countries for 1980–9. Statistically significant evidence of spatial clustering within small census areas has been reported (Alexander *et al.* 1998*a*) but the magnitude is small (extra-Poisson variability, EPV, is just 2% of Poisson variability), and clustering is absent in some countries. The magnitude of the EPV is related to population density. Sub-division by population density revealed uniform excess incidence for density 500–750 person/km^2 with the largest (7%) magnitude of heterogeneity ('clustering') for density 250–500 person/km^2 (Alexander *et al.* 1999). If these are to be interpreted in terms of population micro-epidemics they may suggest an agent having regular epidemics for densities 500–750 person/km^2 and sporadic epidemics for densities 250–500 person/km^2.

The EUROCLUS analysis for Greece has been expanded and reported separately (Petridou *et al.* 1997); these findings are specially strong. EUROCLUS also found evidence of generalised clustering in Sweden; alternative methodologies have, however, not found any such evidence to be statistically significant (Waller *et al.* 1995; Hjalmers *et al.* 1996). Spatial clustering has also been observed in Hong Kong (Alexander *et al.* 1997). This is of particular interest because of, first, differences there in population density and ethnic origin and, second, the availability of high quality diagnostic data which enabled separate analyses to be conducted for ALL and for common-ALL. The clustering was concentrated in common-ALL cases resident in the 'New Territories' which have been described as the largest new town development programme in the world. All of the above related to location at diagnosis. Alternative analyses for the UK covering extended time periods have reported significant spatial clustering for locations at birth, diagnosis, and death (Knox and Gilman 1996). The methodology employed is, however, somewhat obscure, limiting interpretation.

Few analyses of spatial clustering have considered place of birth. Recent data from New Zealand (Dockerty *et al.* 1999) has found statistically significant clustering of older cases (10–14 years) but not other age groups by place of birth.

17.2.6 Clustering around nuclear and other sites

Systematic analyses of clustering around a particular type of putative point source have mainly focused on nuclear sites. Analyses have been conducted in the UK for 1959–80 (Cook-Mozaffari *et al.* 1987) and for England and Wales 1966–87 (Bithell *et al.* 1994). These involved 22 and 23 nuclear installations, respectively. Analyses have also been conducted for France (1968–89) with 13 nuclear sites (Hattchouel *et al.* 1995), West Germany (1980–90) with 13 sites (Michaelis *et al.* 1993), Sweden (1980–90) (Waller *et al.* 1995) with 5 sites, and Kazakhstan (Zarideze *et al.* 1994). The results for the UK confirm some of the reported clusters around nuclear sites (and proposed sites!); the analyses of

Bithell and colleagues found that observed numbers in a 25 km circle around the 23 nuclear sites and 8 control (planned) sites never significantly exceeded expected numbers and a 'linear risk score'—a modification of the method of Bithell and Stone (1989; see also Chapter 9)—gave a significant result only for Sellafield (see Section 17.2.2), Burghfield, and one planned site. Their conclusions were: (i) no evidence of a general increase in risk around nuclear facilities in England and Wales; and (ii) very weak evidence of distance related risk for all sites apart from Sellafield (see Chapter 18).

The results from West Germany give an overall risk ratio of 1.06 for acute leukaemia in the areas around the nuclear facilities compared with national data, although some sub-groups (by site and age) did show statistically significant excesses. The French results are based on leukaemia *mortality* data for 1968–89 which may have been influenced to some degree by prognostic factors in the 1980s and relate to deaths aged < 25 years. The observed cases in 25 km circles around the sites ($O = 69$) did not differ from the expected numbers ($E = 86.15$) and were, indeed *less* than the expected. In the Swedish analysis, the application of 7 focused tests to the 5 sites (35 analyses, not all independent) yielded one result with $p < 0.05$ and one other with $p < 0.1$, both from the same site.

Altogether, these analyses fail to provide convincing evidence of clustering focused on nuclear facilities (including power stations and reprocessing plants). The analyses from Kazakhstan relate to nuclear weapons testing facilities where environmental exposure to ionising radiation may have been more substantial than around the other sites. A significant trend of risk by distance from the nearest site was observed but the magnitude of the distance–risk relationship was small, with risk ratio for residence < 200 km compared with > 400 km being just 1.76. The authors caution that their findings may be affected by confounders, especially urban-rural status and ethnic factors.

Only one other systematic analysis of focused clustering in a national dataset is available in the current literature. This is applied to putative hazards *other than ionising radiation* for UK mortality data for the period 1953–80. Statistically significant evidence of clustering was found, related to proximity to sources of: (i) petroleum-derived volatiles; (ii) kiln and furnace smoke and gases; and (iii) effluents from internal combustion engines (Knox and Gilman 1997). Caution in interpreting these results is required since lack of geographically referenced control data forced the authors to make possibly invalid assumptions regarding, for example, numbers of children per postcode. The fact that the strengths of the associations were similar for leukaemia and for solid tumours suggests that the findings may have been an artefact.

17.3   Conclusions

We conclude that childhood leukaemias do display a general tendency to cluster at place of diagnosis but the magnitude of the extra-Poisson variation is small in general and may only be identified when large datasets are analysed. There is some evidence that the extra-Poisson variation is larger within certain population-density groups. This small magnitude in general may be attributable to:

- the aetiological factor which leads to clustering being a weak determinant of risk and/or itself only slightly clustered,
- dilution of a more substantial effect because (i) children have moved between the time when the causative exposure occurred and the time for which their address was analysed, and/or (ii) children

move around their locality (e.g. to school) or on holiday and the critical exposures need not occur near their current residence,

• case sub-groups having different critical times of exposure.

The literature contains examples of striking individual clusters; it is reasonable to assume some shared aetiology between the cases within these clusters but no environmental pollutant and no infectious agent has ever explained a cluster satisfactorily. To proceed further we need more understanding of the aetiology of childhood leukaemia and this is unlikely to come from scrutiny of cases in any single cluster. It is possible that studying large numbers of clusters (Alexander *et al.* 1998*b*,1999) may contribute to a concerted research effort, which will also include utilising and developing methods discussed in this book.

Meanwhile clusters will continue to be noticed and public concern aroused with consequent need for reassurance. This need is justified. Methods for use by public health specialists are available elsewhere (CDC 1990; Arrundale *et al.* 1997; and see Chapter 8). Finally, the fact that localised clustering of childhood leukaemia does occur provides a note of caution to all those seeking to apply methodology based on the Poisson distribution to map and analyse childhood leukaemia incidence data.

References

Alexander, F. E. (1992). Space-time clustering of childhood acute lymphoblastic-leukaemia—indirect evidence for a transmissible agent. *British Journal of Cancer*, **65**, 589–92.

Alexander, F. E. (1993). Viruses, clusters and clustering of childhood leukaemia: a new perspective? *European Journal of Cancer*, **29A**, 1424–43.

Alexander, F. E. (1997). Is mycoplasma pneumonia associated with childhood acute lymphoblastic leukaemia? *Cancer Causes and Control*, **8**, 803–11.

Alexander, F. E. and Boyle, P. (ed.) (1996). *Methods of investigating localised clustering of disease*, International Agency for Research on Cancer. Scientific Publications 135. IARC, Lyon.

Alexander, F. E. and Cuzick, J. (1992). Methods for the assessment of disease clusters. In *Geographical and environmental epidemiology*, P. Elliot ed. 238–50. Oxford University Press.

Alexander, F. E. and Greaves, M. F. (1998). Ionising radiation and leukaemia potential risks: review based on the workshop held during 10th Symposium on Molecular Biology of Hematopoiesis and Treatment of Leukaemias and Lymphomas, Hamburg, Germany, 5 July 1997. *Leukaemia*, **12**, 1319–23.

Alexander, F. E., McKinney, P. A., Moncrieff, K. C., and Cartwright, R. A. (1992). Residential proximity of children with leukaemia and non-Hodgkins-lymphoma in 3 areas of Northern England. *British Journal of Cancer*, **65**, 583–8.

Alexander, F. E., Chan, L. C., Lam, T. H., Yuen, P., Leung, N. K., Ha, S. Y. *et al.* (1997). Clustering childhood leukaemia in Hong Kong: Association with the childhood peak of common acute lymphoblastic leukaemia and with population mixing. *British Journal of Cancer*, **75**, 457–63.

Alexander, F. E., Boyle, P., Carli, P.-M., Coebergh, J. W., Draper, G. J., Ekbom, A. *et al.*, on behalf of the EUROCLUS project. (1998*a*). Spatial clustering of childhood leukaemia: summary results from the EUROCLUS project. *British Journal of Cancer*, **77**, 818–24.

Alexander, F. E., Boyle, P., Carli, P.-M., Coebergh, J. W., Draper, G. J., Ekbom, A. *et al.*, on behalf of the EUROCLUS project. (1998*b*). Spatial temporal patterns in childhood leukaemia: further evidence for an infectious origin. *British Journal of Cancer*, **77**, 812–17.

Alexander, F. E., Boyle, P., Carli, P.-M., Coebergh, J. W., Ekbom, A., Levi, F. *et al.*, on behalf of the EUROCLUS project. (1999). Population density and childhood leukaemia: results of the EUROCLUS study. *European Journal of Cancer*, **35**, 439–44.

Arnspreger, L. (1905). Endemisches Auftreten von myeloid Leukämie. *München Medizin Wochenschrift*, **52**, 9.

size:

Arrundale, J., Bain, M., Botting, B., Brewster, D., Cartwright, R., Chalmers, J. *et al.*, (1997). *Handbook and guide to the investigation of clusters of diseases.* University Print Services, Leeds.

Bartlett, M. S. (1953). Spectral analysis of two-dimensional point processes. *Biometrika*, **51**, 299–311.

Besag, J. and Newell, J. (1991). The detection of clusters in rare diseases. *Journal of the Royal Statistical Society, Series A*, **154**, 143–55.

Bithell, J. F. and Stone, R. A. (1989). On statistical methods for analysing the geographical distribution of cancer cases near nuclear installations. *Journal of Epidemiology and Community Health*, **43**, 79–85.

Bithell, J. F., Dutton, S. J., Draper, G. J., and Neary, N. M. (1994). Distribution of childhood leukaemias and non-Hodgkin's lymphomas near nuclear installations in England and Wales. *British Medical Journal*, **309**, 501–5.

Black, D. (1984). *Investigation of the possible increased incidence of cancer in West Cumbria.* Report of the Independent Advisory Group. HMSO, London.

Boyle, P., Walker, A. M., and Alexander, F. E. (1996). Historical aspects of leukaemia clusters. In *Methods of investigating localised clustering of disease* (F. E. Alexander and P. Boyle ed.), 1–20, International Agency for Research on Cancer. Scientific Publication 135. IARC, Lyon.

Byers, V. C., Levin, A. S., Ozonoff, D. M., and Baldwin, R. W. (1988). Association between clinical symptoms and lymphocytic abnormalities in a population with chronic domestic exposure to industrial solvent-contaminated domestic water supply and a high incidence of leukaemia. *Cancer Immunology and Immunotherapy*, **27**, 77–81.

Caldwell, G. G. (1990). Twenty-two years of cancer cluster investigations at the centre for disease control. *American Journal of Epidemiology*, **132**, 543–7.

CDC (Centers for Disease Control) (1990). Guidelines for investigating clusters of health events. *Morbidity and Mortality Weekly Report*, **39** (RR-11), 1–23.

Chen, R., Mantel, N., and Klingberg, M. A. (1984). A study of three techniques for time-space clustering in Hodgkin's disease. *Statistics in Medicine*, **3**, 263.

Cliff, A. D. and Ord, J. K. (1981). *Spatial processes: models and applications.* Pion, London.

Cocco, P., Bernardinelli, L., Biddau, P., Montomoli, C., Murgia, G., Rapallo, M. *et al.* (1993). Childhood leukaemia in SouthWest Sardinia (Italy). *Tumori*, **79**, 244–5.

Cocco, P., Bernardinelli, L., Biddau, P., Montomoli, C., Murgia, G., Rapallo, M. *et al.* (1995). Childhood acute lymphoblastic leukaemia: a cluster in South Western Sardinia (Italy). *International Journal of Occupational and Environmental Health*, **1**, 232–8.

COMARE (Committee on Medical Aspects of Radiation in the Environment) (1996). *Fourth report.* HMSO, London.

Cook-Mozaffari, P. J., Ashwood, F. L., Vincent, T., Forman, D., and Alderson, M. (1987). *Cancer incidence and mortality in the vicinity of nuclear installations England and Wales 1959–80.* Studies on Medical and Population Subjects 51. HMSO, London.

Cuzick, J. and Edwards, R. (1990). Spatial clustering for inhomogeneous populations (with discussion). *Journal of the Royal Statistical Society, Series B*, **52**, 73–104.

Dockerty, J. D., Sharples, K. J., and Borman, B. (1999). An assessment of spatial clustering of leukaemias and lymphomas among young people in New Zealand. *Journal of Epidemiqlogy and Community Health*, **53**, 154–8.

Draper, G. J. (1991). *The geographical epidemiology of childhood leukaemia and non-Hodgkin's lymphoma in Great Britain 1966–1983.* HMSO, London.

Draper, G. J., Stiller, C. A., Cartwright, R. A., Craft, A. W., and Vincent, T. J. (1993). Cancer in Cumbria and in the vicinity of the Sellafield nuclear installation, 1963–90. *British Medical Journal*, **306**, 89–94.

Draper, G. J., Little, M. P., Sorahan, T., Kinien, L. J., Bunch, K. J., Conquest, A. J. *et al.* (1997). Cancer in the offspring of radiation workers: a record linkage study. *British Medical Journal*, **315**, 1181–8.

Ford, A. M., Bennett, C. A., Price, C. M., Drum, M. C. A., Van Wering, E. R., and Greaves, M. F. (1998). Fetal origins of the TEL-MAL1 fusion gene in identical twins with leukaemia. *Proceedings of the National Academy of Science USA*, **95**, 4584–8.

Gale, K. B., Ford, A. M., Repp, R., Borkhardt, A., Keller, C., Eden, O. B. *et al.* (1997). Backtracking leukaemia to birth: Identification of clonotypic gene fusion sequences in neonatal blood spots. *Proceedings of the National Academy of Science USA*, **94**, 13950–4.

Gardner, M. J., Hall, A. J., Downes, S., and Terrell, J. D. (1987*a*). Follow-up study of children born elsewhere but attending schools in Seascale, West Cumbria (schools cohort). *British Medical Journal*, **295**, 819–22.

Gardner, M. J., Hall, A. J., Downes, S., and Terrell, J. D. (1987*b*). Follow-up study of children born to mothers resident in Seascale, West Cumbria (birth cohort). *British Medical Journal*, **295**, 822–7.

Gardner, M. J., Sneer, M. P., Hall, A. J., Powell, C. A., Downes, S., and Terrell, J. D. (1990). Results of case-control study of leukaemia and lymphoma among young people near Sellafield nuclear plant in West Cumbria. *British Medical Journal*, **300**, 423–9.

Gilman, E. A. and Knox, E. G. (1991). Temporal-spatial distribution of childhood leukaemias and non-Hodgkin's lymphomas in Great Britain. In *The geographical epidemiology of childhood leukaemia and non-Hodgkin lymphomas in Great Britain, 1966–1983* (G. J. Draper ed.), 77–81. HMSO, London.

Gilman, E. A. and Knox, E. G. (1995). Childhood cancers—space-time distribution in Britain. *Journal of Epidemiology and Community Health*, **49**, 158–63.

Gonzalez, C. A., Borras, J. M., Luna, P., Baixeras, C., Mariano, E., and Pera, G. (1997). Brief communication: childhood leukaemia in a residential town near Barcelona. *Archieves of Environmental Health*, **52**, 322–5.

Greaves, M. F. (1988). Speculations on the cause of childhood leukaemia. *Leukaemia*, **2**, 120–5.

Greaves, M. F. (1997). Aetiology of acute leukaemia. *Lancet*, **349**, 344–9.

Greaves, M. F. and Alexander, F. E. (1993). An infectious aetiology for common acute lymphoblastic-leukaemia in childhood. *Leukaemia*, **7**, 349–60.

Greaves, M. F., Colman, S. M., Beard, M. E. J., Bradstock, K., Cabrera, M. E., Chen, P.-M., *et al.* (1993). Geographical distribution of acute lymphoblastic leukaemia subtypes: Second Report of the Collaborative Group Study. *Leukaemia*, **7**, 27–34.

Gustafsson, B. and Carstensen, J. (1999). Evidence of space-time clustering of childhood acute lymphoblastic leukaemia in Sweden. *British Journal of Cancer*, **79**, 655–7.

Hattchouel, J. M., Laplanche, A., and Hill, C. (1995). Leukaemia mortality around French nuclear sites. *British Journal of Cancer*, **71**, 651–653.

Hjalmers, U., Kuldorff, M., Gustaffason, G., and Nagawalla, N. (1996). Childhood leukaemia in Sweden—using GIS and a spatial scan statistic for cluster detection. *Statistics in Medicine*, **15**, 707–15.

Heath, C. W. and Hasterlick, R. J. (1963). Leukaemia amongst children in a suburban community. *American Journal of Medicine*, **34**, 796–812.

Heath, C. W., Manning, M. D., and Zelkowitz, L. (1964). Case clusters in the occurrence of leukaemia and congenital malformations. *Lancet*, **ii**, 136–7.

Hoffmann, W., Dieckmann, H., and Schmitz Feuerhake, I. (1997). A cluster of childhood leukaemia near a nuclear reactor in Northern Germany. *Archives of environmental Health*, **52**, 275–80.

Lagakos, S. W., Wessen, B. J., and Zelen, M. (1986). An analysis of contaminated well water and health effects in Woburn, Massachusetts. *Journal of the American Statistical Association*, **81**, 583–96.

Lawson, A. B., Waller, L. A., and Biggeri, A. (ed.) (1995). Spatial disease patterns. *Statistics in Medicine* **14**, (Special Issue) 2289–505.

Kinlen, L. J. (1993). Can parental pre-conceptional radiation account for the rise of leukaemia and non-Hodgkin's lymphoma in Seascale? *British Medical Journal*, **306**, 1718–21.

Kinlen, L. J. (1995). Epidemiological evidence for an infective basis in childhood leukaemia. *British Journal of Cancer*, **71**, 1–5.

Kinlen, L. J., Clark, K., and Hudson, C. (1990). Evidence from population mixing in British New Towns 1946–1985 of an infective basis for childhood leukaemia. *Lancet*, **336**, 577–82.

Knox, E. G. (1964). The detection of space-time interactions. *Applied Statistics*, **13**, 25–9.

Knox, E. G. and Gilman, E. A. (1996). Spatial clustering of childhood cancers in Great Britain. *Journal of Epidemiology and Community Health*, **50**, 313–19.

Knox, E. G. and Gilman, E. A. (1997). Hazard proximities of childhood cancers in Great Britain from 1953–80. *Journal of Epidemiology and Community Health*, **50**, 151–9.

Kulldorff, M. and Nagarwalla, N. (1995). Spatial disease clusters: detection and inference. *Statistics in Medicine*, **14**, 799–810.

MacMahon, B. (1968). Epidemiological aspects of acute leukaemia and Burkitt's tumour. *Cancer*, **21**, 558–61.

Michaelis, J., Keller, B., Haaf, G., and Kaatsch, P. (1993). Incidence of childhood malignancies in the vicinity of West German nuclear power plants. In *Childhood cancer and nuclear Installations* (V. Beral, E. Roman, and M. Bobrow ed.), 443. BMJ Publishing, London.

Openshaw, S., Charlton, M., Craft, A. W., and Birch, J. M. (1988). Investigation of leukaemia clusters by the use of a geographical analysis machine. *Lancet*, **1**, 272–3.

Petridou, E., Revinthi, K., Alexander, F. E., Haidas, S., Koliouskas, D., Kosmidis, H. *et al.* (1996). Space-time clustering of childhood leukaemia in Greece—Evidence supporting a viral aetiology. *British Journal of Cancer*, **73**, 1278–83.

Petridou, E., Alexander, F. E., Trichopoulos, D., Revinthi, K., Dessiprys, N., Wray, N. *et al.* (1997). Aggregation of childhood leukaemia in geographical areas of Greece. *Cancer Causes and Control*, **8**, 239–45.

Rogers, C. E., Tomita, A. V., Trowbridge, P. R., Gone, J-K., Chen, J., Zeeb, P. *et al.* (1997). Hair analysis does not support hypothesised arsenic and chromium exposure from drinking water in Woburn, Massachussetts. *Environmental Health Perspectives*, **105**, 1090–7.

Richardson, S., Monfort, C., Green, M., Draper, G., and Muirhead, C. (1990). Spatial variation of natural radiation and childhood leukaemia incidence in Great Britain. *Statistics in Medicine*, **15**, 683–97.

Schwartz, S. O., Greenspan, I., and Brown, E. R. (1963). Leukaemia cluster in Niles iii. *Journal of the American Medical Association*, **186**, 106–8.

Schlehofer, B., Blettner, M., Geletneky, K., Haaf, H. G., Kaatsch, P., Michaelis, J. *et al.* (1996). Sero-epidemiological analysis of the risk of virus infections for childhood leukaemia. *International Journal of Cancer*, **65**, 1–7.

Smith, M. (1997). Considerations on a possible viral aetiology for B-precursor acute lymphoblastic leukaemia of childhood. *Journal of Immunology*, **20**, 89–100.

Statistics in Medicine (1996). Proceedings of conference of statistics and computing in disease clustering, **15** (Issues 7–9), 681–952.

Waller, L. A., Turnbull, B. W., Gustafsson, G., Hjalmars, U., and Andersson, B. (1995). Detection and assessment of clusters of disease—an application to nuclear-power-plant facilities and childhood leukaemia in Sweden. *Statistics in Medicine*, **14**, 3–16.

Zaridze, D. G., Li, N., Men, T., and Duffy, S. W. (1994). Childhood cancer incidence in relation to distance from the former nuclear testing site in Semipalatinsk, Kazakjstan. *International Journal of Cancer*, **59**, 471–5.

18. Geographical variations in childhood leukaemia incidence

J. F. Bithell and T. J. Vincent

18.1 Childhood leukaemia

The pattern of cancer and leukaemia in childhood is quite different from that in adults. Although in developed countries childhood deaths after the first year of life are more common from malignant disease than from any other single disease, they are nevertheless comparatively rare: in the UK, for example, only around one child in 600 can expect to experience some form of malignancy before the age of 15, and the death rate is dropping steadily as survival rates improve (Draper 1995). This is in contrast to the picture in adults, of whom around one in three can expect to develop some form of malignant disease during their lifetime.

Leukaemia as a sub-group also behaves quite differently in children and adults. Although accounting for only around 2% of diagnosed cases of adult malignant disease in the UK, it is much the commonest type of malignancy in children, constituting around a third of all cases. Again, the pattern of leukaemia types differs markedly, with acute lymphocytic leukaemia (ALL) accounting for around 80% of cases in children, but only around 5% in adults (Cartwright *et al.* 1990). It is consequently important that studies of leukaemia incidence differentiate between children and adults.

Perhaps because it is more common than other causes of serious morbidity or mortality in children, childhood leukaemia has attracted a great deal of attention, both in the scientific literature and in the popular news media. In contrast to many adult tumours, its causes are still largely unknown; our understanding at the molecular level is only partial and is largely unrelated to explanatory mechanisms.

Among the latter, the most important are almost certainly genetic. Evidence for this includes: (a) association with various conditions having a clear genetic aetiology, including major chromosomal defects such as Down's syndrome (trisomy 21), in which the risk of childhood leukaemia is increased about 15-fold (Zipursky *et al.* 1992); (b) the fact that certain gene rearrangements are frequently found in children with leukaemia (Greaves 1997); (c) substantial variation between ethnic groups (Parkin *et al.* 1988a); and (d) a degree of familial association (Draper *et al.* 1996).

More significant in the popular consciousness are various environmental pollutants, particularly from the nuclear and chemical industries. Although biochemical pathways for chemical carcinogens have been postulated (Greaves 1997) the epidemiological evidence for a chemical cause of childhood leukaemia is indirect, being mostly in terms of association with specific parental occupations (McBride 1998). Ionising radiation, on the other hand, is known to cause leukaemia in both adults (Weiss *et al.* 1995) and children (Preston *et al.* 1994), while exposure to X-rays in obstetric examinations is now generally believed to carry a small but measurable risk to the fetus (Doll and Wakeford 1997).

Although the evidence is weaker and it attracts less popular attention, a viral aetiology is also a serious possibility. The first reported viral association was related to influenza infection in the mothers of a cohort of children born in March 1958 in the UK (Fedrick and Alberman 1972). These authors observed a ninefold increase in the risk of leukaemia and lymphoma in the affected children, which is statistically highly significant; however, the finding was based on only 13 cases and related to an atypical time period, namely that following a virulent epidemic of the Asian strain. Other studies—mostly of population data—were either negative or indicative of a much lower relative risk (Shore *et al.* 1976) and maternal influenza infection is not currently regarded as a significant cause of childhood leukaemia. More recently, however, various infective mechanisms have been postulated as contributing to the aetiology of childhood leukaemia (Kinlen 1995; Greaves 1991), though there is no evidence to indicate a particular organism.

With the most liberal interpretation of the epidemiological evidence, these possible mechanisms appear to account for only a modest fraction of all cases of childhood leukaemia. It is interesting, however, that they might all be expected to result in geographical variation of some kind and it is this that provides the motivation for studying the geographical epidemiology of the disease. Different mechanisms would be expected to yield variation of different kinds and at different levels of geographical proximity and accordingly we look in turn at international variation, and regional and small-scale variation within the UK.

18.2   International variation

International comparisons are made difficult by: (a) the shortage of good population-based registers; (b) differences in diagnostic practice and completeness of ascertainment; and (c) competing causes of death, notably infectious diseases, which are more likely to be lethal in children whose immune system is affected by leukaemia and which may also mask the underlying malignancy (Kneale 1971).

Currently, the best source for international comparisons is the volume published by the International Agency for Research on Cancer (IARC) (Parkin *et al.* 1988*a*). This was the result of a major collaborative project in which substantial efforts were made to standardise the bases of comparison. The result is a set of comparative rates relating to over 70 registries in some 50 different countries. Small registries were excluded by the criterion that there should be at least 200 cases of childhood cancer over the study period, which was standardised as far as was practicable to the decade 1970–9. Around a quarter of the data-sets had inadequate population data and consequently provided only proportional incidence rates; they have consequently been excluded from our analysis.

The raw data in the IARC volume have subsequently been summarised and interpreted by a number of authors, notably Parkin *et al.* (1988*b*), Linet and Devesa (1991), and Stiller and Parkin (1996). They have generally not taken account of the sampling errors in the rates on the grounds that these are likely to be dominated by non-sampling errors, such as incomplete or inconsistent ascertainment of the cases (Parkin *et al.* 1988*a*).

While acknowledging the importance of the latter factors, we feel, however, that it is helpful to be able to *exclude* from consideration differences that are well within sampling variation, and we have accordingly calculated the standard errors of the rates shown in Table 18.1, and incorporated them into our brief analysis of the data.

Table 18.1 shows the following data, abstracted or recalculated from the IARC volume:

Column 1: The number of person-years at risk covered by the registry (in millions).

Column 2: The number of cases of leukaemia registered under 15 years of age.

Column 3: The ASR (age-standardised annual leukaemia rate) for children in this age range. An asterisk (*) indicates a registry that did not specify a separate rate for infants in the first year of life; for these, the ASRs and their standard errors were computed on a separate basis. Direct standardisation with the world population as standard was utilised.

Column 4: The standard error of the latter rate.

Column 5: The proportion of all leukaemias of specified type that were specified as ALL.

Column 6: The proportion of all leukaemic children registered who were under 5 years of age.

Table 18.1 Age-standardised rates of childhood leukaemia under age 15 (from Parkin *et al.* 1988*a*), with standard errors and other statistics (see text)

Region	Million person-yrs	No. cases	ASR (0–14)	SE	Prop. ALL	Prop. 0–4 yrs
America: *North*						
1 Canada: Atlantic Prov.	6.45	224	37.9	2.58	0.67	0.50
2 Canada: Western Prov.	16.44	649	43.8	1.75	0.82	0.53
3 USA: GDV, whites [1]	16.39	645	42.8	1.72*	0.81	0.47
4 USA: GDV, non-whites [1]	3.70	81	22.4	2.52*	0.75	0.33
5 USA: LA, blacks	3.13	82	27.8	3.11	0.75	0.44
6 USA: LA, Hispanics	6.41	315	50.2	2.83	0.78	0.56
7 USA: LA, Other whites	9.70	428	48.2	2.37	0.83	0.51
8 USA: NY, whites	21.73	928	46.6	1.56	0.76	0.48
9 USA: NY, blacks	4.56	121	28.1	2.59	0.68	0.47
10 USA: SEER, whites [2]	39.60	1591	43.7	1.11*	0.81	0.52
11 USA: SEER, blacks [2]	5.82	141	25.2	2.15*	0.68	0.45
America: *Other*						
12 Brazil: Fortaleza	1.52	64	41.9	5.24	0.78	0.28
13 Brazil: Recife	5.68	143	25.4	2.13*	0.68	0.41
14 Brazil: São Paolo	19.53	643	33.5	1.33	0.61	0.47
15 Colombia	2.17	93	44.1	4.64*	0.82	0.40
16 Costa Rica	3.60	212	59.4	4.09	0.81	0.42
17 Cuba	38.74	1139	29.8	0.89	0.69	0.36
18 Jamaica	2.98	65	22.2	2.77*	0.74	0.48
19 Puerto Rico	10.09	388	40.2	2.06*	0.77	0.51
Asia						
20 China: Shangai	8.21	316	40.8	2.56	0.60	0.22
21 China: Taipei	11.52	306	27.3	1.57	0.70	0.49
22 Hong Kong	8.03	364	47.2	2.54	0.61	0.39

Table 18.1 (*cont.*)

Region	Million person-yrs	No. cases	ASR (0–14)	SE	Prop. ALL	Prop. 0–4 yrs
23 India: Bangalore	3.46	46	12.7	1.90*	0.65	0.24
24 India: Bombay	21.70	493	22.9	1.04*	0.66	0.38
25 Isreal, Jews	8.74	283	32.7	1.94	0.72	0.54
26 Israel, Non-Jews	2.59	67	25.8	3.16	0.67	0.57
27 Japan: Kanagawa	8.16	315	38.3	2.16	0.58	0.55
28 Japan: Miyagi	4.16	160	39.5	3.14	0.56	0.48
29 Japan: Osaka	20.45	776	38.4	1.38	0.65	0.52
30 Kuwait, Kuwaitis	2.05	26	12.9	2.54*	0.92	0.50
31 Kuwait, non-Kuwaitis	1.90	68	34.7	4.22*	0.94	0.50
32 Philippines	6.61	287	43.9	2.59	0.75	0.41
33 Singapore, Chinese	8.05	282	37.8	2.30*	0.68	0.45
34 Singapore, Malay	1.81	69	38.6	4.73*	0.64	0.32
Europe						
35 Czech: Slovak Rep.	12.35	463	38.9	1.82	0.75	0.52
36 Denmark	5.38	193	38.7	2.84	0.81	0.48
37 FRG: CTR	29.89	1168	43.4	1.30	0.84	0.52
38 FRG: Saar	3.80	136	39.7	3.49*	0.78	0.46
39 Finland	10.41	408	42.3	2.13	0.76	0.49
40 France: Bas-Rhin	2.00	69	38.3	4.68*	0.78	0.55
41 France: Paed. Registries	3.22	120	40.3	3.73	0.84	0.54
42 GDR	17.01	525	34.2	1.53	0.73	0.47
43 GB: England & Wales	111.18	3857	37.5	0.61	0.81	0.50
44 GB: Scotland	12.57	438	37.9	1.85	0.78	0.49
45 Hungary	22.79	762	34.3	1.25	0.82	0.57
46 Italy	7.51	351	49.2	2.65	0.80	0.50
47 Netherlands: DCLSG	33.34	1127	37.6	1.14*	0.84	0.52
48 Netherlands: Eindhoven	2.12	78	43.1	5.02*	0.74	0.55
49 Norway	9.44	393	44.6	2.27	0.69	0.56
50 Poland: Warsaw	3.26	95	31.0	3.21	0.07	0.51
51 Spain: Zaragoza	1.86	84	46.5	5.12	0.69	0.45
52 Sweden	21.65	900	44.3	1.49	0.79	0.52
53 Switzerland	1.89	76	43.8	5.11	0.88	0.46
54 Yugoslavia	4.24	139	34.1	2.91	0.66	0.53
Oceania						
55 Australia: NSW	4.17	663	49.9	1.95	0.80	0.55
56 Australia: Queensland	5.30	190	38.0	2.79	0.87	0.52
57 New Zealand, Maoris	1.16	35	32.2	5.49	0.48	0.57
58 New Zealand, Non-Maoris	7.92	342	45.4	2.48	0.73	0.48

[1] GDV, Greater Delaware Valley; [2] SEER, Surveillance, Epidemiology and End Results Program. For details of the registries, see Parkin *et al.* (1998*a*).

It will be seen from Table 18.1 that the largest single registry is the National Registry of Childhood Tumours (NRCT) maintained by the Childhood Cancer Research Group (CCRG) in Oxford. This returned information on 3857 cases of leukaemia in England and Wales over the study period; although the Register covers Scotland also, a separate local register was used to supply Scottish data. A further UK register based in Manchester was also represented; this has been excluded from Table 18.1 on the grounds that the first period considered differed from that used for the other registries, while practically all the cases in the second period are included in the NRCT. The next largest register represented is that of the USA Surveillance, Epidemiology and End Results (SEER) Program, a large inter-state collaborative study initiated in 1972 and covering about 10% of the US population. Indeed, the US registers as a whole account for more cases in the aggregate than the CCRG over the decade considered, though coverage of the country as a whole is far from complete.

Examination of the rates in Table 18.1 with their standard errors reveals substantial differences which cannot be accounted for in terms of sampling error. Although some of these may be due to differences in methods of ascertainment, it seems certain that there are substantial residual differences which cannot be explained in this way.

Table 18.2 compares the rates between registers in certain groups, cross-referenced by index number to Table 18.1, showing a weighted mean and the result of a formal test of significance (based on a chi-square test of the differences between the rates). It will be seen, for example, that the rates for the registers in the UK are quite comparable; their mean of 37.5 ± 0.58 per annum may be considered to provide a benchmark for a predominantly white caucasian population.

Comparison with North American rates reveals a rather higher rate in Canada, the difference between the Atlantic and Western provinces being just significant. Among the (non-Hispanic) whites of the four US registers, the rates are rather higher still (though not

Table 18.2 Comparisons between groups of registers with pooled means and tests for intra-group differences

Comparison	Reference no.*	Mean (SE) (ASR)	Deviance χ^2	p
England and Wales vs. Scotland	43 44	37.5 (0.58)	0.04	0.84
UK and Canada	1 2 43 44	38.2 (0.54)	11.6	0.01
Canada	1 2	41.9 (1.45)	3.6	0.06
USA, Non-Hispanic White	3 7 8 10	44.6 (0.74)	5.8	0.12
Los Angeles	6 7	49.0 (1.82)	0.3	0.59
USA, All White	3 6 7 8 10	45.0 (0.72)	9.5	0.05
South/Central America	12 : 19	31.9 (0.62)	103.1	0.000
Brazil	12 : 14	31.6 (1.09)	14.8	0.000
Caribbean	17 : 19	30.7 (0.78)	33.5	0.000
Latin Europe	48 53	48.6 (2.35)	0.2	0.64
Europe	35 : 54	38.1 (0.35)	117.8	0.000
West Europe mainland, Non-Latin	36 : 41 47 : 49 52 : 53	41.3 (0.61)	22.2	0.014
East Europe, Non-Latin	35 39 42 45 50	35.9 (0.77)	16.9	0.002

*Refer to Table 18.1.

significantly so) but similar to one another ($\chi^2 = 5.8$, 3 d.f.); their mean is 44.6 ± 0.74. Although the rate in the Hispanic whites of Los Angeles (50.2 ± 2.83, Table 18.1) is higher than that for other US whites (44.6 ± 0.74), the difference is not quite significant (SE $= 2.92$, $p = 0.055$).

This rate is in fact only matched by that in Costa Rica, the highest rate recorded in the IARC volume; the latter is tentatively attributed by Linet and Devesa (1991) to the use of high levels of agricultural chemicals in the flower production industry, though not all commentators accept this explanation (Stiller and Parkin 1996). Although rates in the other four South and Central American registers (nos 12–15) are no higher than for other white populations, the variability of the Brazilian rates is suggestive of inconsistent ascertainment and it is interesting that the two highest rates in Europe are recorded in two small registries in Italy and Spain.

The rates in the US registers for blacks, on the other hand, are clearly indicative of a marked ethnic difference. Unfortunately, the African registries in the IARC volume do not have population data adequate for the calculation of absolute rates. It is therefore not possible to determine the rates in predominantly black populations with any precision, though age-standardised rates calculated for Ibadan, Kampala, and Bulawayo using outdated census information are all under 20 per million per annum—even smaller than for American blacks. Comparisons involving African populations would in any case be difficult because of very different patterns of child mortality in developing countries. Most authors have concluded that leukaemia rates in blacks of African origin are indeed lower than in whites and there are clear differences in the patterns of occurrence of different histological types and age distributions (Stiller and Parkin 1996). Other countries which exhibit interesting differences between ethnic groups covered by the same registry include Kuwait and New Zealand.

The rates for mainland Europe are variable to a degree that is certainly not due to sampling errors, even if we exclude the Italian and Spanish registers ($\chi^2 = 69.1$, 15 d.f.). The main feature is the difference between West and East European countries ($\chi^2 = 5.4$, 1 d.f., $p = 0.02$) and the variability of the latter ($\chi^2 = 16.9$, 4 d.f., $p = 0.002$), an observation suggestive of incomplete ascertainment.

18.3   Regional variation in the United Kingdom

We now turn our attention to variation at an intermediate geographical scale using data from the NRCT relating to England and Wales. The size of this single register provides a good opportunity to examine the degree of heterogeneity and the factors affecting the leukaemia risk. The nature and sources of the data have been described by Stiller *et al.* (1991); we have, however, updated the year range considered in this volume from 1966–83 to 1969–88.

There are clearly many different sub-groups that could be analysed, but, partly in the light of the experience of previous analyses (Draper *et al.* 1991), we will restrict our attention to the analysis of registration rates for: (a) all leukaemias under 15 years of age: and (b) ALL in the age range 1 to 4 years. In our subsequent analyses of the former, we used the numbers of registrations under 15 years of age and referred them to an effective population size based on the age-standardised rates (i.e. direct standardisation was used) to eliminate the effect of atypical age distributions; in practice, the results were very similar to those based on the actual 0–14 population, equivalent to using crude registration rates. In (b), the group chosen reflected experience from previous studies, in which the effect of social class on the risk has been observed to be strongest for young children with ALL, while registrations in the first year of life include a number of infant cases whose aetiology is thought to be distinct (Greaves 1997). We examine first the variation at county level.

Table 18.3a shows (first four columns) the age-standardised rate for all leukaemias by county, its rank order, the numbers of cases on which it is based and its standard error. Treating the rates as being approximately normally distributed, we can compute a heterogeneity chi-square statistic of 69.1 with 54 d.f., which is not significant at the 5% level ($p = 0.08$).

Table 18.3a Childhood leukaemia (ages 0–14) by county in England and Wales, 1969–88. Age-standardised rates (with standard errors), their rank order, the numbers of cases, and adjusted rates using an empirical Bayes shrinkage towards the mean (see text)

	ASR	Order	No. cases	SE ASR	Adj. rate	SE Adj. rate
County: England						
Inner London	36.6	23	371	1.90	36.98	1.25
Outer London	37.5	28	647	1.47	37.40	1.10
Greater Manchester	37.3	26	436	1.79	37.29	1.22
Merseyside	33.5	10	231	2.20	35.90	1.33
South Yorkshire	40.4	37	226	2.69	38.15	1.42
Tyne and Wear	41.4	44	202	2.91	38.30	1.45
West Midlands	36.8	24	446	1.74	37.05	1.21
West Yorkshire	34.2	15	311	1.94	35.97	1.26
Avon	41.2	43	154	3.32	38.07	1.49
Bedfordshire	36.0	20	85	3.90	37.08	1.53
Berkshire	41.6	46	127	3.69	38.01	1.52
Buckinghamshire	45.8	53	116	4.25	38.42	1.55
Cambridgeshire	39.1	31	97	3.97	37.55	1.54
Cheshire	34.9	16	144	2.91	36.69	1.45
Cleveland	35.0	17	96	3.57	36.87	1.51
Cornwall	44.5	51	72	5.24	37.94	1.59
Cumbria	37.5	29	73	4.39	37.31	1.56
Derbyshire	40.2	36	153	3.25	37.89	1.48
Devon	38.6	30	138	3.29	37.55	1.49
Dorset	39.6	34	82	4.37	37.58	1.56
Durham	33.2	8	85	3.60	36.56	1.51
East Sussex	32.5	6	72	3.83	36.52	1.53
Essex	36.2	21	228	2.40	36.93	1.37
Gloucestershire	41.1	42	86	4.43	37.76	1.56
Hampshire	35.8	19	226	2.38	36.79	1.37
Hereford & Worcester	36.5	22	97	3.71	37.15	1.52
Hertfordshire	33.1	7	137	2.83	36.20	1.44
Humberside	31.5	4	119	2.89	35.83	1.44
Isle of Wight	34.0	13	14	9.09	37.17	1.64

Table 18.3a *(cont.)*

	ASR	Order	No. cases	SE ASR	Adj. rate	SE Adj. rate
Kent	40.4	38	251	2.55	38.22	1.40
Lancashire	33.9	12	196	2.42	36.19	1.37
Leicestershire	37.4	27	139	3.17	37.31	1.48
Lincolnshire	43.3	49	97	4.40	38.04	1.56
Norfolk	40.8	39	111	3.87	37.83	1.53
Northamptonshire	44.8	52	106	4.35	38.25	1.56
Northumberland	29.8	1	36	4.97	36.52	1.58
North Yorkshire	41.8	47	109	4.00	37.95	1.54
Nottinghamshire	33.8	11	144	2.82	36.38	1.44
Oxfordshire	39.1	32	89	4.14	37.54	1.55
Shropshire	41.4	45	67	5.06	37.69	1.58
Somerset	36.8	25	62	4.67	37.23	1.57
Staffordshire	39.4	33	175	2.98	37.79	1.46
Suffolk	41.0	40	103	4.04	37.82	1.54
Surrey	44.4	50	177	3.34	38.70	1.49
Warwickshire	42.6	48	87	4.57	37.91	1.57
West Sussex	41.0	41	100	4.10	37.81	1.55
Wiltshire	48.5	54	111	4.60	38.58	1.57
County: Wales						
Clwyd	35.3	18	58	4.64	37.05	1.57
Dyfed	33.4	9	44	5.04	36.90	1.58
Gwent	39.8	35	76	4.57	37.58	1.57
Gwynedd	34.0	14	32	6.01	37.05	1.61
Mid Glamorgan	31.2	3	75	3.60	36.21	1.51
Powys	51.2	55	22	0.92	37.60	1.65
South Glamorgan	32.4	5	54	4.41	36.67	1.56
West Glamorgan	30.9	2	47	4.51	36.51	1.56
Total/mean E&W	37.3	–	7839	0.42	37.4	0.50

The weighted mean of the rates is 37.3 ± 0.42. However, even though there appears not to be significant variation, it is likely that there is a natural underlying variation and it may be regarded as appropriate in these circumstances to adjust this figure to take account of this natural variability. This random-effects approach was done using the method of moments to estimate the component of variance due to inter-county variation. In effect we now estimate the mean of the population of county means from which our sample may be considered to have been drawn; this approach gives a slightly adjusted mean of 37.4 ± 0.50, the importance of the adjustment lying in the increased standard error of the estimate.

A similar philosophy underlies the empirical Bayes (EB) approach advocated by Clayton and Kaldor (1987) and now gaining ground (see Chapter 7); here, we argue that the natural variability in the true underlying risks makes it sensible to use information about the overall mean rate to 'shrink' the county rates towards it, effectively damping out the effect of the sampling error in the county rates. The last two columns of Table 18.3a show this adjustment, using an analysis based on the normal distribution, rather than the Poisson approach described by Clayton and Kaldor. It will be seen that all the rates are moved substantially in the direction of the overall mean, while their standard errors have been decreased, to take account of the extra certainty resulting from the use of the overall mean. Which set of estimates should be quoted is a matter of interpretation, but the EB rates are frequently used nowadays and they arguably provide a better estimate of the risk in individual counties. This changes the rank order of areas, such that, for example, Northumberland, which has the lowest rates in the age-standardised analysis, becomes ninth equal ranked in the EB analysis.

Table 18.3b shows the same rates for the other tumour group under consideration, namely ALL at age 1–4 years. Here there is, as expected, appreciably more variation, the heterogeneity chi-square statistic being 90.6. For example, the rates for Gwynedd are shrunk a long way towards the mean of the EB estimation.

Table 18.3b Acute lymphocytic leukaemia (ALL) in children aged 1–4 years by county in England and Wales, 1969–88. Registration rates (with standard errors), their rank order, the numbers of cases, and adjusted rates using an empirical Bayes shrinkage towards the mean (see text)

	Rate	Order	No. cases	SE ASR	Adj. rate	SE Adj. rate
County: England						
Inner London	57.2	30	154	4.61	57.13	3.73
Outer London	59.3	32	267	3.63	58.73	3.15
Greater Manchester	58.8	31	178	4.41	58.21	3.62
Merseyside	49.7	10	86	5.36	52.75	4.09
South Yorkshire	68.2	45	98	6.89	62.13	4.66
Tyne and Wear	79.4	52	99	7.98	65.65	4.96
West Midlands	49.7	11	155	3.99	51.78	3.38
West Yorkshire	55.9	25	132	4.87	56.31	3.86
Avon	63.5	35	61	8.13	59.46	4.99
Bedfordshire	52.6	18	33	9.15	55.58	5.20
Berkshire	65.2	39	52	9.04	59.70	5.18
Buckinghamshire	65.5	40	43	9.99	59.44	5.35
Cambridgeshire	91.3	55	60	1.79	64.68	5.58
Cheshire	45.8	8	48	6.61	51.65	4.57
Cleveland	35.9	2	25	7.18	47.79	4.75
Cornwall	69.7	46	29	2.95	59.45	5.69
Cumbria	70.3	47	35	1.88	59.94	5.59
Derbyshire	65.1	38	64	8.14	60.06	5.00
Devon	66.6	43	61	8.53	60.41	5.08
Dorset	64.1	36	34	0.99	58.77	5.48
Durham	55.0	23	36	9.17	56.36	5.21
East Sussex	42.5	4	24	8.67	51.97	5.11
Essex	56.8	29	93	5.89	56.90	4.31
Gloucestershire	56.6	27	30	0.34	56.90	5.40
Hampshire	52.0	16	85	5.64	54.22	4.21
Hereford & Worcester	52.3	17	36	8.72	55.38	5.12
Hertfordshire	43.1	5	45	6.43	50.16	4.51
Humberside	53.1	19	51	7.43	55.36	4.82

Table 18.3b *(cont.)*

	Rate	Order	No. cases	SE ASR	Adj. rate	SE Adj. rate
Isle of Wight	48.1	9	5	1.51	56.30	6.07
Kent	71.2	48	15	6.64	63.76	4.58
Lancashire	51.2	12	76	5.87	53.89	4.31
Leicestershire	56.7	28	55	7.65	56.88	4.87
Lincolnshire	62.5	34	36	0.41	58.49	5.41
Norfolk	68.1	44	48	9.83	60.26	5.32
Northamptonshire	66.1	41	41	0.32	59.49	5.39
Northumberland	51.6	14	16	2.90	55.96	5.68
North Yorkshire	64.7	37	43	9.87	59.25	5.33
Nottinghamshire	54.0	20	59	7.03	55.66	4.70
Oxfordshire	66.1	42	39	0.59	59.40	5.43
Shropshire	74.1	51	31	3.31	60.16	5.71
Somerset	55.3	24	24	1.28	56.60	5.52
Staffordshire	60.5	33	70	7.23	58.52	4.76
Suffolk	51.5	13	34	8.83	55.14	5.14
Surrey	72.4	50	73	8.48	62.52	5.07
Warwickshire	88.5	54	47	2.91	63.11	5.68
West Sussex	45.2	7	28	8.55	52.83	5.09
Wiltshire	80.4	53	48	1.61	62.37	5.56
County: Wales						
Clwyd	54.9	22	23	1.45	56.51	5.54
Dyfed	39.5	3	13	0.95	52.62	5.48
Gwent	71.5	49	35	2.08	60.13	5.61
Gwynedd	33.6	1	8	1.89	51.84	5.59
Mid Glamorgan	43.4	6	27	8.35	52.04	5.04
Powys	56.4	26	6	3.02	56.96	6.10
South Glamorgan	54.0	21	23	1.26	56.28	5.52
West Glamorgan	51.8	15	20	1.58	55.81	5.55
Total/mean E&W	57.0	–	3057	1.03	57.70	1.43

It has been found in previous analyses (Draper *et al.* 1991; Bithell *et al.* 1995) that at least some of this variability may be explained by an association between childhood leukaemia and socio-economic status though, unusually for childhood illnesses, the risk is higher in higher socio-economic groups. We accordingly modelled the probability of leukaemia as a function of ecological variables describing the social class structure of the different geographical units. However, we used the data relating to the 403 county districts in England and Wales, partly because the higher level of geographical resolution provides extra power and partly for convenience, in that the variables are easily available at this level.

Looking first at the rates for all leukaemias (Table 18.4a), we find again that there is a degree of variation only slightly greater than would be expected by chance (residual deviance = 449.1, 402 d.f., $p = 0.056$). We fitted the Carstairs index (Morris and Carstairs 1992), the degree of urbanisation and the population density, both as single linear terms in the model and also as factors defined by their quintiles. It will be seen from the analyses

Table 18.4a Analysis of deviance for all leukaemias aged 0–14 years, fitting socio-economic variables and county of registration

Model	Residual deviance	d.f.	Deviance due to last term	d.f.
Null	449.1	402	–	–
Carstairs index	434.3	401	14.8	1
Carstairs quintiles	430.9	398	18.2	4
C index + quintiles	426.8	397	6.5	4
Null	449.1	402	–	–
Urban class	436.7	401	12.4	1
C index + quintiles	435.6	397	1.1	4
Null	449.1	402	–	–
Density	443.9	401	5.2	1
C index + quintiles	436.6	397	7.3	4
All above terms	420.5	387	28.6	15
Null	449.1	402	–	–
County	378.6	348	70.5	54
Carstairs index	373.8	347	4.8	1

of deviance in Table 18.4a that the Carstairs index achieves a significant reduction in the deviance ($\chi^2 = 14.8$, 1 d.f.); so too does fitting the quintiles ($\chi^2 = 18.2$, 4 d.f.), though the latter produces only a marginal improvement in fit of the model after fitting the linear term. A similar pattern is observed for the other two variables, though in the case of the degree of urbanisation the quintiles achieve virtually no additional reduction, suggesting that the relationship is very close to linear. It will be seen that the Carstairs index is the variable achieving the best fit when fitted singly. Fitting all the variables achieves a rather modest reduction in deviance after the Carstairs index and it would seem to be satisfactory to use only the latter index in the model. The fit can be improved by fitting the set of 55 counties of England and Wales as a factor and the last three rows of Table 18.4a give the results of doing so. The deviance difference attributable to counties is 70.5 with 54 d.f., which approaches statistical significance ($p = 0.066$). The effect of fitting the Carstairs index, while still significant ($p = 0.029$), is much reduced, indicating that the differences between counties are partly due to the effect of socio-economic differences. The overall fit is now better, with a residual deviance of 373.8 on 347 d.f. ($p = 0.15$).

For ALL at age 1–4 years, the deviance is 475.0 with 402 d.f., a result which is statistically significant ($p < 0.01$). Table 18.4b shows the effect of fitting the ecological variables as before and it will be seen that the effects of these variables are rather less pronounced, at least in terms of statistical significance. This may be due to the smaller number of cases. The relative strengths of the associations with the different variables are the same as for the all leukaemias case and the Carstairs index provides an adequate representation of the socio-economic variables available. The differences between counties are now more pronounced ($\chi^2 = 91.8$, 54 d.f., $p = 0.001$); the effect of the Carstairs index is again reduced by fitting the counties first, though still significant ($p = 0.022$) and the final fit is not significantly bad ($\chi^2 = 378.0$, $p = 0.12$). Fitting the Carstairs index before

Table 18.4b Analysis of deviance for all acute lymphocytic leukaemias (ALL) aged 1–4 years, fitting socio-economic variables and county of registration

Model	Residual deviance	d.f.	Deviance due to last term	d.f.
Null	475.0	402	–	–
Carstairs index	465.7	401	9.3	1
C index + quintiles	464.4	397	1.3	4
Null	475.0	402	–	–
Urban class	469.1	401	5.9	1
C index + quintiles	468.3	397	0.8	4
Null	475.0	402	–	–
Density	471.5	401	3.5	1
C index + quintiles	468.5	397	3.0	4
Null	475.0	402	–	–
All above terms	461.1	387	13.3	15
Null	475.0	402	–	–
County	383.2	348	91.8	54
Carstairs index	378.0	347	5.2	1

the counties gives a deviance reduction due to the latter of 87.7 on 54 d.f. ($p = 0.002$), indicating that there are important between-county differences that are not explained by the Carstairs index. We have a picture therefore of moderately important differences at county level, associated with but not fully explained by socio-economic status, while within counties the districts are relatively homogeneous, though such heterogeneity as exists may be explained by the socio-economic score. These results are closely in line with the results of the modelling described in Draper *et al.* (1991), which we should expect because of the overlap of the periods and consequently of the actual datasets.

18.4   Local-scale geographical variation

Finally, we look at geographical variation at a local scale, again using UK data, but now with a rather different dataset already available at ward level. This set covers all leukaemia and non-Hodgkin's lymphomas (NHL) aged 0–14 years and was constructed for a major study of the risk near nuclear installations (Bithell *et al.* 1994). It takes the form of counts of children in the 9836 wards or equivalent units registered anywhere in Britain in the years 1966–87. The counts are paired with expectations which were computed using data on the populations at risk and also socio-economic ecological variables similar to those described above. Log-linear modelling was used to obtain good models for different sub-groups of the data and the fitted values from these models were used to define the expectations for the various analyses subsequently performed. Further details of the construction of this dataset can be found in Bithell *et al.* (1994) and an associated technical report. As before, we confine the present analysis to the 8801 geographical units located in England or Wales.

In comparing these observed values with their expectations, various possible measures of the discrepancies may be used. The one we favour is the 'deviance contribution', defined by

$$D = 2(e_i - X_i + X_i \log(X_i|e_i)),$$

which is the contribution each unit would make to the log of the likelihood of the data under the assumption that the observations X_i are independent Poisson variates with the computed expectations e_i. An analysis of these deviance contributions for the NRCT dataset reveals that the largest such contribution is due to the village of Seascale near the Sellafield nuclear reprocessing plant; the value of D is 18.7, corresponding to an observed count of 6 cases and an expectation of 0.51. This is to be expected, since this ward was known to have a large excess of cases. The ten largest contributions are shown in Table 18.5 and it will be seen that Seascale stands out as being unequalled in England and Wales in the degree of the excess.

The overall deviance (i.e. the sum of the contributions from the different wards) is likewise a good measure of the extent to which the underlying risks vary. Since the expectations have been constrained to sum to the same value as the observed counts, namely 10 194, the observed value (9113.3) could be compared approximately with a chi-square statistic on 8800 d.f. ($p < 0.01$) were it not for the fact that the expectations are too small for the appropriate asymptotic theory to hold. (The fact that the expectations have been calculated 'internally' using the log-linear model referred to above may be expected to reduce the number of degrees of freedom somewhat, though in a complicated fashion; it would seem likely, however, that this should make only a marginal difference to the interpretation with so many units in the dataset.)

Table 18.5 The ten wards in England and Wales with the biggest discrepancies between observed and expected numbers of childhood leukaemias (0–14) as judged by the deviance or log likelihood. The ordering by the observed significance level (testing the null hypothesis with the Poisson distribution) for the first ten wards is the same as for the deviance contribution

No. cases	Expected no.	Deviance contrib.	Poisson prob.
6	0.506	18.68	0.000015
4	0.266	14.21	0.000169
4	0.274	14.00	0.000188
6	0.867	12.95	0.000281
5	0.574	12.79	0.000324
6	0.940	12.13	0.000430
5	0.678	11.34	0.000682
4	0.404	11.15	0.000805
6	1.092	10.63	0.000934
7	1.527	10.37	0.001024

We can address the question of how significant these results are by 'boot-strapping', or simulating from the underlying Poisson distributions. In practice, we use the multinomial distribution instead, to ensure that the observed counts are constrained as before to sum to 10 194. In a run of 1000 simulations the largest deviance exceeded the observed value of 18.7 in 48 samples, giving an estimated *p*-value of 0.048. In the same run, the simulated value of the total deviance exceeded the observed value in 32 samples, yielding an estimated *p*-value of 0.032.

Rerunning the simulation without Seascale, the estimated *p*-values were 0.40 for the largest deviance contribution and 0.054 for the total deviance.

18.5   Discussion

Interest in the geographical variation in incidence rates of childhood leukaemia is centred partly on the aetiological mechanisms that might be suggested by such variation and partly on the supposed tendency for cases to cluster. The most important distinction between these two phenomena is that we expect variation of risk to apply throughout a given region, while clustering may be localised to only a single location. It follows that the former is best assessed by using tests for heterogeneity or overdispersion, while for the latter tests looking for extremes may be more appropriate. Alternatively, a hierarchical model with heterogeneity and clustering components may be fitted (see Chapter 7).

Our analyses above suggest that there is appreciably more variation of incidence at international level than at the smaller geographical scales of study. Notwithstanding the caveats about differences of ascertainment, the comparatively large variations between different ethnic groups—of the order of two- to threefold variation—are clearly of aetiological interest. It seems likely that genetic differences probably go a long way towards furnishing an explanation, though it would be very hard to quantify this extent. At county level within the UK the variation is much less marked; the deviances in Table 18.4 are consistent with an unexplained variation in relative risk for all leukaemias having a standard deviation between 5% and 8%; for ALL at age 1–4 years the corresponding figures are 10–15%. The level of significance achieved for the dispersion throughout the small-area dataset is indicative of even less important variation at this geographical level.

It must be admitted that merely looking at the dispersion of rates in small areas does not provide a powerful procedure for picking up clustering. A large value of the maximum deviance occurring in a particular small-area could be indicative of clustering, but would be sensitive to it only at one particular scale. We should be wary, therefore, of interpreting the small-area analysis described above as providing much evidence against clustering. On the other hand, analyses using more appropriate tests on the dataset described in Stiller *et al.* (1991) found rather little evidence of widespread clustering (Alexander 1991); see Bithell (1998) for a fuller discussion of the evidence relating to the clustering of childhood leukaemia.

We conclude that geographical variations in childhood leukaemia incidence are generally not as great as is sometimes supposed, and that such as do occur may be due as much to genetic differences as to environmental ones. Certainly, the totality of the evidence relating apparent clusters or variations in risk to a clear aetiological mechanism is very slender. Nevertheless, the possibility remains that better data collection may reveal some important clue to the aetiology and prevention of the disease and interest in the subject is likely to persist.

References

Alexander, F. E. (1991). Investigations of localised spatial clustering, and extra-Poisson variation. In *The geographical epidemiology of childhood leukaemia and non-Hodgkin lymphomas in Great Britain, 1966–83* (G. Draper, ed.), 69–76. Studies on Medical and Population Subjects 53. HMSO, London.

Bithell, J. F. (1998). Leukaemia clusters. In *Encyclopaedia of Biostatistics* (P. Armitage, and T. Colton, ed.). Wiley, New York.

Bithell, J. F., Dutton, S. J., Draper, G. J., and Neary, N. M. (1994). The distribution of childhood leukaemias and non-Hodgkin's lymphomas near nuclear installations in England and Wales. *British Medical Journal*, **309**, 501–5.

Bithell, J. F., Dutton, S. J., Neary, N. M., and Vincent, T. J. (1995). Controlling for socio-economic confounding using regression methods. *Journal of Epidemiology and Community Health*, **49** (Suppl. 2), S15–S19.

Cartwright, R. A., Alexander, F. E., McKinney, P. A., and Ricketts, T. J. (1990). *Leukaemia and lymphoma: an atlas of distribution within areas of England and Wales 1984–1988.* Leukaemia Research Fund, London.

Clayton, D. and Kaldor, J. (1987). Empirical Bayes estimates of age-standardized relative risks for use in disease mapping. *Biometrics*, **43**, 671–82.

Doll, R. and Wakeford, R. (1997). Risk of childhood cancer from fetal irradiation. *British Journal of Radiology*, **70**, 130–9.

Draper, G. (ed.) (1991). *The geographical epidemiology of childhood leukaemia and non-Hodgkin lymphomas in Great Britain, 1966–83.* Studies on Medical and Population Subjects, 53. HMSO, London.

Draper, G. J. (1995) Cancer. In *The health of our children*, (B. Botting ed.), 135–47. HMSO, London.

Draper, G. J., Vincent, T. J., O'Connor, C. M., and Stiller, C. A. (1991). Socio-economic factors and variations in incidence rates between County Districts. In *The geographical epidemiology of childhood leukaemia and non-Hodgkin lymphomas in Great Britain, 1966–83.* (G. Draper, ed.), 37–45. Studies on Medical and Population Subjects 53. HMSO, London.

Draper, G. J., Sanders, B. M., Lennox, E. L., and Brownbill, P. A. (1996). Patterns of childhood cancer among siblings. *British Journal of Cancer*, **74**, 152–8.

Fedrick, J. and Alberman, E. D. (1972). Reported influenza in pregnancy and subsequent cancer in the child. *British Medical Journal*, **ii**, 485–8.

Greaves, M. F. (1997). Aetiology of acute leukaemia. *Lancet*, **349**, 344–9.

Kinlen, L. J. (1995). Epidemiological evidence for an infective basis in childhood leukaemia. *British Journal of Cancer*, **71**, 1–5.

Kneale, G. W. (1971). Excess sensitivity of pre-leukaemics to pneumonia. *British Journal of Preventive and Social Medicine*, **25**, 152–9.

Linet, M. S. and Devesa, S. S. (1991). Descriptive epidemiology of childhood leukaemia. *British Journal of Cancer*, **63**, 424–9.

McBride, M. L. (1998) Childhood cancer and environmental contaminants. *Canadian Journal of Public Health*, **89**, S53–S62.

Morris, R. and Carstairs, V. (1992). Which deprivation? A comparison of selected deprivation indices. *Journal of Public Health Medicine*, **13**, 318–26.

Parkin, D. M., Stiller, C. A., Draper, G. J., Bieber, C. A., Terracini, B., and Young, J. L. (1988a). *International incidence of childhood cancer*, International Agency for Research on Cancer Scientific Publications. IARC, Lyon.

Parkin, D. M., Stiller, C. A., Draper, G. J., and Bieber, C. A. (1988b). The international incidence of childhood cancer. *International Journal of Cancer*, **42**, 511–20.

Preston, D. L., Kusumi, S., Tomonaga, M., Izumi, S., Ron, E., Kuramoto, A. *et al.* (1994). Cancer incidence in atomic bomb survivors. Part III: leukemia, lymphoma and multiple myeloma, 1950–1987. *Radiation Research*, **137**, S68–S97.

Shore, R. E., Pasternack, B. S., and McCrea Curnen, M. G. (1976). Relating influenza epidemics to childhood leukemia in tumor registries without a defined population base: a critique with suggestions for improved methods. *American Journal of Epidemiology*, **103**, 527–35.

Stiller, C. A. and Parkin, D. M. (1996). Geographic and ethnic variations in the incidence of childhood cancer. *British Medical Bulletin*, **52**, 682–703.

Stiller, C. A., O'Connor, C. M., Vincent, T. J., and Draper, G. J. (1991). The National Registry of Childhood Tumours and the leukaemia/lymphoma data for 1966–83. In *The Geographical Epidemiology of Childhood Leukaemia and non-Hodgkin Lymphomas in Great Britain, 1966–83.* (G. Draper ed.), 69–76. Studies on Medical and Population Subjects 53. HMSO, London.

Weiss, H. A., Darby, S. C., Fearn, T., and Doll, R. (1995). Leukemia mortality after X-ray treatment for ankylosing spondylitis. *Radiation Research*, **142**, 1–11.

Zipursky, A., Poon, A., and Doyle, J. (1992). Leukemia in Down syndrome: a review. *Pediatric Hematology and Oncology*, **9**, 139–49.

IV   Exposure and the link to health

19. Exposure assessment

D. J. Briggs

19.1 Introduction

Exposure assessment is an important tool both for epidemiological research and as an aid to health risk protection, policy development, and decision-making. Accurate information on levels and patterns of exposure is essential, for example, in the search for associations between environment and health, and to quantify the dose-response relationships found. It is vital, also, to translate knowledge of such relationships into assessments of risk across the population, for example as a basis for policy-targeting and priority-setting. It is required, equally, to provide early warnings of potential health effects, to evaluate and compare the possible effects of policy or other interventions, to monitor the impacts and effectiveness of policy, and to help inform the public of health risks and support advice on risk avoidance or risk minimisation strategies.

The concept of exposure is nevertheless somewhat elusive and difficult to define. Many definitions specify exposure in terms of 'contact' between an environmental agent (e.g. a pollutant) and the human body. The National Academy of Science (1991), for example, defines exposure as: 'an event that occurs when there is contact at a boundary between a human and the environment with a contaminant of a specific concentration for an interval of time'. Such definitions are certainly widely applicable, especially to environmental pollution: they can thus be applied to most of the examples used elsewhere in this book. They may also be applied to many physical hazards (e.g. flooding, avalanches, or accidents) where direct contact is clearly involved. They are less appropriate, however, to those environmental hazards, such as famine, which affect health more by omission than commission. It is similarly difficult to apply these definitions to many psychological and perceptual health effects that may be generated by the fear, rather than the eventuality, of a hazard (e.g. stress or anxiety caused by fear of exposure to radiation from a nuclear power station, or of physical injury from war).

These definitions are also of limited relevance when health is considered in the broader sense of positive well-being, rather than merely ill-health, as promoted by the World Health Organisation. In this context, aesthetic and perceptual, as well as physical, qualities of the environment—to which individuals may be exposed only remotely or visually—assume importance. Although such exposures may be associated with relatively 'soft', non-clinical health effects, they are none the less significant, not only in terms of the number of people involved, but also in terms of the importance given to them by the public.

For all these reasons, a looser definition of exposure may often need to be applied, which recognises what might be termed 'virtual' environmental encounters, for example, through contact with information about the hazard rather than the hazard itself.

This is not to argue either for fuzzy thinking or lack of precision. In whatever context exposures are being considered, they need to be analysed rigorously, since errors in exposure assessment, however defined, may seriously weaken or bias epidemiological findings (see Chapter 5) and distort or impair policy response. Indeed, it can be argued with some justification that uncertainties in exposure assessment remain one of the major constraints on both environmental epidemiology and effective environmental health protection. The need is to define exposure clearly and precisely in relation to the environmental factors and health outcomes of concern.

19.2   Exposure pathways and processes

Exposure to any environmental hazard or event can occur as a result of many different sources, processes and pathways. Figure 19.1 presents a simple model of the links involved for the example of environmental pollution. Human activities generate pollutants which are emitted into the environment from a variety of different sources. These pollutants are then dispersed via different media and different pathways—for example, in the atmosphere, in ground and surface waters, in the soil, by food. En route, they are subject to a range of processes—including chemical reactions, sorting by size, shape, or mass, deposition and impaction, abrasion, and decay—which change both the character of the pollutants and the environmental concentrations which thereby accumulate. Humans then encounter these pollutants either as they move through or reside within the resulting pollution field, or as they use environmental materials. Exposures mainly occur by three processes: dermal contact, inhalation, or ingestion. Different stages of exposure can thus be seen, depending upon the extent of entry into the body and the specificity of the site concerned. External exposure refers to external contact with the pollutant; the absorbed dose refers to that proportion of the pollutant that enters the body; the target dose is that portion which reaches the human organs where the relevant health effect occurs. These exposures may subsequently lead to a range of health effects, from early and less intense sub-clinical effects, to clinically detectable morbidity and ultimately mortality.

Several important points emerge from this model of exposure. The first is the multiplicity of the processes involved. Exposures may derive from many different sources, both now and in the past. These include not only human activities, such as those depicted in Fig. 19.1, but also natural processes, such as weathering and release of materials from rocks (e.g. radon). Many different pollutants may also be released, which then follow complex and intersecting pathways through the environment. The resulting environmental pollution fields are consequently extremely varied and complex in terms both of their spatial and temporal distribution and their composition. Different individuals, with different time-activity patterns, will encounter these pollutants to differing degrees. Exposures are therefore likely to vary enormously over time and space and between individuals in any population. Exposure assessment thus faces severe methodological challenges.

There arises from this a second implication: that exposures can be parameterised in a wide variety of ways, each of which is liable to give a different picture of exposure levels and histories. They might, for example, be assessed in terms of individual pollutant species, or pollutant mixes; characterised by specific media or pathways (e.g. air or food), or in terms of total exposures; quantified in terms of magnitude ('burden'), frequency, or

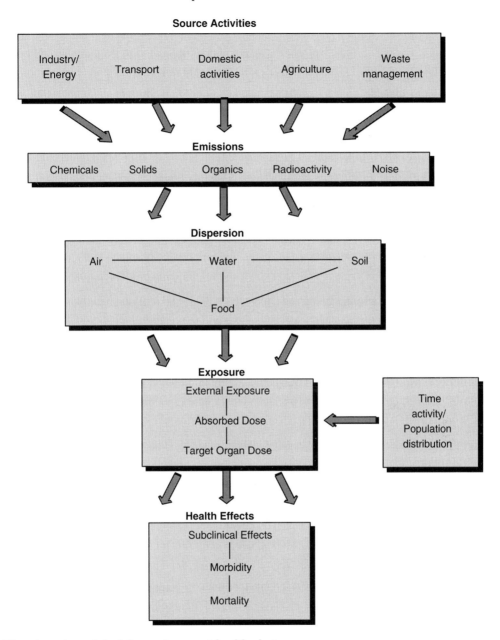

Fig. 19.1 A model of the environment-health chain.

duration; or expressed as lifetime exposures, time-specific exposures, extreme exposures, cumulative exposures above a threshold level, or in many other ways. Which of these is appropriate is likely to depend on the health outcome of concern, the aetiological hypothesis underlying the environmental health risk, the purpose of the analysis, and the available data. What is clear is that different measures will, in many cases, show different patterns of variation across the study population or group, reflecting their different spatial and temporal distributions. Choice of exposure measure may thus have a major influence on the results of any study, although the choice may be limited by the availability of appropriate methodology, and by the resources available to the study.

A third point to emerge from Fig. 19.1 is that exposure may be both assessed and controlled at different points within the environment-health chain: for example, at source, at point of emission, in the open environment, or at point of exposure. In terms of policy and management, different control strategies may be envisaged at different points in this chain (Fig. 19.2). Measures, such as land use policy, selective taxation, or constraints on manufacturing processes, can be used to control source activities. Legislation establishing emission limits or the introduction of clean technologies can restrict releases into the

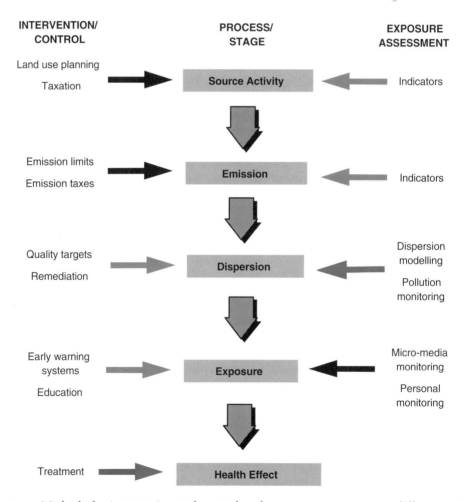

Fig. 19.2 Methods for intervention and control and exposure assessment at different points in the environment-health chain. (*Note:* the density of the horizontal arrows indicates the effectiveness of the method.)

environment. Quality standards may be applied to set targets for environmental con-centrations, and clean-up operations may be used to reduce pollution levels after the event. Educational programmes, early-warning systems, and awareness-raising measures may be used to encourage the public to reduce exposures, either by avoiding polluted environments or by changes in lifestyle. Ultimately, medical intervention may be used after exposure to reduce the target dose or mitigate the health effects (e.g. the use of iodide tablets to minimise the effects of radiation exposure).

The effectiveness of intervening at these different points of control varies considerably, both in terms of the ability to prevent adverse health effects and cost. Generally, upstream interventions (e.g. aimed at source activity or emissions) are likely to be the more effective in reducing health risk, since they are preventative and typically act across the entire population. In contrast, late interventions may not reach many of the individuals at risk. Awareness-raising campaigns and early-warning systems, for example, are often ignored, or not encountered, by large groups of the population—often those who intrinsi-cally are most at risk because of their limited access to resources and information and their specific lifestyle. Action at source, however, often carries a relatively high economic and social cost, for it may involve substantial and far-reaching changes in industrial processes and competitiveness, and may ultimately threaten jobs. Legislation to limit industrial processes or to control emissions may also be seen as anti-competitive, and may thus fall foul of international agreements on freedom of trade (e.g. the Single Market in the European Union, or—as is being demonstrated in relation to genetically modified foods—the World Trade Organisation).

The effectiveness and feasibility of assessing exposures also vary between these dif-ferent points in the environment-health chain (Fig. 19.2). In general, it may be expected that the most reliable assessments occur at the point of exposure (e.g. by measuring external exposures of absorbed dose). In practice, direct assessments of exposure in this way are often difficult due to their potential intrusiveness and cost. Commonly, therefore, expos-ures are assessed at earlier points in the environment-health chain: for example, on the basis of measured or modelled pollution levels, emissions or source activity. Table 19.1 presents examples of exposure measures used in relation to the health effects of traffic-related pollution.

19.3   Methods of exposure assessment

Several different approaches to exposure assessment can be identified, aimed at different points in the environment-health chain (Fig. 19.2):

- personal monitoring,
- micro-media (or micro-environmental) monitoring,
- ambient pollution monitoring,
- dispersion modelling,
- indicator-based methods.

This section reviews each of these methods and considers their relative advantages and disadvantages. Chapters 20 and 21 explore in more detail the use of personal monitoring and dispersion modelling, respectively, as techniques for exposure assessment.

Table 19.1 Examples of exposure measures used in studies of relationships between traffic-related air pollution and health (from de Hoogh 1999)

Location	Exposure measure	Age range	Health outcome	Source
Japan	Distance from main road	Age 4–11	Parental reporting of resp. symptoms	Murakami et al. (1990)
London, UK	Distance from road	Age 2–15	GP diagnosis of asthma	Livingstone et al. (1996)
Birmingham, UK	Distance from road; traffic flow	Age 0–4	Hospital admissions for resp. illness	Edwards et al. (1994)
Münster, Germany	Self-reported truck traffic	Age 12–15	Self-reporting of resp. symptoms	Duhme et al. (1996)
Bochum, Germany	Self-reported index of traffic flow, truck flow, and road type	Age 12–15	Self-reporting of resp. symptoms	Weiland et al. (1994)
Munich, Germany	Traffic flow on busiest road in school district	Age 9–11	Parental reporting of resp. symptoms; measurement of lung function	Wjst et al. (1993)
Six areas near motorways, Netherlands	Distance home/school from motorway; traffic density (trucks and cars); measured NO_2/particulate matter$_{10}$ indoor and outdoor	Age 7–12	Parental reporting of resp. symptoms; measurements of lung function	Brunekreef et al. (1997)
Tokyo, Japan	Distance from road; measured NO_2	Females aged 40–60	Self-reporting of resp. symptoms	Nitta et al. (1993)
Stockholm, Sweden	Modelled outdoor NO_2 concentrations	4 mths–4 yrs	Hospital admissions for resp. symptoms	Pershagen et al. (1995)
Haarlem, Netherlands	Modelled traffic pollution (CAR model)	Age 0–15	Parental reporting of resp. symptoms	Oosterlee et al. (1996)
Huddersfield (UK), Amsterdam (NL), Prague (CR), Poznan (Poland)	Modelled NO_2 concentrations (regression model)	Age 7–11	Parental reporting of resp. symptoms	Briggs et al. (1997); Elliott & Briggs (1998); see also Chapter 22

19.3.1 Personal monitoring

Personal monitoring represents the attempt to quantify exposures directly at the point of exposure (i.e the individual). As Fig. 19.2 indicates, such measurements can be focused on three different stages in the exposure process: external dose, absorbed dose, or target dose. Different methods and sampling designs may be required for each of these types of measurement.

Measuring external exposure

Measurements of external exposure are most widely used in relation to air pollution or occupational exposures, where exposure occurs as a result of daily contact with pollution in a wide variety of environments. It is often monitored using some form of portable personal monitoring device, which can be carried by the individual during their normal activities. This may take the form of either an active or passive sampler. The traditional active sampler comprises a pump sampler, which draws a known volume of air through the sampling medium over a known period of time. The sampling medium varies according to the pollutant under consideration: it may take the form of an absorbent medium, a membrane containing a reagent, or a liquid through which the air is bubbled. The quantity of the measured pollutant is determined in the laboratory using standard chemical procedures. In recent years, a number of active portable analysers have also been developed (e.g. for CO, aerosols), containing sensors which take time-referenced measurements of the target pollutant and store the results until they can be downloaded to a computer for analysis.

Personal active samplers have several advantages compared to other monitoring devices, not least their relative accuracy. Nevertheless, use of such samplers is often inhibited by cost, which means that few studies have been able to obtain replicate results for large sample populations. Their bulkiness may also limit their use in some environments and with some participants (e.g. children), and may inhibit normal behaviour, thereby giving unrepresentative results. CO monitors, however, have been widely used for personal monitoring both indoors and outdoors (Ackland *et al.* 1985; Ott *et al.* 1988; Wallace *et al.* 1988; Alm *et al.* 1994), while portable monitors have also been used to a lesser extent for measuring personal exposures to fine particulates (Wallace *et al.* 1993) and volatile organic compounds (VOCs) (Hartwell *et al.* 1987).

Since they were first devised by Palmes *et al.* (1976), a wide range of passive samplers have also been developed and used for personal monitoring. The main application has been for monitoring NO_2 (Boleij *et al.* 1986; Laxen and Noordally 1987; Bower *et al.* 1991; Hewitt 1991; Song *et al.* 1993; Campbell *et al.* 1994; Spengler *et al.* 1994; Atkins and Lee, 1995). Samplers have also been developed, however, for a range of other pollutants, including SO_2, NH_3, ozone, formaldehyde, and benzene (Williams 1995). Passive samplers are also widely used for measuring exposure to radioactivity (e.g. radon), both in occupational and ambient environments (Henshaw 1993).

The design of passive samplers varies depending upon the pollutant under study and the exposure environment of interest. Many consist of a tube or badge, one end of which is exposed to ambient air while the other contains an absorbent reagent on a membrane. A diffusion zone is created by the body of the monitor, through which air passes into the pollution sink (i.e. the reactive material). The rate of pollution uptake can be controlled by altering the dimensions of the sampler (Palmes *et al.* 1976; Atkins *et al.* 1986).

The principle underlying passive techniques of monitoring is the molecular diffusion of gas in a stationary air layer. This diffusion is described by Fick's law:

$$J = \frac{D * A(C - C_0)}{L},$$

where:

J = mass flux of gas (μg s^{-1}),
D = diffusion coefficient of gas in air (m^2 s^{-1}),
A = reaction area of sampler (m^2),
C = external gas concentration in air (μg m^{-3}),
C_0 = equilibrium concentration at reaction surface (μg m^{-3}),
L = diffusion length (m).

The main advantages of diffusion tubes are their low cost and ease of application. This allows them to be used *en masse*, as a basis for personal monitoring on large population samples. The most important disadvantage is their poor temporal resolution. The detection limits of most passive samplers mean that they must be exposed for several days (typically 5–30) to provide a reliable measure of ambient concentrations. The samplers thus provide data only on relatively long-term average pollution levels, and cannot measure short-term peaks. The long exposure time also means that they must be worn for relatively long durations, increasing the risk of damage, loss, or misuse.

Sampling problems caused by meteorological conditions and interference of other pollutants are also possible disadvantages. These may lead to significant bias in the measurements. Studies by the US National Bureau of Standards and Warren Spring Laboratory in the UK showed that accuracy for NO_2 was better than $\pm 10\%$ for a 1-week sampling period (Boleij *et al.* 1986). Heal and Cape (1997), however, reported that the tubes overestimated actual concentrations by up to 28% at urban sites in the summer, and by 8–14% at rural sites and at urban sites in the winter. This overestimation was believed to be a result of chemical reaction between NO and O_3 inside the diffusion tube. In a study of the effects of wind speed and turbulence on the performance of diffusion tubes, Gair and Penkett (1995) reported overestimation by up to 40%, apparently because wind-induced turbulence at the mouth of the sampler shortened the effective diffusion path along the tube. Campbell *et al.* (1994) found a 26% over-estimation of tubes against chemiluminescent monitoring for NO_2. Precision, however, is relatively good. Boleij *et al.* (1986) reported precision of $< 4\,\mu$g/m^3; Atkins *et al.* (1986) and Goldsmith (1986) gave coefficients of variation between duplicate tubes of 5–8%. Van Reeuwijk *et al.* (1998) found a detection limit of $3.7\,\mu$g/m^3 and a coefficient of variation (CV) of 8% from duplicate NO_2 diffusion tubes, in four European cities.

Measuring absorbed or target dose

Measurement of external exposure often provides only a relatively crude assessment of the effective dose received by individuals, which does not directly allow for the effects of differences in physical activity or actual intake of the pollutant. Such measurements also tend to be restricted to specific exposure pathways. For many purposes, therefore, it is more appropriate to assess exposures in terms of the absorbed or target organ dose.

These are normally assessed by some form of biological sampling or biomarker. Common targets for sampling include exhaled breath (e.g. for nicotine or chloroform), blood (e.g. for blood-lead analysis), urine (e.g. for analysis of urinary excreted cadmium or arsenic), and hair (e.g. for heavy metals). Tollerud *et al.* (1983), for example, used analysis of lead in both hair and blood to assess levels of exposure of tunnel and turnpike workers to road traffic pollution. Siegel and Siegel (1985) measured mercury in hair to examine exposures to emissions from the hotsprings in the geothermal area of Rotorua, New Zealand. Raaschou-Nielsen *et al.* (1996) analysed urinary concentrations of two polycyclic aromatic hydrocarbon (PAH) metabolites—1-hydroxypyrene and β-napthyl-amine—as measures of exposures to mutagens from road traffic. Järup *et al.* (1995) used determination of *N*-acetyl-β-glucosaminidase (NAG) in urine to assess levels of cadmium exposure in and around a cadmium battery plant in Sweden (see also Chapter 23). Other examples of the use of biomarkers, for assessing exposures to water- and soilborne pollutants, are discussed by Niewenhuijsen in Chapter 20.

Use of biomarkers such as these clearly has the advantage of providing a measure both of internal and total exposure. Media with clear growth patterns, such as hair, also have the benefit of being able to provide time-sequenced measurements of exposure over periods of weeks or even longer. Nevertheless, biomarkers also suffer from two main problems. The first is the relative intrusiveness of the methods, which may require tight ethical scrutiny and control. The second is the cost and time-consuming nature of sampling, which may limit analysis to relatively small population samples (often, those known to be at risk).

19.3.2 Micro-media monitoring

Micro-media (or micro-environmental) monitoring is in many ways a close alternative to personal exposure monitoring. Rather than measuring exposures on or in the individual, however, it involves detailed measurement of pollution levels in their immediate exposure environment or pathway: for example, in different parts of the home or work environment (in the case of air pollution) or in different foodstuffs (in the case of foodborne exposures). Estimates of total exposure can then be obtained by aggregating the measured concentrations, with a weighting if appropriate for their relative contribution (e.g. reflecting residence times in different micro-environments, or consumption of different foodstuffs).

This approach to exposure assessment is most widely used in relation to air pollution, especially in studies of occupational or indoor exposure (e.g. Quackenboss *et al.* 1986; Song *et al.* 1993). Linaker *et al.* (1996) used Palmes tubes in the kitchen and living room of children's homes, and in the classroom and playground of their school, to assess levels and patterns of exposure to NO_2. Results were compared with data from personal monitoring. Significant correlations were found in most cases between exposures measured with the personal sampler and levels monitored in the two home environments, though the relationship was far from exact. In India, Saksena *et al.* (1992) monitored CO concentrations in indoor and outdoor cooking areas, bedrooms, and the outdoor ambient environment as a basis for modelling personal exposures of villagers in the Himalayas. Time-activity data, collected through personal interviews, were used to weight the contribution from each environment.

Micro-media monitoring clearly provides relatively detailed and individual level assessments of exposures, which can often be readily validated by personal monitoring. It has a major advantage over personal monitoring in that it is less intrusive to the individuals concerned. It also reduces the risks of interference with, or misuse of, the samplers which may occur in personal monitoring. Like personal monitoring, however, the approach suffers from a number of problems. Use of low-cost passive samplers allows relatively large numbers of sites to be monitored simultaneously, but, as noted previously, these provide only averaged concentrations over relatively long exposure times. Continuous sampling, on the other hand, is often limited by cost. Micro-media monitoring is therefore most appropriate either as a means of obtaining estimates of average exposures for an entire population, or as part of relatively small (e.g. case-control or panel) epidemiological studies. It is less appropriate for large ecological studies, where the need is to obtain individual or small-group estimates of exposures across a large population.

19.3.3   Ambient pollution monitoring

For many large population studies, the opportunity to carry out purpose-designed measurements of exposures, either through personal or micro-media monitoring, is limited. In these cases, recourse usually has to be made either to readily available data, or to more limited sampling campaigns, aimed at characterising concentrations in the ambient environment.

Routinely available data

The use of routinely available monitoring data clearly has many attractions. It can help to reduce study costs; it allows results from the study more easily to be extended to other areas; and in many cases it provides the opportunity both to assess past exposures (based on historic monitoring data) and to continue monitoring into the future. In recent decades, the opportunities to use routinely available pollution data have in many cases increased, as national and regional monitoring networks have been expanded in response to growing public concern and the demands of policy. In Europe, for example, well-established monitoring networks exist in almost all countries for air pollution, surface freshwater quality, bathing water quality, and drinking water quality. These provide valuable, yet often underutilised, sources of information from which to assess exposures to a wide range of pollutants, via a range of pathways. Table 19.2 illustrates the extent of several routine networks in the UK.

Nevertheless, use of routinely available data also faces several serious difficulties. One of the most important is the limited spatial coverage and density of most routine monitoring networks. Many networks have been set up to comply with policy requirements, and as such are targeted at specific environments (e.g. at areas of known industrial pollution, or at sites of ecological importance). They may therefore provide a far from representative coverage of the wider environment. Costs, and a tendency to adopt a somewhat minimalist approach to policy compliance, also mean that many networks are relatively sparse, especially when compared to the complex local variation which can occur in environmental pollution. Urban air pollution, for example, may vary several-fold over distances of tens or hundreds of metres, yet most urban monitoring networks comprise only a few sites in any city. The range of pollutants covered by these networks is also limited, typically to those considered to be of greatest policy concern, so often data are scarce for new pollutants, or for pollutants not previously considered to be hazardous to the environment or health.

Table 19.2 Examples of routine environmental data available in the UK*

Medium	Pollutants/indicator	Source	Description	Frequency of update
Atmospheric emissions	SO_2, NO_x, NMVOCs, CO, PM_{10}	AEA Technology	Emission estimates for $1 km^2$ grid across UK; from road, industrial, domestic, and other point sources	Annual
Air quality	SO_2 conc.	AEA Technology	64 automatic sites (57 urban, 7 rural); circa 220 non-automatic sites (acid titration) (urban); 38 automatic sites (rural)	Annual
	Black smoke conc.		Circa 220 non-automatic sites (smoke reflectance from a filter)	Annual
	Fine particulate conc.		50 automatic sites (47 urban, 3 rural)	Annual
	NO_2 conc.		83 automatic sites (76 urban, 7 rural); circa 1100 diffusion tube sites	Annual
	Lead conc.		25 non-automatic sites (filtration)	Annual
	O_3 conc.		71 automatic sites (52 urban, 19 rural)	Annual
	CO conc.		61 automatic sites (urban)	Annual
Stream water quality	Biological water classification	Environment Agency	All stream segments classified on A (good)–D (poor) scale, macro based on the invertebrate species present in the streams	Annual
	General water quality classification		All major streams classified on A (good)–F (bad) scale, based on measurements of biological oxygen demand (BOD), dissolved oxygen, and ammonia concentration	Annual
Surface water pollution incidents	No. of pollution incidents	Environment Agency	No. of incidents by source, severity and outcome (by site)	Annual

Table 19.2 (*cont.*)

Medium	Pollutants/indicator	Source	Description	Frequency of update
Bathing water quality		Environment Agency	Status of bathing waters for circa 486 sites in UK, measuring faecal coliforms, mineral oils, surface-active substances, and phenols	Annual
Drinking water quality		Water companies	Statistical results of water testing (at pumping stations) for water company area	Annual

Sources: Department of Environment (1998); http://www.aeat.co.uk/netcen/airqual/networks/; http://www.aeat.co.uk/netcen/airqual/welcome.html/; http://europa.eu.int/water/water-bathing/report/uk.html.

Another problem is the lack of consistency which can occur between different networks. This is most apparent at the international level, but even municipal or regional networks may not be wholly comparable, due for example to differences in monitoring equipment, laboratory techniques, monitoring frequencies, and protocols for site location (Briggs 1995). Air pollution networks, for example, may monitor different size fractions of particulates, in terms of mass, number, or blackness. Stream water quality monitoring sites tend to be deliberately located upstream of major urban areas in some networks, and downstream in others, leading to different biases in the monitored concentrations. Frequencies of stream water quality monitoring in national networks may vary from continuous to only once or twice per year. Studies which make use of data from different networks or laboratories need to consider these potential sources of error carefully.

Low-cost sampling methods

Given the limitations of routine monitoring networks, there is clearly often a need to use alternative sources of data on pollution levels. With the development of low-cost sampling technology (e.g. passive samplers), one possible approach is to undertake purpose-designed surveys in the area of interest. This was the approach used in the SAVIAH (Small Area Variations in Air quality and Health) study (Briggs *et al.* 1997; Elliott and Briggs 1998; Fischer *et al.* 1998; see also Chapter 22). In this case, four surveys each of two weeks were undertaken using duplicate passive samplers for NO_2 or SO_2 at 80 sites in each of four urban areas (Amsterdam, Huddersfield, Poznan, Prague). Comparison of the results from these surveys with sites monitored on a continuous basis in each study area showed that they gave a good estimate of the annual mean concentration. Subsequent application of the same approach in other study areas, has confirmed that reliable estimates of the annual mean can be obtained from a small number (3–6) of short-term surveys using passive samplers. In the UK, also, a national passive sampler network has been established, comprising almost 1100 sites, which provides a valuable source of data on NO_2 concentrations (Table 19.2; Campbell *et al.* 1994).

Although passive samplers undoubtedly provide a low-cost means of obtaining data on ambient pollution levels, they cannot satisfy every epidemiological need. In particular, passive samplers are currently available for only a relatively limited range of pollutants, and for some of these accuracy and precision are still poor. Alternative means of low-cost sampling do, however, exist for some pollutants, such as moss bags for heavy metals (Archibold and Crisp 1983), corrosion plates to assess atmospheric acidity (Yocum 1962), and plastic track detectors for radon (Henshaw 1993).

Various natural monitors also exist, which can provide valuable sources of information on ambient pollution levels. Aquatic animal species provide biological indicators of freshwater pollution: indeed, this is the basis of many national water quality classifications (e.g. the Belgian Biotic Index and the Irish Streamwater Quality Classification). In the case of air pollution, one of the most extensively used natural monitors is lichen. Different lichen species show different sensitivities to air pollutants (especially SO_2). Mapping of lichen species can thus provide a measure of pollution levels (Gilbert 1974; Hawksworth and Rose 1976; Nyangababo 1987). It has also been shown that the plant symmetry is sensitive to air pollution and may thus be used to map concentrations of air pollutants. Freeman *et al.* (1993), for example, reported clear correlations between leaf asymmetry in a range of plant species (including both trees and perennial herbs) and distance (up to 5 km) from major chemical sites in the Ukraine and northern Russia. They also showed systematic variation in the symmetry of leaflets of soybean with distance (to circa 100 metres) from high voltage transmission lines in Ohio.

These absorption samplers, as they are known, are clearly cheap and easy to use, but they have a number of important limitations for exposure monitoring, not least the long (and often indeterminate) exposure times, substrate sensitivity (in the case of many biological samplers), and the relatively poor accuracy of the methods. Nonetheless, they do provide a simple and fast means of undertaking preliminary surveys in new study areas, and as such can help to target and design more detailed sampling campaigns. They can also be used, perhaps, as ancillary information to help interpolate pollution estimates between monitoring sites.

Spatial interpolation

Whatever method is used, most pollution monitoring provides only point estimates for a sample of locations across an area. For the purposes of exposure assessment, however, estimates are needed at locations defined not by the distribution of available sampling points, but by the distribution of the study population. Typically, therefore, estimates of pollution levels must be made for unsampled sites. The process of making these estimates, on the basis of monitored data from surrounding locations, is known as spatial interpolation. The accuracy of such interpolations is often one of the most important determinants of any attempt at exposure assessment based on ambient pollution data.

Spatial interpolation can be conducted on the basis of many different assumptions and by many different methods. The simplest—and perhaps the most often used—is to assume that the pollution level at any unsampled site is best described by that at the nearest available monitoring site, or by the average of the surrounding sites. Implicitly, this is the assumption often made in many acute epidemiological studies, or in broad-scale ecological studies, where measured concentrations at the available monitoring stations are used to give a measure of pollution across an entire city. This assumption is defensible where the variation of interest (whether spatially, between cities, or temporally, from day to day) is large compared to the spatial variation within any one study area. Even in these cases, however it may lead to considerable exposure misclassification, and inevitably results in underestimation of the amount of variation in exposure across the study population. It can also lead to the ecological fallacy (see Chapter 5). Where monitoring stations are located on the basis of different criteria in different cities (e.g. in industrial areas in the more polluted city, but in residential areas in the less polluted) it may also lead to systematic bias in the exposure estimates. Muschett (1981) showed that simple averaging of data from monitoring sites in US cities overestimated mean annual concentrations by up to 12% compared with area-weighted averages. Table 19.3 shows similar comparisons for Antwerp and Brussels.

For many studies—and especially for small-area or individual-level studies—more sophisticated methods of interpolation are clearly required. With the advent of geographical information systems (GIS), a wide range of techniques have become available. These can usefully be divided into global interpolators, such as trend surface analysis, which fit a smoothed surface through all the data points, and local interpolators, which attempt to fit locally optimal surfaces to the data, taking account only of nearby points. For the purpose of exposure assessment, local interpolation methods are generally the more appropriate.

Table 19.3 Effects of averaging method on estimates of mean annual air pollution level: Antwerp and Brussels

	Concentration (μg/m³)	
	Antwerp (11 sites)	Brussels (12 sites)
Particulates		
Arithmetic mean	14.3	14.8
Area-weighted mean	10.5	12.5
Sulphur dioxide		
Arithmetic mean	51.1	26.1
Area-weighted mean	40.8	21.0

They include geostatistical techniques, such as kriging (Isaaks and Srivastava 1989; see also Chapter 10), spline interpolation techniques (Hutchinson and Bischof 1983), and moving window approaches (Collins 1998).

In recent years, kriging, especially, has been increasingly used to map and model spatial variation in environmental pollution and exposure, in a wide range of media, albeit with variable success (Lefohn *et al.* 1988; Vincent and Gatrell 1991; Wartenberg 1993; Liu and Rossini 1996; Anh *et al.* 1997; Collins 1998). Liu and Rossini (1996), for example, used ordinary kriging to model twelve-hour mean ozone levels in Toronto, Canada. They found that the method gave considerably better predictions of ozone levels at reference points than obtained on the basis of the nearest monitoring station. Wartenberg (1993) used kriging to estimate exposures to organic chemicals in underground drinking waters and microwave radiation from a radar facility in the Cape Cod area of the USA. The limited number of data points and, for the microwave radiation especially, the spatial clustering of the data limited the reliability of the results. Similarly, Vincent and Gatrell (1991) used kriging to investigate the spatial variability of radon gas in Lancaster, UK. Although radon gas was measured at 391 homes, they concluded that levels of spatial variation were too great to provide accurate interpolation. Collins (1998) and de Hoogh (1999) have also used kriging in the attempt to map traffic-related air pollution in urban areas. Both concluded that, while the technique works well in urban background areas, where spatial variation in pollution levels is relatively smooth, it is unable to model the steep pollution gradients and pollution hotspots close to roads, without an exorbitant number of sample points.

A number of attempts have been made to compare the performance of kriging and other interpolation methods under field conditions (e.g. Dubrule 1984; Laslett *et al.* 1987; El Abbass *et al.* 1990; Knotters *et al.* 1995). In general, all the methods perform relatively well where the data density is high and relatively uniform across the study area. Most methods, however, tend to be less effective where data points are sparse relative to the underlying level of spatial variation in the pollution field. In these cases, one potentially useful approach is to use ancillary data as predictors of pollution levels. One method for doing this is co-kriging. In trying to model radon levels, for example, factors such as geology, soil type, and housing age might be used as covariates within a co-kriging model. Similarly, data on traffic volume or road density might be used to help model patterns of traffic-related air pollution. Again, attempts to use these approaches for pollution modelling have met with mixed success. de Hoogh (1999), for example, found that co-kriging using data on traffic volume and distance to road as covariates did not improve estimates of pollution levels at sample points in London compared to ordinary kriging.

One alternative approach which has met with more success is regression mapping. In this case, empirically based relationships are defined between predictor variables (e.g. measures of source density or activity) and measured pollution levels for a small sample of 'training' sites. These can then be used to predict pollution levels in the study area. This approach was used by Briggs *et al.* (1997) to model exposure to traffic-related pollution in three urban areas, as part of the SAVIAH study. Relationships were first established between NO_2 concentrations and traffic volume and land cover within a 300 metre zone of each site, and site altitude, for a sample of 80 sites at which passive samplers had been deployed. The resulting equation was then used to model pollution levels for a fine $(10 \times 10$ metre) grid across each study area, within a GIS. Predictions from the model were validated against measured concentrations for 8–10 independent reference sites, and were found to be accurate to ± 3–$5 \mu g/m^3$ (circa 10% of the mean). Exposure estimates were then derived for study subjects (< 5000 schoolchildren) in each area, by dropping the place of residence on to the pollution map. Further details are given in Chapter 22.

This approach is clearly highly empirical, and cannot be automatically transferred to other areas without local recalibration and revalidation, or necessarily to other pollutants such as PM_{10}. Recently, however, the SAVIAH method has been applied in a number of other study areas, including Northampton, Sheffield, and part of London, with consistent results. With local calibration against as few as 10–20 monitoring sites, it thus seems that the method can be used to map NO_2 concentrations across a wide range of urban environments.

19.3.4   Dispersion modelling

The use of dispersion modelling for the analysis of local patterns of pollution and for environmental management is now widely established. Dispersion models, however, have only rarely been used to date for exposure assessment (see Section 21.5). Examples include the use of the CAR model by Oosterlee *et al.* (1996) to assess NO_2 concentrations in Oslo, and the use of the CALINE model to map traffic-related pollution in Huddersfield (Collins 1997, 1998).

Several reasons may be suggested for their limited use. In part, it probably reflects understandable anxiety about the reliability of the models and also problems of data acquisition. In addition, many of the models are limited because they provide pollution estimates only within a relatively narrow zone around the emission source and thus do not give direct measures of exposure in more remote, background areas; this can lead to gaps in the exposure map. More generally, however, the main constraint on their use seems to have been epidemiologists' lack of familiarity with the models. Certainly, they would seem to have far greater potential as a basis for exposure assessment than their current level of usage would suggest. One key advantage of dispersion models is that they use data on source activity and other environmental conditions, both of which tend to be relatively widely accessible; they are thus relatively unconstrained by the availability of monitoring data—though some monitoring data are generally required for local validation or calibration of the models. Second, the models are explicitly predictive over both time and space; they can thus be used to estimate both past and future pollution levels and exposures provided that the relevant input data are available. Third, they can be relatively easily adapted both to different pollutants and to different environments, without the need for extensive field work.

In recent years a wide range of dispersion models have been developed for environmental pollution. Atmospheric dispersion models are, perhaps, the most advanced, and these will be the focus of attention here. Numerous models also exist, however, for analysing the dispersion of pollutants through the soil (e.g. Burns 1980) and in streams (e.g. Revitt *et al.* 1990; Wilson *et al.* 1997), as well as broader-scale inter-compartmental flows (e.g. van de Meent 1990).

Atmospheric dispersion models take a wide variety of forms; for most epidemiological investigations, point- and line-source models are of most relevance, since these are ostensibly capable of measuring local variations in pollution to a reasonably high degree of accuracy. Area-source models are more appropriate for broadscale (e.g. regional) modelling. Point-source models are those which model dispersion away from individual stacks or other point sources. Examples include the ISC models, developed for the US Environmental Protection Agency (USEPA 1995), the more recent AERMOD, also developed for USEPA (Perry *et al.* 1994), and the COSYMA model designed to predict dispersion of radionuclides from nuclear installations (National Radiological Protection Board and Forschungszentrum Karlsruhe 1995). Line-source models are those which model dispersion from roadways or other line sources. These include the CALINE suite of models (Benson 1992), CAR-International (Eerhens *et al.* 1993), HIWAY (Zimmerman and Thompson 1974) and SBLINE (Namdeo and Colls 1996). The recently available ADMS model (CERC Ltd 1999) provides both a point- and line-source model, within an integrated package which links to the ArcView GIS.

Most of these models are designed to model dispersion from one, or a few, individually defined sources, over distances of a few tens to several thousand metres. Many assume that dispersion occurs as a plume exhibiting Gaussian properties (i.e. in which the vertical and horizontal distribution of the pollutant follows a normal distribution). This assumption holds reasonably well for simple situations, in which there is little deposition from the plume at ground level, little effect from surface roughness, and limited variation in windspeed. However, it provides only a rough approximation of reality in more complex environments, such as street canyons or large urban areas with a wide range of sources and variable topography.

Data inputs for these models are also broadly similar. The main requirements are for data on source activity (e.g. emission rate, height, and temperature), meteorology (e.g. windspeed, wind direction, temperature, and atmospheric stability), and surface topography. The models vary, however, in a number of characteristics, including the way in which they model atmospheric boundary layer conditions and turbulence. Indeed, much of the recent effort to enhance these models has focused on improving these parameters (see Chapter 21).

Performance of the different models inevitably varies, depending to a large extent on the conditions under which they are run. There have also been surprisingly few rigorous comparisons of the models, and those that have been undertaken have tended to highlight inadequacies in many of the models when applied under field conditions. Choosing between them is therefore not easy. Noll *et al.* (1978), for example, compared three early line-source models (HIWAY, CALINE-2, and the California Line-Source model) and found that all three tended to overestimate concentrations for parallel wind directions (in some cases by a factor of two or three), but underestimate them for oblique or crosswind directions. Rao *et al.* (1980) compared seven models—four Gaussian and three numerical models. In general, the Gaussian models (GM, HIWAY, AIRPOL-4, and CALINE-2) performed better, with 49–95% of the predictions being within a factor of two of the observed concentrations. Only 1–12% of predictions, however, were within 5% of observed levels. Of the Gaussian models, the GM (General Motors) model was the most reliable—though notably the validation was run using data collected at the General Motors proving ground. Rodden *et al.* (1982) compared six line-source models (two versions of CALINE, two versions of TRAPS, HIWAY, and AIRPOL-4a) and found that all performed poorly. De Hoogh (1999) assessed the performance of three models—the simple DMRB (Design Manual for Roads and Bridges) model, CALINE-3 and ADMS—as a basis for mapping mean annual and two-week average NO_2 concentrations in Sheffield, UK. Notwithstanding its simpler structure and assumptions (it does not take account of meteorological factors), the DMRB significantly out-performed the other models.

19.3.5   Indicator-based methods

Despite the availability of these many different methods for monitoring or modelling exposures to pollution, probably the majority of studies still rely on simpler, more indirect indicators of exposure. These are typically based on the principle that levels of exposure are broadly related either to the level of source activity which is responsible for pollution, or the distance of individuals from that source. Thus, the UK Small Area Health Statistics Unit (SAHSU) has traditionally used distance from source as a proxy for exposure in analysing health effects around point sources (Elliott *et al.* 1992; see also Chapter 9). Many studies of traffic-related pollution have used similar exposure indicators such as distance from the nearest main road, road type, traffic volume on the nearest road, or a self-reported measure of traffic density in the neighbourhood (see Table 19.1).

The main advantage of exposure indicators such as these is that they are easy to cal-culate, whether manually, by use of GIS, or through self-reporting by participants. They nevertheless have serious limitations. They provide only crude and semi-quantitative measures of exposure; they take little account of the actual distribution of pollution levels; they are for the most part non-specific; and in many cases they are relatively poorly defined. Partly for this reason, perhaps, results from the studies of chronic health effects of traffic-related pollution, which have often used these measures, have been somewhat inconsistent.

19.4   Time-activity analysis

Monitoring or modelling of pollution levels, or estimation of indicators of source activity, clearly provide a means both of generating point estimates of exposure and of construct-ing exposure maps. None of these approaches is likely to give wholly reliable estimates of exposure, however, if the individuals to whom they are meant to relate are represented by static locations, such as the place of residence or workplace. In reality, the process of exposure is far more complex. It occurs as individuals move through the changing pollution field, passing as they do so through a potentially wide range of pollution environments, characterised by different pollution levels and different pollution mixes.

In order to take account of these effects in exposure assessment, information is clearly needed on the time activity and movement patterns of individuals in any study. In practice, this poses immense difficulties. Local surveys of time activity have been conducted (Saksena *et al.* 1992; Silvers *et al.* 1994; Farrow *et al.* 1997), often using questionnaires or time-activity diaries, but in general little information is available on time activity patterns, in a form suitable for exposure assessment. Time-activity patterns are also extremely varied, both across members of any population and for any one member over time. The extent to which information from specific surveys can be generalised to the wider population (or even for the individuals concerned) is uncertain. Methods to use this information for the purpose of exposure assessment have, until recently, also been poorly developed. An early attempt at developing an exposure model to take account of time activity was the SHAPE (Simulation of Human Air Pollution Exposures) model, devised by Ott *et al.* (1988). With the development of GIS, the capability to carry out complex time-activity modelling has been considerably enhanced. Using GIS techniques, it is now possible either to trace the pathway of any individual, or to simulate movements of a population group, through the environment, across a time-changing model of the pollution field, and thus to obtain integrated measures of exposure.

19.5   What makes a good exposure measure?

Surprisingly, few attempts seem to have been made to evaluate exposure methods or measures before they have been applied; too often, it seems that the choice of methodology has been driven either by readily available data or by previous practice. In recent years, however, a number of studies have begun to explore and compare the relative performance of different exposure measures, specifically in relation to traffic-related pollution. Collins (1997, 1998), for example, compared the use of different spatial interpolation and modelling methods for the assessment of traffic-related pollution levels in Huddersfield, UK. By comparing predictions from these various methods with independent measures of NO_2 concentrations at monitoring sites, she showed that geostatistical methods performed relatively poorly; dispersion modelling (CALINE3) gave intermediate results; and the locally calibrated regression mapping method performed the best. Broadly similar results have been found by Wills (1998) working in London and de Hoogh (1999) in both London and Sheffield. Wills (1998) applied ten measures—including eight exposure indicators, the CALINE-3 dispersion model and the SAVIAH regression method—to 500 sites in central London, and compared the results in terms of their quintiles of exposure. In general, only 20–30% of sites were ranked in the same quintile by any pair of methods—little better than would be achieved by chance. Different exposure measures thus tend to give markedly different results, and the choice of exposure indicator can have a marked effect on the outcomes of any study.

In the light of this, an important question arises: how can exposure best be assessed? In reality, in addressing this question many different, and often conflicting, considerations have to be taken into account. On the one hand, for example, there is a need for accuracy of exposure assessments at the individual level; this, however, must be set against the need for large population estimates if exposures with small relative effects are being investigated. Spatial precision is important if exposure assessments are to cope with the large degree of local variation present in many urban environments. Nevertheless, exposure does not occur at single, fixed points, but across a complex web of locations as people move through the pollution field. Single point measurements may thus be overprecise. Real-time measurements of exposure are clearly useful, since they can be related to individual activity and can be validated. For many health outcomes, however, long latency periods may occur between exposure and the appearance of symptoms. Assessment of historic exposures may therefore be needed, and these inevitably often require use of different methods, which may be less easy to validate. Exposure indicators are often needed which are pollutant-specific, so that reliable estimates of the dose-response relationship can be made. Yet this ignores the potential influence of pollutant mixes and synergistic effects, and may thus underestimate the health impacts of the total pollution load from any specific source.

It also needs to be noted that, while the needs for reductionism in epidemiology may focus attention on specific pollutants, many policy actions and interventions are far broader in their attack. Attempts to tackle problems of road congestion and traffic pollution, for example, might involve generic measures such as road pricing or fuel taxation.

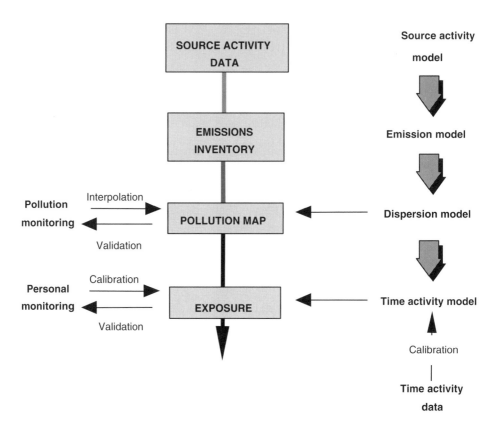

Fig. 19.3 An integrated approach to exposure assessment. (*Note*: interpolation/calibration and validation should be done with independent datasets.)

These may offer solutions not only to health problems associated with one specific pollutant (e.g. the impact of fine particulates on respiratory health), but to a wide range of other air pollutants, as well as noise, vibration, road accidents, and community severance. Similarly, adjustments to the system of agricultural prices and subsidies aimed at reducing agricultural intensity, although non-specific, may do far more to reduce problems of exposure to pesticides and fertilisers, as well as livestock wastes and occupational accidents, than a wide array of problem-specific interventions. To inform policy interventions of these types requires the use of much more diverse exposure measures.

There is, therefore, no single or optimal method of defining and assessing exposures. Much depends upon the specific circumstances of the study: the pollutant and the sources under investigation, the scale of analysis, the study design, the specific aetiological hypothesis which motivates it, and the purposes of the study. Fitness for purpose must therefore be the key criterion in choosing methods of exposure assessment. What is also clear is that, for many applications, no single method will be optimal. Instead, the way forward would seem to be to use a combination of different methods, as shown in Fig. 19.3. Dispersion modelling, or monitoring and spatial interpolation, may be used, for example, to generate pollution maps, which can then be validated against independent monitoring data. Exposures can then be modelled by simulating the time activity patterns of people living in, or moving through, these pollution fields. Field-based time-activity data can be used to inform these models, and personal monitoring or micro-environment monitoring to calibrate or validate the modelled results. Such an approach is clearly challenging, but with the development of GIS it is now achievable in many studies. Certainly, exposure assessment is worth the effort, for accurate exposure measures are essential if the complex relationships between environment and health are to be understood.

References

Ackland, G., Hartwell, T., Johnson, T., and Whitmore, R. (1985). Measuring human exposure to carbon monoxide in Washington, DC and Denver, Colorado, during the winter of 1982–1983. *Environmental Science and Technology*, **19**, 911–18.

Alm, S., Repnone, A., Mukala, K., Pasanen, P., Tuomisto, J., and Jantunen, M. J. (1994). Personal exposures of preschool children to carbon monoxide: roles of ambient air quality and gas stoves. *Atmospheric Environment*, **28**, 3577–80.

Anh, V., Duc, H., and Shannon, I. (1997). Spatial variability of Sydney air quality by cumulative semivariogram. *Atmospheric Environment*, **31**, 4073–80.

Archibold, O. W. and Crisp, P. T. (1983). The distribution of airborne metals in the Illawara region of New South Wales, Australia. *Applied Geography*, **3**, 331–44.

Atkins, D. H. F. and Lee, D. S. (1995). Spatial and temporal variation of rural nitrogen dioxide concentrations across the United Kingdom. *Atmospheric Environment*, **29**, 223–39.

Atkins, D. H. F., Sandalls, J., Law, D. V., Hough, A. M., and Stevenson, K. (1986). *The measurement of nitrogen dioxide in the outdoor environment using passive diffusion tube samplers.* United Kingdom Atomic Energy Authority Report, AERE R-12133. Harwell Laboratory, Oxfordshire.

Benson, P. E. (1992). A review of the development and application of the CALINE3 and CALINE4 models, *Atmospheric Environment*, **26B**, 379–90.

Boleij, J. S. M., Lebret, E., Hoek, F., Noy, D., and Brunekreef, B. (1986). The use of Palmes tubes for measuring NO$_2$ homes. *Atmospheric Environment*, **20**, 596–600.

Bower, J. S., Broughton, G. F. J., Dando, M. T., Lees, A. J., Stevenson, K. J., Lampert, J. E. *et al.* (1991). Urban NO$_2$ concentrations in the UK in 1987. *Atmospheric Environment*, **25B**, 267–83.

Briggs, D. J. (1995). Environmental statistics for environmental policy: genealogy and data quality. *Journal of Environmental Management*, **44**, 39–54.

Briggs, D. J., Collins, S., Elliott, P., Fischer, P., Kingham, S., Lebret, E., *et al.* (1997). Mapping urban air pollution using GIS: a regression-based approach. *International Journal of Geographical Information Science*, **11**, 699–718.

Brunekreef, B., Janssen, N. A. H., Hartog, J. de, Harssema, H., Knape, M., and Vliet, P. van (1997). Air pollution from truck traffic and lung function in children living near motorways. *Epidemiology*, **8**, 298–303.

Burns, I. G. (1980). Influences of the spatial distribution of nitrate on the uptake of N by plants: a review and model for rooting depth. *Journal of Soil Science*, **31**, 155–73.

Campbell, G. W., Stedman, J. R., and Stevenson, K. (1994). A survey of nitrogen dioxide concentrations in the United Kingdom using diffusion tubes, July–December (1991). *Atmospheric Environment*, **28**, 477–86.

CERC (1999). *ADMS-Urban. An urban air quality management system. User Guide*. CERC Ltd, Cambridge.

Collins, S. (1997). Modelling urban air pollution using GIS. In *Geographic information research. Bridging the Atlantic* (M. Craglia and H. Couclelis ed.), 427–40. Taylor & Francis, London.

Collins, S. (1998). Modelling spatial variations in air quality using GIS. In *GIS and health. GISData 6* (A. Gatrell and M. Loytonen ed.), 81–95. Taylor & Francis, London.

Department of Environment (1998). *Digest of environmental protection and water statistics, 1997*. HMSO, London.

de Hoogh, C. (1999). Estimating exposure to traffic-related pollution within a GIS environment. Unpublished Ph.D. thesis, University College Northampton and University of Leicester.

Dubrule, O. (1984). Comparing splines and kriging. *Computers and Geosciences*, **10**, 327–8.

Duhme, H., Weiland, S. P., Keil, U., Kraemer, B., Schmid, M., Stender, M. *et al.* (1996). The association between self-reported symptoms of asthma and allergic rhinitis and self-reported traffic density on street of residence in adolescents. *Epidemiology*, **7**, 578–82.

Edwards, J., Walters, S., and Griffiths, R. K. (1994). Hospital admissions for asthma in preschool children: Relationship to major roads in Birmingham, United Kingdom. *Archives of Environmental Health*, **49**, 223–7.

Eerhens, H. C., Sliggers, C. J., and van den Hout, K. D. (1993). The CAR model: the Dutch method to determine city street air quality. *Atmospheric Environment*, **27B**, 389–99.

El Abbass, T., Jallouli, C., Albony, Y., and Diament, M. (1990). A comparison of surface fitting algorithms for geophysical data. *Terra Nova*, **2**, 467–75.

Elliott, P. and Briggs, D. J. (1998). Recent developments in the geographical analysis of small area health and environmental data. In *Progress in public health* (G. Scally ed.), 101–25. Royal Society of Medicine Press, London.

Elliott, P., Kleinschmidt, I., and Westlake, A. J. (1992). Use of routine data in studies of point sources of environmental pollution. In *Geographical and environmental epidemiology: methods for small-area studies* (P. Elliott, J. Cuzick, D. English, and R. Stern ed.), 106–14. Oxford University Press.

Farrow, A., Taylor, H., and Golding, J. (1997). Time spent in the home by different family members. *Environmental Technology*, **18**, 605–13.

Fischer, P. H., Kriz, B., Martuzzi, M., Wojtyniak, B., Lebret, E., van Reeuwijk, H. *et al.* (1998). Risk factors indoors and prevalences of childhood respiratory health in four countries in western and central Europe. *Indoor Air*, **8**, 244–54.

Freeman, D. C., Graham, J. H., and Emlem, J. M. (1993). Developmental stability in plants: symmetries, stress and epigenesis. *Genetica*, **89**, 97–119.

Gair, A. J. and Penkett, S. A. (1995). The effects of wind speed and turbulence on the performance of diffusion tube samplers. *Atmospheric Environment*, **29**, 2529–33.

Gilbert, O. L. (1974). An air pollution survey by school children. *Environmental Pollution*, **60**, 174–80.

Goldsmith, A. (1986). *Measurements of nitrogen dioxide at rural sites using diffusion samplers*. Warren Spring Laboratory Report, 582 (AP) M. Warren Spring Laboratory, Hatfield UK.

Hartwell, T. D., Pellizzari, E. D., Perrit, R. L., Whitmore, R. W., Zelon, H. S., Sheeldon, L. S. *et al.* (1987). Results from the total exposure assessment methodology (TEAM) study in selected communities in northern and southern California. *Atmospheric Environment*, **21**, 1995–2004.

Hawksworth, D. L. and Rose, F. (1976). *Lichens as pollution monitors*. Edward Arnold, London.

Heal, M. R. and Cape, J. N. (1997). A numerical evaluation of chemical interferences in the measurement of ambient nitrogen dioxide by passive diffusion samplers. *Atmospheric Environment*, **31**, 1191–23.

Henshaw, D. L. (1993). Radon exposure in the home: its occurrence and possible health effects. *Contemporary Physics*, **34**, 31–48.

Hewitt, C. N. (1991). Spatial variation in nitrogen dioxide concentrations in an urban area. *Atmospheric Environment*, **25B**, 429–34.

Hutchinson, M. F. and Bischof, R. J. (1983). A new method for estimating the spatial distribution of mean seasonal and annual rainfall applied to the Hunter Valley, New South Wales. *Australian Meteorological Magazine*, **31**, 117–84.

Issaks, E. H. and Srivastava, R. M. (1989). *An introduction to applied geostatistics*. Oxford University Press, New York.

Järup, L., Carlsson, M. D., Elinder, C. G., Hellström, L., Persson, B., and Schütz, A. (1995). Enzymuria in a population living near a cadmium battery plant. *Occupational Environmental Medicine*, **52**, 770–2.

Knotters, M., Brus, D. J., and Oude Voshaar, J. H. (1995). A comparison of kriging, co-kriging and kriging combined with regression for spatial interpolation of horizon depth with censored observations. *Geoderma*, **67**, 227–46.

Laslett, G.M, McBratney, A. B., Pahl, P. J., and Hutchinson, M. F. (1987). *Journal of Soil Science*, **38**, 3250–73.

Laxen, D. P. H. and Noordally, E. (1987). Nitrogen dioxide distribution in street canyons. *Atmospheric Environment*, **21**, 1899–1903.

Lefohn, A. S., Knudsen, H. P., and McEvoy Jr. L. R. (1988). The use of kriging to estimate monthly ozone exposure parameters for the southeastern United States. *Environmental Pollution*, **53**, 27–42.

Liu, S. L. -J. and Rossini, A. J. (1996). Use of kriging models to predict 12-hour mean ozone concentrations in metropolitan Toronto—a pilot study. *Environment International*, **22**, 677–92.

Linaker, C. H., Chauhan, A. J., Inskip, H., Frew, A. J., Sillence, A., Coggon, D. *et al*. (1996). Distribution and determinants of personal exposure to nitrogen dioxide in school children. *Occupational and Environmental Medicine*, **53**, 200–3.

Livingstone, A. E., Shaddick, G., Grundy, C., and Elliot, P. (1996). Do people living near inner city main roads have more asthma needing treatment? Case control study. *British Medical Journal*, **312**, 676–7.

Murakami, M., Ono, M., and Tamura. K. (1990) Health problems of residents along heavy-traffic roads. *Journal of Human Ergology*, **19**, 101–6.

Muschett, F. D. (1981) Spatial distributions of urban atmospheric particulate concentrations. *Annals of the Association of American Geographers*, **71**, 552–65.

Namdeo, A. K. and Colls, J. J. (1996). Development and evaluation of SBLINE, a suite of models for the prediction of pollution concentrations from vehicles in urban areas, *The Science of the Total Environment*, **189/190**, 311–20.

National Academy of Science (1991). *Human exposure assessment for airborne pollutants. Advances and opportunities* National Academy Press, Washington, DC.

National Radiological Protection Board and Forschungszentrum Karlsruhe (1995). *PC Cosyma. EUR 16420 En* (NRPB-SR280), ECSC-EEC-EAEC. Brussels–Luxembourg.

Nitta, H., Nakai, S., Maeda, K., Aoki, S., and Ono, M. (1993). Respiratory health associated with exposure to automobile exhaust. I: Results of cross-sectional studies in 1979, 1982 and 1983. *Archives of Environmental Health*, **48**, 53–8.

Noll, K. E., Miller, T., and Claggett, M. (1978). A comparison of three highway line-source dispersion models. *Atmospheric Environment*, **12**, 1323–9.

Nyangababo, J. T. (1987). Lichen as monitors of aerial heavy metal pollution in and around Kampala. *Bulletin of Environmental Contamination and Toxicology*, **38**, 91–5.

Oosterlee, A., Drijver, M., Lebret, E., and Brunekreef, B. (1996). Chronic respiratory symptoms in children and adults living along streets with high traffic density. *Occupational and Environmental Medicine*, **53**, 241–7.

Ott, W., Thomas, J., Mage, D., and Wallace, L. (1988). Validation of the simulation of human activity and pollutant exposure (SHAPE) model using paired days from the Denver, CO, carbon monoxide field study. *Atmospheric Environment*, **22**, 2101–13.

Palmes, E. D., Gunnison, A. F., DiMattio, J., and Tomczyk, C. (1976). Personal sampler for nitrogen dioxide. *American Industrial Hygiene Association Journal*, **37**, 570–7.

Perry, S. G., Cimorelli, A. J., Fee, R. F., Paine, R. J., Venkatram, A., and Weil, J. C. (1994). *AERMOD: a dispersion model for industrial source applications*. USEPA Report 94-TA23.04. Boulder Co.

Pershagen, G., Rylander, E., Norberg, S., Eriksson, M., and Nordvall, S. L. (1995). Air pollution involving nitrogen dioxide exposure and wheezing bronchitis in children. *International Journal of Epidemiology*, **24**, 1147–53.

Quackenboss, J., Spengler, J., Kanarek, M., Letz, R., and Duffy, C. (1986). Personal exposure to nitrogen dioxide: relationship to indoor/outdoor air quality and activity patterns. *Environmental Science and Technology*, **20**, 775–83.

Raaschou-Nielsen, O., Olsen, J. H., Hertel, O., Berkowicz, R., Skov, H., Hansen, A. M. *et al.* (1996). Exposure of Danish children to traffic exhaust fumes. *The Science of the Total Environment*, **189/190**, 51–5.

Rao, S. T., Sistia, G., Keenan, M. T., and Wilson, J. S. (1980). An evaluation of some commonly used highway dispersion models. *Journal of the Air Pollution Control Association*, **30**, 239–46.

Revitt, D. M., Hamilton, R. S., and Warren, R. S. (1990). The transport of heavy metals within a small urban catchment. *The Science of the Total Environment*, **93**, 359–73.

Rodden, J. B., Green, N. J., Messina, A. D., and Bullin, J. A. (1982). Comparison of roadway pollutant dispersion models using the Texas data. *Journal of the Air Pollution Control Association*, **32**, 1226–8.

Saksena, S., Prasad, R., Pal, R. C., and Joshi, V. (1992). Patterns of daily exposure to TSP and CO in the Garhwal Himalaya. *Atmospheric Environment*, **26A**, 2125–34.

Siegel, B. Z. and Siegel, S. M. (1985). Mercury in human hair: uncertainties in the meaning and significance of 'unexposed' and 'exposed' in sample populations. *Water, Air and Soil*, **26**, 191–9.

Silvers, A., Florence, B. T., Rourke, D. L. and Lorrimer, R. J. (1994). How children spend their time: a sample survey for use in exposure and risk assessments. *Risk Analysis*, **15**, 931–44.

Song, R., Wang, G., and Zhou, J. (1993, July). Study on the personal exposure level to nitrogen dioxide for housewives in Beijing. In *Indoor Air '93. Proceedings of the 6th International Conference on Indoor Air Quality and Climate* (M. J. Jantunen, P. Kalliokoski, E. Kukkonen, K. Saarela, O. Seppänen, and H. Vuorelma ed.), 377–42. Helsinki, Finland. Gummerus, Jyväsklä, Finland.

Spengler, J., Schwab, M., Ryan, P. B., Billick, I. H., Colome, S., Wilson, A. L., and Becker, E. (1994). Personal exposure to nitrogen dioxide in the Los Angeles basin. *Journal of Air and Waste Management Association*, **44**, 39–47.

Tollerud, D. J., Speizer, F. E., Weiss, S. T., Ferris, B., and Elting, E. (1983). The health effects of automobile exhaust. VI: Relationship of respiratory symptoms and pulmonary function in tunnel and turnpike workers. *Archives of Environmental Health*, **38**, 334–40.

USEPA (1995). *User's guide for the industrial source complex (ISC3) dispersion models*. Vol I: *user instructions*. Report EPA-454/B-95-003a. USEPA, Triangle Park, NC.

van de Meent, D. (1990). Modelling intercompartmental transfers of pollutants: the case of lead. *Science of the Total Environment*, **90**, 41–54.

van Reeuwijk, H., Fischer, P. H., Harssema, H., Briggs, D. J., Smallbone, K., and Lebret, E. (1998). Field comparison of two NO_2 samplers in a dense network. *Environmental Monitoring and Appraisal*, **50**, 37–51.

Vincent, P. and Gatrell, A. (1991, April). The spatial distribution of radon gas in Lancashire (UK): a kriging study. In *Proceedings of the Second European Conference on Geographical Information Systems* (J. Harts, H. Ottens, H. Scholten ed.), 1179–86. EGIS Foundation, Brussels, Belgium.

Wallace, L., Thomas, J., Mage, D., and Ott, W. (1988). Comparison of breath CO, CO exposure and Coburn model predictions in the US EPA Washington–Denver study. *Atmospheric Environment*, **22**, 2183–93.

Wallace, L., Özkaynak, H., Spengler, J., Pellizzari, E., and Jenkins, P. (1993, July). Indoor, outdoor and personal air exposures to particles, elements and nicotine for 178 southern California residents. In *Indoor Air '93. Proceedings of the 6th International Conference on Indoor Air Quality and Climate* (M. J. Jantunen, P. Kalliokoski, E. Kukkonen, K. Saarela, O. Seppänen, and H. Vuorelma ed.), 445–50. Helsinki, Finland. Gummerus, Jyväsklä, Finland.

Wartenberg, D. (1993). Some epidemiological applications of kriging. *Geostatistics Troia '92*, **5**, 911–22.

Weiland, S. K., Mundt, K. A., Ruckmann, A., and Keil, U. (1994). Self-reported wheezing and allergic rhinitis in children and traffic density on street of residence. *AEP*, **4**, 243–7.

Williams, M. L. (1995). Monitoring of exposure to air pollution. *The Science of The Total Environment*, **168**, 169–74.

Wills, J. (1998). The development and use of environmental health indicators for epidemiology and policy applications: a geographical analysis. Unpublished Ph.D. thesis, University College Northampton and University of Leicester.

Wilson, D. A., Butcger, D. P., and Labadz, J. C. (1997). Prediction of travel times and dispersion of pollutant spillages in non-tidal rivers. In *Proceedings of the British Hydrological Society 6th National Symposium*, 4.13–4.19. Salford, UK.

Wjst, M., Reitmeir, P., Dold, S., Wulff, A., Nicolai, T., Freifrau von Loeffelholz-Colberg, E. *et al.* (1993). Road traffic and adverse effects on respiratory health in children. *British Medical Journal*, **307**, 596–600.

Yocum, J. E. (1962). Effects of air pollution on materials. In *Air pollution*, Vol. 1. (A. C. Sterm ed.), 199–219. Academic Press, London.

Zimmerman, J. L. and Thompson, R. S. (1974). *HIWAY: a highway air pollution model.* National Environmental Research Center, Research Triangle Park, NC.

20. Personal exposure monitoring in environmental epidemiology

M. J. Nieuwenhuijsen

20.1 Introduction

Exposure assessment for environmental epidemiology and risk assessment in general is attracting increasing interest and is becoming more refined. In the past, the estimation of exposure levels for various populations was often fairly crude: for example, by using fixed site monitors for air pollution monitoring, by comparing chlorinated with non-chlorinated water sources in studies of trihalomethanes in drinking water, or on the basis of soil sampling in investigations of land contamination by arsenic. Recently, although not always for epidemiological purposes, there has been a trend towards more sophisticated exposure assessments, in an attempt to obtain more accurate individual-level exposure estimates. Thus, personal monitors are increasingly being used to estimate exposure to a range of air pollutants, including PM_{10}, $PM_{2.5}$, VOCs, ozone, metals, CO, and NO_2 (Lioy *et al.* 1990; Clayton *et al.* 1993; Brauer and Brook 1995; Nakai *et al.* 1995; Hoteit *et al.* 1996; Linn *et al.* 1996; Ozkaynak *et al.* 1996; Monn *et al.* 1997, 1998; Janssen 1998; Jantunen *et al.* 1998; Leung and Harrison 1998). Waller *et al.* (1998) and Gallagher *et al.* (1998) estimated trihalomethane intake by modelling concentrations in tapwater, and people's daily consumption. Exposures to metals and other long-lasting pollutants are being assessed using biomarkers—such as metabolites of arsenic (As(III), As(V), MMA, DMA)—in urine, blood, or hair (Bencko and Symon 1977; Valentine *et al.* 1979; Lin *et al.* 1985; Bencko 1995; Kavanagh *et al.* 1998).

The use of personal monitoring of exposure has been especially widely accepted in occupational epidemiology (Nieuwenhuijsen 1997). It is also, increasingly, regarded as more informative and more representative than fixed site monitoring for environmental epidemiological purposes (see Chapter 19). Quantification of the relation between environmental pollution and adverse human health effects requires the use of exposure estimates which are accurate, precise, and biologically relevant, and show a range of exposure levels in the population under study. In practice, these ideals are often not met, and exposure estimates do not reflect the 'true' exposure, or more importantly, the dose, of the target individual(s), and show large exposure variance. This can lead to attenuation of risk estimates in the exposure-response relation in epidemiological studies and dilute any relationships which exist (Armstrong and Oakes 1982; Armstrong 1990; Armstrong *et al.* 1992; Thomas *et al.* 1993a; Nieuwenhuijsen 1997; Heederik and Miller 1999; see also Chapter 5). Personal monitoring is generally labour-intensive, costly, and difficult to carry out. These factors often restrict its use, though the information obtained is generally more informative and relevant than other approaches (depending on the circumstances) and increases the scientific value of epidemiological studies.

Exposure to any pollutant is determined by the concentration of the pollutant in the environment, its specific character (e.g. its chemical form or particle size), and the duration and frequency of contact. Estimates of these characteristics can generally be obtained instrumentally (i.e. using a monitoring device), via questionnaires, through direct observation, or through the use of biomarkers. These methods are complementary. Which is used often depends on the circumstances of the study. The emphasis in this chapter is on the measurement of personal exposure with instruments or biomarkers; these provide information mainly on the level of exposure. Information on duration, frequency, and pattern of exposure is generally obtained by questionnaire or observation. Various approaches and problems related to personal monitoring will be discussed and examples given. The chapter is not intended to be exhaustive; other information regarding exposure assessment, and more information on personal monitoring, can be found elsewhere (e.g. see Hering 1989; NRC 1991; Armstrong *et al.* 1992; Keith 1996; Wallace 1996; and the brief overview in Chapter 19).

20.2   Generic issues in personal monitoring

Once the decision has been made to use personal monitoring for an epidemiological study, a comprehensive sampling strategy needs to be designed. In the process, a number of choices need to be made which will fundamentally affect the way in which the study is carried out and the reliability of the results. These include whether to adopt a group or individual approach, the number of measurements needed, the duration of monitoring and appropriate averaging time, the type of monitor or method to be used, and how the data will be analysed and used for the epidemiological study. Crucial to these choices is the fact that, in most circumstances, marked variation occurs in exposure levels, both over time for any individual and between individuals for any given time. Thus, a single 'best estimate' of the average exposure level may not be appropriate; instead, data are needed on levels of variations in exposure.

20.2.1   Group versus individual approach

To obtain exposure estimate(s) for a population in an epidemiological study, two main approaches are available: the individual approach and the group approach. In the individual approach, every member of the population is monitored either once or repeatedly, and data are obtained at the individual level. In the group approach, the group is first split into smaller subpopulations based on specific determinants of exposure. Subpopulations might be defined, for example, on the basis of presence or absence of an exposure source (e.g. gas cooker, or smoker in the house), distance from an exposure source (e.g. roads or factories), or activity (e.g. commuting by car or by bus). Subsequently, a representative sample of members from each subpopulation is monitored, either once or repeatedly. If the aim is to estimate mean exposure, the average of the exposure measurements is then assigned to all the members in that particular subpopulation. A weighted average can also be obtained for the population as a whole.

Intuitively, one would expect the individual approach to give the best exposure esti-mates. This is often not true, however, because of variability in exposure. In general, in epidemiological studies, the individual approach leads to attenuated, though more precise, health risk estimates than the group approach, although one must be wary of the eco-logical fallacy (see Chapter 5 for a discussion of this issue). The group approach, in contrast, results in less attenuation of the risk estimates, provided that sufficient meas-urements are taken of a large enough sample of subpopulation members adequately to characterise each group (Heederik *et al.* 1996; Kromhout *et al.* 1996; Seixas and Sheppard 1996; Nieuwenhuijsen 1997). These differences can be explained by Classical and Berkson type error models (Thomas *et al.* 1993*a*; see also Chapter 5).

20.2.2   Variance components

Epidemiological studies require relatively large variations in exposure between subjects or groups, but high precision and accuracy in the exposure estimates, if effects on health are to be reliably detected. Knowledge of the variability in exposure is therefore extremely important in designing studies. Variability can derive from a number of different sources. It may occur either between or within subjects, and may be either temporal or spatial. Between subject variance relates to systematic variation in average exposure levels between subjects, for example as a result of behavioural factors or differences in activities. Within subject variance is largely due to day-to-day variations in exposure as a result of different patterns of activity. Where subpopulations are being studied, variation also occurs both within and between subpopulations and is referred to as within and between subpopula-tion variance. Variation in exposure can also occur due to analytical errors (e.g. during laboratory analyses). These, however, are generally very small compared to variation caused by environmental factors (Nicas *et al.* 1991).

Wherever possible, a pilot study should be carried out to obtain estimates of variability in exposure in the population under study. This information can be used to help select the optimal exposure measurement strategy, to define subpopulations, to determine the number of samples needed to characterise each subpopulation and to assess the accuracy and precision of the resulting health risk estimates. The measurement strategy used in the full study should also, ideally, be designed to provide information on variance com-ponents. This requires repeated measurements of subjects or subpopulations. Variance components can then be estimated using statistical analysis of variance techniques (Liu *et al.* 1978; Searle *et al.* 1992; Kromhout *et al.* 1996; Nieuwenhuijsen 1997).

20.2.3   Number of subjects and measurements

From the previous discussion, it is clear that the number of subjects to be measured and the number of measurements to be taken on each subject depends on the chosen strategy and the distribution of the variability in exposure across the population. In the case of the individual approach, every subject will be monitored. Repeated measure-ments are highly recommended in these cases to provide estimates of variation (both within and between subjects) and to reduce attenuation in health risk estimates. The optimal number of measurements can be calculated from, and is dependent on, the ratio of within and between subject variance and the level of attenuation (Liu *et al.* 1978). The use of errors-in-variables modelling allows the number of samples per subject to be reduced, but with the need to assess certain distributional assumptions (see Chapter 5). In the group approach, the optimal number of measurements depends on the between group variance (or between subpopulation variance) and the required precision of the estimated mean for each group. The number of subjects required to be monitored can be calculated in various ways, using conventional statistical design techniques. Again, however, repeated measurements on the subjects are highly recommended in order to estimate variance components (within and between subject variance and between subpopulation variance), although they contribute less to the overall precision of the subgroup mean (Leidel *et al.* 1977; WHO 1991; Kromhout *et al.* 1996; Nieuwenhuijsen 1997).

20.2.4 Duration of sampling

The duration of the sampling period (or averaging period) depends on the health outcome of interest in the epidemiological study, the detection limits of the measurement technique and the levels of the pollutant in the environment.

Chronic disease outcomes (e.g. the effects of potential carcinogens on cancer prevalence) generally require long sampling durations. Studies of acute disease outcomes (e.g. relationships between ammonia and irritant effects) require shorter sampling durations. Relatively long sampling times may also be necessary for less sensitive measurement and analysis techniques (e.g. use of passive samplers to measure exposure to nitrogen dioxide), or where low exposure concentrations are being investigated (e.g. $PM_{2.5}$). Sampling duration will also depend on the relevant exposure measure, for example, daily average/daily maximum.

20.3 Personal air pollution measurements

Personal monitoring is perhaps most fully developed in relation to air pollution. Many air pollutants (e.g. PM_{10}, $PM_{2.5}$, VOCs, O_3, CO, NO_2) have the ability to cause adverse human health effects given a sufficient level of exposure. To estimate exposures, a range of methods are available, including the measurement of personal airborne exposures, and biomarkers of exposure in exhaled breath, blood, or urine (e.g. for certain VOCs). The emphasis here is on personal airborne exposure measurements.

20.3.1 Active or passive sampling

To take personal airborne samples, equipment is needed which is light enough to be carried around without undue inconvenience to the subject and which will not significantly alter their usual behaviour patterns. Ideally, the sampler should be placed such that it takes a sample of the inhaled air of the subject, or what is called the breathing zone (within around 30 cm of the nose and mouth). Both active and passive samplers are available for this purpose.

For active sampling, air is drawn by a sampling pump through a collection unit (e.g. a sampling head with a filter inside for PM_{10}, or a Tenax tube for VOCs). The sampling flow is dependent on the requirements of the collection unit and may vary from less than

100 ml/min for VOC sampling to over 4 litres/min for particle sampling. The exposure concentration in air is determined by dividing the difference in the measured amount of the substance before and after the sampling period (e.g. for particles, the weight on the filter before and after sampling, adjusted for control measurements) by the volume of air drawn through the collection unit.

Passive sampling is based on the principle of diffusion and does not require a sampling pump. It is widely used for gaseous substances, such as NO_2. Passive samplers for particulates are in the design stage (Brown *et al.* 1994). A problem in sampling environmental pollutants using passive samplers is often the low concentration of pollutants present, relative to the detection limits of the samplers. This implies the need for relatively long sampling durations and means that the samplers typically provide measures only of long-term average concentrations (e.g. over a week or longer period). There are also problems of accuracy and precision; the widely used Palmes tube (Palmes *et al.* 1976), for example, has been quoted as overestimating NO_2 concentrations by up to 40% compared to active samplers (Gair and Penkett 1995). On the other hand, passive sampling is generally less labour-intensive and costly than active sampling. This provides the possibility of taking more measurements for the same cost and of carrying out relatively intense spatial and temporal sampling (e.g. for use of estimating variance components). Recent advances in the design of passive samplers, the application of strict sampling protocols (including repeat measurements at each site), and the use of validation studies comparing passive samplers with more conventional methods, all offer the scope to improve the performance of passive sampling.

20.3.2   Continuous or average sampling

Depending on the collection unit used, exposure measurements can take the form either of continuous readings or an average over the sampling period. Continuous measurements are provided by direct reading instruments, such as the MINIRAM or GRIMM monitor for particulate sampling and the Langran CO Enhanced Measurer T15 monitor for CO.

Information from direct reading instruments can be stored in data loggers and downloaded to a computer, where they can be graphed and analysed. Although direct reading instruments can provide an informative picture of the variation in exposure over the sampling period, they are relatively rarely used for epidemiological studies. The instruments are often expensive, they are sometimes not very specific, and accurate calibration is of considerable importance. Also, in the case of chronic disease, short-term variations in exposure may not be considered important. More commonly, therefore, monitoring is aimed at providing estimates of average concentrations over a relatively long measurement period (e.g. a day or a few days). As noted above, time-averaged data of this type are provided by passive sampling devices, such as the Palmes tube, or active particle monitors discussed later.

20.3.3   Size selective sampling

In recent years, increasing epidemiological attention has focused on airborne particulates. The health hazard from airborne particulates varies with their physical, chemical, and/or biological properties. An important property is the aerodynamic diameter, which determines how deeply the particle is likely to penetrate into the respiratory system. Particles have thus been categorised according to which region they are likely to reach in the respiratory system; to measure different size fractions, a personal sampler with different sampling heads is needed (Lippman 1989; ACGIH 1998). The inhalable particle fraction is the fraction that enters the nose and the mouth, and has a 50% cut-point diameter of 100 μm (i.e. the distribution of inhalable particles has a median of 100 μm). This fraction is often measured in the workplace, but rarely in the general environment (ACGIH 1998). The thoracic fraction is the fraction that enters the thorax, and has a 50% cut-point diameter of 10 μm; it is therefore often referred to as PM_{10}. The PM_{10} is often measured in the general environment, but rarely in the workplace. To measure this fraction, a special PM_{10} sampling head is required, the most frequently used to date being that designed by Buckley *et al.* (1991) which runs at an airflow rate of 4 litres/min. The respirable fraction is the fraction that enters the lungs (the alveolar region). This has a 50% cut-point diameter of 4 μm. $PM_{2.5}$, particles with a 50% cut-point diameter of 2.5 μm, is the fraction that goes deep into the alveolar region. In environmental studies, cyclones are used to measure this fraction: for example, the GK2.05 cyclone, which runs at 4 litres/min, designed by BGI Inc., Waltham, MA, USA for the EXPOLIS study (Jantunen *et al.* 1998).

20.4   Examples of personal air pollution measurement studies

20.4.1   Nitrogen dioxide

Nitrogen dioxide (NO_2) is one of the most widely monitored substances in environmental epidemiological studies of air pollution. This is partly due to its potential adverse health effects and its use as a marker for traffic. It is also relatively cheap and easy to monitor, using passive samplers such as the Palmes tube (Palmes *et al.* 1976) or the Willems badge (van Reeuwijk *et al.* 1998). Nitrogen dioxide is absorbed on metal grids, coated with triethanolamine, then extracted with sulphonic acid and NEDA which produces a coloured product that can be analysed in a photometer. Nitrogen dioxide is an air pollutant generated mainly by combustion. It occurs both in homes, primarily from gas stoves or heaters, and in the outdoor environment, primarily as a result of emission from road vehicles.

A growing number of studies of exposure to NO_2, using passive samplers, have now been completed. Monn *et al.* (1998), for example, took personal (1 week) indoor and outdoor NO_2 measurements of 500 subjects using diffusion tubes in different Swiss cities. Overall, they found NO_2 exposure levels of 21, 27, and 31 μg/m³ for indoor, personal, and outdoor exposure levels respectively, though the levels varied by city. Nitrogen dioxide outdoor levels during the winter were about 25–40% higher than during the summer. Winter indoor NO_2 levels were in the range of summer levels. There were no significant differences between summer and winter personal NO_2 levels, possibly because people spend 80–90% of their time indoors. Personal NO_2 levels of subjects living in homes with gas cooker were on average 4–7 μg/m³ higher than NO_2 levels in homes with electric cookers. Smokers also had significantly higher personal NO_2 levels (approximately $2\,\mu g/m^3$). The correlation between indoor and personal NO_2 levels was 0.72, and between outdoor and personal NO_2 levels 0.58, suggesting that indoor levels are a better predictor for personal NO_2 levels than outdoor levels, even though a large proportion of the indoor NO_2 comes from outdoor sources. Other larger-scale personal NO_2 measurement studies have been carried out by Quackenboss *et al.* (1986), Spengler *et al.* (1994), and Alm *et al.* (1998).

20.4.2 Particulate exposure

Personal particulate sampling has a long history in the workplace environment. In recent years, however, it has also become widespread in environmental epidemiology. This is partly due to the increased interest in the adverse health effects of particulates, such as respiratory and cardiovascular disease, and partly to realisation that fixed point outdoor monitors do not necessarily provide reliable estimates of exposure to particulates. Also, environmental particulate exposure levels are generally much lower than particulate exposure levels in the workplace, which makes it harder to obtain accurate and precise personal measurements. Examples of large-scale studies using personal particulate exposure methods are the PTEAM study (Clayton *et al.* 1993; Thomas *et al.* 1993*b*; Ozkaynak *et al.* 1996), the THEES study (Lioy *et al.* 1990), and the EXPOLIS study (Jantunen *et al.* 1998).

Some of the issues involved in personal particulate sampling can be illustrated by results from a study of personal exposure of children and adults in the Netherlands, conducted by Janssen (1998). She took repeated personal measurements of PM_{10} with a commonly used PM_{10} sampling head running at an airflow rate of 4 litres/min (Buckley *et al.* 1991), and of fine particulates using a Casella cyclone at 4 litres/min (Casella Ltd, London, UK; 50% cut-point approximately $3\,\mu m$). Results were compared with measurements obtained by fixed point outdoor monitors (Janssen 1998). As expected, PM_{10} exposure levels were higher than fine particulate levels (Table 20.1). Children had higher PM_{10} exposure levels than adults, mainly due to high classroom concentrations of coarse particles and/or suspension of soil material, caused by the presence and activity of the children. Personal particulate exposure levels were higher than ambient exposure levels (Table 20.1), as has often been observed, except perhaps in cases where the ambient exposure levels are very high (Wallace 1996). Higher personal PM_{10} exposure levels have commonly been attributed to the 'personal dust cloud' which is generally not observed with finer particulates (Wallace 1996). The results also showed that personal particulate exposure levels were considerably lower in adults and children not exposed to environmental tobacco smoke (ETS) than for the population as a whole; this confirms that environmental tobacco smoke is one of the main sources of indoor air particulate exposure (Wallace 1996).

Janssen (1998) observed that the correlation between personal particulate exposure levels and outdoor fixed point exposure measurements was low in the whole population when only one personal and one fixed point outdoor exposure measurement was used. The correlation was considerably higher, however, for people not exposed to ETS, especially for fine particulates. Using repeated measurements of personal and fixed point outdoor exposure measurements for each subject increased the correlation, in particular for subjects not exposed to environmental tobacco smoke and for fine particulates. The median of the individual correlation coefficients was 0.9, suggesting that fixed point outdoor monitors might be a good indicator of personal exposure to fine particulates in

Table 20.1 Average levels of personal and outdoor concentrations, and the correlation between personal and outdoor concentrations in Dutch children and adults (after Janssen 1998)

Population	Size fraction	n	Mean personal[1] ($\mu g/m^3$)	Mean ambient[1] ($\mu g/m^3$)	Median individual correlation	Cross sectional correlation[2]
All subjects						
Adults	PM_{10}	37	62	42	0.50	0.34
Children	PM_{10}	45	105	39	0.63	0.28
Children	FP	13	28	17	0.86	0.41
Non-ETS exposed						
Adults	PM_{10}	23	51	41	0.71	0.50
Children	PM_{10}	25	89	40	0.73	0.49
Children	FP	9	23	18	0.92	0.84

[1] mean of individual averages.
[2] Estimated cross-sectional R, by randomly selecting 1 measurement per subject.
  FP, fine particulate; ETS, environmental tobacco smoke; n, number of samples.

epidemiological time series studies, where one links day-to-day variation in particulate exposure levels with day-to-day variation in health end-points. The moderate to high correlation between repeated personal and fixed point outdoor measurements can be explained by the exclusion of 'fixed' indoor air particulate sources such as smoking and gas cookers, which are likely to change little from day to day compared to outdoor levels.

It is not only the particulate mass that might be important in the development of adverse health effects but also the composition of the particulates. It is therefore often useful to analyse particulate samples for their elemental composition. A range of techniques are available for this purpose, including X-ray fluoresence (XRF), inductively coupled plasma-mass spectrometry (ICP-MS), gas chromatography-mass spectrometry (GC-MS), gas chromatography-flame ionisation detection (GC-FID), gas chromatography flame absorption spectrometry (GFAAS), electron scanning microscopy or reflectance methods.

20.4.3 Other gaseous exposures

Other common gaseous exposures, such as ozone (O_3), carbon monoxide (CO), and volatile organic compounds (VOCs—compounds with a boiling point between 50 and 250°C, such as benzene, toluene and trichloroethene), can be measured (semi) personally with active and passive samplers (Hering 1989; Brauer and Brook 1995; Dor *et al.* 1995; Hoteit *et al.* 1996; Jantunen *et al.* 1998; Leung and Harrison 1998). Brauer and Brook (1995) used a nitrite-coated filter passive personal sampler developed by Koutrakis *et al.* (1993) to measure 24-hour personal ozone levels. Liu *et al.* (1995) used the same method to compare outdoor, indoor, and personal exposures to ozone in Toronto. They found that personal and indoor ozone exposure levels were comparable but that outdoor levels were much higher (Table 20.2). Also, ozone levels in the summer were higher than in the winter.

Table 20.2 Ozone levels (ppb) in Toronto (after Liu *et al.* 1995)

	n	Mean	SD
Winter (weekly)			
Home outdoor	72	15.4	6.0
Home indoor	114	1.6	4.1
Workplace	38	0.7	0.7
Personal	71	1.3	2.9
Summer (12 h)			
Home outdoor (D)	199	19.1	10.8
Home outdoor (N)	160	9.4	10.2
Home indoor (D)	199	7.1	12.6
Home indoor (N)	160	6.2	9.5
Workplace (D)	93	10.0	11.6
Personal (D)	424	8.2	8.7

n, number of samples; SD, standard deviation; D, day; N, night.

Hoteit *et al.* (1996) carried out active sampling with stainless steel tubes with an absorbent with Carbopack-B to measure personal VOC exposure levels of commuters in London. They found the highest levels of VOCs among car users with levels of 55.2 $\mu g/m^3$ for benzene and 177.9 $\mu g/m^3$ for toluene in the morning. Using active personal sampling with sorbent tubes with Tenax TA, Leung and Harrison (1998) found average personal exposure levels to benzene of 4.69 ppb during the day for urban volunteers in Birmingham, UK and 2.98 ppb for non-urban volunteers from surrounding Birmingham; night-time concentrations were lower.

Carbon monoxide can be measured using active continuous samplers. Dor *et al.* (1995), for example, used a portable monitor—the PAC II CO (Draeger Industry)—to study exposure levels during commuting. They reported average CO levels of 12 ppm inside the car. Jantunen *et al.* (1998) used a CO Enhanced Measurer T15 (Langan Products Inc., San Francisco, USA) to measure CO levels. Fernandez-Bremauntz (1993) and Fernandez-Bremauntz and Ashmore (1995) measured exposure to CO in Mexico City commuters with the commonly used General Electric COED-1 detector (General Electric). Highest levels were recorded among car users (up to 66 ppm) compared with users of the bus and metro. The in-vehicle CO levels were higher than fixed monitor point levels.

20.5 Examples of personal exposure measurements in water

Disinfection by-products in drinking water, such as the trihalomethanes (THMs), have attracted considerable attention in recent years because of their suspected health effects (see Chapter 24). THMs are formed when chlorine reacts with organic matter in the water. The four major THMs are chloroform, bromodichloromethane (BDCM), dibromochloromethane (DBCM), and bromoform. Chloroform is the main THM and makes up around 75% of the total THMs (typically *c.* 40–50 $\mu g/litre$). BDCM tends to make up about 20% of total THMs, DBCM 3% and bromoform 2%. The composition can vary, however, depending on water source and environmental conditions (Keegan 1998). THMs are routinely measured in the drinking water supply, and total THM levels are generally below the exposure standard of 100 µg/litre.

In the past, epidemiological studies tended to analyse associations between THM and health outcome by comparing populations drinking ground water (low THM levels) with those using surface water (higher THM levels), or different treatment method (e.g. chlorine versus ozone treatment). Recently, however, there has been a trend towards estimating the actual intake of THM through ingestion, by estimating the consumption of tapwater (both hot and cold, at home and away from home) and multiplying this by estimated or measured THM levels (Savitz *et al.* 1995; Cantor *et al.* 1998; Hildesheim *et al.* 1998; Waller *et al.* 1998). A drawback of some of these studies is that they have summed concentrations of the four different THMs to create an estimate of total THM concentration. This may be misleading, since the different THMs may have different toxicities and be associated with different health effects. Variations in water composition also mean that total THM levels are generally not a good marker for individual THM levels (Keegan 1998).

THMs have been associated with a number of health effects, including cancers, in particular bladder and rectal cancer (Morris *et al.* 1992), and more recently reproductive outcomes (Reif *et al.* 1996). Waller *et al.* (1998) found an increased risk of spontaneous abortions (odds ratio = 1.8, 95% confidence interval 1.1–3.0) with the consumption of 5 glasses or more a day of water with 75 µg/litre or more total THMs. In analyses of individual THMs, however, an increased risk was found only for BDCM exposure (5 glasses or more and 18 µg/litre or more BDCM).

It is important to note that ingestion is not the only pathway of THM uptake. THMs are volatile and can also enter the body through inhalation or dermal exposure during showering, bathing, and swimming and this needs to be taken into account in epidemiological studies to avoid exposure misclassification. Recent studies have shown that uptake through routes other than ingestion could well make the largest contribution to the total uptake of THMs, particularly chloroform. This can be determined by biomonitoring: for example, by measuring chloroform in the bloodstream, or more easily in the exhaled breath (Jo *et al.* 1990; Weisel and Jo 1996). Uptake of chloroform through a 10-minute shower or half-hour bath is similar to ingestion of 2 litres of water, the estimated average daily consumption (Jo *et al.* 1990; Weisel and Jo 1996). Swimming, similarly, might be an important route of uptake (Levesque *et al.* 1994). Dermal absorption appears to be temperature-dependent, with 30 times higher uptakes in a 40°C bath compared with a 30°C bath (Gordon *et al.* 1998). Also, ingested chloroform appears to be metabolised completely in the liver before it can enter the bloodstream, while uptake through dermal and inhalation exposure appears in the bloodstream (Weisel and Jo 1996).

20.6   Examples of personal exposure measurement in soil

Soil represents an important pathway of exposure, through handling of soil materials (e.g. during play or work), through contact with soil-derived dust, and through foodstuffs. Exposures to arsenic have attracted particular concern, and several studies

Table 20.3 Arsenic (As) in soil, house dust, and urine in the southwest
of England (after Kavanagh *et al.* 1998)

	Cargreen	Gunnislake	Devon GC	Ratios between sites
Soil (µg/g)	37	365	4500	1 : 10 : 122
House dust (µg/g)	49	217	1167	1 : 4 : 24
Urine (µg/g creatine)				
Total As	4.7	9.2	10.0	1 : 2 : 2
Arsenite (As III)	< LOD	1.7	0.9	
Arsenate (As V)	< LOD	0.9	1.3	
DMA	4.7	5.6	8.5	
MMA	< LOD	0.3	0.7	

GC, Great Consols; < LOD, below limit of detection; DMA, dimethylarsinic acid; MMA, monomethylarsinic acid.

have suggested an association between soil arsenic and cancer of, for example, the skin, lung, and bladder. This is mainly attributed to the inorganic form of arsenic (Chen *et al.* 1997). The acute toxicity of inorganic arsenic is reduced by methylation in mammals, including humans, forming monomethylarsinic acid (MMA) and dimethylarsinic acid (DMA) (Buchet and Lauwerys 1994). Arsenic uptake is most likely through inhalation and digestion of soil and house dust, including hand-to-mouth contact, but also through ingestion of contaminated vegetables, fish and water, and smoking.

Arsenic and its species can be measured in soil, house dust, and by biomonitoring in hair, urine, blood, and toenails (Bencko and Symon 1977; Kavanagh *et al.* 1998). Mining and smelting have left certain areas of southwest England with high arsenic levels in soil. Kavanagh *et al.* (1998) measured arsenic levels in soil, house dust, and urine of residents in three areas: two exposed areas (Gunnislake and Devon Great Consols) and one unexposed area (Cargreen) (Table 20.3). Arsenic species in urine were determined using high pressure liquid chromatography-induced coupled plasma-mass spectrometry (HPLC-ICP-MS). High levels of arsenic were found in the soil and, to a lesser extent, in house dust. Marked variations were evident, however, between the different areas. For the soil, concentrations in the exposed areas were up to 122 times those in the unexposed; for house dust, concentrations were up to 24 times higher; in urine, there was only a twofold difference in arsenic levels between the areas. This suggests that the actual uptake of arsenic from soil and house dust is relatively low. Moreover, biomonitoring needs to be undertaken to obtain good estimates of personal arsenic uptake, since soil or house dust samples cannot be relied on to provide a reliable dose estimate. The study also suggested that arsenic speciation is important, for inorganic arsenic levels in the control village were below the detection limit, while in the other two areas they were measurable.

20.7 Conclusions

The examples of personal monitoring in air, water, and soil presented here provide only an illustration of the methods and potential for exposure assessment using personal monitoring. Many other exposures are also of undoubted interest in terms of their health effects, and many pose particular opportunities and challenges for personal monitoring. Examples include noise, electromagnetic fields, and radioactivity.

Personal monitoring is inevitably often labour-intensive and expensive. It is nevertheless a valuable technique, for it can dramatically improve exposure assessment in epidemiological studies, and thereby add to the scientific credibility of the studies. Intuitively, personal monitoring should provide more accurate exposure estimates than other methods. As has been shown, however, this is highly dependent on the quality and rigour of sampling and the variability in exposure levels in the study population. Good exposure assessment thus requires careful design of personal monitoring campaigns. Estimates of average exposure levels also provide only one perspective on exposures; equally important are the sources and pathways of exposure and the distribution of variability in exposure levels. In many cases, an understanding of the major determinants of exposure can be as informative as measures of the exposure levels themselves.

References

ACGIH (1998). *TLVs and BEIs: Threshold limit values for chemical substance and physical agents.* ACGIH, Cincinnati, OH.

Alm, S., Mukala, K., Jantunen, M. J., Pasanen, P., Tiitanen, P., Ruuskanen, J. *et al.* (1998). Personal NO₂ exposures of preschool children in Helsinki. *Journal of Exposure Analysis and Environmental Epidemiology*, **8**, 79–100.

Armstrong, B. G. and Oakes, D. (1982). Effects of approximation in exposure assessments on estimates of exposure response relationship. *Scandinavian Journal of Working Environmental Health*, **8**, 20–3.

Armstrong, B. (1990). The effects of measurement errors on relative risk regressions. *American Journal of Epidemiology*, **13**, 1176–84.

Armstrong, B. K., White, E., and Saracci, R. (1992). *Principles of exposure measurement in epidemiology.* Oxford University Press, New York.

Bencko, V. and Symon, K. (1977). Health aspects of burning coal with a high arsenic content. I: Arsenic in hair, urine and blood in children residing in a polluted area. *Environmental Research*, **13**, 378–85.

Bencko, V. (1995). The use of hair as a biomarker in the assessment of exposure to pollutants in occupational and environmental settings. *Toxicology*, **101**, 29–39.

Brauer, M. and Brook, J. R. (1995). Personal and fixed-site ozone measurements with a passive sampler. *Journal of the Air and Waste Management Association*, **45**, 529–37.

Brown, R. C., Wake, D., Thorpe, A., Hemingway, M. A., and Roff, M. W. (1994). Preliminary assessment of a device for passive sampling of airborne particulate. *Annals of Occupational Hygiene*, **38**, 303–18.

Buchet, J. P. and Lauwerys, R. (1994). Inorganic arsenic metabolism in humans. In *Arsenic exposure and health effects* (W. R. Chappell, C. O. Abernathy, and C. R. Cothern ed.), 181–96. Science and Technology Letters, Northwood, USA.

Buckley, T. J., Waldman, J. M., Freeman, N. C. G., Lioy, P. J., Marple, V. A. *et al.* (1991). Calibration, intersampler comparison and field application of a new PM-10 personal air sampling impactor. *Aerosol Science and Technology*, **14**, 380–7.

Cantor, K. P., Lynch, C. F., Hildesheim, M. E., Dosemeci, M., Lubin, J., Alavanja, M. *et al.* (1998). Drinking water source and chlorination by products. I: Risk of bladder cancer. *Epidemiology*, **9**, 21–8.

Chen, C. J., Hsueh, Y. M., Chiou, H. Y., Hsu, Y. H., Chen, S. Y., Horng, S. F. *et al.* (1997). Human carcinogenicity of inorganic cancer. In *Arsenic, exposure and health effects* (C. O. Abernathy, R. L. Calderon, and W. R. Chappell ed.), 232–42, Chapman & Hall, London.

Clayton, C. A., Perritt, R. C., Pellizzari, E. D., Thomas, K. W., Whitmore, R. W., Wallace, L. A. *et al.* (1993). Particle total exposure assessment methodology (PTEAM) 1990 study: distributions of aerosol and elemental concentrations in personal, indoor and outdoor air samplers in a southern California community. *Journal of Exposure Analysis and Environmental Epidemiology*, **3**, 227–50.

Dor, F., Le Moullec, Y., and Festy, B. (1995). Exposure of city residents to carbon monoxide and monocyclic aromatic hydrocarbons during commuting trips in the Paris metropolitan area. *Journal of the Air and Waste Management Association*, **45**, 103–10.

Fernandez-Bremauntz, A. A. (1993). Commuters' exposure to carbon monoxide in the metropolitan area of Mexico City. Unpublished Ph.D. thesis, Centre for Environmental Technology, Imperial College, University of London.

Fernandez-Bremauntz, A. A. and Ashmore, M. R. (1995). Exposure of commuters to carbon monoxide in Mexico city. I: Measurement of in-vehicle concentrations. *Atmospheric Environment*, **29**, 525–32.

Gair, A. J. and Penkett, S. A. (1995). The effects of wind speed and turbulence on the performance of diffusion tube samplers. *Atmospheric Environment*, **29**, 2529–33.

Gallagher, M. D., Nuckols, J. R., Stallones, L., and Savitz, D. (1998), Exposure to trihalomethanes and adverse pregnancy outcomes. *Epidemiology*, **9**, 484–9.

Gordon, S. M., Wallace, L. A., Callahan, P. J., Kenny, D. V., and Brinkman, M. C. (1998). Effects of water temperature on dermal exposure to chloroform. *Environmental Health Perspectives*, **106**, 337–45.

Heederik, D. and Miller, B. (1988). Weak associations in epidemiology: adjustment for exposure estimation error. *International Journal of Epidemiology*, **17**, 970–4.

Heederik, D., Kromhout, H., and Braun, W. (1996). The influence of random exposure estimation error on the exposure-response relationship when grouping into homogeneous exposure categories. *Occupational Hygiene*, **3**, 229–41.

Hering, S. V. (1989). *AGGIH air sampling instruments for evaluation of atmospheric contaminants* (7th edn). ACGIH, Cincinnati, OH.

Hildesheim, M. E., Cantor, K. P., Lynch, C. F., Dosemeci, M., Lubin, J., Alavanja, M. *et al.* (1998). Drinking water source and chlorination by products. II: Risk of colon and rectal cancer. *Epidemiology*, **9**, 29–35.

Hoteit, J. A., Gee, I. L., and Sollars, C. J. (1996). Commuters' exposure to VOCs in London. Paper presented to the Conference on Current Research Trends in Air Quality, London, Society of Chemical Industry.

Janssen, N. (1998). Personal exposure to airborne particles. Validity of outdoor concentrations as a measure of exposure in time series studies. Unpublished Ph.D. thesis, Wageningen Agricultural University.

Jantunen, M. J., Hanninen, O., Katsounyanni, K., Knoppel, H., Kuenzli, N., Lebret, E. *et al.* (1998). Air pollution in European cities: the EXPOLIS study. *Journal of Exposure Analysis and Environmental Epidemiology*, **8**, 495–518.

Jo, W. K., Wiesel, C. P., and Lioy, P. J. (1990). Routes of chloroform exposure and body burden from showering with chlorinated tap water. *Risk Analysis*, **10**, 575–80.

Kavanagh, P., Farago, M. E., Thornton, I., Goessler, W., Kuehnelt, D., Schlagenhaufen, C. *et al.* (1998). Urinary arsenic species in Devon and Cornwall residents, UK. *The Analyst*, **123**, 27–30.

Keegan T. (1998). Trihalomethane levels in the North of England 1992–1996. Unpublished M.Sc. thesis, Imperial College of Science, Technology and Medicine, University of London.

Keith, L. H. (1996). *Principles of environmental sampling* (2nd edn). American Chemical Society, Washington.

Koutrakis, P., Wolfson, J. M., Bunyaviroch, A., Froehlich, S. E., Hirano, K., and Mulik, J. D. (1993). Measurement of ozone using nitrite coated filter. *Analytical Chemistry*, **65**, 209–14.

Kromhout, H., Tielemans, E., Preller, L., and Heedrik, D. (1996). Estimates of individual dose from current measurements of exposure. *Occupational Hygiene*, **3**, 23–9.

Leidel, N. A., Busch, K. A., and Lynch, J. R. (1977). *Occupational exposure sampling strategy*. NIOSH Publication. 77–173. NIOSH, Cincinnati, OH.

Leung, P.-L. and Harrison, R. M. (1998). Evaluation of personal exposure to monoaromatic hydrocarbons. *Occupational and Environmental Medicine*, **55**, 249–57.

Levesque, B., Ayotte, P., LeBlanc, A., Dewailly, E., Prudhomme, D., Lavoie, R. *et al.* (1994). Evaluation of dermal and respiratory chloroform exposure in humans. *Environmental Health Perspectives*, **102**, 1082–7.

Lin, S. M., Chang, C. H., and Yang, M. H. (1985). Arsenic concentration in urine of patients with Blackfoot disease and Bowen's disease. *Biological Trace Element Research*, **8**, 11–8.

Linn, W. S., Shamoo, D. A., Anderson, K. R., Peng, R.-C., Avol, E. L., Hackney, J. D. *et al.* (1996). Short-term air pollution exposures and responses in Los Angeles area schoolchildren. *Journal of Exposure Analysis and Environmental Epidemiology*, **6**, 449–72.

Lioy, P. J., Waldman, J. M., Buckley, T., Butler, J., and Pieterinen, C. (1990). The personal indoor and outdoor concentrations of PM-10 measured in an industrial community during the winter. *Atmospheric Environment*, **24B**, 57–66.

Lippman, M. (1989). Size selective health hazard sampling. In *ACGIH air sampling instruments for evaluation of atmospheric contaminants* (7th edn), (S. V. Hering ed.), 163–98. ACGIH, Cincinnati, OH.

Liu, K., Stamler, J. A., Dyer, A., McKeever, J., and McKeever, P. (1978). Statistical methods to assess and minimize the role of intra individual variability in obscuring the relationship between dietary lipids and serum cholesterol. *Journal of Chronic Disease*, **31**, 399–418.

Liu, L. J. S., Koutrakis, P., Leech, J., and Border, I. (1995). Assessment of ozone exposures in greater metropolitan Toronto area. *Journal of the Air and Waste Management Association*, **45**, 223–34.

Monn, C., Fuchs, A., Hogger, D., Junker, M., Kogelschatz, D., Roth, N. *et al.* (1997). Particulate matter less than 10 mm (PM10) and fine particles less than 2.5 mm (PM2.5): relationships between indoor, outdoor and personal concentrations. *Science of the Total Environment*, **208**, 15–21.

Monn, C., Brandli, O., Schindler, C., Ackermann-Liebrich, U., and Leuenberger, P. (1998). Personal exposure to nitrogen dioxide in Switzerland. *Science of the Total Environment*, **215**, 243–51.

Morris, R. D., Audet, A. M., Angelillo, I. F., Chalmers, T. C., and Mosteller, I. F. 1992). Chlorination, chlorination by-products and cancer: a meta-analysis. *American Journal of Public Health*, **82**(7), 955–63.

Nakai, S., Nitta, H., and Maeda, K. (1995). Respiratory health associated with exposure to automobile exhaust. II: Personal NO_2 exposure levels according to distance from the roadside. *Journal of Exposure Analysis and Environmental Epidemiology*, **5**, 125–36.

NRC (National Research Council) (1991). *Human exposure assessment for airborne pollutants. Advances and opportunities*. National Academy of Science, Washington, DC.

Nicas, M., Simmons, B. P., and Spear, R. C. (1991). Environmental versus analytical variability in exposure measurements. *American Industrial Hygiene Association Journal*, **52**, 553–7.

Nieuwenhuijsen, M. J. (1997). Exposure assessment in occupational epidemiology: measuring present exposures with an example of occupational asthma. *International Archives of Occupational and Environmental Health*, **70**, 295–308.

Ozkaynak, H., Xue, J., Spengler, J., Wallace, L., Pellizzari, E., and Jenkins, P. (1996). Personal exposure to airborne particles and metals: results from the particle team study in Riverside, California. *Journal of Exposure Analysis and Environmental Epidemiology*, **6**, 57–78.

Palmes, E. D., Gunnison, A. F., Dimattio, J., and Tomczyk, C. (1976). Personal sampler for nitrogen dioxide. *American Industrial Hygiene Association Journal*, **37**, 570–7.

Quakenboss, J., Spengler, J., Kanarek, M., Letz, R., and Duffy, C. (1986). Personal exposure to nitrogen dioxide: relationship to indoor/outdoor air quality and activity patterns. *Environmental Science and Technology*, **20**, 775–83.

Reif, J. S., Hatch, M. C., Bracken, M., Holmes, L. B., Schwetz, B. A., and Singer, P. C. (1996). Reproductive and development effects of disinfection by products in drinking water. *Environmental Health Perspectives*, **104**, 1056–61.

Savitz, D. A., Andrews, K. W., and Pistore, L. M. (1995). Drinking water and pregnancy outcome in central North Carolina: source, amount and trihalomethane levels. *Environmental Health Perspectives*, **103**, 592–6.

Searle, S. R., Casella, G., and McCulloch. C. E. (1992). *Variance components*. Wiley, New York.

Seixas, N. S. and Sheppard, L. (1996). Maximizing accuracy and precision using individual and grouped exposure assessments. *Scandinavian Journal of Environment and Working Health*, **22**, 94–101.

Spengler, J., Schwab, M., Ryan, P. B., Billick, I. H., Colome, S., Wilson, A. L. *et al.* (1994). Personal exposure to nitrogen dioxide in the Los Angeles basin. *Journal of the Air and Waste Management Association*, **44**, 39–47.

Thomas, D., Stram, D., and Dwyer, J. (1993a). Exposure measurement error: influence on exposure-disease relationships and methods of correction. *Annual Review of Public Health*, **14**, 69–93.

Thomas, K. W., Pellizzari, E. D., Clayton, C. A., Whitaker, D. A., Shores, R. C., Spengler, J. D. *et al.* (1993b). Particle total exposure assessment methodology (PTEAM) 1990 study: method performance and data quality for personal, indoor and outdoor monitoring. *Journal of Exposure Analysis and Environmental Epidemiology*, **3**, 203–26.

Valentine, J. L., Kang, H. K., and Spivey, G. (1979). Arsenic levels in human blood, urine and hair. *Environmental Research*, **20**, 24–32.

van Reeuwijk, H., Fischer, P. H., Harssema, H., Briggs, D. J., Smallbone, K., and Lebret, E. (1998). Field comparison of two NO_2 passive samplers to assess spatial variation. *Environmental Monitoring and Assessment*, **50**, 37–51.

Wallace, L. (1996). Indoor particles: a review. *Journal of the Air and Waste Management Association*, **46**, 98–126.

Waller, K., Swan, S. H., DeLorenze, G., and Hopkins, B. (1998). Trihalomethanes in drinking water and spontaneous abortion. *Epidemiology*, **9**, 134–40.

Weisel, C. P. and Jo, W. K. (1996). Ingestion, inhalation, and dermal exposures to chloroform and trihalomethane from tap water. *Environmental Health Perspectives*, **104**, 48–51.

WHO (World Health Organisation) (1991). *An introductory guide to human exposure field studies— Survey methods and statistical sampling*. WHO, Geneva.

21. Dispersion modelling

R. Colvile and D. J. Briggs

21.1 Introduction

This chapter is concerned with the processes and mechanisms by which human populations are exposed to environmental contaminants. A number of physical and chemical
processes can cause the concentration, and sometimes the nature, of pollutants to change
after emission. These processes, which operate on different length- and time-scales,
interact with the spatial distribution of sources and the time-history of emissions to
produce a characteristic geography and temporal variation of a given pollutant in any
specific situation. The action of a given process also typically depends on factors that
vary in time and space. The most important such process, to which every material pollutant is subject, is dispersion by turbulent diffusion. This forms the focus for much of
this chapter. Other processes are considered in Section 21.4. We discuss these processes
mainly in relation to air pollution; many of the basic principles involved, however, are
applicable to other environmental media, such as water or soil. In Section 21.5, we
discuss the problems and limitations of the approach, including the availability of data,
while in Section 21.6 we address the use of dispersion modelling in exposure assessment
for epidemiological study, including the link to GIS-based systems.

21.2 Dispersion processes

Within the context of this chapter, it is necessary to specify the term 'material pollutant'.
In most cases, when considering dispersion, one is dealing either with gases mixed, or
particles suspended, in the air. There are, however, other atmospheric pollutants, such as
electromagnetic radiation or noise which, though propagated through the air, are not
actually subject to turbulent diffusion.

The term 'turbulent diffusion' also needs defining. Two forms of diffusion can, in fact,
be distinguished. Molecular diffusion is the process by which two miscible fluids of
similar density in different halves of a closed box will, after sufficient time has elapsed,
end up being homogeneously mixed throughout the box. This is due to thermal motion
of individual molecules in a gaseous or liquid fluid, so the process operates in a perfectly still medium. It occurs at length-scales of the distance between molecules (10^{-8} m)
and is effective over distances of centimetres to metres. Turbulent diffusion, in contrast,

only occurs when the fluid moves in bulk. Like thermal molecular motion, turbulent motion has a random nature. The smallest turbulent motions, however, are performed by parcels of air centimetres in size containing approximately 10^{18} molecules moving together. This random motion is therefore on a much larger scale than thermal motion, and so turbulent diffusion acts over much larger distances than molecular diffusion. While both kinds of diffusion can be described by identical mathematics—the diffusion equation—turbulent diffusion is significantly more complicated because it depends on, and is superimposed upon, the larger-scale motion of the fluid. It is this interaction between large-scale advection and small-scale turbulence that causes a time-based process (diffusion) to manifest itself as a spatial variation in pollutant concentration (dispersion).

It is possible to have bulk movement of a fluid without turbulence occurring. Flow that occurs slowly or which is confined to have a small cross-section or a thin layer can be entirely predictable and regular. As the speed of flow increases, however, or as the depth of the flow increases, a transition to turbulent flow takes place. The point at which this transition occurs can be defined by the Reynolds number: this is calculated by taking a length-scale characteristic of the flow, multiplying it by the flow speed and dividing by the viscosity of the fluid. A small value defines regular, predictable laminar motion, while at large Reynolds numbers the flow tends to become turbulent and any inhomogeneity introduced into the fluid is quickly mixed across the flow. In the atmosphere, we are dealing with a fluid (air) that has low viscosity moving at several metres per second in layers ranging from several metres to kilometres in depth, giving rise to large Reynolds numbers. Nearly all atmospheric flows, therefore, have the potential to become highly turbulent, and it is impossible to predict the detailed path that will be followed by a single molecule of pollutant after it is emitted into the atmosphere.

Even when the Reynolds number is very large, laminar flow may nevertheless occur if the surfaces that bound the flow are extremely smooth. The relevant parameter describing this is the roughness length of the surface. This is not directly equal to the size of the roughness elements of which that surface is composed (e.g. the length of the blades of grass which make up a grassland surface), but tends to be somewhat smaller and is a function of both the shape of the roughness elements and their distance apart. Table 21.1

Table 21.1 Typical surface roughness for different land covers (based on CERC 1999)

Land cover	Surface roughness (mm)
Cities	1000
Woodland	1000
Parkland	500
Open suburbia	500
Arable crops	200–300
Root crops	100
Open grassland	20
Short grassland	5
Sandy desert	1

gives roughness lengths for a range of different surfaces. Increasing roughness leads to increased levels of turbulence. Pollutants will therefore be diluted by dispersion somewhat more rapidly over a rough urban surface than over a smoother rural one.

Treating an urban area as a rough surface is to ignore the detail of individual buildings and to consider only their effect en masse. This adequately describes the processes operating some distance above the rooftops—two or three times the building height. In the near-surface layers, however, turbulence is generated at individual edges and vertices. Regions of highly chaotic flow occur downwind of bluff obstacles as the air becomes unable to follow the outline of the obstacle and detaches from its surface to form separated flow regions and wakes. This can have a variety of effects on pollution levels. On the one hand, pollution can be dispersed more rapidly because of the enhanced levels of turbulence; on the other hand, it can become trapped as it gets caught up in a recirculation zone from which it only slowly leaks out. The rate of leakage in this latter case is determined by details of the turbulence at the interface with the surrounding flow.

In addition to surface characteristics, processes in the atmosphere itself can also reduce or enhance turbulence. One of the most important is the effect of temperature variations. If a cool parcel of air near the ground on a clear night rises slightly due to the turbulence of the flow it will encounter warmer surrounding air and its upward motion will be impeded by the cooler air's greater density. The temperature gradient within the atmosphere thus dampens down turbulence to a certain extent. Small eddies can persist, but the larger ones disappear. In this condition, the atmosphere is said to be stable (Fig. 21.1a). The vertical height at which turbulence is inhibited can be estimated by calculating a parameter called the Monin–Obukhov length (L_{MO}), which is proportional to the surface wind speed cubed and inversely proportional to the flux of heat at the ground.

Conversely, instability occurs where the ground surface is hotter than the air above it, as on a sunny day with a cool gentle breeze. A parcel of warm air from near the ground rising into the cooler air above will be less dense than its surroundings and will therefore be encouraged to rise further. Turbulence is enhanced, and over vertical distances larger than L_{MO} it is then not the surface roughness that dominates the generation of turbulence but the heating of the air by its contact with the ground. The variation of temperature with height can thus cause overturning motions as deep as several hundreds of metres to be generated.

In intermediate conditions, between stable and unstable, the thermal stratification of the atmosphere is defined as neutral. These conditions are found when the earth is thermally insulated both from the heat of the sun and from the cold of outer space, for example by an unbroken layer of thick cloud in the presence of a weak sun, and when the wind is strong (Fig. 21.1b). Thermal equilibrium is thus established, and air temperature falls at a rate of about 9.8 °C per kilometre of height. This is the simplest situation, for turbulence is generated solely by the flow of air over the roughness of the earth's surface. In these conditions, L_{MO} becomes infinite and meaningless. The amount of turbulence is intermediate between the inhibited mixing of stable conditions and the enhanced overturning of unstable conditions.

The dispersion of pollution is related directly to the level of turbulence. Dilution therefore occurs most rapidly in unstable conditions and least rapidly in stable conditions. For sources close to the ground, ground-level concentrations at a given distance downwind

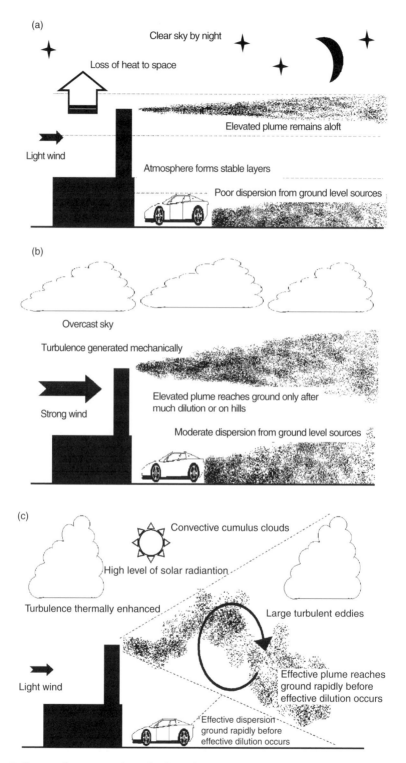

Fig. 21.1 Pollutant dispersion from high and ground-level sources under different meteorological conditions: (a) stable conditions; (b) intermediate conditions; (c) unstable conditions.

will be highest in stable conditions. The same does not apply, however, to an elevated source such as the pollution from a tall chimney. Under stable conditions, the dilution is slight, but the spread of the plume is also slight so the pollution remains aloft (Fig. 21.1a). Under unstable conditions, in contrast, large turbulent eddies transport the plume down to the ground close to the source. Averaged over several minutes, the plume assumes the shape of a broad fan that intercepts the ground close to the source. Over shorter time-scales, fluctuating concentrations occur at any location, as the plume loops up and down under the influence of turbulent eddies that are larger than the plume itself (Fig. 21.1c).

Where obstacles to the flow are large enough for these temperature effects to be significant on vertical scales comparable with the height of the obstacle, surface and thermal effects can interact with each other. Most buildings are too small to do this, but even moderately small hills can have temperature differences of several degrees Celsius between the valley floor and the summit. In stable conditions, air has difficulty rising up the windward slope of a hill. If the hill is isolated, the air upwind will be deflected around the sides of the hill. In the case of a continuous ridge, however, air will stagnate upwind of the hill and any pollution emitted into that air will be trapped there. This is what causes the notorious pollution problems of cities that are situated in basins surrounded by hills. For cities with mountains on one side and sea on the other, such as Los Angeles or Athens, the problem can be even worse, for then pollution which is carried out to sea during the morning tends to return in the afternoon, on the sea breeze.

The layer of air through which pollutants can be dispersed is, in fact, limited. The influence of the Earth's surface exchanging heat with the air above and generating turbulence is limited to a boundary layer that has quite different properties to the free troposphere above. At the top of the boundary layer, marked discontinuities tend to occur in most of the parameters that describe the atmosphere—temperature, windspeed, wind direction, and turbulence parameters. It is significantly less easy for pollution to be transported across this discontinuity than it is for material to be dispersed within the turbulent boundary layer itself.

The height of the top of the boundary layer may vary substantially. During a still night the boundary layer may be as shallow as only a few metres. In these conditions, pollution thus tends to be trapped close to the ground, both by the thermal stratification of the air and by the shallowness of the boundary layer. As the sun rises and wind starts to blow, turbulence gradually causes this shallow boundary layer to grow as air is pulled in from above. Typically, therefore, a depth of several hundred metres may be reached by mid afternoon in conditions of neutral atmospheric stability. In unstable conditions, especially in summer when the longer day provides more time for boundary-layer growth than in winter, depths in excess of a kilometre can be attained.

Boundary-layer depths can also vary geographically. For example, a deeper, more turbulent boundary layer can develop over a very rough surface than over a smoother one. Just as the maximum daytime boundary-layer depth is limited by the number of hours since dawn, however, so the influence of an increase in surface roughness is limited by the distance downwind of the roughness change. As a result, internal boundary layers develop within the wider boundary layer, as shown in Fig. 21.2. In the internal boundary layer, turbulence parameters are determined by the properties of the surface below, while higher up the flow is influenced by the surface further upwind.

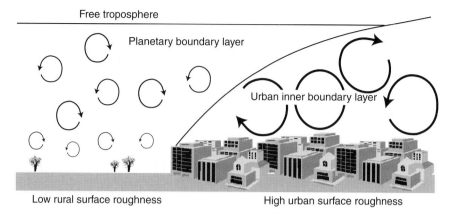

Fig. 21.2 Geographical variations in the internal boundary layer across a rural-urban area.

21.3   Dispersion modelling

The most simplistic approach to modelling atmospheric dispersion is simply to write a computer code encapsulating the mathematical equations that govern the dispersion and advection of pollutants from source to sink in a given geographical area. For input, such a model takes the spatial and temporal distribution of emissions plus values for fundamental meteorological parameters, such as the upper atmosphere windspeed, direction, pressure, and temperature. Assuming that the equations can be solved (and that the necessary processing power is available), maps can then be generated of the pollutant concentration and deposition values, windspeed and direction, temperature and turbulence parameters.

Unfortunately, the computational difficulties inherent in this approach limit its applicability. A process known as discretisation has to be carried out, in which the mathematical description of the continuum of the atmosphere is mapped on to a discrete grid in space (a Eulerian grid) and solved by stepping from one snapshot in time to another. Any process that occurs on length-scales smaller than the grid size, or on time-scales shorter than the stepping interval, cannot therefore be considered explicitly. Even with discretisation, the numerical methods face the problem of indeterminacy: the number of unknown parameters which need to be solved is larger than the number of equations of motion available.

To narrow down the model output to a single set of calculated parameter values, it is therefore necessary to make assumptions about the relationships between some of the unknown parameters. Most importantly (in all except the most recent large eddy resolving models) turbulence needs to be parameterised as a process occurring on smaller length-scales than the model grid. A widely used turbulence model of this type, especially at small length-scales such as for flow around buildings, is the k–ε model. This consists of empirical relationships, expressing the rate of production of turbulence, k, and its rate of dissipation, ε, as functions of the mean flow velocity and vertical and horizontal gradients therein. In this way, the model captures approximately how turbulence generated in one place (e.g., at the corner of a building) is transported in the direction of the mean flow and can then influence dispersion some distance away before the turbulence dies away.

In simple topographic environments, (e.g. in open fields and gently rolling hills), it is possible to use simpler turbulence models. Turbulence that is generated in one place tends not to persist for any significant distance downwind, so the turbulence in the flow at a point is determined by the topography at that point. It is therefore possible to use a single empirical relationship to calculate the amount of turbulence at a point from the properties of the flow at that point. This is called local equilibrium of turbulence.

The success (and complexity) of the Eulerian gridded approach thus depends on the complexity of the geographical features that one wishes to represent. Flow and dispersion over a gentle hill can be modelled in a few seconds assuming local equilibrium of turbulence for a given set of meteorological conditions using a personal computer. The complexities of flow and dispersion around a small group of buildings can be resolved in one hour or more using a k–ε model on a powerful desktop workstation. But the detailed flow and dispersion across a complex range of mountains or a whole urban area can keep a supercomputer busy for run times that vary between minutes and several hours.

One application of such large Eulerian models is not pollution dispersion but operational weather forecasting. These models currently calculate only the meteorological parameters of interest to forecasters, but they can be adapted for air pollution modelling if sufficient computational power is available. As interest in air quality grows and ever more powerful computers become available, it is likely that air pollution parameters will be calculated routinely in operational models and will be available alongside rainfall, temperature, and wind parameters in every weather forecast. Currently, leading global weather circulation models include a realistic treatment of sources, dispersion, transformation, and loss of sulphur dioxide from major fossil fuel, volcanic and biological sources, so that the significant effects of these on climate can be studied. Many major cities worldwide have also had their air quality assessed using much finer resolution but equally detailed Eulerian models covering only the city and its immediate surroundings, of which the USEPA's urban airshed model (UAM) is a well-known example (USEPA 1993).

For many atmospheric dispersion problems, however, it is possible to make even more drastic assumptions than the local equilibrium of turbulence closure assumption mentioned above. This allows the computational resources required to model pollutant dispersal to be very greatly reduced. For a source of pollution over flat terrain, for example, it can be assumed that turbulence in the atmosphere is the same everywhere. Under this assumption, the pollution concentration from a single point source is represented by a regular geometrical plume with a Gaussian cross-section (Fig. 21.3). This approach considerably simplifies the computational process and underlies many widely used dispersion models, such as the ICS3 suite of models developed for the US Environmental Protection Agency (USEPA 1995) and the CALINE line-source model (Benson 1992). In addition to information on the source strength, for short-range calculations data on only four meteorological parameters are required as minimum input to the formula. These are windspeed and direction and two parameters which provide a measure of the vertical and horizontal plume spread (σ_y and σ_z).

A crucial factor in these determinations is atmospheric stability. As noted earlier, variations in stability can cause marked differences in rates and scales of turbulent diffusion. Atmospheric stability is often classified in terms of the Pasquill stability classes (Turner 1969): classes A and B refer to unstable conditions, C and D are close to neutral,

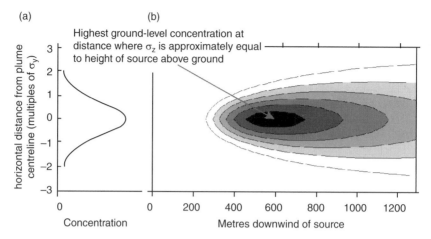

Fig. 21.3 Pollutant concentrations around a single point source, modelled as a Gaussian plume: (a) cross-sectional pollutant profile; (b) plan.

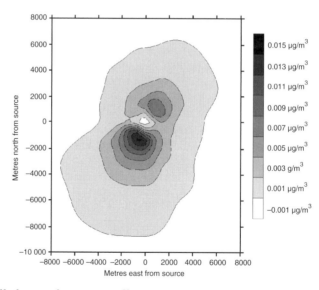

Fig. 21.4 Modelled annual average pollutant concentration around a point source, using a plume dispersion model.

E and above are stable stratification. Given sufficient meteorological measurements to estimate the stability class, values of σ_y and σ_z can be obtained from simple graphs. By carrying out Gaussian plume model calculations repeatedly with windspeed and direction and stability class distributions typical of a year's weather, it is then possible to build up a map of annual average ground-level concentration, such as that shown in Fig. 21.4. The characteristic zero of concentration near the source in this figure is caused by the height of the stack, as was shown in Fig. 21.1, while the asymmetry of the distribution further away is caused in this example by a deep valley which channels the wind preferentially in two directions. The effect of the hills has not been taken into account in the modelling itself, where flat terrain has been assumed, but the effect of the hills on the wind is included as local meteorological measurements have been used to provide input to the model.

The Pasquill stability classification system and Gaussian plume model have been in use now for several decades, during which time understanding of atmospheric turbulence has increased significantly. This has led to the development of a second generation of plume dispersion models that are similar in principle to the simple Gaussian formulation but which incorporate some refinements. The Pasquill scheme for determining plume spread is tending to be replaced by a scaling based on the Monin–Obukhov length (L_{MO}) that was mentioned in Section 21.2. In unstable conditions, the fact that levels of turbulence increase with height away from the ground and then decrease again close to the top of the boundary layer means that a plume may be modelled more realistically by allowing its vertical profile to assume a skewed Gaussian concentration distribution. Examples of these second-generation models, include UK-ADMS (CERC 1999) and the new USEPA model AERMOD (USEPA 1998). These are computationally more complex and costly than the earlier Gaussian models, but modern software typically includes many additional utilities such as the ability to map not only short- and long-term average concentrations but also specified percentile concentrations, so the extra computation required to calculate the more complex source-receptor relationships is a small price to pay for potentially much improved accuracy.

In addition to point sources, line, area, and volume sources can be analysed by these models. This is achieved by integrating the contributions of emissions from point-source elements to which the Gaussian-type formulae can be applied. Complex topography, such as industrial buildings and city streets, are treated by empirical formulae to modify the Gaussian plume without having to turn to the computational expense and unreliability of a k–ε or similar models (see also Section 21.4). The UK-ADMS software package also includes a linear airflow model (i.e. one that assumes local equilibrium of turbulence) to compute plume spread parameters over gentle hills, while some other modelling systems include more empirical approaches. Further details may be found in Colvile *et al.* (1999).

21.4 Other atmospheric processes and how to model them

In many situations, dispersion is only one of several atmospheric processes that influence pollutant concentrations. Other processes must therefore be considered as well if accurate assessments are to be made of pollution levels.

21.4.1 Wet and dry deposition

All pollutants will, sooner or later, be removed from the atmosphere. Gases and particles stick to solid surfaces such as the ground and vegetation, and soluble pollutants are lost in a similar fashion at water surfaces. In dry air, the same turbulence that produces dispersion also transports pollutants to the ground: in the lowest few centimetres of the atmosphere, molecular diffusion completes the process of dry deposition. The rate at which pollutants are lost to a surface may be described by a deposition velocity. A highly reactive gaseous pollutant, such as nitric acid, may have a deposition velocity of tens of centimetres per second, while for less reactive gases, such as nitrogen dioxide, rates of millimetres per second are typical. Deposition velocities are also affected by the character of the deposition surface. Ozone, for example, is chemically reactive but not very soluble in water. As a result, it has a high deposition velocity over land but a low deposition velocity over the sea. Aerosol particles have deposition velocities that are a function of particle size. Large particles deposit at a speed equal to the gravitational settling velocity; very fine particles (only a few nanometres in diameter) are also deposited rapidly because they undergo molecular diffusion close to the ground surface and are then strongly held on the ground surface by electrostatic forces. Particles of intermediate size are too large to be subject to molecular diffusion, yet too small to undergo gravitational settling, so deposition rates are low. These materials thus tend to accumulate in the atmosphere and are referred to as accumulation mode aerosol. It is simple to model the effect of dry deposition, as the flux of pollutant to a surface is equal to the concentration multiplied by the deposition velocity. The rate of change of concentration throughout the boundary layer as a whole may then be estimated by dividing the flux by the boundary-layer depth.

When rainfall occurs, soluble pollutants can be removed from the atmosphere by washout, while insoluble pollutants remain airborne. This wet deposition can be an order of magnitude more rapid than dry deposition for a highly soluble gas. Snow is even more efficient than rain at cleaning the air, because of the large surface area of snow-flakes on to which pollutants can stick, especially if the snow is wet. Formation of cloud and fog is another highly efficient way of dissolving water-soluble pollutants, because of the long time available during which a growing water droplet is in contact with the surrounding air. Concentrations of highly soluble gases in cloud can drop essentially to zero in a few seconds when cloud or fog forms, while less soluble gases such as sulphur dioxide can be significantly depleted in several minutes. Cloud droplets are then deposited to the ground very efficiently wherever the cloud is in contact with the ground (e.g. as fog or hill cloud).

21.4.2   Chemical reactions

The other major process of pollutant loss is chemical reaction. The rate of a chemical reaction can be calculated by multiplying the concentrations of the reagents by a reaction rate coefficient. Many reactions involve the action of sunlight, with the result that reaction rates vary with time of day, season, latitude, and cloud cover. The chemical reactions that destroy most common air pollutants occur on time-scales of hours to days; many global pollutants, such as carbon dioxide and chlorofluorocarbons, are far less reactive and have lifetimes ranging from several weeks to many centuries for the most chemically stable. The atmosphere also contains very low concentrations of highly reactive species, such as hydroxyl radicals, that have lifetimes of only seconds or minutes.

Chemical reactions do not only cause the removal of pollutants. They can also be sources of atmospheric pollutants. The most notable example of this is the generation of ozone. This is not emitted directly in significant quantities from any source, but is a secondary pollutant produced through chemical reaction with nitrogen oxides. Reaction rates for these processes are measured in terms of seconds to minutes.

Chemical reactions involving atmospheric aerosol particles are especially complex. Chemical reactions can occur on the particle surfaces, while sticky gases or high boiling point vapours can condense onto the surfaces of these particles. Gases have difficulty reaching the surface of the smallest nanometre-sized particles, while large particles are often too few and far between to have much effect, but the accumulation-mode particles, of a fraction of a micrometre in size, can scavenge vapours, such as nitric acid and certain organic molecules, quite effectively in several minutes if the particle loading is high. Particles can also interact with each other. One example of this is the coagulation of the very small particles in diesel exhaust; this results in the rapid growth of particles from a few nanometres to several tens of nanometres within seconds of emission at the very high concentrations very close to the source. For larger particles, and at lower concentrations, coagulation is much slower, and other processes become more important.

21.4.3 Modelling deposition and chemical processes

The spatial variability in pollution levels produced by chemical reactions and deposition processes depends on two main factors: the rate of reaction; and the speed of movement of the air parcel in which they occur. An indication of the scales involved can be gained by assuming an atmospheric transport rate of about one metre per second. In this situation, the fastest chemical reactions, occurring over time-scales of seconds, will result in spatial variations in pollutant composition over length-scales of metres; the slower processes of dry deposition will show variations only over distances of several tens of kilometres or more. From the point of view of mapping pollutant concentrations, therefore, a crucial difference can be emphasised between the treatment of dispersion (as outlined in Sections 21.2 and 21.3) and the treatment of deposition and chemical reaction. Dispersion can be mapped easily using source-receptor relationships in a Gaussian model. Some basic treatment of deposition and chemical reaction can be included in the Gaussian formulation, using simple correction factors, for example, an attenuation factor that reduces the amount of material in the plume with increasing distance from the source. However, it rapidly becomes difficult to model increasingly complicated chemistry, such as that of ozone, in this way. As soon as more than one or two chemical reactions are identified, the simple relationship between source geography and concentration map is lost, and the much greater complexity of a grid model is required, or empirical relationships have to applied with great care.

21.4.4 Building and downwash effects

When a source of pollution is situated close to a building, it is possible for part of the plume to become caught up in the extremely complex turbulent flow pattern around the building. This can cause the pollution to reach the ground as it is pulled down in the building-induced eddies, in a similar fashion to the action of large thermally induced eddies in unstable conditions over flat ground. The Apsley and Robins buildings effects model (Apsley and Robins 1994) is an empirical method of treating this effect when one is using a Gaussian plume model. The fraction of the plume that is caught up behind the building is estimated using the distance from source to building and details of the building size and windspeed. The strength of the real source is then reduced according to this fraction, and an additional virtual source is considered to be the effective origin of the remainder of the

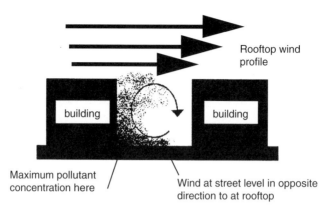

Rooftop wind
profile

building

building

Maximum pollutant
concentration here

Wind at street level in opposite
direction to at rooftop

Fig. 21.5   The effect of a street canyon on pollutant dispersion.

plume, at some point within the recirculation zone close to the ground downwind of the
building. It is this virtual source that gives rise to the increased ground-level concentrations caused by the building. These effects can be calculated using the usual Gaussian
formula, modified to take account of increased turbulence in the building wake.

Some of the most important effects of buildings and downwash occur in street canyons
(i.e. in roads bounded on both sides by tall buildings). Here, a special effect occurs due to
the interaction of buildings in close proximity to each other. When the wind blows
across the canyon, a characteristic recirculation pattern is established, as shown in Fig. 21.5.
This causes pollutants emitted by road traffic at the bottom of the canyon to pile up
against the side of the street in an upwind direction relative to the wind at rooftop level.
Variations in concentration of a factor of three or more can easily result from one side of
the street to the other under these conditions, with the trapping effect of the buildings
maintaining street-level concentrations an order of magnitude higher than they would be
alongside an open road. When the wind blows along the street, the dispersion behaves
more like a Gaussian plume but with its lateral dimensions constrained by the buildings.
For intermediate wind directions, a superposition of the two dispersion patterns may be
expected. This situation has been studied in detail by several workers in wind tunnels and
in the field, and the information collected together in several empirical or semi-empirical
models, of which OSPM (Berkowicz *et al.* 1994) and CAR-International (Eerhens *et al.*
1993) are examples.

Both the OSPM street canyon model and the Apsley and Robins building effects model
are combined with a second-generation Gaussian-type dispersion model in the ADMS-
Urban modelling system (CERC Ltd 1999). Similar functionality is also offered by other
software packages such as those incorporating the USEPA Gaussian model ISC3
(USEPA 1995).

21.5   Problems and limitations

Modern computer software packages produce such effective graphical output that it is
often tempting to accept the results of dispersion modelling or mapping and ignore the
assumptions and approximations which had to be made to produce them. This problem

was recognised several years ago by the then UK Department of the Environment and the Royal Meteorological Society. In an attempt to prevent modelling from becoming discredited by widespread bad practice, these organisations set up an expert group to publish guidelines for good practice in dispersion modelling and reporting of its results (Britter *et al.* 1995). Similar guidance is available in the United States (e.g., USEPA 1997); the situation there is slightly different, however, in that modelling is applied in a more rigid fashion as part of the strict regulatory procedures. Even in this situation, however, modelling faces a number of problems, not least the limitations of the available input data.

Particular difficulties arise in acquiring reliable emissions data. The emissions data used in dispersion modelling have usually been initially collected for the quite different purpose of regulation. Features of interest to a modeller may not, therefore, be accurately represented in the data; for example, details of particle size distribution or diurnal variations in emissions. For smaller sources, emissions estimation becomes increasingly problematic. Emissions from a small boiler or industrial process are commonly calculated by multiplying some measure of activity, such as energy use, by an emissions factor. Emissions estimates for domestic sources may rely on applying similar emission factors to whole areas, using regional data on fuel type and consumption and population. The precision of such estimates is clearly open to doubt.

Similar problems occur in estimating emission from road traffic. Again, these tend to be assessed by extrapolating from test data (e.g. data obtained from selected 'drive cycles' or from manufacturers' data) to an entire road length or area, on the basis of traffic flows and fleet composition or vehicle type. Vehicle emissions estimated on the basis of such data, however, can be seriously in error unless account is taken of the fact that a large fraction of pollutants from road traffic come from the small fraction of vehicles that are not properly maintained. By the very nature of these vehicles, it is extremely difficult to know what emissions factor should be used. Even if emissions are known for constant speed travel on flat roads, emissions during acceleration uphill are strongly dependent on that most unpredictable factor of all: the human driver. These problems are especially acute in the case of particulate emissions. Direct emissions from road traffic exhaust depend strongly on driver behaviour and vehicle maintenance. In addition, however, many other emission sources may be of importance, including road dust and tyre wear; these depend on a host of factors—such as the type of road surface, its state of wear, wetness, etc.—for which data are rarely available. For a large urban area as a whole over a period of several weeks or longer, good traffic flow monitoring and modelling can provide activity data sufficiently accurate for errors in the emissions factors to be the largest source of emissions uncertainty. For an individual road, however, or over a short averaging time, traffic flow might be known no more accurately than within a factor of three, with errors as great as a factor of ten not unexpected, especially for minor roads where large numbers or people typically live.

The second important area of input data is meteorology. In this context, several problems occur. Most weather stations make measurements only a few metres above the ground, which is relevant for dispersion from ground-level sources at that point but may provide little information about a plume aloft from an elevated source. The second-generation Gaussian-type models (as discussed in Section 21.3) are a little more problematic in this respect than older models, as they require a good measure or estimate of boundary-layer height if the more accurate model formulation is to give any advantage over the simpler models. Even for ground-level sources, a weather station several kilo-metres away may provide measurements that are difficult to relate to local conditions, especially in the urban environment or in complex hilly terrain. It is possible to correct for differences in land surface roughness between the modelling site and the meteorological station, but more complex effects, such as reduced windspeeds in valleys and among buildings, are much more difficult to take into account.

One way of assessing the accuracy of dispersion modelling is by local validation of the model. In fact, this is not possible in many routine applications, as the model is required to predict the impact of emissions from a source that has not yet commenced operation. The models are therefore validated through field experiments, in which especially detailed measurements of meteorological conditions, source characteristics and the resulting concentration field are made. The validation thus provided is then used as a basis for applying the dispersion model elsewhere, or at other times, for which no air quality measurements are made. This practice needs to be followed with caution, for it relies on the assumption that the model is being applied in similar conditions to those in which it was tested. This assumption needs to be verified. In many cases, significant differences in the field conditions will exist, for model validation is usually carried out either in unusually simple situations (e.g. very large flat fields) or in more complex situations which by their very nature are unique. Validation is also performed in con-ditions of well-controlled data. Field applications, on the other hand, often rely on less accurate input data. In these cases, sensitivity analyses ought to be performed to assess the extent to which differences in the field conditions, or data quality, might affect the model results.

Most dispersion models have been developed not as a means of assessing exposure to air pollution, but for regulatory purposes. Validation is thus undertaken with this purpose in mind. A common means of validating regulatory dispersion models, for example, uses not point-by-point comparison between calculations and measurements, but quartile-quartile plots (e.g. Gryning and Millan 1994; Kretzschmar and Cosemans 1997). In such a validation exercise, the modelled and measured time-series and/or map points are each separately ranked from the highest concentration to the lowest before scatter-plotting one against the other. A regulatory model may need to err on the side of overestimating the peak concentration and the higher percentiles; it may be relatively unimportant if it underestimates lower percentiles, or even if it predicts high concentra-tions in completely the wrong places or at completely the wrong times of day or year. In the case of exposure assessment, however, systematic misclassifications of exposure of this type are likely seriously to bias the analysis (see Chapter 5). Great care is therefore needed in using models validated for regulatory regimes for the purpose of exposure assessment.

A key step in air pollution modelling is to check that the model is fit for the purpose for which it is being applied. This relates both to the specific situations that it is designed to handle and the conditions under which it has been validated. An especially widespread example of this problem is that of low windspeeds or still conditions. The Gaussian plume model predicts infinite concentrations at zero windspeed, which is clearly nonsensical as dispersion processes other than turbulence and advection will cause some spreading of the plume. When the model is used to estimate long-term average con-centrations, this may not be overly important, for very light wind conditions are likely to be relatively rare. A model that assumes some cut-off wind speed will therefore not be significantly in error. When shorter-term concentrations are being modelled, or data are needed on maxima or high percentile concentrations, the effect may be far more serious. Just how serious is difficult to assess, however, for meteorological measurements are made predominantly at locations where the instrumentation is well exposed. As a result, the available data may not adequately characterise more sheltered (e.g. urban) areas, where very light winds are more common.

21.6 Dispersion modelling for exposure assessment

Dispersion models have been used only remarkably rarely for the purpose of exposure assessment as part of epidemiological studies. This reflects a number of factors, including lack of suitable input data and caution about the validity or appropriateness of the models, but more generally, a lack of understanding by epidemiologists both about the potential utility of spatial modelling of exposures and the methods available to do so. This situation certainly needs to be redressed, for so long as exposure assessments are based on inadequate methods, doubts will remain about the findings of epidemiological studies.

One of the areas in which dispersion modelling has been used is in the investigation of the health effects of traffic-related pollution (see also Table 19.1). Raaschou-Nielsen *et al.* (1996), for example, used the operational street pollution model (OSPM) (Berkowicz *et al.* 1994) to estimate concentrations of outdoor NO_2 concentrations, as a marker for traffic-related pollution, at the homes of 19 000 children as part of a case-control study of cancers in Denmark. To validate the accuracy of the model, modelled concentrations were compared with measurements taken using passive samplers, outside the homes of 200 children (100 in central Copenhagen, 100 in rural areas 20–50 km outside Copenhagen), though as yet full results have not been reported. Oosterlee *et al.* (1996) applied the Dutch CAR model (Eerhens *et al.* 1993) to estimate exposures to NO_2 pollution for 673 adults and 106 children (age 0–15 years) living in busy streets in Haarlem, the Netherlands. A control group of 812 adults and 185 children was also chosen living along quiet streets. Data on health outcome, including prevalence of chronic cough, episodes of cough with phlegm, wheeze, dyspnoea, attacks of dyspnoea with wheeze, and doctors diagnosis of asthma were obtained through a questionnaire survey. Questions were also asked about respondents' use of respiratory medication and potentially confounding variables such as lifestyle, living circumstances, housing conditions, and habits. Comparisons between high-exposed and low-exposed groups showed significant adjusted odds ratios for both wheeze (OR = 2.1) and respiratory medication used (OR = 4.8) in children. When analysed separately, however, significant odds ratios were only found for girls: OR 2.9–15.8, compared to no significant ratios for boys. In adults, no clear association was found with respiratory conditions.

One of the most detailed attempts to investigate the use of dispersion models for exposure assessment is that by de Hoogh (1999). He used a range of methods, including the simple Design Manual for Roads and Bridges (DMRB) model (Department of Transport 1994), the Gaussian plume dispersion model CALINE-3 (Benson 1992) and the ADMS-Urban model (CERC 1999) to estimate exposures to NO_2 for a sample of 1800 children in Sheffield, UK for whom data on respiratory symptoms were available (Strachan and Carey, 1995). Model results were validated by comparing predicted concentrations with measurements at 28 sites, using passive samplers, deployed for five two-week periods over a year. The results showed that all three dispersion models gave good, relative predictions of monitored NO_2 levels at the sample sites, with Spearman correlation coefficients of 0.83 (CALINE) to 0.93 (DMRB). However, both CALINE-3 and ADMS-Urban showed non-linear relationships between modelled and monitored concentrations, and ADMS-Urban substantially underestimated concentrations at the monitoring sites. Modelled concentrations at the place of residence and school (both separately and combined) were compared with respiratory symptoms using logistic regression, with and without control for confounding. No significant associations were found.

   Collins (1998) has also compared the use of a dispersion model (an adapted form of the CALINE-3 model, developed to run within a GIS) and other methods for exposure assessment (including kriging, a moving window method, and regression mapping). Exposures were estimated for the place of residence of 4357 children, age 9–11, in Huddersfield, UK, as part of the SAVIAH (Small-Area Variation in Air Quality and Health) study (Briggs *et al.* 1997; Elliott and Briggs 1998; see also Chapter 22). Performance of the various methods was assessed by comparing modelled concentrations with mean annual NO_2 levels, monitored at eight sites using consecutive passive samplers. The regression method gave the most reliable estimates ($r^2 = 0.82$, SEE = $3.68\,\mu g/m^3$); dispersion modelling and the moving window approach performed rather less well ($r^2 = 0.63$ and 0.67, respectively; SEE = 5.25 and $4.92\,\mu g/m^3$, respectively); kriging performed the least well ($r^2 = 0.44$, SEE = $6.45\,\mu g/m^3$). The methods were also compared by estimating the proportion of children likely to be exposed to NO_2 concentrations in excess of the National Air Quality Strategy mean annual standard of $37.6\,\mu g/m^3$. Results showed a 2.8-fold variation in the estimated proportion of exposed population, from 2.9% (using the moving window approach) to 8.0% (using kriging). Collins concludes that choice of method may fundamentally affect exposure estimates, and have significant effects on attempts to explore relationships with health outcome. The study thus highlights the need both for care in selecting methods of exposure assessment, and for local validation of the methods used.

21.7   Conclusions

Dispersion modelling clearly provides a potentially powerful tool for exposure assessment, though one which has, as yet, been relatively rarely applied. Several recent developments in dispersion modelling, notably the development of the second-generation Gaussian dispersion models, the closer links which are now available to GIS and the improved visualisation which this provides, would seem greatly to enhance the capability of dispersion models in epidemiological research. Nevertheless, as with any tool, caution is needed in their implementation. As has been noted, most models have been developed with specific applications in mind, and for specific environmental situations. Use of the models beyond these situations needs to be carried out with care. The added complexity inherent in the new generation models also means that they cannot be treated naively: it is incumbent on users, in whatever field, to understand the assumptions on which they are based, and adequately to meet their data needs.

   This said, there is clearly a growing opportunity and need to apply dispersion models for exposure assessment. It is widely recognised that weaknesses in exposure classification remain one of the major constraints to the investigation of environment-health relationships. In the large majority of studies, relatively simple exposure measures continue to be used (see Chapter 9). Only rarely are methods used that can properly characterise both the spatial and temporal variations in pollution levels which occur across a population. Misuse of dispersion modelling undoubtedly needs to be avoided; but the adaptation and application of dispersion models to tackle problems of environmental-health, in the context of closer collaboration between atmospheric scientists and epidemiologists, must surely be encouraged.

References

Apsley, D. D. and Robins, A. G. (1994). *Modelling of building effects in UK-ADMS*. ADMS Technical Specification. UK-ADMS 1.0 P16/01K/94. Cambridge Environmental Research Consultants Ltd.

Benson, P. E. (1992). A review of the development and application of the CALINE3 and CALINE4 models. *Atmospheric Environment*, **26B**, 379–90.

Berkowicz, R., Hertel, O., Sørensen, N. N., and Michelsen, J. A. (1994, March) Modelling air pollution from traffic in urban areas. *Proceedings of the IMA Conference on Flow and Dispersion Through Groups of Obstacles*, University of Cambridge.

Briggs D. J., Collins S., Elliott P., Fischer P., Kingham S., Lebret E. *et al.* (1997). Mapping urban air pollution using GIS: a regression-based approach. *International Journal of Geographical Information Science*, **11**, 699–718.

Britter, R., Collier, C., Griffiths, R., Mason, P., Thomson, D., Timmis, R. *et al.* (1995). *Atmospheric dispersion modelling: Guidelines on the justification of choice and use of models, and the communication and reporting of results*. Policy statement. Royal Meteorological Society, Reading.

CERC (1999). *ADMS-Urban. An urban air quality management system. User guide*. CERC Ltd, Cambridge.

Collins, S. (1998). Modelling spatial variations in air quality using GIS. In *GIS and health. GISData 6* (A. Gatrell and M. Loytonen ed.), 81–95. Taylor & Francis, London.

Colvile, R. N., Scaperdas, A. S., Hill, J. H., and Smith, F. B. (1997). *Review of models for calculating air concentrations when plumes impinge on buildings or the ground*. In Atmospheric Dispersion Modelling Liaison Committee, Annual Report 1996/97. NRPB-R302. National Radiological Protection Board, Chilton, Didcot.

de Hoogh, C. (1999). Estimating exposure to traffic-related pollution within a GIS environment. Unpublished Ph. D. thesis, University College Northampton and University of Leicester.

Department of Transport (1994). *Design manual for roads and bridges*, Vol. 11: *Environmental assessment*, Section 3, Part 1: *Air quality*. HMSO, London.

Eerhens, H. C., Sliggers, C. J., and van den Hout, K. D. (1993). The CAR model: the Dutch method to determine city street air quality. *Atmospheric Environment*, **27B**, 389–99.

Elliott, P. and Briggs, D. J. (1998). Recent developments in the geographical analysis of small area health and environmental data. In *Progress in public health* (G. Scally ed.), 101–25. Royal Society of Medicine Press, London.

Gryning, S.-E. and Millan, M. M. (ed.) (1994). In Air pollution modelling and its application. In *Proceedings of the Twentieth NATO/CCSM International Technical meeting on Air Pollution Modelling and its Application*, 29 November–3 December 1993, Valencia, Spain. Plenum, New York.

Kretzschmar, J. and Cosemans, G. (1997). Foreword. *Fourth workshop on Harmonisation within Atmospheric Dispersion Modelling for Regulatory Purposes*, 6–9 May 1996, Ostend, Belgium. *International Journal of Environment and Pollution*, (Special Issue), **8**, 237–8.

Oosterlee, A., Drijver, M., Lebret, E., and Brunekreef, B. (1996). Chronic respiratory symptoms in children and adults living along streets with high traffic density. *Occupational and Environmental Medicine*, **53**, 241–7.

Raaschou-Nielsen, O., Olsen, J. H., Hertel, O., Berkowicz, R., Skov, H., Hansen, A. M. *et al.* (1996). Exposure of Danish children to traffic exhaust fumes. *The Science of the Total Environment*, **189/190**, 51–5.

Strachan, D. P. and Carey, I. M. (1995). Home environment and severe asthma in adolescence: a population based case-control study. *British Medical Journal*, **311**, 1053–6.

Turner, D. B. (1969). *Workbook of atmospheric diffusion estimates.* US Environmental Protection Agency Report, 999-AP-26. USEPA, Washington, DC.

USEPA (1993). *UAM model user's guide.* USEPA, Research Triangle Park.

USEPA (1995). *User's guide for the industrial source complex (ISC3) dispersion models.* Vol. I: User instructions. Report EPA-454/B-95-003a. USEPA Research Triangle Park, NC.

USEPA (1997). *Guideline on air quality models. Appendix W to Part 51.* 40 CFR, Ch. 1, 1 July. USEPA, Research Triangle Park, NC.

USEPA (1998). *AERMOD: description of model formulation.* USEPA, Research Triangle Park, NC.

22. Combining models of health and exposure data: the SAVIAH study

N. G. Best, K. Ickstadt, R. L. Wolpert, and D. J. Briggs

22.1 Introduction

Over the last two decades the rate of respiratory illnesses, particularly in children, has shown an apparent increase in almost all countries in the Western world, and in many developing countries (Anderson *et al.* 1994; Burney 1988; Burney *et al.* 1990). In view of the inexorable rise in traffic volume and associated emissions of urban air pollutants, this has intensified the search for possible environmental causes for these conditions, including a putative effect of traffic-related air pollution. The evidence for a link between respiratory illness and air quality remains equivocal, however, due in part to major problems of measuring or estimating exposure.

Studies have used a range of markers to quantify the exposure to air pollution: some studies have focused on fine particulates (Schwartz 1993; Dockery *et al.* 1993; Pope *et al.* 1995), some have used either measured (Nitta *et al.* 1993) or modelled (Osterlee *et al.* 1996; Pershagen *et al.* 1995) nitrogen dioxide $(NO)_2$ levels, while others have relied on less specific exposure indicators, such as proximity to roads (Edwards *et al.* 1994; Murakami *et al.* 1990), living in streets with high levels of traffic (Wjst *et al.* 1993), or self-reported exposure to truck traffic (Duhme *et al.* 1996; Weiland *et al.* 1994). See also Table 19.1 in Chapter 19.

Many previous studies have focused on the *acute* effects of exposure to air pollution in individuals (e.g. Committee of Medical Effects of Air Pollution 1995*a,b*; Schwartz 1994; Pope *et al.* 1995). To what extent, if any, the findings of the acute studies can be extrapolated to predict the effects of chronic exposure to lower levels of ambient air pollution is unknown.

Viewing ambient air pollution as an ecological phenomenon that affects whole populations suggests a *population* approach to the study of air pollution and health. This public health dimension is important because of the large number of people exposed: the population risk of respiratory illness attributable to road pollution may be large, even if the excess relative risk to the individual from low levels of traffic pollutants is small.

Unfortunately, population studies of the health effects of chronic exposures tend, per force, to be ecological in design, aggregating cases over geographical regions. Methodological difficulties associated with such studies include the problem of controlling for confounding by both known factors and unmeasured confounders, some of which may vary spatially (Chapters 5 and 11). The potential for bias arising from approximation and aggregation in the data is also a major problem (Chapter 11), often compounded by the fact that the health, exposure, and reference population data available for such studies are typically measured at different, non-nested geographical scales.

In the light of these concerns there is a clear need for improved methods of assessing exposure to traffic-related air pollution and for modelling the potential links to human health. In this chapter we describe a regression-based approach to air pollution mapping, developed as part of the European Union-funded SAVIAH (Small-Area Variations In Air quality and Health) project (Elliott and Briggs 1998). The approach involves the use of monitored NO_2 concentrations as a marker for traffic-related pollution, integrated with data about road networks, traffic volume, and topography within a geographical information system (GIS) environment, and feeding a regression model to predict air pollution across the study area.

We then present a Bayesian spatial regression model to relate prevalence of respiratory illness in children to the modelled pollutant (NO_2) concentrations. This model features an *identity link* Poisson regression (leading to a linear dose-response relationship). Such a model is not commonly used because it may require parameter constraints to ensure non-negative risk estimates. However, it has the attractive property of being consistent under aggregation or refinement of the geographical areas taken as the units of analysis. This allows direct interpretation of the regression coefficients in terms of area- *or individual-level* risk (see Chapter 11, Section 11.2.1). Unmeasured confounders are accommodated by introducing correlated random effects that allow for possible spatial dependence between these latent covariates.

In Section 22.2 we provide some background to the SAVIAH study, and introduce the data. In Section 22.3 we describe the methods used to characterise exposure to traffic-related air pollution, including NO_2 concentration monitoring, integration within a GIS, multiple regression modelling of the data, and validation of the predicted exposure surface. In Section 22.4 we briefly review some common approaches for analysing the link between health and environmental exposure, including a discussion of the problems of unmeasured confounding, aggregation consistency, and information loss when modelling area-level data. This discussion motivates our use of an identity link spatial Poisson regression model, which is introduced in Section 22.4.1. Results are presented in Section 22.5 and a discussion of the modelling approaches for both the exposure and health data appears in Section 22.6.

22.2   The SAVIAH study

The SAVIAH study was a European multicentre study funded by the European Union (EU) in 1993–4 to develop and test methodologies for collecting and analysing environmental epidemiological data. The study was carried out in four centres: Huddersfield (UK), Amsterdam (the Netherlands), Prague (Czech Republic) and Poznan (Poland). In this chapter, we focus only on a subset of the data for Huddersfield.

Data collection for the SAVIAH study involved two main phases:

1. Monitoring of air pollution data (specifically NO_2 concentrations).
2. Surveys of childhood respiratory ailments and potential confounding variables.

Air pollution monitoring was carried out via intensive and replicated surveys using low-cost Palmes diffusion tubes as passive samplers (Palmes *et al.* 1976; see also Section 19.3.1

in Chapter 19). A dense network of 80 fixed and 40 variable monitoring sites was established. These were selected to represent different degrees of expected traffic impact (regional background, urban background, and street level) to obtain maximum variation in pollutant levels. Duplicate Palmes tubes were exposed at each site for four two-week periods between June 1993 and June 1994, timed to reflect different seasonal/synoptic conditions. In addition, eight reference sites were monitored continuously on a monthly basis over the study period for validation purposes.

Health data were collected using questionnaire surveys of the parents or guardians of all local schoolchildren aged 7–9 years. The questionnaires contained items on chronic respiratory disease, based on the WHO (Florey and Leeder 1973) and ISAAC (Pearce *et al.* 1993) standard parent-administered questionnaire. Questions relating to potentially confounding variables, such as parental smoking, damp housing, socio-economic factors etc., were also asked. Valid questionnaires were completed for 4437 children in Huddersfield, giving a 90.1% response rate. A number of questions on respiratory wheeze and cough were chosen at the outset as key outcomes under study. In this chapter, we focus on the outcome *frequent cough*: children were deemed to have a positive response if their parents reported that they usually suffered from a cough in the morning in the autumn–winter season. This gave 826 cases, which were georeferenced to the centroid of the postal code of the home address. Figure 22.1 presents a map of the study region showing the locations of the 597 distinct postcodes in which cases occurred, 438 with only a single case and 159 with multiple (2–6) cases.

While demographic variation in the total number of 7- to 9-year-old children at risk is small over periods of a few years, the spatial distribution of children in this age range does change noticeably from year to year. We model both the overall population of 7- to 9-year-old children at risk and the frequent cough cases in Huddersfield at any given time as independent inhomogeneous Poisson processes, with uncertain spatially varying mean

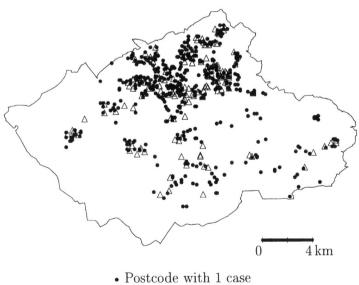

・ Postcode with 1 case

△ Postcode with > 1 case

Fig. 22.1 Frequent cough cases in the study region, located by postcode centroid.

intensities $100 \cdot N(x)$ and $\lambda(x)$, respectively (overall population density $N(x)$ is given in *hundreds*, but case density $\lambda(x)$ is measured by individuals). Under the null hypothesis of uniform risk the mean intensities would be proportional, $\lambda(x) = p \cdot N(x)$, where p is the expected number of cases per 100 population. Environmental or other influences may lead to spatially varying risk $p(x) = \lambda(x)/N(x)$.

One approach to making inference about $p(x)$ is to *condition* on the observed postcode locations of children at risk and model the cases using binomial methods (under the uniform-risk null hypothesis each child would have identical probability p of being a case). In this approach the postcode locations are treated as a marked point process with marks (labels) indicating whether the child living at each postcode is a case or not, leading to a spatial binary regression model for the case-control labels (Diggle and Rowlingson 1994; Kelsall and Diggle 1998; see also Chapter 6). However, the narrow range of ages in the present study leads to a sparse cohort distribution (about 7–8 children per km², on average) that leaves large areas with no recorded cases or controls, and many others with only one or two children. Even Bayesian smoothing methods would struggle to produce sensible risk estimates for these areas using binomial regression.

Our approach is *not* to condition on the cohort distribution, but instead to treat the cases directly as an inhomogeneous Poisson process with intensity $\lambda(x) = p(x) \cdot N(x)$ proportional to the long-term or typical mean density (in hundreds) of 7- to 9-year-old children. We estimate $N(x)$ from the 1991 census count (in hundreds) of children aged 0–14 years, scaled by a factor of 3/15 to accommodate the difference of age ranges. We neglect the sampling variability in this estimate (this will typically be small relative to uncertainty about $p(x)$), and treat the population density $N(x)$ as known.

Figure 22.2 shows maps of the study region with (a) census Enumeration districts (EDs), and (b) an arbitrary 750 m × 750 m grid shaded according to the observed prevalence of frequent cough in cases per 100 children.

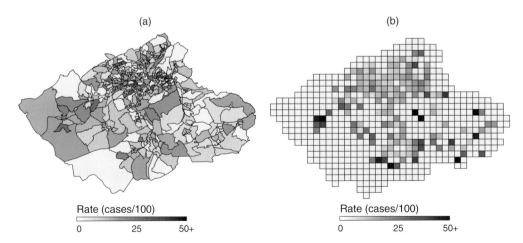

Fig. 22.2 Empirical prevalence (in cases/100 children): (a) in each enumeration district; (b) on an arbitrary grid.

22.3   Exposure mapping

The development in recent years of GIS and geostatistical techniques has led to the availability of a wide range of methods for air pollution mapping (see Chapter 19). Broadly speaking, these may be classified into: (a) indicator-based methods; (b) spatial interpolation; and (c) dispersion modelling. The first of these uses data on either source activity (e.g. traffic volume) or distance from source (e.g. distance to nearest main road) as proxies for exposure. Spatial interpolation includes global methods, such as trend surface analysis, which fit a single surface to the entire dataset of pollution measurements, and local methods, such as kriging and spline interpolation, which are based on a series of local estimates using nearby measurements. Dispersion models attempt to predict the dispersion process of the pollutant directly, taking into account factors, such as source activity, topography, and meteorological conditions, which are likely to influence the ultimate pollution concentration field.

In practice, all these methods suffer from difficulties when applied to estimate exposures at the individual or small-area level, across large populations in urban environments. Most indicators, for example, are imprecise and difficult to define in consistent and meaningful terms. Spatial interpolation methods are limited by the sparsity of monitored data, relative to the often complex and local patterns of spatial variation in the pollution surface. They thus tend to produce oversmoothed pollution maps. Line dispersion models, whilst relatively accurate when used at the site level in conjunction with reliable and local meteorological and emission data, often perform rather poorly when applied across entire urban areas, because of uncertainties in the input data (for further discussion of these methods see Chapters 19 and 21).

The SAVIAH study considered an alternative approach to mapping air pollution, namely regression mapping. This method was designed to exploit the capability of GIS to extract and link information from a variety of relevant datasets in order to develop a predictive model of the NO_2 pollution surface for each of the four SAVIAH study centres. Full details are given in Briggs *et al.* (1997) and Elliott and Briggs (1998); here we summarise the method used for mapping NO_2 in the UK centre of Huddersfield.

22.3.1   Pollution monitoring and data collection

The datasets available for the regression mapping included exogenous information on digitised road networks (based on aerial photography), mean traffic flow for each road segment (based on automatic and manual counts for major roads and local knowledge for other roads), plus factors, such as land cover and altitude, which may affect dispersion of the pollutant. Monitored NO_2 concentration measurements were also collected specifically for the SAVIAH study as described above in Section 22.2.

22.3.2   Estimation of mean annual NO_2 at each monitoring site

One of the aims of the SAVIAH study was to develop a marker of *chronic* exposure to traffic-related pollution. The data from the four pollution surveys therefore needed to be combined to give an estimate of the mean annual NO_2 concentration at each site. These estimates were obtained by using a mixed effects model to adjust for spatial and temporal

variation within and between sites and to accommodate missing data for some sites and
surveys (Lebret *et al.* 1999):

$$X_{itk} \sim N(\eta_{itk}, \sigma_\epsilon^2)$$
$$\eta_{itk} = \alpha_i + \beta_t + \gamma_{it}$$
$$\gamma_{it} \sim N(0, \sigma_\gamma^2)$$

where X_{itk} is the measured NO_2 concentration (in $\mu g \, m^{-3}$) at site i, survey t, and replicate
k; α_i and β_t are fixed site and survey effects; and γ_{it} are random site/survey interaction
effects. Estimation was carried out using maximum likelihood and the fitted values
$\hat{X}_i = \hat{\alpha}_i$ were calculated to obtain estimates of average annual NO_2 concentrations at
each site i.

22.3.3   Regression mapping of NO_2 pollution

In order to develop estimates of ambient NO_2 pollutant levels in the proximity of the
home addresses of each child in the SAVIAH study, the next stage of the exposure
modelling process was to generalise the estimated mean NO_2 concentration at each of the
80 monitoring sites to create a pollution map on a $10 \, m \times 10 \, m$ grid for the entire
Huddersfield area. This was achieved using regression mapping methods carried out in
the GIS package ARC/INFO (ESRI 1996). The method is outlined below.

1. GIS coverages of the four main datasets (modelled annual NO_2 concentrations, road traffic, land
   cover, and altitude) were compiled.
2. Buffer zones of 20 m width to a distance of 300 m were defined around each monitoring site.
   Weighting factors for the traffic and land use variables were then calculated for each buffer zone
   and an optimum model constructed by comparing predicted concentrations with monitored
   concentrations at the 80 fixed monitoring sites. Initially, multiple regression analyses of traffic
   volume against the modelled annual NO_2 concentrations ($\hat{X}$) gave a traffic volume factor of

$$\text{Tvol}_{300} = 15 \, \text{Tvol}_{(0-40)} + \text{Tvol}_{(40-300)}$$

   where $\text{Tvol}_{(0-40)}$ is the hourly average number of vehicle kilometres travelled within 0–40 metres
   from the monitoring site, and $\text{Tvol}_{(40-300)}$ is the hourly average number of vehicle kilometres
   travelled in the range of 40–300 metres from the monitoring site. The land cover factor was then
   estimated by regressing land cover variables for different distance bands against the residual
   from the previous model. This gave a land cover factor of

$$\text{Land}_{300} = 1.8 \, \text{HDH}_{(0-300)} + \text{Ind}_{(0-300)}$$

   where $\text{HDH}_{(0-300)}$ is the area (in hectares) of high density housing within 300 metres from the
   monitoring site, and $\text{Ind}_{(0-300)}$ is the area (in hectares) of industrial land within 300 metres from
   the monitoring site.
3. The weighted factors Tvol_{300} and Land_{300} were then entered into a step-wise multiple linear
   regression model with altitude (variously transformed), sampler height, site exposure (mean angle
   to visible horizon at each monitoring site), and topographical exposure (mean difference in
   altitude between each $10 \, m \times 10 \, m$ grid cell and the eight surrounding cells), using the fitted

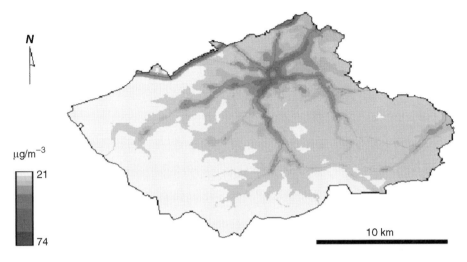

N

μg/m⁻³

21

74

10 km

Fig. 22.3 Annual NO$_2$ concentrations for Huddersfield estimated on a 10 m × 10 m grid.

annual NO$_2$ concentrations at each site, $\hat{X}_i$, as the dependent variable. Only variables significant at the 5% level were retained, giving the following regression equation

$$\hat{X} = 11.83 + 0.00398 \text{ Tvol}_{300} + 0.268 \text{ Land}_{300} - 0.0355 \text{ RSAlt} + 6.777 \text{ Sampht} \qquad (22.1)$$

where RSAlt $= 1/\text{sine(altitude)}$ and Sampht is the sampler height in metres above the ground surface. This model explained 64% of the variation in fitted NO$_2$ values ($r^2 = 0.64$).

4. Equation (22.1) was then used to compute the estimated annual NO$_2$ concentration on a fine grid of 10 m × 10 m cells across Huddersfield, as shown in Fig. 22.3.

5. Validation of the estimated NO$_2$ pollution map was carried out by regressing the arithmetic mean of the monthly measured NO$_2$ concentrations at each of the 8 independent reference sites against the concentrations predicted by the model (22.1) for these sites. This gave a value of $r^2 = 0.82$ with a standard error for the estimated concentration of 3.69 µg m^{-3}, suggesting that the regression mapping model gave extremely good predictions.

22.4 Modelling the association between pollution and health

A variety of statistical models can be used to relate the estimated NO$_2$ concentrations shown in Fig. 22.3 to the health event data shown in Fig. 22.2. One approach is to exploit the case-control design of the SAVIAH study to carry out an individual-level logistic regression analysis relating the frequent cough probability to the estimated NO$_2$ concentration at the location of each child's home postcode. This approach was adopted by Elliott *et al.* (1997) for modelling the risk of frequent cough and other respiratory illnesses using the SAVIAH data. They found a moderately increased risk of frequent cough associated with modelled NO$_2$ concentration at residence although this was not statistically significant (odds ratio = 1.30; 95% confidence interval 0.87–1.94 after adjusting for individual-level confounders). None of the other respiratory outcomes considered showed any association with NO_2 concentration. However, such models make no allowance for *spatial dependence* in the health events or the exposure data, which may distort the analysis, and offer no possibility of discovering an association of frequent cough with unmeasured, possibly spatially varying, confounders. Here, we employ Bayesian multilevel (or hierarchical) models which facilitate the inclusion of spatial structure.

The most common multi-level Bayesian approach to disease mapping and ecological regression is to adopt a Markov random field (MRF) model, such as the three-stage hierarchical model described in Chapter 7 (see also Chapter 11, Section 11.3.3, and Chapters 15 and 16). In this approach the aggregated numbers of disease cases in each geographical area are modelled as Poisson random variables with a log-linear model relating area level relative risks to the average exposure in those areas, as well as to both spatially structured and unstructured random effects. Spatial dependence in these models is typically introduced through a Gaussian conditional autoregressive (CAR) prior for the structured random effects (Besag *et al.* 1991).

Implicit in the use of such MRF models is the requirement that health outcomes, exposure estimates and population data all be aggregated to some common area level, which will usually be coarser than the scale at which the data arise naturally. In our example, the health outcomes (cases of frequent cough) are originally given by postcode and the exposure estimates (NO_2 concentrations) are given on a 10 m × 10 m spatial grid; both would need to be further aggregated to the ED level (at which the population data are available) in this approach.

The disadvantage of such aggregation is that the relationship between disease prevalence and average exposure in each area may be quite different from the disease-exposure relationship for individuals. Different aspects of this problem have been described by a number of authors, under a number of different names: the terms *ecological bias*, *ecological fallacy*, *aggregation bias*, and the *modifiable areal unit problem* have all been used (Robinson 1950; Openshaw 1984; Fotheringham and Wong 1991; Greenland 1992; King 1997; Chapter 11; Chapter 14). In a spatial modelling problem the phenomenon has three different aspects:

- *Confounding*: if an important unobserved covariate differs across aggregation units, then the baseline risk and/or exposure-response gradient will vary between units. This can lead to biases in estimating exposure effects which would not be present in an individual-level analysis (Richardson 1992).

- *Non-linearity*: if the response depends nonlinearly on some exposure of interest, then individual-level response will not be the same as linearly averaged response across aggregation units (see Chapter 11, Section 11.2).

- *Information loss*: whenever variables are aggregated to a coarser resolution the rounding entails a loss of information and a distortion of the exposure-response relationship, especially if within-area variability is large. In the present study, for example, averaging estimated NO_2 concentrations over each ED would distort the exposure of individuals in that ED since all information about fine-scale spatial variability of NO_2 would be lost; similarly marginal summaries of the overall prevalence of frequent cough aggregated to ED level would result in information loss if individual risk is heterogeneous within EDs. Comparing Fig. 22.4(a) and 22.4(b), showing the estimated NO_2 concentrations averaged over each ED and over an arbitrary grid of 750 m × 750 m cells, with Fig. 22.3 showing the original data (given on a 10 m × 10 m grid), demonstrates the information loss.

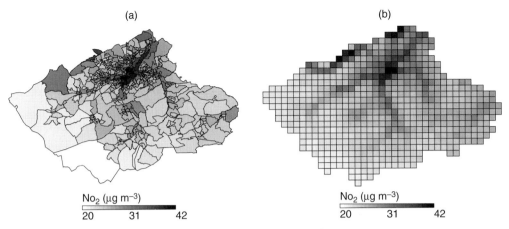

Fig. 22.4 Average estimated NO_2 concentrations (in $\mu g\,m^{-3}$): (a) in each enumeration district; (b) on an arbitrary $750\,m \times 750\,m$ grid.

Some of the deleterious effects of ecological bias can be minimised or eliminated by using statistical models that are consistent under different levels of aggregation (King 1997: 249–55). For example, the log-linear dose-response relationship implied by the usual Poisson-log Gaussian MRF models leads to products rather than sums for the Poisson means under aggregation of the areal units. This represents a violation of aggregational consistency, making parameters and their estimates in such models meaningful only for the specific geographical partition for which they were constructed. In contrast, a *linear* model for the dose-response relationship is aggregation consistent, and in particular leads to the same relationship at the individual level as for an arbitrary area level provided the true dose-response relationship is (nearly) linear (Greenland 1992; Chapter 11, Section 11.2.1). In the present analysis we achieve a linear dose-response relationship by abandoning the logarithmic link in favour of a Bayesian hierarchical Poisson regression model with *identity* link and reduce information loss by using each data source at a low level of aggregation. The method can be extended to a continuous model that minimises information loss by eliminating all aggregation, using each data source at its finest level of aggregation (Best *et al.* 1998). We also overcome the problem of unmeasured confounders by modelling them as spatially varying latent (or random) effects (see Chapter 11, Section 11.3.1).

22.4.1   Identity-link spatial regression models

We now construct a multi-level model for the case counts in geographical areas. If we were to condition on knowing the true population of 7- to 9-year-old children in each area, then the observed cases would follow a binomial distribution (e.g. see Martuzzi and Elliott 1996). However, since the population at any given time is not known exactly, we prefer to model the case counts marginally, without conditioning. This leads to independent Poisson distributions with uncertain (and therefore *random*, in the Bayesian paradigm) means for the number of cases in each area. These Poisson means are parameterised as the product of a disease rate and the estimated population of 7- to 9-year-old children per area (based on the pro-rated 1991 census counts). We achieve a linear dose-response relationship by modelling the disease rates as linear combinations of area-level risk factors, both observed and latent; gamma prior distributions are assumed for the linear coefficients, leading to non-negative predicted values. As a special case in which the latent terms are treated as independent and there are no observed covariates, this includes the conjugate Poisson-gamma models described in Section 7.2.2 of Chapter 7. However, here our interest lies in the spatial dependence of risk.

Let χ denote the Huddersfield region and let $\{Y_i\}_{i \in I}$ be the numbers of reported cases of frequent cough among 7- to 9-year-old Huddersfield children grouped by geographical area $\{A_i\}_{i \in I}$ such as EDs or an arbitrary partition of Huddersfield into quadrats. We model the numbers of reported cases in these areas as independent random variables with Poisson distributions $Y_i \sim Po(\lambda_i)$, with means $\lambda_i = N_i \times p_i$ proportional to the estimated long-term average population (in hundreds) N_i of 7- to 9-year-old children in the area.

In our identity-link Poisson regression model the disease rate p_i in area $A_i \subset \chi$, measured in cases per 100 expected population, is expressed as a sum of linear terms

$$p_i = \beta_0 + \beta_1 X_i + \beta_2 \sum_{j \in J} k_{ij} \gamma_j$$

$$= p_{i0} + p_{i1} + \sum_{j \in J} p_{ij}$$

(22.2)

where $p_{i0} = \beta_0$ is a constant representing the baseline rate of disease, $p_{i1} = \beta_1 X_i$ is proportional to the excess NO_2 concentration X_i in A_i (measured in $\mu g\,m^{-3}$ above the Huddersfield baseline NO_2 concentration of approximately $20\,\mu g\,m^{-3}$), and $p_{ij} = \beta_2 k_{ij} \gamma_j$ is a collection (indexed by $j \in J$) of latent quantities representing the effect in area A_i of unobserved spatially distributed risk factors for frequent cough associated with regions B_j in or near χ or with specific locations $s_j \in B_j$. The regions B_j might again be census EDs or an arbitrary partition of Huddersfield into quadrats. They may also cover an area bigger than Huddersfield; in our analysis we use quadrats covering a rectangle containing the Huddersfield study region plus a 2 km surrounding buffer zone. It is possible (and perfectly reasonable), especially in sparsely populated areas, for the number of cases in some years to exceed the average population. Constraints may be introduced on the parameters in (22.2) to avoid estimating Poisson rate $p_i > 100$, but they were not needed in our analysis.

We regard the coefficient vector $\boldsymbol{\beta} = \{\beta_0, \beta_1, \beta_2\}$ in this linear expansion as an uncertain quantity of interest: β_0 indicates the baseline disease rate, β_1 indicates how large an increase in the disease rate is associated with each $\mu g\,m^{-3}$ increase in NO_2, and β_2 indicates how much variation is explained by other spatial factors; the latter may also be interpreted as a scale factor for the latent random effects. The latent quantities γ_j are also uncertain. We take the kernel matrix k_{ij} governing the influence in A_i arising from latent influences in β_j to be of parametric Gaussian form

$$k_{ij} = \frac{1}{2\pi\rho^2} e^{-|x_i - s_j|^2 / 2\rho^2},$$

with distance scale $\rho > 0$ governing how rapidly the influences k_{ij} decline with increasing distance $|x_i - s_j|$ from the centre x_i of A_i to the centre s_j of B_j.

This model is governed by a number of uncertain parameters: the regression coefficient vector $\boldsymbol{\beta} = \{\beta_0, \beta_1, \beta_2\}$, the latent risk factors $\boldsymbol{\gamma} = \{\gamma_j\}_{j \in J}$, and (possibly) the distance scale ρ. We make inference about these parameters and derived quantities such as the disease rates $\{p_i\}_{i \in I}$ by employing a Bayesian analysis with independent prior distributions given in Table 22.1, where $Ga(\alpha, \tau)$ denotes the gamma distribution with mean α/τ and variance α/τ^2. The parameters of the gamma prior distributions for the three regression coefficients were chosen so that, with 90% prior probability, the number of cases of frequent cough associated with each of the three risk categories (baseline, NO_2-related, and unobserved spatial) would lie between one-tenth and ten times a nominal equal attribution; this was achieved by choosing a shape parameter $\alpha_k = 0.575$ in each case (giving a factor of 100 for the ratio of the 95th to 5th percentiles of a gamma distribution) and setting the value of the prior mean (α_k/τ_k) for each regression coefficient β_k such that the contribution of each risk category $(k = 0, 1, 2)$ would be equal to one third of the overall observed disease rate in the Huddersfield region, a priori.

The prior shape parameters α_{γ_j} and precision parameter τ_γ for the latent risk factors $\{\gamma_j\}_{j \in J}$ were chosen so that each γ_j would have prior mean $\alpha_{\gamma_j}/\tau_\gamma = |B_j|$, the area in km^2 of the region B_j; this makes the model spatially extensible in the sense that coarse or fine partitions $\{B_j\}$ will lead to identical probability distributions for the sums of γ_js over any set, and for kernel sums like our latent risk factor $\sum_{j \in J} k_{ij} \gamma_j$. The degree of uncertainty we express about this spatially varying latent random effect can be adjusted by setting the value of the parameter τ_γ; our uncertainty about its spatial distribution is about the same as if we had to infer a priori the value of this spatially varying function by observing the locations of points randomly scattered with the same distribution, at a density of about τ_γ points per km^2. A small value of τ_γ, would express the prior belief that the spatial variation of the latent risk factors may be high; a large value reflects prior beliefs that there is little spatial variation in the latent variables, that is, that they are close to their (uniform) prior mean. Here, we set $\tau_\gamma = 1.0/km^2$ to give $1.0 \times 30 \times 20 = 600$ 'prior' points over the 30 km $\times$ 20 km Huddersfield region: this represents the prior belief that the latent risk factors exhibit moderate spatial variability.

For the distance scale ρ we employ a point mass prior of $\rho \equiv 1$ km. It would be possible to allow an uncertain prior on this parameter but this complicates the computational implementation; instead, we considered several different fixed values for ρ (ranging from zero to 15 km) and reported our results for the value most consistent with the data. Readers are referred to the Appendix for further computational details such as the

Table 22.1 Prior distributions for model parameters. $\bar{X}$ denotes the population-weighted average excess NO_2 concentration (about 8.8 µg m^{-3} in Huddersfield), and $\bar{Y}$ the approximate overall disease rate (here about 10.2 cases per hundred population)

Baseline Coefficient	$\beta_0 \sim Ga(\alpha_0, \tau_0)$	$\alpha_0 = 0.575$	$\tau_0 = 3\alpha_0/\bar{Y}$
[NO_2] Coefficient	$\beta_1 \sim Ga(\alpha_1, \tau_1)$	$\alpha_1 = 0.575$	$\tau_1 = 3\alpha_1\bar{X}/\bar{Y}$
Latent Coefficient	$\beta_2 \sim Ga(\alpha_2, \tau_2)$	$\alpha_2 = 0.575$	$\tau_2 = 3\alpha_2/\bar{Y}$
Latent Risk Factors	$\gamma_j \sim Ga(\alpha_{\gamma j}, \tau_\gamma)$	$\alpha_{\gamma j} = \tau_\gamma|B_j|$	$\tau_\gamma = 1.0/km^2$
Distance Scale	$\rho \equiv 1$ km		

likelihood function, the posterior distributions of all uncertain quantities, and the partial likelihood for the distance scale parameter ρ.

22.4.2 Implementation

We studied frequent cough rates aggregated both by EDs, where the $\{Y_i\}$ represent the total case counts for residents of the 427 EDs in the study region, and aggregated to a grid of 750 m $\times$ 750 m square quadrats, 605 of which intersect Huddersfield. To compute disease incidence rates we also needed the population (in hundreds) of children aged 7–9 in each aggregation unit A_i. For the ED level analysis we used the pro-rated 1991 UK census population counts discussed in Section 22.2, which are given directly at the required ED level. For the grid analysis we took area-weighted averages of ED-level population values. In both cases, we used a grid of approximately 3 km $\times$ 3 km square quadrats for $\{B_j\}$ (the regions associated with the latent spatial risk factors) covering a rectangle that contains all of Huddersfield and a 2 km buffer zone surrounding it.

Estimation was carried out using Bayesian Markov chain Monte Carlo methods (for an overview see Gilks *et al.* 1996 and Brooks 1998), implemented in a prototype of an upcoming version of the WinBUGS statistical software package (Spiegelhalter *et al.* 1998). This simulation-based approach generates large samples from the posterior joint distribution of all uncertain quantities, from which we can estimate posterior means, histograms, and related summaries for the quantities of interest. Our software, which relies on features not yet available in the distributed version of WinBUGS, is available on request.

22.5 Results

Figure 22.5 shows the posterior distribution, with median and central 90% credible intervals indicated, for the rates of frequent cough in the ED-level analysis associated with: (a) overall baseline, (b) traffic pollution (NO_2), and (c) latent spatial risk factors, in cases per hundred population. Since the baseline (model intercept) term can be regarded as a *non-spatial* latent effect reflecting unobserved risk factors which are constant across the study region, we may combine the estimates of disease rate for the baseline and latent spatial effects to obtain an estimate of the disease rate associated with all latent (unobserved) factors. The posterior distribution for this combined term is shown in Fig. 22.5(d). Table 22.2 gives the medians and central 90% credible intervals of these quantities for both ED-level and grid-level analyses.

Evidently, very little of the risk is attributable to traffic-related pollution such as NO_2 for the ED analysis (0.299 cases per 100 is only about 3% of the total rate); traffic pollution accounts for somewhat more of the risk for the grid-level analysis (about 27%), although there is considerable posterior uncertainty about this estimate. The latter result is more in line with the findings of Elliott *et al.* (1997), who reported a moderate but non-significant excess risk of frequent cough associated with NO_2 concentration at the place of residence in an individual-level analyses of these data. The somewhat different findings for the ED and grid level analysis may well be due to the problem of information loss under data aggregation discussed in Section 22.4. The patterns of NO_2 concentrations and prevalence of frequent cough more closely reflect those of the original data when

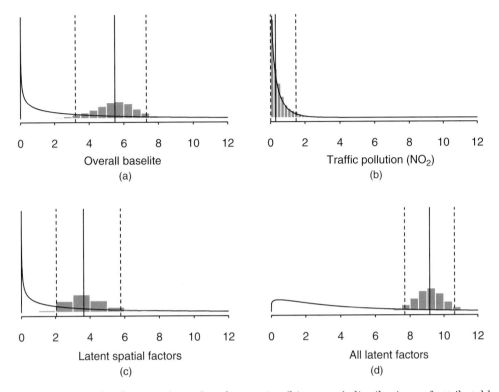

Fig. 22.5 ED-level risk: prior (curve) and posterior (histogram) distributions of attributable risk, in cases per 100 population, with medians (solid vertical lines) and 90% intervals (dashed lines) indicated.

Table 22.2 Summary of posterior distributions of risk attribution for the ED-based and grid-based analyses (cases per 100 population)

Risk factor	Enumeration districts		750 m grid cells	
	Median	90% interval	Median	90% interval
Overall baseline	5.497	[3.195, 7.30]	0.946	[0.016, 3.77]
Traffic pollution (NO_2)	0.299	[0.005, 1.49]	2.821	[0.860, 4.65]
Latent spatial factors	3.628	[2.057, 5.77]	4.920	[3.082, 7.10]
All latent factors	9.157	[7.691, 10.62]	6.210	[4.414, 8.35]

aggregated over the 750 m × 750 m grid than over EDs (see Figs 22.1–22.4), suggesting that less information was lost under the grid-level analysis.

Figure 22.6 gives the posterior mean of the latent spatial risk factors in the form of an image plot to illustrate their spatial distribution under (a) the ED-level analysis and (b) the grid-level analysis using the same shading scale as for the maps of observed rates

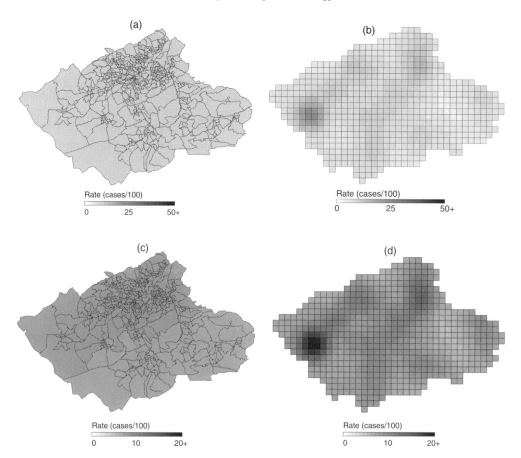

Fig. 22.6 Posterior expected rate (in cases/100 children attributed to the latent spatial covariate: (a) in each enumeration district; (b) on a 750 m × 750 m grid; (c) in each enumeration district (shaded using a narrower range); (d) on a 750 m × 750 m grid (shaded using a narrower range).

(Fig. 22.2); the posterior mean maps are repeated in Fig. 22.6(c) and (d), respectively, using a shading scale with a narrower range.

For the ED-level analysis, the latent spatial factors show virtually no spatial variation, suggesting that no unobserved spatially varying risk factor is associated strongly with frequent cough; this makes the spatial factor similar to the (non-spatial) baseline factor, and the model nearly indifferent about to which of these the risk should be assigned. Each has a median of about 3.6–5.5 cases per hundred (about 38–58% of the total risk), with wide ranges for central 90% intervals. Their sum, the total risk attributed to sources other than NO_2, is much less uncertain, with a median of 9.16 cases per hundred (96% of the total risk) and central 90% range of 7.7–10.6 cases.

By contrast, the latent spatial factors show more pronounced spatial variation under the grid-level analysis: regions with a high latent rate are identified in the west and (to a much lesser extent) north of Huddersfield, although the number of cases per 100 children attributed to the latent spatial term remains nearly constant across the rest of the study

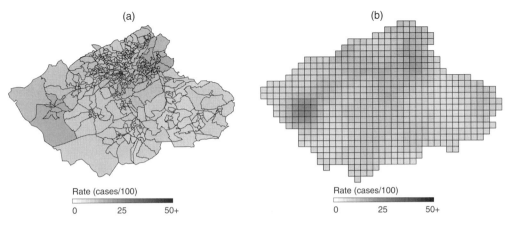

Fig. 22.7 Posterior total expected rate (in cases/100 children): (a) in each enumeration district; (b) on an arbitrary grid.

region. This pattern suggests that there may be localised unobserved risk factors which were missed under the ED-level analysis due to the coarser aggregation units in the more rural outer edges of the study region. Alternatively, the apparent excess number of cases attributed to the latent spatial factors in the west of Huddersfield may be an artefact of the method used to attribute ED populations to each 750 m × 750 m quadrat for the grid-level analysis. Our use of area-weighted averages of ED-level population values assumes that the population is evenly distributed throughout the ED. This is unlikely to be the case for rural EDs where the population tends to cluster in villages within the ED. Hence, the grid-level population values will tend to underestimate the actual population in cells where the postcoded cases are located, leading to artificially high disease rates in those cells. Improved methods for allocating ED-level populations to arbitrary grids are discussed in Section 22.6 (e.g. see Mugglin and Carlin 1998).

22.5.1   Shrinkage

A comparison of the raw case rates of Fig. 22.2 and the posterior mean estimates of frequent cough rate presented in Fig. 22.7 shows that the latter are less variable than the former. The extremes for the raw rates, both high and low, arise from areas with low populations where small chance variations in case counts lead to large swings in rates. These are precisely the rates about which the data are least informative and the likelihood is most diffuse, and whose Bayesian posterior distributions are most strongly shrunk towards the prior mean.

We illustrate this phenomenon in Fig. 22.8, with raw disease rates shown on the left and posterior mean rates on the right for a representative selection of 50 of the 605 Huddersfield 750 m × 750 m quadrats, connected by a line segment. The thick line segments on the left have length proportional to the quadrat populations; evidently the raw data and posterior means are quite similar for the more populous areas, the line segments of which are nearly horizontal, while for the less populous areas the lines slope towards the overall mean of 10.2 cases per hundred.

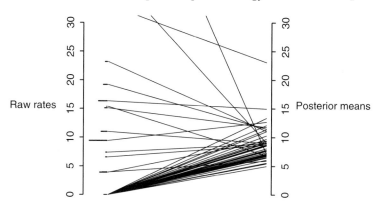

Fig. 22.8 Raw rates and posterior mean risk of frequent cough, in cases/100 population, for selected 750 m × 750 m grid cells, with relative populations indicated by horizontal bars left.

22.6 Discussion

In this chapter we have presented a regression-based approach for mapping ambient air pollution and combining the resulting exposure estimates with health data to study the association between traffic-related air pollution and frequent cough in children. A variety of alternative methods are available for both the exposure modelling and the health data modelling which have been used with varying success in other applications. However, there are a number of problems which may limit their usefulness in the present context. Our methods represent one attempt to address some of these difficulties.

The regression-based methods for exposure modelling used in this study clearly performed well, in that they provided relatively accurate assessments of pollution levels across the study area (as indicated by the results of the validation analysis). Comparisons between the SAVIAH method and a range of other methods (including the CALINE line dispersion model, kriging, and a moving window technique) in the Huddersfield area also showed that it gave consistently the most accurate results (Collins 1998). Similar results have been found in comparisons between a slightly modified version of the SAVIAH model and a range of indicator methods, dispersion models, and spatial interpolation techniques in other cities, including part of London (Wills 1998) and Sheffield (de Hoogh 1999). Briggs *et al.* (2000) show that, with calibration at as few as 10–20 monitoring sites, the method can readily be applied in other areas, or to other years, with equal levels of accuracy. The method can thus be seen as a simple, rapid, and transportable method both for air pollution mapping and exposure assessment. To date, the main application has been to assess long-term (e.g. mean annual) NO_2 concentrations, as measures of chronic exposure to traffic-related pollution. Some potential does seem to exist, however, to apply the methodology for shorter periods (e.g. to estimate 2- to 4-week averages) by incorporating meteorological data (Briggs *et al.* 2000). Nevertheless, although the variables used in the model have been chosen to represent the main source and dispersion factors influencing levels of traffic-related pollution, the model does not explicitly take account either of traffic behaviour or atmospheric processes. It cannot, therefore, be expected to provide reliable estimates of short-term (e.g. hourly or daily) variations in air pollution, as might be used to analyse acute health effects.

Our latent random effects model using a distance-based Gaussian kernel $\{k_{ij}\}$ is similar in spirit to the joint formulation of the conditional autoregressive (CAR) prior model described in Chapter 7, in which the covariance matrix for the spatial Gaussian random effects is specified as a function of distance between area centroids. One difference is, however, that our latent quantities γ_j need not be specified on the same geographical units as the case counts. This provides considerable extra flexibility, since the latent effects are intended to reflect unmeasured spatial confounders which will not necessarily arise at, or vary over, the same aggregation units as the health event data. As with the CAR prior models, metrics other than distance could be used to define the kernel for the latent random effects, or an adjacency-based kernel could be employed. The Gaussian kernel could also be replaced by alternative parametric forms such as the Matérn class (see Chapter 7, Section 7.2.2).

In Section 22.4 we presented an identity link spatial Poisson regression model for the health data. In contrast to the usual individual-level regression models, this approach allows for incorporating spatial dependence via a gamma mixture model for the latent random effects. Our model is thus able to account for possibly spatially varying unmeasured confounders which, if ignored, could lead to bias in the estimates of other model parameters.

In contrast to Poisson-log Gaussian MRF models typically used for spatial modelling of small-area disease counts (see Chapters 7, 11, 15 and 16), our identity link spatial regression model uses a *linear* exposure-response relationship and thus reduces the potential for errors due to mathematical aggregation bias. Being aggregation-consistent, the method can be extended to a *continuous* model that minimises information loss by eliminating all aggregation, using each data source at its finest level of aggregation: for example, using cases at the postcode level and treating NO_2 as an individual-level covariate or as a spatially referenced observed risk factor on a fine grid. Such a model may be achieved by further refining both the areas, A_i, which partition the study region χ, and the regions, B_j, upon which the latent spatial risk factors are defined, until in the limit, both the case locations and latent spatial random effects may be represented by continuous random fields. This version of the model also permits the inclusion of individual-level covariates (if present) by representing the case locations as a marked point process. Best *et al.* (1998) use such a model for an analysis of the respiratory outcome *severe wheeze*, including parental smoking and home dampness as individual covariates.

In our analysis we do not investigate the effect of gender. This is more likely to act as a *modifying* risk factor which influences each child's susceptibility to respiratory illness, rather than as a possible 'cause' of illness to which cases may be attributed. Modifying risk factors act multiplicatively on risk, whereas our identity-link model assumes additive risk factors. We could include a modifying factor in our model by multiplying each p_i in Equation 22.2 by a factor of $\exp(\beta_3 G_i)$ where covariate G_i represents the ratio of boys to girls in each area A_i, and $\exp(\beta_3)$ may be interpreted as a relative risk. However, this leads to a loss of the feature of aggregation consistency (the exposure-response relationship is no longer linear) and might introduce ecological bias (see Chapter 11) in the discrete versions of the models used in this chapter.

One issue that emerged in our grid-based analysis was the need to reallocate the population of 7- to 9-year-old children, originally given on EDs, onto the $750\,\text{m} \times 750\,\text{m}$ grid cells. Here, we proportion the populations according to area. Whilst this approach works well for homogeneously populated regions, including the densely populated areas where the majority of our cases were observed, population is unevenly distributed in the large but sparsely populated rural areas and our uniform allocation scheme may be expected to distort modelled exposure rates in those areas (see Section 22.5). Other approaches, such as realigning ED populations in proportion to the number of postcode centroids in each $750\,m \times 750\,m$ grid cell, might be more meaningful in the low-populated parts of the EDs at the outer boundary of Huddersfield. It would also be possible to use the land cover map available within the GIS for Huddersfield to redistribute population within each ED, for example, using dasymetric mapping (i.e. where counts are redistributed while preserving marginal ED totals; see Langford *et al.* 1990) or weighted control zone techniques (Flowerdew and Green 1994). Another approach, introduced by Mugglin and Carlin (1998), would be to construct a Bayesian hierarchical model for interpolating and smoothing population counts over misaligned zones.

In this analysis, we have coupled two separate regression models: one for predicting exposure to traffic pollutants including NO_2, and a separate one for predicting health effects of exposure. The exposure model expresses NO_2 concentration as a linear combination of local geographical and traffic-related covariates (within a $300\,m$ buffer zone), with uncorrelated Gaussian error terms, while the health effects model expresses incidence counts as Poisson variables whose means are linear combinations of NO_2 exposure and latent spatially correlated covariates.

This approach ignores exposure measurement error (the present exposure estimates have a standard error of $\pm 3.69\,\mu g\,m^{-3}$; see Section 22.3). To better accommodate both measurement uncertainty and the variability of children's NO_2 exposure during their daily activities, the two models may be synthesised into a single model with exposure treated as a second latent spatially varying random effect, with a kernel, k_{ij}^*, reflecting children's exposure at school and during transit as well as at home. This is the approach we are taking in work now in progress.

Appendix

From Equation (22.2) we see that each Poisson mean $\lambda_i = N_i \times p_i$ is a sum $\lambda_{i0} + \lambda_{i1} + \sum_{j \in J}\lambda_{ij}$ of terms associated with the intercept, with NO_2, and with the latent factors, so each Y_i is identical in distribution to the sum $Y_i = \sum_{j \in J^+} Y_{ij}$ of independent random variables $Y_{ij} \sim Po(\lambda_{ij})$ for $i \in I, j \in J^+ \equiv \{0, 1\} \cup J$, with $\lambda_{ij} \equiv N_i p_{ij}$ and $\boldsymbol{p_i} = \{p_{ij}\}_{j \in J^+}$ given in (22.2). The likelihood function for the augmented data $\{Y_{ij}\}$ is

$$L(\boldsymbol{\beta}, \boldsymbol{\gamma}, \rho) = \prod_{i \in I} \left\{ \frac{(\beta_0 N_i)^{Y_{i0}} e^{-\beta_0 N_i}}{Y_{i0}!} \frac{(\beta_1 N_i X_i)^{Y_{i1}} e^{-\beta_1 N_i X_i}}{Y_{i1}!} \right\}$$

$$\times \prod_{i,j \in I, J} \left\{ \frac{(\beta_2 N_i k_{ij} \gamma_j)^{Y_{ij}} e^{-\beta_2 N_i k_{ij} \gamma_j}}{Y_{ij}!} \right\}$$

$$= (\beta_0^{Y_{i0}} e^{-\beta_0 N_I})(\beta_1^{Y_{i1}} e^{-\beta_1 \sum_{i \in I} N_i X_i})(\beta_2^{Y_{ij}} e^{-\beta_2 \sum_{i,j \in I, J} N_i k_{ij} \gamma_j})$$

$$\times \left(\prod_{i \in I} N_i^{Y_i} X_i^{Y_{i1}} \right) \left(\prod_{i,j \in I, J} k_{ij}^{Y_{ij}} \right) \left(\prod_{j \in J} \gamma_j^{Y_{ij}} \right) \left(\prod_{i,j \in I, J^+} Y_{ij}! \right)^{-1} \qquad (22.3)$$

Table 22.3 Complete conditional distributions for model parameters

Baseline coefficient	$\beta_1\vert\cdots \sim \mathrm{Ga}(\alpha_0 + Y_{I0}, \tau_0 + \sum_{i\in I} N_i)$
(NO$_2$) coefficient	$\beta_1\vert\cdots \sim \mathrm{Ga}(\alpha_1 + Y_{I1}, \tau_1 + \sum_{i\in I} N_i X_i)$
Latent coefficient	$\beta_2\vert\cdots \sim \mathrm{Ga}(\alpha_2 + Y_{IJ}, \tau_2 + \sum_{i,j\in I,J} N_i k_{ij}\gamma_j)$
Latent risk factors	$\gamma_j\vert\cdots \sim \mathrm{Ga}(\alpha_j + Y_{Ij}, \tau_j + \beta_2\sum_{i\in I} N_i k_{ij})$
Augmented data	$Y_{ij}\vert\cdots \sim \mathrm{MN}(Y_i, \boldsymbol{p_i})$

where subscripts I and J indicate sums over $i\in I$ and $j\in J$, respectively. With the prior distributions given in Table 22.1 the complete conditional distributions of each parameter, given the augmented data and all other parameters (indicated by '$\vert\cdots$'), are those given in Table 22.3, where $\mathrm{MN}(Y_i, \boldsymbol{p_i})$ denotes the multinomial distribution with sample size Y_i and probability vector proportional to $\boldsymbol{p_i} = \{p_{ij}\}_{j\in J^+}$ (see Equation (22.2)).

Each conditional distribution is simple to sample numerically, making the problem suitable for the Gibbs Sampler variation of Markov chain Monte Carlo (Gelfand and Smith 1990; Tierney 1994).

It would be possible to make inference about the distance scale ρ as well, instead of treating it as certain as we do here. While the likelihood function is a complicated function of ρ, making Gibbs unsuitable, nevertheless one may include a Metropolis–Hastings step for ρ based on the partial likelihood

$$L_P(\rho) \propto \prod_{i,j\in I,J} \left\{ k_{ij}(\rho)^{Y_{ij}} \right\} e^{-\beta_2 \sum_{i,j\in I,J} N_i k_{ij}(\rho)\gamma_j}$$

$$\propto \rho^{-2Y_I} \exp\left\{ -\frac{1}{2\rho^2} \sum_{i,j\in I,J} \left(Y_{ij}\vert x_i - s_j\vert^2 + \frac{\beta_2 N_i \gamma_j}{\pi} e^{-\vert x_i - s_j\vert^2/2\rho^2} \right) \right\}. \tag{22.4}$$

Acknowledgements

This work was partially supported by the Deutsche Forschungsgemeinschaft (supporting K. Ickstadt), a US N.S.F. grant DMS-9626829 (supporting R. Wolpert), a Wellcome Research Travel grant (supporting N. Best), and an equipment grant from the Wellcome Trust (0455051/Z/95/Z).

The authors would like to thank Andrew Thomas for invaluable assistance in implementing the models in the WinBUGS software.

The authors are also indebted to the team of researchers involved in the SAVIAH project. This was a multi-centre project, funded under the EU Third Framework Environment Programme, grant number EV5V-CT920209. It was led by Prof. Paul Elliott (Department of Epidemiology and Public Health, Imperial College of Science, Technology and Medicine, London, UK—formerly at the London School of Hygiene and Tropical Medicine) and co-principal investigators were Prof. David Briggs (Department of Epidemiology and Public Health, Imperial College of Science, Technology and Medicine,

London, UK—formerly at the University of Huddersfield), Dr Erik Lebret (Environmental Epidemiology Unit, National Institute of Public Health and Environmental Protection, Bilthoven, the Netherlands), Pawel Gorynski (National Institute of Hygiene, Warsaw, Poland), and Prof. Bohumir Kriz (Department of Public Health, Charles University, Prague, Czech Republic). Other members of the project were: Marco Martuzzi and Chris Grundy (London School of Hygiene and Tropical Medicine, London, UK); Susan Collins, Emma Livesley, and Kirsty Smallbone (University of Huddersfield, UK); Gerda Doornbos, Caroline Amaling, Paul Fischer, Luuk Gras, Hans van Reeuwijk, and Andre van der Veen (National Institute of Public Health and Environmental Protection, Bilthoven, NL); Bogdan Wojtyniak and Irene Szutowiez (National Institute of Hygiene, Warsaw, Poland); Martin Bobak, Hynek Pikhart, Martin Celko, and Jana Danova, (National Institute of Public Health, Prague, CR), Karel Pryl (City Development Authority, Prague, CR), and Jan Pretel (Czech Hydrometerological Institute); Hendrik Harssema (Wageningen University, NL). Thanks are also due to the local authorities and health authorities in the study area for their assistance in carrying out this research.

References

Anderson, H. R., Butland, B. K., and Strachan, D. P. (1994). Trends in prevalence and severity of childhood asthma. *British Medical Journal*, **308**, 1600–4.

Besag, J., York, J., and Mollié, A. (1991). Bayesian image restoration, with applications in spatial statistics (with discussion). *Annals of the Institute of Statistical Mathematics*, **43**, 1–59.

Best, N. G., Ickstadt, K., and Wolpert, R. L. (1998). Spatial Poisson regression for health and exposure data measured at disparate resolutions. Technical Report No. 98–36. Institute of Statistics and Decision Sciences, Duke University, Durham, NC, USA.

Briggs, D. J., Collins, S., Elliott, P., Fischer, P., Kingham, S., Lebret, E. *et al.* (1997). Mapping urban air pollution using GIS: a regression-based approach. *International Journal of Geographical Information Science*, **11**, 699–718.

Briggs, D. J., de Hoogh, C., Gulliver, J., Wills, J., Elliott, P., Kingham, S., and Smallbone, K. (2000). A regression-based method for mapping traffic-related air pollution: application and testing in four contrasting urban environments. *The Science of the Total Environment* (in press).

Brooks, S. P. (1998). Markov chain Monte Carlo method and its application. *The Statistician*, **47**, 69–100.

Burney, P. (1988). Asthma deaths in England and Wales 1931–85: evidence for a true increase in asthma mortality. *Journal of Epidemiology and Community Health*, **42**, 316–20.

Burney, P., Chinn, S., and Rona, R. J. (1990). Has the prevalence of asthma increased in children? Evidence from the national study of health and growth 1973–86. *British Medical Journal*, **300**, 1306–10.

Collins, S. (1998). Modelling spatial variations in air quality using GIS. In *GIS and health. GIS Data 6* (A. Gatrell and M. Loytonen ed.), 81–95. Taylor and Francis, London.

Committee on Medical Effects of Air Pollution. (1995*a*). Asthma and outdoor air pollution. HMSO, London.

Committee on Medical Effects of Air Pollution. (1995*b*). Non-biological particles and health. HMSO, London.

de Hoogh, C. (1999). Estimating exposure to traffic-related pollution within a GIS environment. Unpublished Ph.D. thesis. University College Northampton and University of Leicester.

Dockery, D. W., Pope, C. A. III, Xiping, X., Spengler, J., Ware, J., Fay, M. *et al.* (1993). An association between air pollution and mortality in six US cities. *New England Journal of Medicine*, **329**, 1753–9.

Duhme, H., Weiland, S. K., Keil, U., Kraemer, B., Schmid, M., Stender, M. *et al.* (1996). The association between self-reported symptoms of asthma and allergic rhinitis and self-reported traffic-density on street of residence in adolescents. *Epidemiology*, **7**, 578–82.

Edwards, J., Walters, S., and Griffiths, R. K. (1994). Hospital admissions for asthma in preschool children: relationship to major roads in Birmingham, United Kingdom. *Archives of Environmental Health*, **49**, 223–7.

Elliott, P., and Briggs, D. J. (1998). Recent developments in the geographical analysis of small area health and environmental data. In *Progress in public health* (G. Scally ed.), 101–25. FT Healthcare, London.

Elliott, P., Briggs, D. J., Lebret, E., Gorynski, P., and Kriz, B. (1997). Small Area Variations in Air quality and Health (the SAVIAH study): Relationship of childhood respiratory symptoms to road traffic pollution. Technical Report: Department of Epidemiology and Public Health, Imperial College School of Medicine, London.

ESRI (1996). *Understanding GIS: The ARC/INFO method*. Environmental Systems Research Institute (ESRI), Redlands, CA, USA.

Florey, C. du V., and Leeder, S. R. (1973). *Methods for cohort studies of chronic airflow limitation*, European Series 12. WHO Regional Publications, Copenhagen.

Flowerdew, R., and Green, M. (1994). Areal interpolation and types of data. In *Spatial analysis and GIS* (S. Fotheringham and P. Rogersen ed.), 121–45. Taylor and Francis, London.

Fotheringham, A. S., and Wong, D. W. S. (1991). The modifiable areal unit problem in multivariate statistical analysis. *Environment and Planning*, **23**, 1025–45.

Gelfand, A. E., and Smith, A. F. M. (1990). Sampling-based approaches to calculating marginal densities. *Journal of the American Statistical Association*, **85**, 398–409.

Gilks, W. R., Richardson, S., and Spiegelhalter, D. J. (1996). *Markov chain Monte Carlo in practice*. Chapman and Hall, New York.

Greenland, S. (1992). Divergent biases in ecologic and individual-level studies. *Statistics in Medicine*, **11**, 1209–23.

Kelsall, J. E., and Diggle, P. J. (1998). Spatial variation in risk: a non-parametric binary regression approach. *Applied Statistics*, **47**, 559–73.

King, G. (1997). *A solution to the ecological inference problem*. Princeton University Press, Princeton.

Langford, M., Uniwin, D., and Maguire, D. J. (1990). Generating improved population density maps in an integrated GIS. In: EGIS '90. *Proceedings of the First European Conference on Geographical Information Systems* (J. Harts, H. F. L. Ottens, and H. J. Scholten ed.), 651–60. EGIS Foundation, Utrecht.

Lebret, E., Briggs, D., Collins, S., van Reeuwijk, H., Fischer, P., Smallbone, K., Hendrick, H. *et al.* (1999). Small area variations in ambient NO_2 concentrations in four European countries. *Atmospheric Environment*, **34**(2), 177–85.

Martuzzi, M., and Elliott, P. (1996). Empirical Bayes estimation of small area prevalence of non-rare conditions. *Statistics in Medicine*, **15**, 1867–73.

Mugglin, A. S., and Carlin, B. P. (1998). Hierarchical modeling in geographic information systems: population interpolation over incompatible zones. *Journal of Agricultural, Biological and Environmental Statistics*, **3**, 111–30.

Murakami, M., Ono, M., and Tamura, K. (1990). Health problems of residents along heavy-traffic roads. *Journal of Human Ergology*, **19**, 101–6.

Nitta, H., Sato, T., Naliai, S., Maeda, K., Aoki, S., and Ono, M. (1993). Respiratory health associated with exposure to automobile exhaust. 1: Results of cross-sectional studies. *Archives of Environmental Health*, **48**, 53–8.

Openshaw, S. (1984). *The modifiable areal unit problem. Concepts and techniques in modern geography, No. 38*. Geo Books, Norwich, England.

Osterlee, A., Drijver, M., Lebret, E., and Brunekreef, B. (1996). Chronic respiratory symptoms in children and adults living along streets with high traffic density. *Occupational Environment Medicine*, **53**, 241–7.

Palmes, E. D., Dunnison, A. F., DiMattio, J., and Tomczyc, C. (1976). Personal sampler for nitrogen dioxide. *American Industrial Hygiene Association Journal*, **37**, 570–7.

Pearce, N., Weiland, S., Keil, U., Langridge, P., Anderson, H. R., Strachan, *et al.* (1993). Self-reported prevalence of asthma symptoms in children in Australia, England, Germany and New Zealand: an international comparison using the ISAAC protocol. *European Respiratory Journal*, **6**, 1455–61.

Pershagen, G., Rylander, E., Norberg, S., Eriksson, M., and Nordell, S. L. (1995). Air pollution involving nitrogen dioxide exposure and wheezing bronchitis in children. *International Journal of Epidemiology*, **24**, 1147–53.

Pope, C. A., Thun, M. J., Namboodiri, M. M., Dockery, D., Evans, J., Speizer, F. *et al.* (1995). Particulate air pollution as a predictor of mortality in a prospective study of US adults. *American Journal of Respiratory Critical Care Medicine*, **151**, 669–74.

Richardson, S. (1992). Statistical methods for geographical correlation studies. In *Geographical and environmental epidemiology*: *Methods for small-area studies* (P. Elliott. J. Cuzick, D. English, and R. Stern ed.), 181–204. Oxford University Press.

Robinson, W. S. (1950). Ecological correlations and the behaviour of individuals. *American Sociological Review*, **15**, 351–7.

Schwartz, J. (1993). Particulate air pollution and chronic respiratory disease. *Environmental Research*, **62**, 7–13.

Schwartz, J. (1994). Air pollution and daily mortality: a review and meta-analysis. *Environmental Research*, **64**, 36–52.

Spiegelhalter, D. J., Thomas, A., and Best, N. G. (1998). *WinBUGS user manual, version 1.1.1*. Medical Research Council Biostatistics Unit, Cambridge. (Available from http://www.mrc-bsu.cam.ac.uk/bugs)

Tierney, L. (1994). Markov chains for exploring posterior distributions (with discussion). *Annals of Statistics*, **22**, 1701–62.

Weiland, S. K., Mundt, K., Ruckmann, A., and Keil, U. (1994). Self-reported wheezing and allergic rhinitis in children and traffic density on street of residence. *Annals of Epidemiology*, **4**, 243–7.

Wills, J. (1998). The development and use of environmental health indicators for epidemiology and policy applications: a geographical analysis. Unpublished Ph.D. thesis. University College Northampton and University of Leicester.

Wjst, M., Reitmeir, P., Dold, S., Wulff, A., Nicolai, T., Freifrau von Loeffelholz-Colberg, E. *et al.* (1993). Road traffic and adverse effects on respiratory health in children. *British Medical Journal*, **307**, 596–600.

23. The role of geographical studies in risk assessment

L. Järup

23.1 Introduction

Modern society uses a vast number of chemicals, supposedly for human benefit. Several hundred thousand chemicals are employed daily and thousands of new compounds are added each year, while others may cease to be used. Many of them may have toxic properties and—if present in the air, water, or food—may constitute potential health hazards. Evaluation of the toxicity of these chemicals is therefore essential in order to protect people from exposure to harmful substances.

The risk assessment process includes several different methods, including the evaluation of existing experimental data as well as epidemiological evidence. The potential health effects should be characterised and dose-response relationships should be computed whenever possible. Furthermore, exposure should be characterised and the uncertainty in each step of the analysis should be evaluated. The risk assessment process may lead to recommendations of acceptable concentrations in air, water, or food.

Risk patterns usually have both spatial and temporal components. It is well known that exposure and disease are unevenly distributed geographically. It is equally well-recognised that diseases may occur in regular (e.g. yearly influenza epidemics) or irregular time intervals (most non-infectious diseases). The reasons for the spatial distribution of disease are often unclear, particularly if the temporal component is of the order of many years, which commonly is the case for chronic diseases such as cancer. Thus, the nature of the risk assessment process implies that many different skills are needed to produce good risk evaluations. Industrial or environmental hygienists are needed to estimate exposures, whereas occupational or environmental health specialists should characterise the potential health effects. Epidemiologists and statisticians should carry out the necessary population-based studies to assess exposure response relationships. Specialists in geographical information systems (GIS), with training in epidemiology, may assist in producing maps of the spatial distribution of exposure and/or disease to reveal any underlying geographical patterns (Vine *et al.* 1997).

Geographical approaches to risk assessment involve the integration and analysis of several different sets of information, each of which may be subject to errors and uncertainties. The basis for risk assessment is a thorough characterisation of exposure. However, sampling and analysis of environmental contaminants are expensive and few spatial locations are normally used. Thus, air pollutants are usually measured in one or a few selected places in a town or a region, even though the distribution of air pollution is often spatially irregular. Spatial patterns of pollution are also often complex, for example because of meteorological and topographic conditions (see Chapter 20). The limited distribution and number of sample points, in both time and space, mean that it is often necessary to make interpolations of pollution data in order to assess exposures and health risks. The quality of the results clearly depends on the accuracy of these interpolations.

A detailed assessment of health outcomes is equally vital for risk assessment. Health data, however, may also be sparse and of uneven quality. The reporting of a disease, such as congenital malformations, may vary between regions and over time (see Chapter 2). Geographical patterns of disease may also be used to infer possible associations between environmental pollutants and health and to detect potentially harmful agents. Estimates of the number of cases associated with an exposure may also be made by overlaying maps of exposures and populations at risk or, more formally, by statistical modelling. Again, however, there are several pitfalls in such studies that need to be addressed, such as latency between exposure and disease incidence, the effects of using spatially aggregated data to represent disease or population patterns, and inherent errors in the source data and the models used (see Chapter 5).

The difficulties of dealing with spatial data, and the wish to avoid presenting misleading information, may contribute to this hesitancy amongst risk professionals to map risk. In the case of groundwater contamination, for example, the subsurface geology, which is often unknown, has profound effects on subsurface flow and movement of contaminants. In the face of such complex factors, most risk professionals have chosen to present results without a spatial component. Nevertheless, risk assessment may benefit greatly from a spatial approach, and GIS may thus be a powerful tool in risk analysis. Although there are difficulties and problems in the spatial analysis of risk, it may be a better—and more conservative—strategy openly to present these details and assumptions spatially, rather than allowing them to remain implicit. It has been argued that 'risk professionals will not mislead by presenting maps—they mislead by not presenting maps' (Hargrove *et al.* 1996).

23.2   Historic examples

The ability to link exposure and disease as part of the risk assessment process depends on the certainty which can be attached to the exposure as well as the time between exposure and disease outbreak (the latency time). The definition of exposure is discussed in more detail later in this chapter, but essentially contact must have been made between the agent under suspicion and the human body. The longer the latency time, the more difficult it will be to associate exposure with disease, since levels and patterns of exposure may have changed considerably over time and/or the population may have changed due to migration. Some of the issues raised can be illustrated through two well-known historic examples.

23.2.1   The cholera epidemics in London

One of the classic examples of geographical risk assessment was that of John Snow, in the 1850s. Snow discovered the association between contaminated river water and cholera risk by mapping both exposure (household usage of water pumps) and disease (cholera cases) in a part of London (Snow 1855) (Fig. 23.1a). In this particular case, he could be reasonably certain that exposure had taken place, since the household members used the locally obtained water for drinking and cooking. There was also a relatively short time (a few days) between exposure and outbreak of disease (latency time). Thus, he was able to draw inferences which provided a sound basis for preventive actions.

Snow made his findings in the pre-computer era. He thus mapped the data as simple point locations. If he had tried to analyse the data using choropleth maps, however—as would now be much easier with modern computers and GIS technology—he may well have missed the connection between the water pump at Broad Street and the cholera cases clustering around that particular pump. Choropleth maps would probably have completely distorted the picture, depending on how the area boundaries were chosen (Fig. 23.1b). The lesson to be learned from this is that the arbitrary boundaries (e.g. counties, health authorities, or other administrative areas), which are often used to map diseases, may result in incorrect risk assessment and inappropriate choice of preventive

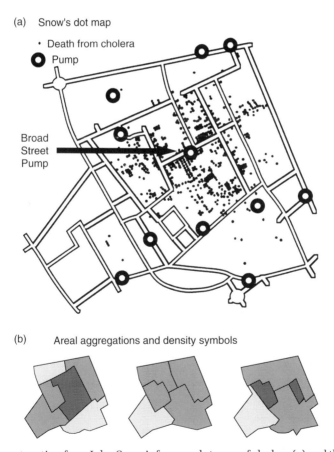

Fig. 23.1 A reconstruction from John Snow's famous dot map of cholera (a) and three choropleth maps (b) produced by different areal aggregation of this part of London (from Monmonier, M. (1996) *How to lie with maps*. The University of Chicago Press, Chicago and London).

actions. This problem has been termed the 'modifiable area unit problem' (Openshaw 1984; see also Chapter 14) and is fundamental in all attempts to map disease using aggregated statistics.

23.2.2   The itai-itai disease in Japan

Approximately one hundred years after Snow's study, a clustering of a hitherto unknown bone disease was recognised in the Jinzu river basin in western Japan. The disease was characterised by severe skeletal pain, due to the distortion of the long bones, and pathological fractures. The disease soon became known as the 'itai-itai' (or the 'ouch-ouch') disease (Hagino and Kono 1955). A local physician, Dr Hagino, noted that the cases were distributed in the Jinzu river basin irrigation area. The irrigation water was taken from the Jinzu river, which was contaminated by cadmium being discharged from the zinc mines in the adjacent mountains.

Measurements of soil cadmium showed very high concentrations in the areas covered by the irrigation system (Fig. 23.2). Analyses of locally grown rice also showed very high concentrations of cadmium. Hagino realised that the itai-itai patients came from areas where cadmium concentrations in rice were high, and he concluded that cadmium-contaminated rice was the likely cause of the disease. He knew that his patients were exposed to cadmium, since most people ate locally grown rice. There was a long latency time (several years) between exposure and disease, but the stability of the population—with virtually no migration—made it possible to draw the aetiological conclusion. After several years, results from risk assessments finally led to the decision to replace the topsoil layer in the area to prevent further exposure to cadmium.

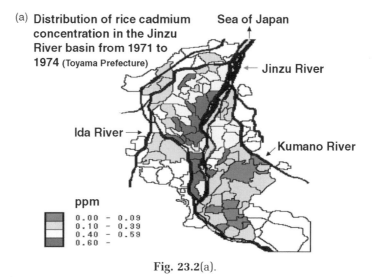

Fig. 23.2(a).

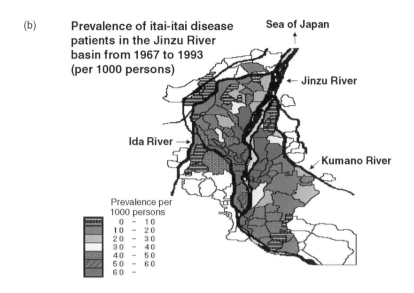

(b) **Prevalence of itai-itai disease patients in the Jinzu River basin from 1967 to 1993 (per 1000 persons)**

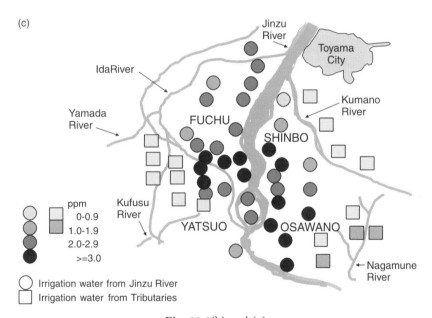

Fig. 23.2(b) and (c).

Fig. 23.2 (a) The Jinzu river basin in Toyama, Japan. Cadmium concentrations in soil (a) and rice (b) and the prevalence of itai-itai disease (c). (Figure kindly provided by Professor K Nogawa, Chiba University, Japan.)

23.3   Exposure mapping

The assessment of exposure and dose is of vital importance in risk assessment. It is important, however, to keep in mind the definition of exposure. A person is considered exposed to an (environmental) agent if the agent in question has been in contact with a body surface (Berglund *et al.*, in press). The main point of contact is usually the mucous membrane of the respiratory or the gastrointestinal tract, although it may also be the skin. The key word in this definition is 'contact': the National Academy of Science, for example, defines exposure as follows: 'an event that occurs when there is contact at a boundary between a human and the environment with a contaminant of a specific concentration for an interval of time' (NAS 1991). Nevertheless, sometimes exposure is said to have occurred merely because the allegedly exposed population has lived in a contaminated environment, even though no contact between the environmental pollutants and the individuals living there may have occurred. Such careless use of the term 'exposure' should be avoided.

The following section considers various routes of exposure. Examples are drawn mainly from the United Kingdom and Sweden.

23.3.1   Oral route of exposure

Exposure via the oral route commonly takes place via ingestion of contaminated food-stuffs or drinking water. The soil in an area may, for example, be contaminated with chemical waste material, such as heavy metals and other persistent substances. Indirect exposure may then occur, if the soil is used for growing vegetables or cereals, or if there is a leakage of chemicals to the groundwater which may pollute adjacent wells. Soil contaminants may also find their way into the human body through a longer chain of events, if animals used for food have been grazing in the polluted area. Most residents in the contaminated area will not be exposed, but small children especially may be exposed by direct ingestion of soil or licking their contaminated fingers while playing. GIS has been used quite extensively to map soil contamination, in particular, heavy metals. Using such data as a basis for estimating exposures, however, needs to be carried out with care, as the following examples show.

Cadmium in soil, feed, and pig kidneys

Reports from several countries have indicated an increase of cadmium in soil (up to 50%) during the last century. Similar increases have been shown for wheat and other crops. A recent Swedish study thus revealed a correlation between cadmium in soil, feed, and pig kidneys (Grawe *et al.* 1997). During the period 1984–92, a large number of pig kidney samples were analysed for cadmium. Statistical analysis showed that the cadmium concentration in pig kidney had increased by 2% annually. Geographical trends in cadmium concentration of pig kidney were analysed using GIS and correlated to cadmium levels in moss and pH in soil. These latter two parameters explained 60% of the random variation in cadmium levels in pig kidney. The authors concluded that an increase in cadmium body burden in pigs may be an indicator of an increase in human cadmium exposure. The data may be used as an argument to decrease cadmium in soil, with the aim of reducing cadmium levels in crops, and thus lowering cadmium levels in grazing animals and meat.

Cadmium in vegetation

It has been claimed that geochemical data, such as heavy metal concentrations in certain plants, may be used for human exposure assessment. In a recent study of cadmium-induced health effects, an attempt was therefore made to evaluate the possible use of cadmium in moss and stream vegetation for human exposure assessment. It has been claimed that the moss contents mirror airborne cadmium deposited during the previous few years (Tyler 1970), whereas cadmium in stream vegetation would reflect the concentration in subsoil water (Grip and Rhode 1985).

A cadmium-emitting battery factory in the south of Sweden operated from the beginning of the twentieth century until 1974. Data on cadmium in moss and stream vegetation in the vicinity of the factory were obtained from the Swedish Geological Survey in 1989, the earliest year for which such data were available. Figure 23.3 shows the cadmium concentration in moss mapped using ordinary kriging (see Chapter 10).

Cadmium in urine has a biological half-life of 10–15 years and provides a good estimate of the body burden. Urinary cadmium was determined for 904 persons in the area close to the battery factory. Geographical coordinates for the addresses where the test subjects lived were linked to the cadmium concentrations in the moss and stream vegetation. The participating individuals had lived at the same address for more than five years.

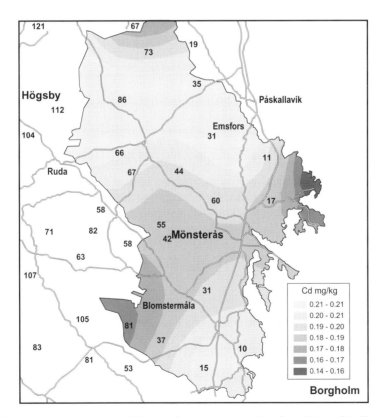

Fig. 23.3 Cadmium in moss, 1995, Mönsterås community, Sweden. (Figure kindly provided by Dr Lennart Hellström, County Council of Kalmar, Sweden.)

No correlation was found between cadmium in moss and urinary cadmium. This is not surprising, since the cadmium levels in urine were most likely heavily influenced by the previous exposure (before 1974) to airborne cadmium emissions from the nearby battery factory. It is also not entirely clear to what extent moss concentrations really reflect the airborne cadmium concentrations. Nor was a correlation found between cadmium in stream vegetation and urinary cadmium. This suggests that cadmium contents of stream vegetation do not indicate actual human intake through water, since most people in the area did not consume local wellwater. Thus, even if cadmium in stream vegetation is a good indicator of the subsoil water concentration of cadmium, it is probably less useful for human exposure assessment. On the basis of this example, therefore, it is evident that caution should be exercised in using data from geochemical surveys for exposure assessment. How reliable these data are as indicators of exposure clearly depends on the extent to which they reflect actual levels of contact and uptake.

23.3.2   The respiratory route of exposure

The natural route of exposure to airborne pollutants is the respiratory system. Since everyone must breathe, there is almost always contact between the air pollutant and the human respiratory mucosa, such that exposure inevitably takes place. The level of exposure may vary, however, depending on many different circumstances: for example, the proportion of time spent indoors and outdoors, recent levels of rest and exercise, or whether respirators have been used for protection.

Ambient air pollution

In the past, relatively simple measures have often been used to provide indicators of exposure to air pollution (e.g. based on distance from the emission source). Most studies of the relationship between traffic-related pollution and respiratory health, for example, have used distance from the nearest main road, or traffic volume on the nearest road, as the exposure indicator (Brunekreef *et al.* 1997; Livingstone *et al.* 1996). The Small-Area Health Statistics Unit (SAHSU) at Imperial College in London has performed several studies around point sources of pollution, such as industrial plants. As a surrogate for exposure, circular areas have traditionally been drawn around the point-source at different distances from the source to define potential exposure zones (see Chapter 9). This provides a somewhat crude estimate of exposure, and does not take into account variations due to meteorological conditions or topography. In a recent study of health effects around cokeworks in England and Wales, the health outcomes—in particular asthma and other (acute) respiratory illness—were assessed in zones at 2 km and 7.5 km distance from the plants (Aylin *et al.* 1998).

Potentially better exposure estimates can be obtained by modelling pollution patterns within a GIS. One of the most powerful techniques is dispersion modelling: a wide range of both point- and line-source models have been developed in recent years (Henriques and Briggs 1998). Nevertheless, modelled air pollution data have rarely been used in epidemiological studies or for risk assessment. One limiting factor is that valid models are available for only a few pollutants (e.g. CO, NO_2 and, more recently, PM_{10}). The accuracy of many existing models is also questionable, and few are able consistently to predict actual concentrations within a factor of two under field conditions (Henriques and Briggs 1998; see also Chapters 19 and 21). Data are also usually available only for the current exposure situation, which makes assessment of chronic health outcomes difficult. Nevertheless, studies of acute health effects (i.e. health outcomes with short latency times), which are thus interested primarily in current or recent exposures, may well benefit from the use of dispersion models. The cokeworks study mentioned above, for example, is currently being further developed by using dispersion models to estimate levels of air pollution around the plants.

A recent case-control study of ambient air pollution and lung cancer used GIS to assess exposure to nitrogen dioxide and sulphur dioxide (Nyberg *et al.*, in press). More than 1000 cases were identified from the regional cancer register in Stockholm, between 1985 and 1990. Over 2000 control individuals were selected. Information on individual exposures was collected via questionnaires including questions on place of residence since 1950. The study thus covered the period of relevant exposure, taking into consideration the long latency time for lung cancer (30 years or more). All places of residence where the case/control had lived for more than one year were recorded, and the addresses transformed into geographical coordinates (geocoded).

Exposure to air pollution (SO_2 and NO_2) was assessed for three different decades (the 1960s, 1970s, and 1980s) using a GIS-based air pollution dispersion model (AIRVIRO). Nitrogen dioxide was used as an indicator of air pollution from road traffic, while SO_2 concentration was used as an indicator for air pollution from heating. Databases were compiled, describing emissions of SO_2 and NO_2 for the different time periods. The results from the dispersion model were validated by comparisons with measured data for all three decades for SO_2, and for the 1980s for NO_2. Figures 23.4a and b show the SO_2

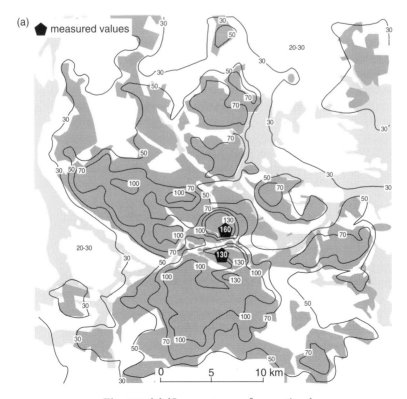

Fig. 23.4(a) (See next page for caption.)

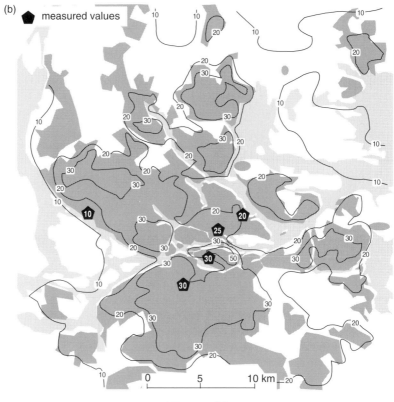

Fig. 23.4(b).

Fig. 23.4 (a) Annual mean concentrations of SO_2, Stockholm, 1960–70. (b) Annual mean concentration of SO_2 ($\mu g/m^3$), Stockholm 1980–90. (Figure kindly provided by the Stockholm Environment and Health Protection Administration, SLB-analys.)

concentrations for 1960–70 and 1970–80. As can be seen in the figure, the estimated concentrations from the dispersion calculations were in good agreement with the measured data. Predicted concentrations at monitoring stations were within the class interval ±20% of the measured data.

The air pollution data were then linked to the individual address coordinates for the relevant time intervals to give exposure indices for each of the air pollution indicators for each decade. In this study it was reasonable to assume that the calculated air pollution concentrations reflected exposure, since all study subjects had to breathe the surrounding air. Furthermore, the collection of addresses and emission information more than 30 years before the onset of disease ensured that the long latency time associated with lung cancer was taken into account.

The resulting exposure data were then compared with health outcome. Results showed small, but statistically significant, increased smoking-adjusted relative risks for lung cancer associated with exposure to NO_2, but not to SO_2. They thus suggest that the elevated risks of lung cancer in a city like Stockholm is associated with road traffic rather than emissions from heating systems.

Ground radon

Airborne radon is a well-known lung carcinogen. In order to assess the risk of radon exposure in a Swedish county (Östergötland), local communes have carried out risk assessments, providing radon maps indicating areas with different levels of exposure (Kohli *et al.* 1997). The areas were classified as having low, normal, or high risk. The classifications took into account measured concentrations of radon (where available), type of soil, and soil permeability.

The annual population registration records and the national property register were used to determine the locations of the persons living in the county. By linking the address in the population register to the property register, each individual was mapped to the centroid of a property. By combining the population data with the radon maps, the populations living in high-, normal-, or low-risk areas were identified. The results show large variations between different areas in the county. Some communes had no population in high radon risk areas, whereas in others as much as 35% of the population lived in high-risk areas.

These data need to be interpreted with caution. It should be noted that individuals living in areas defined as 'high risk' may not necessarily experience high levels of exposure, since the correlation between ground radon and airborne radon is relatively weak. Indeed, marked variations in radon concentrations occur from house-to-house and even from room-to-room within any individual dwelling. Mapped radon areas are thus likely to mask major local variations in exposure. Nevertheless, data on ground radon may be used to guide monitoring programmes for a more detailed assessment of individual risk of exposure.

23.3.3 Other routes of exposure: electromagnetic fields

The previous examples have focused on well-defined routes of exposure (e.g. via ingestion or inhalation). Sometimes the route of exposure is less well defined. This is particularly true for exposure to electromagnetic fields. Partly for this reason, the association between living in the vicinity of powerlines and the risk of cancer (particularly leukaemia) remains controversial.

Relatively little quantitative information on public exposure to magnetic fields generated by high-voltage power lines is available. A recent Finnish report, however, described residential exposure to magnetic fields from high voltage powerlines at the national level (Valjus *et al.* 1995). A GIS was used to identify buildings located near powerlines. The distances between the lines and the place of residence were then determined and data on line load currents were used to estimate the magnetic fields. The magnetic field estimates were then linked to the residents by means of a central population register. Around 10% of all buildings in Finland were found to be located within 500 m of high voltage powerlines and it was estimated that 0.3% of the population was exposed in their homes to an annual average magnetic field from power lines, that was higher than 0.1 microTesla. On the basis of these results, the authors concluded that the problem of magnetic field exposure generated by high voltage lines concerns only a small fraction of the total population in Finland. They also note that the size of the 'population at risk' remains somewhat arbitrary, since there is no clear biological mechanism for any health effect and the importance of duration of exposure is unknown.

23.3.4   Integrated dose via several exposure pathways

It is rarely possible to map dose (i.e. the internal concentration of an agent resulting from external exposure) with any degree of accuracy. Where possible, however, dose mapping may be a valuable tool for identifying sources of exposure. One example of this is provided by a GIS-based study of environmental exposures to lead in the USA (Guthe *et al.* 1992). Available GIS databases on industrial lead-emitting sites and hazardous waste sites were used, together with data on traffic volume, to define areas of potential environmental exposure to lead. Blood screening data were then entered into the GIS and geocoded on the basis of the reported addresses. Other data associated with each geographical point (e.g. age, sex, and date of blood sampling) were also recorded. Spatial data on the lead sources and patterns of high blood lead were then compared. A strong correlation was found between sources of lead and elevated blood levels in children.

23.3.5   Acute hazards

Transport of hazardous material through densely populated areas is a common problem in most large cities. GIS may be used to assess risks associated with these activities in different ways. For primary prevention, simulations of the probability of accidents may be useful in order to select optimal routes. Once an accident has occurred, on the other hand, it is vital to make a rapid assessment of the dispersion of hazardous chemicals, in order to minimise the exposure of the population. The examples below illustrate both these aspects of acute hazard risk assessment and management.

Simulation of hazardous transports

The London Waste Regulatory Authority records liquid hazardous waste transport, with information of the origin and destination, though not the route followed during transportation. Lovett *et al.* (1997) used a GIS to forecast the routes used, on the basis of different routing criteria and characteristics of the available road network. Data on population distribution and variables indicating potential pollution of groundwater (mainly hydrological and geological characteristics) were collected, in order to evaluate the potential consequences of a waste discharge during transport.

Four different routing scenarios were implemented to identify road sections with a constant load of heavy traffic. Two scenarios were based on the assumption that tanker drivers would try to find the least-cost path through the area (e.g. by minimising travel time). The other two scenarios aimed to alleviate hazards by limiting tanker traffic on roads in densely populated areas. Data were generated on average length of journey time, population living close to the chosen routes, tanker traffic over zones with extreme groundwater vulnerability, and time interval (years) between cargo threatening accidents. It was shown that, while one type of hazard might be reduced, this might lead to an increase in another hazard. For example, the avoidance of routes through densely populated areas led to a substantial increase of traffic over vulnerable groundwater zones. The simulations thus illustrated that some interventions could lead to risk trade-off and displacement of hazards rather than hazard alleviation.

Early warning system

As an example, transport of hazardous chemicals is common along certain roads in the centre of Stockholm. The surrounding areas are densely populated and an accident with

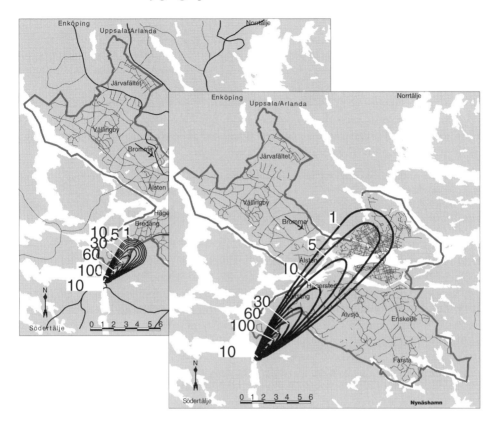

Fig. 23.5 Distribution of concentrations of ammonia from a continuous gas leak after 30 and 120 minutes when the wind is blowing from southwest at 2 metres per second. (Figure kindly provided by the Stockholm Environment and Health Protection Administration, SLB-analys.)

leakage of chemicals would potentially have serious health consequences. An early warning system has thus been designed, aimed at rapidly assessing the dispersion of chemicals, so that advice can be given within minutes of any accident. The system is designed to handle several potentially hazardous chemicals including ammonia, chlorine, propane, vinyl chloride, and methane. Continuous leakage of gases or liquids, as well as tanker lorry accidents, can be handled by the system.

The system uses GIS and a dispersion model to predict the area where potentially hazardous pollution will occur. Figure 23.5 shows an example of dispersion calculations for ammonia following a hypothetical accident, where gas is leaking continuously. The maps show the distribution of concentrations after 30 and 120 minutes, assuming that the wind is blowing from the southwest at 2 metres per second.

23.4 Disease mapping

Geographical approaches to risk assessment are not limited to the assessment and mapping of exposure. Disease mapping is also a valuable part of the risk assessment process. It can help, for example, to identify possible disease clusters, to define and monitor epidemics, to provide baseline data on health patterns, and to show changing patterns of health over time. Disease mapping may also be useful in exploring causal relationships with exposure, in particular for acute health effects. Caution should, however, be exercised when interpreting apparent associations between environmental exposures and health effects for several reasons. One of these has already been referred to—namely, the modifiable area unit problem (MAUP) (Openshaw 1984; see also Chapters 14 and 22). Another important problem is that of latency time. The longer the period between an exposure and the onset of a disease, the more difficult will it be to establish an association, in particular, if migration in the study area has been extensive (see Chapter 5).

23.4.1   Latency

For many infectious diseases the time between exposure to an infectious agent and the outbreak of the disease is short—a few days to a week is common. As noted earlier, this was a key to John Snow's success in discovering the relationship between the exposure to bacterially contaminated water and the outbreak of cholera in London. For most chronic diseases, however, there is a long latency time. Typical latency times for cancers are in the order of decades: the latency time for lung cancer, for example, has been estimated to be more than thirty years. The latency times for other chronic diseases are usually less well known, but are probably in the order of several years.

Latency is thus an important consideration in investigations of associations between exposure and chronic diseases. Current disease patterns may have been caused by exposures decades ago, whereas current exposure levels may lead to disease many years from now. Investigators without epidemiological training sometimes neglect this. In particular, some investigators have used GIS to map and compare current exposures and current disease prevalence, failing to recognise that previous, not current, exposures have caused today's diseases.

23.4.2   Infectious diseases

Traditionally, maps have been used to describe the prevalence of infectious diseases. Since the days of John Snow, cholera, tuberculosis, malaria, and other vectorborne diseases have been mapped in the attempt to forecast the spread of the diseases so that preventive actions may be taken. With the development of the GIS technique, such maps may more readily be produced, thereby enhancing the possibilities for intervention (see Chapter 14).

Malaria

Nearly half of the world's population lives in areas where they are at risk of vectorborne diseases; over two billion people are at risk of malaria alone. Several systems for the surveillance of malaria have therefore been developed, many of which use conventional techniques that are time-consuming and expensive. Recently, however, the use of GIS techniques for malaria risk assessment has begun to increase.

Beck *et al.* (1994), for example, used remote sensing and GIS techniques to discriminate between villages in Mexico which were at high and low risk of malaria. The subtropical climate and vegetation of this region provides a good breeding environment for mosquitoes and thus for malaria transmission. Remotely sensed satellite data for an area in Mexico were digitally processed to generate a map of landscape elements, particularly emphasising pastures and swamps, which are known mosquito areas. Data on mean mosquito numbers were collected in randomly selected villages for different sampling periods.

The GIS was used to determine the proportion of mapped landscape elements surrounding villages where malaria mosquito abundance data had been collected. The relationships between vector abundance and the proportional area of the landscape elements were then analysed using regression methods. Results indicated that the most important landscape elements in terms of explaining vector abundance were transitional swamp and unmanaged pasture. The authors concluded that this approach, which integrated remotely sensed data and GIS capabilities to identify villages with high contact risk, provided a promising tool for malaria surveillance programmes. In principle, similar approaches could also be applied to other vectorborne diseases in areas where the landscape elements critical to vector survival are known and these elements can be detected with remote sensing techniques. Examples include the study of lyme disease (Glass *et al.* 1995) and LaCrosse encephalitis (Kitron *et al.* 1997).

The Onchocerciasis Control Programme in West Africa (OCP)

Onchocerciasis ('river blindness') is a dreaded disease, once blinding thousands of Africans. The OCP has worked to exterminate the vectors (flies) that spread the disease by spraying insecticides in areas of vector abundance. The programme has also treated the population against the parasite causing the illness.

To help target and monitor action, a GIS is used to map insect and epidemiological data (http://www.esri.com/library/usercanf/proc97/proc97/to200/pap182/). Both current and historical data are mapped. Thematic maps based on epidemiological surveys are combined with entomological data, and the system is designed so that graphs of the trend of prevalence for any village can be obtained, by selecting the village on screen. Similarly, clicking on a catching point displays the trend of the annual transmission potential. This information is used to decide whether insecticide treatment should continue or be stopped.

23.4.3 Chronic diseases

Some of the most important diseases for public health in the developed countries are cancers and cardiovascular and respiratory diseases. Environmental factors are considered to play a major role in the development of such chronic diseases, although for most of these diseases the exposure-response relationships are largely unknown.

At the International Agency for Research on Cancer (IARC), maps of cancer incidence and mortality are computed on a global scale. The maps are displayed on the IARC website (http:/www.iarc.fr) and maps for a particular cancer diagnosis and gender can be selected. For example, the map at (http://www-dep.iarc.fr/java/globocan/images/map11f.-html) shows female breast cancer incidence in 1990. It is clear from the map that breast cancer is a disease affecting the affluent parts of the world, whereas the incidence is low in developing countries.

Several other countries have produced similar maps (see Chapter 12). In the USA, for example, the National Cancer Institute (NCI) has published atlases of cancer mortality since 1950 (Pickle *et al.* 1990). The NCI is currently making cancer mortality maps (for the period 1970–92) available on the Internet (http://www-dceg.ims.nci.nih.gov/MRG/index.html). Maps of more than thirty cancers (displayed by race and gender) will be

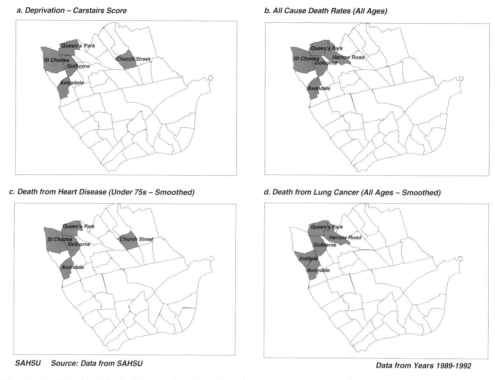

a. Deprivation – Carstairs Score

b. All Cause Death Rates (All Ages)

c. Death from Heart Disease (Under 75s – Smoothed)

d. Death from Lung Cancer (All Ages – Smoothed)

SAHSU   Source: Data from SAHSU

Data from Years 1989-1992

Fig. 23.6 Wards with the highest levels of deprivation, death rates, death from heart disease, and death from lung cancer, 1989–92. (From the Kensington & Chelsea and Westminster Annual Report, 1997; maps produced by the Small Area Health Statistics Unit, Imperial College, London.)

available. As an example, the web-page (http://www-dceg.ims.nci.nih.gov/MRG/ example.html) shows breast cancer mortality for white US women.

At the Small-Area Health Statistics Unit (SAHSU), Imperial College in London, a computerised system has been set up for the rapid production of maps illustrating the differences in relative risk of disease between different areas. The technique has been used, for example, to produce risk of coronary heart disease by electoral wards of the Kensington & Chelsea and Westminster (KCW) Health Authority in London. One of the main topics of the KCW Annual Public Health Report was to address health inequalities within the district, showing maps for specific conditions. Figure 23.6a shows the five wards within KCW with the highest levels of deprivation (measured via the Carstairs index—see Chapter 4); Figs. 23.6b–d show the wards with the highest death rates from all causes, heart disease, and lung cancer. There is a striking similarity between the distributions, implying that variations in heart disease within KCW Health Authority are associated, at least indirectly, with socio-economic conditions.

23.5 Risk assessment

It is clear that the overlay of maps of exposure and disease cannot normally provide reliable estimates of the number of cases that are likely to occur in an exposed

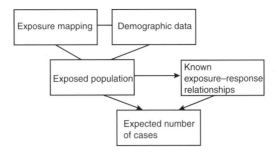

Fig. 23.7 Schematic presentation of the calculation of expected cases caused by exposure to an environmental pollutant.

population. In particular, the accuracy of the exposure estimates and the latency period mean that such estimates are likely to be misleading. GIS can nevertheless be used to estimate the number of expected cases, as schematically shown in Fig. 23.7. This procedure is most suitable for estimating the number of cases caused by air pollution. First, exposure maps may be produced (e.g. by using air pollution dispersion models). Second, these may then be combined with demographic data to produce an estimate of the number of people exposed to certain levels of the pollutant under study. Third, previously established data on exposure-response relationships may be used to compute the number of individuals expected to develop the disease at each exposure level. Such methods are, however, highly sensitive both to the pollution model used, the nature and site of the assumed exposure-response relationship, and to the level of spatial aggregation of the population data. Collins (1998), for example, compared estimates of the residential area (and by implication the proportion of the population living in these areas) above a mean annual NO_2 concentration of $33 \mu g/m^3$ in Huddersfield, UK, using different modelling techniques. Estimates varied from 9% for a method based on the CALINE dispersion model, to 17% using the SAVIAH regression model (Briggs *et al.* 1997; and see Chapter 22) to 35% using ordinary kriging. As these results show, considerable margins of uncertainty are likely to occur around any risk estimate based upon simple mapping and overlay techniques (see Chapter 19).

23.6 Strengths and weaknesses in using GIS for risk assessment

As the examples in this chapter have shown, the use of GIS at all stages in the risk assessment process—for exposure assessment, for disease mapping, and for estimating the number of people at risk—has both strengths and weaknesses.

In the case of *exposure assessment* one of the main strengths is the possibility of modelling exposure geographically so that individual exposure may be estimated without costly and cumbersome measurements. Another obvious advantage is that populations at risk can be estimated for various levels of exposure. It is, however, very important to bear in mind the definition of exposure as stated above: namely, that contact must occur between the agent of concern and the population. It is all too easy to use GIS to describe the distribution of a contaminant on the assumption that this represents exposure, regardless of whether contact actually takes place. It is also crucial to consider the data and other limitations involved in exposure modelling within GIS. As has been seen, many of the models used for pollution modelling are subject to considerable uncertainties, especially when applied across large areas (see the discussion of errors-in-variables modelling in Chapter 5). The spatial resolution and coverage of environmental data are also often poor. These problems should not be lightly dismissed: misuse of GIS for exposure estimation may lead to completely erroneous risk assessment.

Mapping of disease is becoming increasingly popular, perhaps above all to show inequalities in health between regions. Provided that the methods used are valid and the input data are correct, disease mapping may indeed be a valuable means of assessing and displaying geographical differences in health. Nevertheless, as discussed elsewhere in this volume (e.g. see Chapters 5, 7, and 14) great care is needed in interpretation. There may be variations in data quality that produce spurious spatial patterns. The boundaries of the areas to be studied are often administrative and may not necessarily be ideal for mapping health outcomes, while the choice of boundaries themselves may well have a major influence on the results. The importance of using appropriate methods of standardisation also needs to be emphasised and should be recognised in any attempt to map relative risks of diseases, so that valid comparisons may be made.

GIS also provide potentially valuable tools for *estimating the number of cases* associated with an exposure of interest. Unfortunately, two contradictory problems face such an approach. On the one hand, established exposure-response relationships are only available to date for very few pollutants; for many of these, such as PM_{10} good exposure models and methods of exposure assessment are still not obtainable. On the other hand, where reasonably reliable methods of exposure assessment exist (e.g. for NO_2), data on exposure-response relationships tend to be sparse. There are relatively few contaminants, therefore, that can be analysed by this approach. In this area, also, the issues of model and data accuracy noted above are crucial, since errors in any one of the datasets involved (in levels of exposure, or in the distribution of the population of interest) may have an important impact on the results. Before the full potential of GIS in risk assessment can be exploited, therefore, significant advances will need to be made in pollution modelling, in the knowledge of exposure-response relationships and in the availability of high resolution population and demographic data.

References

Aylin, P., Wakefield, J., Grossinho, A., Elliott, P., Colvile, R., and Bottle, A. (1998). Hospital admissions for respiratory disease near cokeworks. *Epidemiology*, 4(Suppl.), S33.

Beck, L. R., Rodriguez, M. H., Dister, S. W., Rodriguez, A. D., Rejmankova, E., Ulloa, A. *et al.* (1994). Remote sensing as a landscape epidemiologic tool to identify villages at high risk for malaria transmission. *American Journal of Tropical Medicine and Hygiene*, 51, 271–80.

Berglund, M., Elinder, C.-G., and Järup, L. (in press). *Human exposure assessment—an introduction* World Health Organisation, Geneva.

Briggs, D. J., Collins, S., Elliott, P., Kingham, S., Fisher, P., Lebret, E. *et al.* (1997). Mapping urban air pollution using GIS: a regression-based approach. *International Journal of Geographical Information Science*, 11, 699–718.

Brunekreef, B., Janssen, N. A. H., de Hartog, J., Harssema, H., Knape, M., and van Vliet, P. (1997). Air pollution from truck traffic and lung function in children living near motorways. *Epidemiology*, 8, 298–303.

Collins, S. (1998). Modelling spatial variations in air quality using GIS. In *GIS and health.* *GISData 6.* (A. Gatrell and M. Loytonen ed.), 81–95. Taylor & Francis, London.

Glass, G. E., Schwartz, B. S., Morgan, J. M., Johnson, D. T., Noy, P. M., and Ebenezer, I. (1995). Environmental risk factors for lyme disease identified with geographical information systems. *American Journal of Public Health,* **85**, 944–8.

Grawe, K. P., Thierfelder, T., Jorhem, L., and Oskarsson, A. (1997). Cadmium levels in kidneys from Swedish pigs in relation to environmental factors—temporal and spatial trends. *The Science of the Total Environment,* **208**, 111–22.

Grip, H. and Rhode, A. (1985). *Vattnets väg från regn till bäck.* Forskningsrådens förlagstjänst, Stockholm.

Guthe, W. G., Tucker, R. K., Murphy, E. A., England, R., Stevenson, E., and Luckhardt, J. C. (1992). Reassessment of lead exposure in New Jersey using GIS technology. *Environmental Research,* **59**, 318–25.

Hagino, N. and Kono, M. (1955). A study on the cause of itai-itai-disease, (in Japanese). *Proceedings, 17th Meeting of the Japanese Society of Clinical Surgeons.*

Hargrove, W. W., Levine, D. A., Miller, M. R., Coleman, P. R., Pack, D. L., and Durfee, R. C. (1996). *GIS and risk assessment: a fruitful combination.* Web page, last modified 17/4/1996: www.esri.com/library/userconf/proc96/TO50/PAP028/P28.HTM

Henriques, W. D. and Briggs, D. J. (1998) Environmental modelling in the NEHAP process. In *Environmental health for all. Risk assessment and risk communication in National environmental health action plans* (D. J. Briggs, R. M. Stern, and T. Tinker, ed.), 113–32. Kluwer, Dordrecht.

Kitron, U., Michael, J., Swanson, J., and Haramis, L. (1997). Spatial analysis of the distribution of LaCrosse encephalitis in Illinois, using a geographical information system and local and global spatial statistics. *American Journal of Tropical Medicine and Hygiene,* **57**, 469–75.

Kohli, S., Sahlen, K., Lofman, O., Sivertun, A., Foldevi, M., Trell, E. *et al.* (1997). Individuals living in areas with high background radon: a GIS method to identify populations at risk. *Computer Methods and Programs in Biomedicine,* **53**, 105–12.

Livingstone, A. E., Shaddick, G., Grundy, C., and Elliott, P. (1996). Do people living near city main roads have more asthma needing treatment? Case-control study. *British Medical Journal,* **312**, 676–7.

Lovett, A. A., Parfitt, J. P., and Brainard, J. S. (1997). Using GIS in risk analysis: a case study of hazardous waste transport. *Risk Analysis,* **17**, 625–33.

Monmonnier, M. (1996) *How to lie maps.* University of Chicago Press, Chicago and London.

NAS (National Academy of Science) (1991). *Human exposure assessment for airborne pollutants. Advances and opportunities.* National Academy Press, Washington, DC.

Nyberg, F., Gustavsson, P., Järup, L., Bellander, T., Berglind, N., and Pershagen G. (in press) Urban air pollution and lung cancer.

Openshaw S. (1984). *The modifiable areal unit problem. CATMOG No 38.* Geo Books. Norwich.

Pickle, L. W., Mason, T. J., Howard, N., Hoover, R., and Fraumeni, J. F. Jr. (1990). *Atlas of US cancer mortality among nonwhites: 1950–1980.* US Government Printing Office, Washington, DC.

Snow, J. (1855). *On the mode of communication of cholera.* London, Churchill Livingstone.

Tyler, G. (1970). Moss analysis—a method for surveying heavy metal deposition. In *Proceedings of the Second International Clean Air Congress* (H. M. Englund and W. T. Berry ed.). Academic Press, New York.

Valjus, J., Hongisto, M., Verkasalo, P., Jarvinen, P., Heikkila, K., and Koskenvuo, M. (1995). Residential exposure to magnetic fields generated by 110–400 kV power lines in Finland. *Bioelectromagnetics,* **16**, 365–76.

Vine, M. F., Degnan, D., and Hanchette, C. (1997). Geographical information systems: their use in environmental epidemiologic research. *Environmental Health Perspective,* **105**, 598–605.

24. Water quality and health

M. Kanarek

24.1 Introduction

There has been a long history of mapping drinking water parameters and linking them to human population disease states. The studies of cholera by John Snow in London in the late 1840s to mid 1850s are often regarded as classic examples. Even before the scientific discovery of the cholera bacterium, Snow mapped cholera cases in the Broad Street Pump area of London (see Chapter 23, Fig. 23.1) to help identify the source of contamination and mapped cholera victims according to their service by different water distribution companies to gain an epidemiological understanding of waterborne cholera epidemics (Snow 1936).

Environmental epidemiology took a great leap forward in the mid 1970s in the USA, as a result of the landmark mapping of 1950–69 cancer mortality by county, by the National Cancer Institute (Mason *et al.* 1974). Page *et al.* (1976) subsequently used these data to seek correlations between mapped cancer mortality and the amounts of Mississippi River water used as a drinking water source. Their provocative results, showing higher cancer rates in areas that used more river water, raised concern over organic contaminants in drinking water sources which eventually led to many cancer epidemiology studies of trihalomethanes (THMs) and other chlorine disinfection by-products in drinking water. More work has since been done on this topic than any other in the research field of drinking water and cancer.

Considering the ubiquity and importance of the exposure involved, mainstream epidemiology has devoted surprisingly limited resources to the possible links between drinking water and disease. This is partially due to inherent problems in environmental epidemiology in the modern world. The mobility of the modern population makes it very difficult to assess exposures and track outcomes. In addition, the epidemiologist must try to assess and allow for the many potential intervening confounders and co-factors, over the many years involved in the latent periods for non-infectious diseases such as cancer. Advances in mapping techniques due to improvements in modelling, geographical information systems (GIS), and disease registries will surely make these tasks easier and lead to improved studies in the future.

In this chapter, the focus will be on mapping non-infectious diseases. This is largely because the long latent period under consideration for these diseases makes them more amenable to mapping. Nevertheless, it must be borne in mind that infectious diseases are more important from an overall public health perspective. This is amply illustrated by the 1993 cryptosporidiosis outbreak in Milwaukee, Wisconsin, where 400 000 fell ill in a waterborne outbreak to a previously ignored protozoan agent (Mackenzie *et al.* 1994).

This Milwaukee outbreak is a clear signal that, even in highly industrialised societies, we will never wholly be rid of concern about infection via drinking water.

24.2 Data sources

24.2.1 Monitoring networks

Globally, there have been several national efforts to map water parameters, notably in the USA and Europe. These efforts have typically focused on gathering, storing, and mapping data on surface and/or groundwater parameters for policy and management purposes; rarely have these databases been utilised for health studies.

In Europe, almost all countries run national surface water quality networks to monitor compliance with water quality standards and to track trends in water quality. Results from these are mapped on a routine basis. In the UK, for example, the General Water Quality Classification is used to classify and map all major streams (circa 100 000 km) on a scale from A (good) to F (bad), based on measurements of biochemical oxygen demand (BOD), dissolved oxygen, and ammonia concentration. Additional data are also collected for about 230 sites, mainly at the tidal limits of rivers, as part of the Harmonised Monitoring Scheme. The systems of water quality classification and monitoring regimes used in different countries tend to vary, however, so that inter-country comparisons need to be made with care (Newman 1988). Under the EU Surface Water Quality Directive, 18 water quality parameters are routinely monitored according to a common protocol at sites across Europe. Determinants include metals (Cd, Hg, Cu), faecal and total coliforms, BOD, chemical oxygen demand, nitrates and phosphates. Monitoring started in the mid 1970s, since when the number of sites in the network has grown to about 250, on all the main European rivers (Stanners and Bordeau 1995). More detailed monitoring is also undertaken on international waterways, such as the Rhine and Danube. Similarly, the EU Bathing Water Directive, adopted in 1974, obliges all member states to undertake routine monitoring of all designated bathing sites, in both coastal and freshwaters. Monitoring of nine parameters—including total and faecal coliforms, enteroviruses, and phenols—is mandatory; a further 10 parameters are monitored on a voluntary basis. In 1997, monitoring was carried out over 13 000 coastal sites and more than 6000 freshwater sites across Europe (Directorate General for the Environment 1998). A bathing water atlas, showing compliance with the standards, is also produced annually to help tourists select holiday destinations. To date, these data have not been used for epidemiological purposes, but they offer a potentially rich source of information for health studies.

Patrick *et al.* (1996) describe the UK Acid Waters Monitoring Network (AWMN) in England, which was established in 1988. It utilises 11 lake and 11 stream sites designed primarily to track acidification for the ultimate purpose of freshwater biology study. The principal objective is to provide a long-term, high quality chemical, biological, and palaeolimnological record which, in conjunction with the UK precipitation monitoring networks, will facilitate the assessment of trends within UK surface waters. However, since it also provides data on trace metals and other chemicals, such as calcium and sulphate, the AWMN is of potential utility to epidemiologists. The data comprise an excellent baseline with which future changes may be compared. In addition, AWMN sites provide data to develop and validate critical loads models and dynamic models of acidification, and could also be used to monitor the impact of other air pollutants, such as trace metals and persistent organic compounds, on the freshwater environment.

During the past thirty years, the US Geological Survey (USGS) has operated two national stream water-quality networks (Alexander *et al.* 1998): the Hydrologic Benchmark Network (HBN) and the National Stream Quality Accounting Network (NASQAN). In these networks, the USGS systematically monitors streams in watersheds throughout the United States to provide national and regional descriptions of stream water-quality conditions and trends. The HBN—which consists of 63 relatively small, minimally disturbed watersheds—provides data for investigating naturally induced changes in streamflow and water quality and the effects of airborne substances on water quality. NASQAN, consisting of 618 larger, more land use-influenced watersheds, provides information for tracking water-quality conditions in major US rivers and streams. The watersheds in both networks include a diverse set of climatic, physiographic, and land use characteristics. Data from the networks have been used to describe geographical variations in water-quality concentrations, quantify water-quality trends, estimate rates of chemical flux from watersheds, and investigate relations of water quality to the natural environment and anthropogenic contaminant sources.

Pebesma (1996) describes the Netherlands national groundwater quality monitoring network (NGM) which was established in 1978. As part of this network, 370 permanent wells spread evenly throughout the Netherlands have been sampled yearly for 19 variables. In more recent years the number of wells has nearly doubled and the number of variables increased to 25. The programme was begun as an effort to map groundwater quality to assess the current state and temporal changes, and the utility of statistical mapping techniques in tracking environmental health exposure parameters. Despite large estimation inaccuracies in the collected data, it was found possible to map to a spatial resolution of $4\,km^2$ blocks. This resolution provides the opportunity to use these data for relatively detailed exposure assessment. Nevertheless, stratification of the data by soil type and land use, and inclusion of data on groundwater flow, would greatly improve the maps. This would allow modelling of groundwater quality, based on actual measurements of soil type, land use, and flow, and would thereby provide a better characterisation of the variation in exposure to pollutants experienced across heterogeneous populations. In this context, the use of airborne reconnaissance also has particular potential. As Jupp *et al.* (1994) show, this offers major improvements in mapping resolution, for example, in the detection, identification, and mapping of algal species, cyanobacteria, and other factors such as turbidity. The improved mapping resolution available from these techniques can help to reduce exposure misclassification and provide more reliable estimates of exposure at the small-area scale.

24.2.2 Modelling

Modelling for mixed contaminants in drinking water aquifers and the use of predicted contaminant levels in groundwater for human health risk assessment needs considerable development (Piver *et al.* 1997). Contaminant transport models from the aquifer to the surface for eventual human consumption are necessarily complex if the essential multiphase, multi-contaminant, and energy transport equations are included. However, no matter how sophisticated the model, its reliability is inevitably constrained by the quality of the input data. These are often limited by the spatial variability of contaminant transport parameters. As a result, exposure assessment is the weakest part of the human cancer risk assessment in relation to groundwaters. Statistical optimisation methods are being developed to provide better estimates of aquifer parameters given limited data. Some progress has also been made over the last few years in methods to reduce uncertainty in single contaminant predictions for heterogeneous aquifers that are fairly uniform (without large fractures that alter transport dynamics). Much more research is, however, needed in situations of complex aquifers with multiple contaminants and multiple phase transport. Models also need to be supported by much more extensive and reliable groundwater monitoring data. Immunoassay methods have been developed for monitoring contaminant levels in water, soil, food, and tissues. It is hoped that data from these assay systems, along with standard chromatography/mass spectroscopy chemical analytical methods, will make it possible to develop more accurate transport models for predicting specific transport behaviour in contaminated aquifers, as a basis for human population exposure assessment (Piver *et al.* 1997).

24.2.3 Exposure assessment techniques

More than good mapping of current levels of contamination is needed for assigning accurate exposures in drinking water epidemiology studies. Many of the health effects of concern have long latency periods, so estimation of past as well as present exposure is necessary. The need to estimate past exposures, based on inadequate data, makes this kind of disease detective work especially frustrating. Levels of exposure also depend on the extent to which the population comes into contact with the water, and this may vary depending on patterns of water supply and individual behaviour. Aral *et al.* (1996) demonstrate how geographical information systems (GIS), coupled with census data and spatial environmental data, can help to quantify this variation. They apply a computational model to a water supply system to estimate the distribution of volatile organic compounds in pipelines in Connecticut. This complex analysis showed the inadequacy of the common approach of drawing a circle of a constant radius around a source of contamination, and that in fact there is substantial spatial variation in levels of exposure if a more advanced computational model is applied.

24.3   Relationships with health

Thornton (1993) reviewed the applications of geochemical mapping to human epidemiological studies. Despite the well-documented difficulties in attempting to fit spatial geochemical patterns with disease patterns, there have been some successes, for example: (i) the relation between fluoride content of drinking water and human fluorosis and its protection for dental caries; (ii) the relation between endemic goitre and lack of iodine in food; and (iii) the relation between low selenium in parts of the People's Republic of China and the prevalence of Keshan and Kaschin–Beck diseases.

A range of pollutants in drinking water have been linked to cancer mortality and incidence, including asbestos, arsenic, chlorination by-products, nitrates, and radium (NRC 1977; Cantor 1997). Here, we will focus on just a few as examples. Generally, the earliest studies for any class have been ecological, where exposures categorised by geographical area are correlated with area-wide cancer rates gathered from death certificates or cancer incidence reporting systems. There have also been studies of other non-infectious diseases (e.g. the effects of drinking water hardness as a protective factor for heart disease) (Marx and Neutra 1997), and there is now a growing impetus to study the potential reproductive effects of drinking water contaminants.

24.3.1   Disinfection by-products

Chlorination by-products in drinking water have been a cause for concern as potential carcinogens since 1974 (Bellar *et al.* 1974; Rook 1974). The by-products, such as THMs, generally result from the interaction of chlorine used for drinking water disinfection with organic chemicals present in the drinking water, usually from natural sources. As a consequence of concern over possible cancer causation, there have been a number of epidemiological studies since the 1970s seeking to link contaminants of drinking water and disease incidence or mortality in various populations around the world (Cantor 1997).

The first tier of studies mostly utilised the mapped NCI 1950–69 cancer by county data (Mason *et al.* 1974), coupled with routine water utility measurements. Cech *et al.* (1987) conducted a typical ecological study. The end-point was urinary cancer mortality by census tracts, compiled by using death certificates and census population data for denominators. Exposure was estimated from geographical distributions of modelled surface water parameters, including chlorination and contaminant levels. Confirmation of the estimates was made by measuring THMs in historically relevant sections of the distribution system and comparing the measurements to historical data on THMs from 1978 to 1987. A series of trend-surface maps to estimate THM concentrations in the drinking water was made for individual census tracts and for census tract aggregations. In 1954, Houston changed from lightly chlorinated to heavily chlorinated drinking water and the investigators did not find a correlation with urinary mortality and chlorination.

The next tier of studies comprised mainly case-control studies, utilising death certificates and routinely collected water quality parameters. The National Research Council (NRC 1980) reviewed the first 14 of these mortality studies and found some consistency of association for bladder, colon, and rectal cancer mortality and indicators of drinking water trihalomethanes.

A third tier of studies (NRC 1986) used cancer incidence reporting registries to sample cancer cases, which were compared with controls for exposure to differing drinking water sources. Using questionnaires or telephone interviews, these incidence studies were able to delve into detail on life history and drinking water consumption, and generally confirmed the earlier positive findings for cancers of the bladder, colon, and rectum.

Generally, the more rigorous studies are done with individual data on exposure based on individual residence history and more detailed monitoring information. The ecological and mortality studies often lack specific information over time as to both the drinking water exposure and exposure to potential confounding factors such as cigarette smoking, occupational exposures, or nutritional factors. Because of the well-documented problems in exposure and confounder assessment in drinking water epidemiology, regulators prefer to extrapolate from animal study results in order to set drinking water standards. It is still surprising how few epidemiological studies have been conducted, and how little public policy impact they have had, considering the potential public health impact of a drinking water exposure compared to the major non-infectious diseases like cancer. Morris (1995) concludes that the use of chlorine as a drinking water disinfectant to reduce infectious disease may account for a substantial burden of cancer risk: 5000 new bladder and 8000 new rectal cases in the US each year. The trade-off between protection of the public health against infectious disease transmission by drinking water disinfection, and the potential cancer worry, may lead ultimately to the adoption of different disinfection techniques other than chlorination. Nevertheless, many of the more recent, individual-level studies have tended to confirm results from the earlier ecological investigations. This suggests that, for an exposure like drinking water which is often reasonably uniform within a small geographical area, ecological studies may be worthwhile.

Current concern over disinfection by-products in drinking water extends to adverse pregnancy outcomes. Gallagher *et al.* (1998) conducted a retrospective cohort study in Colorado where birth certificates were linked to historical water supply data. There was a small, yet provocative association between low birthweight and trihalomethane exposure during the third trimester of pregnancy. Swan and Waller (1998) review a number of studies over the years with different study designs (ecological, case-control, cohort); several have implied a small risk for fetal growth retardation. Amounts and sources of exposure misclassification in these studies vary (see Chapter 5), and the actual aetiological agents among the disinfection by-product mix is still a mystery. Future studies, involving personal exposure measurements to specific chemical species among the mix, may be needed in view of the relative ubiquity of the exposure and birth outcomes in question.

24.3.2 Nitrates

Nitrates are increasing in drinking water sources as a result of increased use of nitro-genous fertilisers worldwide in the twentieth century (Johnson and Kross 1990). Most adult nitrate intake tends to be via vegetables, but a substantial contribution can come from drinking water, especially when nitrate-nitrogen concentrations in the source supplies exceed 10 mg/litre (Chilvers *et al.* 1984). Ingested nitrate is converted to nitrite in the oral cavity (Eisenbrand *et al.* 1980) and can interact with secondary amines and amides in the stomach to form *N*-nitrosamines and *N*-nitrosamides, both of which are strong carcinogens (IARC 1978).

Since the 1970s, areas with high groundwater nitrates have been investigated for elevated stomach and other cancer rates. Most of these studies have been ecological in design. In the UK, for instance, Hill *et al.* (1973) found elevated gastric cancer mortality in Worksop, which has high water nitrate concentrations, compared to similar places with lower nitrate levels. Several other ecological studies have sought to link aggregate exposure to nitrate in drinking water with mortality or disease incidence rates. Most have used contemporary measures to estimate past exposures. Given the long latency period, and subsequent large possibilities for exposure misclassification, it is likely that many potential associations could have been missed.

Individual-level case-control studies have had mixed results. In an interview study of 276 stomach cancer cases versus 276 controls in Columbia, Cuello *et al.* (1976) found significant risk elevations for birthplace in a region with high nitrate concentrations in wells compared to birthplaces with low nitrate wells. In Wisconsin, where there are substantial areas of high nitrates in the groundwater as a result of using nitrate fertilisers in sandy agricultural soils, no associations were found between nitrate concentration in the well and stomach cancer mortality (Rademacher *et al.* 1992).

Cancer sites other than of stomach need further investigation. In Nebraska, Ward *et al.* (1996) found that non-Hodgkin's lymphoma was associated with nitrates in community drinking water supplies, estimated over a 35-year period, in a case-control study. Other non-infectious diseases have also been linked with high nitrate levels in drinking water. Kostraba *et al.* (1992) used a diabetes registry to compute county incidence rates of insulin dependent diabetes mellitus (IDDM). A weighted average of nitrate levels from each water district within each county was calculated. Even though nitrate levels are generally low in Colorado (< 10 mg/litre), the counties with the higher levels (0.77–8.2 mg/litre) had significantly elevated risk of IDDM. Parslow *et al.* (1997) conducted an ecological study comparing nitrate levels in drinking water wells, mapped at the small-area scale, and a population-based IDDM registry. Results showed significant positive associations.

These diabetes findings illustrate the stimulating possibilities of small-area ecological studies in eliciting new leads in disease aetiology. More generally, however, the message from the nitrate studies is that indirect measures, based on pollution mapping, have in the past been too coarse to detect the often subtle effects in health outcome with any degree of certainty. Smaller-area ecological studies, or individual studies, may be necessary to quantify exposure and elicit the health effects adequately.

24.3.3 Infectious diseases

Many serious infectious agents are transmitted in drinking water, including bacteria, protozoa, viruses, and worms (Savitz and Moe 1997). In terms of the size of the populations affected, the paramount concern with infectious agents in drinking water worldwide is acute gastrointestinal illness. Generally, mapping of microbiological water quality is a much more difficult problem than for non-infectious diseases. For infectious agents, the aetiological exposure is less likely to be the steady, low level presence of microbiological pathogens, but instead short-term exposure to a bolus of faecal contamination in the water supply system.

Studies of water quality and health in developing countries have most often used ground versus surface water comparisons as proxies for microbiological monitoring. This can lead to serious misclassification of exposure, since surface water is not necessarily more microbiologically contaminated than groundwater. In addition, untreated water supplies, such as those in many developing countries, can have a large variability in levels of microbiological contamination. Seasonal changes in water temperature and rainfall, for example, can lead to marked variations in faecal contamination and pathogen survival in the water supply system. In industrialised countries, it is often appropriate to compare areas of groundwater or surface water source type or general treatment categories, such as whether there is filtration/disinfection or coagulation/flocculation. Indicators of microbial content, such as the faecal coliform test, are of very limited accuracy in predicting outbreaks; for instance in the Milwaukee cryptosporidium outbreak, mentioned above, the water met the faecal coliform standard for quality. Many alternative indicator organisms have been proposed, though overall it is clear that no one organism will suffice as an indicator (WHO 1993). Mapping of indicator test results may, however, be useful in the future if further development is done on multiple indicator test systems for microbial drinking water quality.

24.4 The past and present: problems in drinking water epidemiology studies

Many common problems plague researchers in conducting studies of drinking water and health. As is evident from the discussion above, the most pervasive is the problem of inaccurate exposure assessment.

Human exposures to contaminants in drinking water are primarily through the inges-tion route and vary largely depending on levels of treatment at the supply source or tap, contamination during distribution, and the effects of cooking, water consumption habits and other factors. Public health estimates of exposure to microbes or chemical contam-inants are usually only very crude, with a wide margin of uncertainty.

In the rare, isolated cases of high dose exposures to single contaminants, such as arsenic (I'Cheng and Blackwell 1968), identifying the public health consequence (in this case, Blackfoot disease) is relatively simple. However, the more common situation—and one which perplexes epidemiologists studying drinking water—is of mixtures of low dose agents, such as trihalomethanes (THMs) and other disinfection by-products. Additional problems occur because many of the contaminants in drinking water, such as lead or nitrates, have other exposure pathways to humans, for example via the air, diet, or soil.

As in other areas of environmental epidemiology, a natural progression can be seen in studies of disinfection by-products and their possible relations to cancer. The first studies in the 1970s were ecological in nature: large geographical areas, such as counties in the USA, were compared in terms of their level of exposure to chlorination of drinking water and cancer mortality or incidence rates. These showed small, but provocative, effects. Subsequent studies refined these investigations by using case-control designs. Cancer deaths or cases of certain sites (bladder, colon, rectum) were compared with controls for individual drinking water chlorination exposure histories. Further refinement came with the use of questionnaires or interviews to collect data on residential histories and con-sumption patterns which, combined with water supply data, gave a much more accurate exposure assessment. These approaches also allowed data to be gathered on confounders and potential effect modifiers, such as cigarette smoking and alcohol consumption. The shift to individual-level studies also allowed latency to be considered. For instance, in the Wisconsin studies of colon cancer (Kanarek and Young 1982; Young *et al.* 1987), expos-ure was considered by deciles of life. This suggested that the most important exposures to consider were those of 20–30 years before the cancer became evident.

Direct data on the actual dose of water and contained contaminants ingested is not and, in the foreseeable future, will not be available to investigators. Instead, estimates must be based on more indirect measures such as measuring the agent in samples from the water supply or at the tap and extrapolating to the larger study population, modelling contaminant levels based on water source and treatment characteristics, or estimating individual exposure via home measurements and questionnaires about consumption, mobility, and residence history.

Mixtures make the exposure situation exceedingly complex. Surrogate chemicals are often used as markers for a wider set of contaminants (e.g. chloroform as a marker for disinfection by-products). Often, however, it will not adequately reflect the toxicity of the species it is intended to represent. Long periods of exposure (decades) are also involved in health effects, such as cancer, so most studies by necessity ignore variations in exposure due to seasonal, short-term, or distribution system effects. Nevertheless, these sources of variation can be substantial. For instance, lead can accumulate in pipes overnight, thus resulting in the recommendation that cold tapwater be allowed to run for one minute in the morning 'to get the lead out'. Marked variations may thereby occur from day-to-day or home-to-home depending on user behaviour. Equally, in-home devices are being increasingly used which can affect exposures to both infectious and non-infectious agents. Nor is drinking water the only source of exposure for many contaminants of interest. For volatile agents such as the THMs, inhalation and dermal routes can make important contributions to total exposure. In addition, recreational swimming and other individual behaviours, such as use of bottled water, can greatly affect exposure.

Drinking water epidemiology studies on both infectious and non-infectious agents are a necessary component of modern public health research. To date, however, mainstream epidemiology has not paid enough attention to this potential source of disease, and drinking water epidemiology studies have been somewhat underfunded by national agencies. Much of the reason for the lack of progress lies in the frustrating difficulty of drinking water studies, especially in terms of exposure assessment. The ubiquity of potential population exposures to drinking water contaminants means that this is a situation which cannot be allowed to persist. It is time that the Cinderella of drinking water studies was allowed to go to the ball!

References

Alexander, R. B., Slack, J. R., Ludtke, A. S., Fitzgerald, K. K., and Schertz, T. L. (1998). *Data from selected U. S. geological survey national stream Water-Quality Monitoring Networks* (WQN). USGS Digital Data Series DDS-37, www:http://www.rvares.er.usgs.gov/wqn96/.

Aral M. M., Maslia, M. L., Ulirsch, G. V., and Reyes, J. J. (1996). Estimating exposure to volatile organic compounds from municipal water supply systems: use of a better computational model. *Archives of Environmental Health*, **51**, 300–9.

Bellar, T. A., Lichtenberg, J. J., and Kroner, R. C. (1974). The occurrence of organohalides in chlorinated drinking water. *Journal of the American Water Works Association*, **66**, 703–6.

Cantor, K. P. (1997). Drinking water and cancer. *Cancer Causes and Control*, **8**, 292–308.

Cech, I., Hoguin, A. H., Littell, A. S., Henry, J. P., and O'Connell, J. (1987). Health significance of chlorination byproducts in drinking water: the Houston experience. *International Journal of Epidemiology*, **16**, 198–207.

Chilvers, C. Inskip H. Caygill C, Bartholomew, B., Fraser, P., and Hill, M. (1984). A survey of dietary nitrate in well-water users. *International Journal of Epidemiology*, **13**, 324–31.

Cuello, C., Correa, P., Haenszel, W., Gordillo, G., Brown, C., Archer, M. *et al.* (1976). Gastric cancer in Columbia. I: Cancer risk and suspect environmental agents. *Journal of the National Cancer Institute*, **57**, 1015–20.

Directorate General for the Environment (1988). *Bathing water quality in the European Union.* www:http://europa.eu.int/water/water-bathing/index-en.html.

Eisenbrand, G., Speiglehalder, B., and Preussmann, R. (1980). Nitrate and nitrite in saliva. *Oncology*, **37**, 227–31.

Gallagher, M. D., Nuckols, J. R., Stallones., R., and Savitz, D. A. (1998). Exposure to trihalomethanes and adverse pregnancy outcomes. *Epidemiology*, **9**, 484–9.

Hill, M. J., Hawksworth, G. M., and Tattersall, G. (1973). Bacteria, nitrosamines and cancer of the stomach. *British Journal of Cancer*, **28**, 562–7.

I'Cheng, C'I. and Blackwell, R. Q. (1968). A controlled retrospective study of Blackfoot disease: an epidemic of peripheral gangrene disease in Taiwan. *American Journal of Epidemiology*, **88**, 7–24.

IARC (International Agency for Research on Cancer) (1978). *Some N-nitroso compounds. IARC Monograph.* Vol. 17: *Evaluating carcinogen risk in humans.* IARC, Lyon.

IARC (International Agency for Research on Cancer) (1991). *Chlorinated drinking-water; chlorination by-products; some other halogenated compounds: cobalt and cobalt Compounds. IARC Monograph.* Vol. 52: *Evaluating carcinogen risks in humans.* IARC, Lyon.

Johnson, C. J. and Kross, B. C. (1990). Continuing importance of nitrate contamination of groundwater wells in rural areas. *American Journal of Industrial Medicine*, **18**, 449–56.

Jupp, D. L. B., Kirk, J. T. O., and Harris, G. P. (1994). Detection, identification and mapping of Cyanobacteria—using remote sensing to measure the optical quality of turbid inland waters. *Australian Journal of Marine Freshwater Resources*, **45**, 801–28.

Kanarek, M. S. and Young, T. B. (1982). Drinking water treatment and risk of cancer death in Wisconsin. *Environmental Health Perspectives*, **46**, 179–86.

Kostraba, J. N., Gay, E. C., Rewers, M., and Hamman, R. F. (1992). Nitrate levels in community drinking waters and risk of IDDM: An ecological analysis. *Diabetes Care*, **15**, 1505–8.

Mackenzie, W. R., Hoxie, N. J., Proctor, M. E., Gradus, M. S., Blair, K. A., Peterson, D. E. *et al.* (1994). A massive outbreak in Milwaukee of Cryptosporidium infection transmitted through the public water supply. *New England Journal of Medicine*, **331**, 161–7.

Marx, A. and Neutra, R. R. (1997). Magnesium and drinking water and ischemic heart disease. *Epidemiologic Reviews*, **19**, 259–72.

Mason, T. H., McKay, F. W., Hoover, R., Blot, W. J., and Fraumeni, J. F. (1974). *Atlas of cancer mortality for U.S. counties: 1950–1969*. USDHEW National Institutes of Health, Washington, DC.

Morris, R. D. (1995). Drinking water and cancer. *Environmental Health Perspectives*, **103**, 225–32.

NRC (National Research Council) (1977). *Drinking water and health*. National Academy Press, Washington, DC.

NRC (National Research Council) (1980). *Drinking water and health*, Vol. 3. National Academy Press, Washington, DC.

NRC (National Research Council) (1986). *Drinking water and health*, Vol. 6. National Academy Press, Washington, DC.

Newman, P. J. (1988). *Classification of surface water quality*. Heinemann, Oxford.

Page, T., Harris, R. H., and Epstein, S. S. (1976). Drinking water and cancer mortality in Louisiana. *Science*, **193**, 55–7.

Parslow, R. C., McKinney, P. A., Law, G. R., Staines, A., Williams, R., and Bodansky, H. J. (1997). Incidence of childhood diabetes mellitus in Yorkshire, northern England, is associated with nitrate in drinking water: an ecological analysis. *Diabetologia*, **40**, 550–6.

Patrick, S., Battarbee, R. W., and Jenkins, A. (1996). Monitoring acid waters in the U.K.: an overview of the U.K. Acid Waters Monitoring Network and summary of the first interpretative exercise. *Freshwater Biology*, **36**, 131–50.

Pebesma, E. J. (1996). *Mapping groundwater quality in the Netherlands*. Nederlandse Geografische Studies 199, Universiteit Utrecht.

Piver, W. T., Jacobs T. L., and Medina, M. A. Jr. (1997). Evaluation of health risks for contaminated aquifers. Environmental Health Perspectives, **105**(Suppl. 1), 127–43.

Rademacher, J. J., Young, T. B., and Kanarek, M. S. (1992). Gastric cancer mortality and nitrate levels in Wisconsin drinking water. *Archives of Environmental Health*, **47**, 292–7.

Rook, J. J. (1974). Formation of haloforms during chlorination of natural waters. *Journal of the Society of Water Treatment Examiners*, **23**, 234–43.

Savitz, D. A. and Moe, C. L. (1997). Water: chlorinated hydrocarbons and infectious agents. In *Topics in environmental epidemiology* (K. Steenland and D. A. Savitz ed.), 89–118. Oxford University Press, New York.

Snow J. (1936). On the mode of communication of cholera. In *Snow on cholera*. The Commonwealth Fund, New York.

Stanners, D. and Bordeau, P. (ed.) (1995). *Europe's environment. The Dobrís assessment*. European Environment Agency, Copenhagen.

Swan, S. H. and Waller, K. (1998). Disinfection by-products and adverse pregnancy outcomes: what is the agent and how should it be measured? *Epidemiology*, **9**, 479–81.

Thornton, I. (1993). Environmental geochemistry and health in the 1990s: a global perspective. *Applied Geochemistry*, 1993, Suppl. 2, 203–10.

Ward, M. H., Mark, S. D., Cantor, K. P., Weisenberger, D. D., Corea, A., and Zahm, S. H. (1996). Drinking water nitrate and risk of non-Hodgkin's lymphoma. *Epidemiology*, **7**, 465–71.

WHO (World Health Organisation) (1993). *Guidelines for drinking water quality*. Vol. 1: *Recommendations* (2nd edn). WHO, Geneva.

Young, T. B., Wolf, D. A., and Kanarek, M. S. (1987). Case-control study of colon cancer and drinking water trihalomethanes in Wisconsin. *International Journal of Epidemiology*, **16**, 190–7.

25. Climate change and human health: mapping and modelling potential impacts

A. J. McMichael, P. Martens, R. S. Kovats, and S. Lele

25.1 Introduction

The phrase 'global environmental change' refers to large-scale environmental perturbations, including climate change, occurring because of the enormous aggregate load that humankind is now placing upon the world's biophysical systems. The main changes comprise alterations in the gaseous composition of the lower and middle atmospheres, worldwide degradation of arable land, depletion of freshwater, and loss of biodiversity. The unprecedented scale and the potentially long time-horizons of these changes pose special, even unusual, challenges to scientists attempting to assess the current and, particularly, the future health impacts. Yet, these are tasks that, increasingly, policy-maker and public are asking scientists to address.

The potential health impacts of global environmental change are diverse. The simpler and more certain health impacts include those resulting from the likely increase in thermally stressful summertime episodes due to climate change and the elevated risk of skin cancer from increased ultraviolet irradiation due to stratospheric ozone depletion. Less simple are the processes that would alter the geographical range of various vectorborne infections in response to changes in climate, land-use patterns, biodiversity, and socio-demographic conditions (including urbanisation). Various other potential health impacts would arise via complex, interactive, and often indirect pathways such as the range of nutritional, infectious disease, and mental health problems afflicting populations displaced by rising sea levels or declining agricultural productivity. These various influences on population health reflect changes in the systemic conditions of the ecological and social environments in which humans live; our health is profoundly affected by the productivity and processes of various natural systems such as the ecology of pests and pathogens, food supplies, water supplies, climatic conditions, and weather patterns.

In this chapter, we examine the methods being used to describe and forecast the health impacts of global climate change. Of the various global environmental change processes, most scientific attention has to date been focused on climate change and its consequences. Human-induced global climate change is being caused by changes in the concentration of energy-trapping gases in the lower atmosphere, principally due to fossil fuel combustion and the depletion of the world's carbon sinks (such as forests). The UN Intergovernmental Panel on Climate Change (IPCC) has concluded that anthropogenic climate change

Table 25.1 Components of future global climate change: derived from global climate model experiments and assessed by the Intergovernmental Panel on Climate Change (IPCC) (from IPCC, 1996)

- Global mean temperature rise of 1–3.5 °C by 2100.
- Global mean sea level rise of 50 cm (range 13–94 cm) by 2100.
- Increase in number of very hot days, decrease in number of very cold days.
- Disproportionate increase in minimum temperatures (i.e. night-time temperatures rise faster than daytime; winter means rise faster than summer means).
- Intensification of global hydrological cycle, with altered pattern of floods and droughts. More droughts in drought-prone areas.
- Changes in the frequency and/or intensity of hurricanes (tropical cyclones) globally is unknown but regional changes are likely.
- Warming likely to be greater on land than in the ocean.
- Warming likely to be greatest at higher latitudes.
- Greatest uncertainty refers to future socio-economic and technological factors which affect fossil fuel consumption

has already begun—that 'on the balance of evidence, there is a discernible human influence on global climate' (IPCC 1996: 4). Therefore, whatever the immediate outcome of agreements under the UN Climate Change Convention, and given the long inertial processes in the climate system, the world is already committed to a significant amount of climate warming, along with, as yet, uncertain changes in climate variability (Table 25.1).

Disturbances of the basic environmental systems that underpin population health such as food production and freshwater availability often result from a chain of antecedent environmental change processes. The assessment of health outcomes in relation to those primary environmental disturbances (e.g. climate change) is therefore a complex task. The assessment must accommodate the multiple uncertainties that compound across those antecedent environmental and social changes (McMichael and Martens 1995). These uncertainties in assessment of the health impact of global environmental change reflect three other distinctive features: (i) the large spatial scale (i.e. regional or global versus local impacts); (ii) the potentially long temporal scale; and (iii) the level of complexity in the systems being studied (by comparison with simpler, direct, locally acting cause-effect relationships).

The assessment of the health impacts of climate change refers predominantly to processes likely to occur over future decades. For some types of impact it may be possible to observe early impacts. For example, if the trend of increasing world temperature, evident since the 1970s, continues then statistically detectable trends in annual heatwave-attributable deaths may soon emerge. Otherwise, however, the predominantly 'future study' time-frame moves us substantially out of the comfort zone of empirical observation and health risk assessment, and directs our attention to future environmental scenarios and their possible health consequences (McMichael 1993). We are obliged to use current knowledge and theory (even though we cannot be sure that they apply to future, as yet unencountered, conditions) to forecast the likely range of population health outcomes. This we can do via mathematical modelling or other systematic models of health risk assessment.

This chapter addresses the research methods applicable to assessing the potential health impacts of global climate change. The most important methods are:

- empirical studies of climate/health relationships, useful as analogues for aspects of future climate change,
- predictive modelling,
- generalised assessments of the range of health consequences of complex demographic, social and economic disruptions, for example, expert judgement. (This third method is not considered any further in this chapter.)

In epidemiological terms, the climate 'exposure' is either a direct measure of climate or weather (e.g. precipitation, temperature) or an indirect measure of the impact of climate on ecological or social systems that affect health. Such climatic exposures can be described in three broad temporal categories (Smit *et al.* 2000): long-term changes in means or norms; inter-annual (or decadal) variability; and isolated extreme events such as floods, droughts, or storms. These categories are not independent. Extreme events are a function of climate variability and any shift in the mean will, for a given distribution, affect the frequency of extreme events.

Table 25.2 illustrates the basic types of methods used in climate change and health research. Integrated health risk assessment uses any or all of these methods, to forecast the net impact of the coexistent processes of environmental change, societal change and policy response upon human health.

25.2 Empirical (analogue) studies

Empirical studies of the relationship between climate and health outcomes are the basis of any formal attempt to forecast future impacts associated with climate change. The accumulated knowledge from empirical studies can eventually form the accepted theory used in process-based models described below.

Certain situations that simulate anticipated aspects of future climate change can be considered as a type of climate change 'scenario' (see Box 1). These 'analogue' situations can therefore be studied empirically in order to obtain an estimate, by 'preview', of the health impacts of that particular aspect of climatic change or variation. There are three basic types of analogue studies (Parry and Carter 1998):

- historical trend analogues (e.g. local warming trend),
- historical event analogues (e.g. extreme weather events such as floods or drought),
- geographical analogues (e.g. one location is compared with another, thereby simulating a comparison of present and *future* climate).

The recent trends of local climate warming illustrate the opportunity to use this 'analogue' situation to look for associated changes in the incidence of climate-sensitive diseases. For example, an analysis of recent historical malaria data in the highland region of Ethiopia demonstrated an increasing trend in malaria mortality and morbidity between the 1970s and 1990s (Tulu 1996). Further, analyses over the most recent decade indicate that increases in malaria outbreaks in Ethiopia were mainly due to the observed increase in night-time temperatures. This regional climate change appeared to be the cause of the extension of malaria transmission to higher altitudes, while also increasing

Table 25.2 Methods used to understand and forecast potential health impacts of climate change

Analogue studies (non-predictive)

Empirical-statistical	Description of basic or recurrent climate/health relationship (e.g. inter-annual variation in malaria correlated with minimum November temperature).
	Analogue of a warming trend (e.g. changes in malaria incidence in highland area correlated with a trend in warming).
	Analogue of extreme event (e.g. assessment of mortality impact of a heatwave—episode analysis).
	Geographical analogue (e.g. comparsion of vector activity in similar locations, the second location has a climate similar to that forecast for the first location).

Predictive models

Empirical-statistical models	Extrapolation of climate/disease relationship in time (e.g. monthly temperature and Salmonella food-poisoning in England and Wales).
	Extrapolation of climate/disease relationship in time and space (e.g. change of distribution of vectors with change in climate).
Process-based models	Models derived from accepted theory; can be applied universally (e.g. vectorborne disease risk forecasting with model based on mathematically defined vectorial capacity).
Integrated assessment models	Comprehensive linkage of process-based models. Linkage may entail 'vertical' linkage of the sequence of affected systems in the causal chain and 'horizontal' linkage of the influences of concurrent changes in other sectors: e.g. population growth, urbanisation, trade regimes. (Examples include modelling the impact of climate change on agricultural yield, and hence on food supplies and the prevalence of hunger, taking into account coexistent trends in economic development, trade, and population growth.)

the rate and duration of transmission in areas that were previously epidemic-prone (e.g. converting a seasonal pattern of malaria to year-round transmission).

Studies of the impacts on health of extreme weather events have primarily focused on the mortality associated with weather-related disasters (Noji 1997). However, non-catastrophic extreme events can also have significant impacts on health. For example, although major floods drown and injure thousands, minor floods are more frequent and increase the risk of infectious disease via the spread of faecal contamination. Another

Box 1 Climate change scenarios

When assessing the impacts of climate change on ecological or social systems, a specified future climate change scenario must be used. Such scenarios should not be treated as forecasts or predictions, but only as plausible representations of future climates. There are several types of climate change scenario:

- Analogue scenarios are current or past periods of observed climate change that simulate anticipated aspects of future climate change.

- Arbitrary scenarios assume that climate variables change by an arbitrary amount, with no change in climate variability. For example, one could assume that temperatures increase by 3 °C, or that precipitation increases by 10%.

- Global climate model (GCM) scenarios. Dynamic mathematical models simulate the physical processes of the atmosphere and oceans. GCM outputs depend on scenarios of future emissions of greenhouse gases (GHGs) which, in turn, are modelled based on projections of population growth, energy demand, and the availability of non-fossil fuels. Future GHG emissions are the most significant source of uncertainty associated with projections of future climate change.

fruitful analogue situation is the occurrence of heatwaves in the UK which are likely to increase in frequency with climate change (Barrow and Hulme 1996) and which can be shown to have an appreciable effect on daily mortality (Rooney *et al.* 1998).

Assessments of the health impacts of short-term climate variability can provide useful information about weather/health relationships. Annual fluctuations in malaria intensity in northeast Pakistan were positively correlated with the variation in mean November temperature during the 1980s (Bouma *et al.* 1994). Marked increases in the incidence of malaria were observed, particularly in a highland area, during atypically hot, wet weather in Rwanda in 1987 (Loevinsohn 1994).

Worldwide climatic fluctuations associated with the Pacific-based El Niño Southern Oscillation (ENSO) phenomenon, especially the aperiodic 'El Niño events', induce widespread changes in precipitation patterns. El Niño events are correlated with interannual variation in the number of people affected by natural disasters and this relationship is particularly strong for those affected by famine and drought (Bouma *et al.* 1997). Particular attention has been paid to ENSO and variations in outbreaks of mosquito-borne infectious diseases. Examples include the approximately fivefold increase in risk of malaria epidemics in northern Pakistan in the year following an El Niño (Bouma and van der Kaay 1996) and the strong positive correlation between the Southern Oscillation index (a key parameter of ENSO) and dengue outbreaks in the Pacific islands (Hales *et al.* 1996, 1999).

The use of ENSO studies to forecast the impact of anthropogenic climate change is not straightforward. ENSO studies do show, however, that weather anomalies associated with short-term climate variations can have far-reaching and strong effects on epidemic disease (Kovats *et al.* 1999). These studies do not refer to an analogue of future climate change; rather, they are relevant to future changes in climate variability. The extent of future changes in climate variability remains highly uncertain, and, indeed, *past* changes in patterns of variability are difficult to ascertain with limited time series data since instrumental meteorological data records began only about a hundred years ago and corresponding historical epidemiological data series are rare.

A geographical analogue study can sometimes be used to explore the effect of a change in temperature on important vector species. For example, a 5 °C temperature differential between two adjacent valleys in California, USA, provided a natural laboratory in which to study, by analogy, climate change impacts (Reeves *et al.* 1994). The study illustrated the importance of ambient temperature on the seasonal activity of the main mosquito vector of Western equine encephalitis and St. Louis encephalitis in the USA. Although other factors, such as the timing and quantity of agricultural irrigation, influence vector abundance, temperature is the main determining factor with respect to transmission of a viral agent by a vector (Reisen *et al.* 1993).

25.2.1   Understanding the relationships between climate, weather, and disease

Geographical information systems (GIS) are becoming an increasingly important tool for describing and understanding the relationship between weather, climate and disease, especially vectorborne disease. Satellite or remote sensing (RS) data are also being used to identify habitats of the kind that are known to foster high survival rates for disease vectors such as ticks, tsetse flies, and mosquitoes (Hay *et al.* 1996). Subsequent GIS analysis of vector habitats, in combination with demographic and other data, can then establish the geographical patterns for human risk of infection. Combinations of spatial data can become very complex and new spatial statistical tools are therefore being developed (for a detailed discussion see Section II of this volume and also Chapter 19).

Lyme disease is an important tickborne disease in the United States and Europe. Local transmission is often associated with the availability of hosts (deer and deer mice) and vegetation (Glass *et al.* 1994). Das *et al.* (1998) have developed an intuitively appealing and simple method of identifying the environmental factors associated with the distribution of tick abundance and of using these factors to forecast changes in the risk of infection. Tick data, in the form of counts from dead deer, were mapped using GIS. Tick abundance, as a continuous variable, can be modelled using the kriging formulation (Cressie 1993; Chapter 10). However, as tick data were only available as counts (an indicator of abundance), generalised linear mixed models (GLMM) were used (Clayton and Kaldor 1987; Chapter 7). Tick counts were modelled as Poisson random variables with the mean representing the abundance at each location. This model was then used to extrapolate tick abundance outside the study region as a function of land use patterns (agricultural, residential), slope and whether on the edge of the forest.

In recent decades, the frequency of heavy rainfall events has increased in several regions of the USA (IPCC 1996). Such extreme weather events have been associated with the contamination of the public water supply, and, therefore, have the potential to affect very large numbers of people. An outbreak of the waterborne disease cryptosporidiosis in Milwaukee, USA, affected over 400 000 people in 1993 (MacKenzie *et al.* 1994; Chapter 24). It has been shown using a permutation test (Mantel 1967) that many reported outbreaks of waterborne disease in the USA over recent decades were related to the occurrence of an extreme rainfall event (Rose *et al.* 2000). It is nevertheless important that other (non-climate) factors are included in such models, such as agricultural practice, type of filtration plants, and other seasonal effects. In this particular study, the statistical approach for addressing these questions was again based on GLMMs but in this case the data were point patterns. Cox point process models can be modified, with the intensity function itself being a realisation of a Gaussian random field (Cressie 1993).

An important question is whether these statistical models can be used to extrapolate the risk outside the geographical range where the sampling was conducted (Das *et al.* 1998; Levin *et al.* 1997). Further, can these models be used to extrapolate disease risk into the future under conditions of climate change? These issues are discussed in the next section.

25.3   Predictive modelling of global climate change and health

Modelling is often used by epidemiologists, for example, to gain insights into the under-lying dynamics of observed infectious disease epidemics. In the estimation of future health impacts of anticipated climate change, several modelling approaches are used. Among the most important ones are empirical-statistical models, process-based models, and integrated models (Parry and Carter 1998). The choice of model will depend on several factors, such as the purpose of the study and the type of data that are available.

Empirical-statistical predictive models are based on the previously documented statistical relationships observed between climate and health (or health-related) outcome. They may range from applying simple indices of risk (e.g. identifying the minimum temperature threshold for malaria transmission) to using complex multivariate models that combine various important environmental factors which affect risk. Where these models are founded on good empirical observation and where there are good grounds for extrapolation (see discussion below), they can be useful tools in climate change health impact assessment. Empirical-statistical models are often simpler to use and may be less data-demanding than process-based models.

Process-based models draw entirely or substantially on accepted theory (the product of previously accumulated, coherent research findings). The models incorporate mathematical equations that represent processes that can be applied universally to similar systems in different environments. For example, an index which encapsulates many of the important processes in the transmission of vectorborne diseases is the vectorial capacity, which may apply to a range of environmental circumstances. Although process-based models incorporate more insights into the underlying processes than do empirical-statistical models, they may also be more data-demanding.

An *integrated modelling approach* is the most comprehensive treatment of the inter-actions between atmospheric changes and society (Carter *et al.* 1994). In general, integrated assessment models try to describe quantitatively as much as possible of the cause-effect relationship of a phenomenon (vertical integration), and the cross-linkages and inter-actions between different contextual circumstances and processes (horizontal integration), including feedbacks and adaptations. Feedback processes can amplify or dampen important aspects of the system. For example, an important determinant of the number of people infected by malaria is the level of immunity within the target population. Hence, in highly endemic regions with a high prevalence of immunity, the impact of a climate-related increase in the malaria transmission potential of the mosquito population will be low (and will soon be counteracted by the further boost in immunity).

The major advantages of integrated assessment models are: (i) the simplified nature of the linked modules in integrated models, which permits rapid development of new concepts and exploration of their implications; (ii) the realistic inclusion of interactions and feedback mechanisms; and (iii) the enhancement of communication between scientists of many disciplines, and between scientists and decision-makers (van Asselt *et al.* 1996). Furthermore, integrated assessment models may serve as a repository of what is known about the elements of a system and their relationships, and can thus augment simple extrapolation from historical data.

The limitations and drawbacks of all three types of predictive model include (Rotmans *et al.* 1996):

- the high level of aggregation;
- the absence of stochastic behaviour;
- the limited possibilities for validation;
- the inadequacy of knowledge;
- the necessary simplifications in methodology.

The accumulation of uncertainties is an unavoidable component of integrated assessment modelling. This multi-layered compounding (or 'cascading') of uncertainties from other disciplines and sectors is illustrated in Fig. 25.1. Thus, the projections about environmental changes (temperature increase, ozone depletion rates, etc.) embody inherent scientific uncertainties. These may be narrowed as a result of new scientific research or more

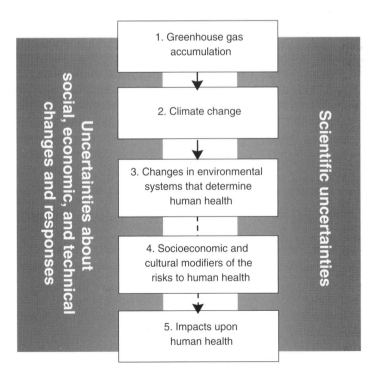

Fig. 25.1 'Cascading' of uncertainties in climate health impact modelling.

detailed/appropriate modelling. Further scientific uncertainties arise from incomplete knowledge about the first-order impact of these environmental changes upon biophysical systems (e.g. flooding, vector abundance, and food yields) which then affect human health. Yet further uncertainties exist in relation to the environment-health relationships (e.g. the dose-response curve between thermal stress and mortality, or between ultraviolet radiation and skin cancer incidence). Social and economic uncertainties arise from the inherent unpredictability of future geopolitical, socio-economic, demographic, and technological evolution. Model evaluations should therefore include some form of uncertainty analysis (McMichael and Martens 1995). Qualitative reasoning modelling and simulation, using the formalism of qualitative differential equations (QDE), may also be helpful.

25.3.1 Modelling the impact of climate change on vectorborne infectious diseases

Worldwide, vector-borne infectious diseases are a major cause of illness and death (Table 25.3). The distribution of vectorborne diseases is limited by the climatic tolerance of their vectors and by biological restrictions that limit the survival of the infective agent in the vector population. In addition, certain human activities that help to prevent the spread of pathogens and reduce vector populations restrict the distribution of many diseases in countries that can afford to do so. However, climate can play a dominant role in determining the distribution and abundance of insects, either directly or indirectly through its effects on host plants and animals. Therefore, it is anticipated that climate change will

Table 25.3 Major tropical vectorborne diseases and the likelihood of change with climate change (from McMichael *et al.* 1996)

Disease	Vector	Present distribution	Likelihood of altered distribution with climate change
Malaria	Mosquito	Tropics/subtropics	+++
Schistosomiasis	Water snail	Tropics/subtropics	++
Dengue	Mosquito	All tropical countries	++
Yellow fever	Mosquito	Tropical South America and Africa	++
Onchocerciasis (river blindness)	Blackfly	Africa/Latin America	++
American trypanosomiasis (Chagas disease)	Triatomine bug	Central and South America	+
Leishmaniasis	Phlebotomine sandfly	Asia/southern Europe/Africa/ Americas	+
African trypanosomiasis (sleeping sickness)	Tsetse fly	Tropical Africa	+
Lymphatic filariasis	Mosquito	Tropics/subtropics	+
Dracunculiasis (Guinea worm)	Crustacean (copepod)	South Asia/Arabian peninsula/Central-West Africa	?

+, likely; ++, very likely; +++, highly likely; ?, unknown.

have a significant effect on the geographical range of many vector species (McMichael *et al.* 1996). Past events also teach us that local human-made environmental change, either directly or via changes in the local climate, can have an important effect on vector abundance and disease transmission. Deforestation, agriculture, and water resource development are all important factors in this context (Lines 1993; Lindsay and Martens 1998). How best to untangle these relationships in order to find a climate change 'signal' in observed changes in insect distributions is the subject of much current debate. For example, there is some suggestive evidence that mosquitoes, and malaria itself may have spread in highland regions as a result of global climate change (Epstein *et al.* 1998).

25.3.2 Mapping arthropod vectors of disease

Models incorporating a range of meteorological variables have been developed to describe a specific 'bioclimate envelope' for a particular vector or pest species. Multivariate statistical techniques can be used to select predictive variables (whether meteorological or environmental, ground-based or remotely sensed; see above). For example, Rogers *et al.* (1996) developed a statistical model to map the distribution of tsetse flies in West Africa using meteorological satellite data. Models that match the presence of a particular species with a discrete range of temperature and precipitation parameters can then be used to project the effect of climate change on vector redistribution.

The CLIMEX model, developed by Sutherst *et al.* (1995), maps the translocation of species between different areas as they respond to climate change. CLIMEX analyses indicate that the indigenous vector of malaria in Australia would be able to expand its range 330 km south under one typical scenario of climate change (Bryan *et al.* 1996). However, these studies clearly cannot include all factors which affect species distributions. For example, local geographical barriers and interaction/competition between species are important factors which determine whether species colonise the full extent of suitable habitat (Davis *et al.* 1998).

Some mosquito species have now been successfully mapped in Africa using meteorological data (e.g. Lindsay *et al.* 1998). Satellite data are often used as surrogates for instrumental meteorological data; weather variables are usually measured at ground level but coverage can be relatively sparse or inappropriate, especially in developing countries (Hay *et al.* 1996). In addition, more complex indices may be useful: the normalised difference vegetation index (NDVI) correlates with the integrated outcome of photosynthetic activity of plants, rainfall, and saturation deficit (a measure of the drying power of air). In eastern Africa, NDVI has been used to predict tsetse fly abundance (Rogers and Randolph 1991). The validity of the predictive model was established using data from a fully documented field survey.

Changes in the distribution of three important disease vectors (ticks, tsetse flies, and mosquitoes) have been mapped in southern Africa under three climate change scenarios (Hulme 1996). The results indicate that there would be significant changes in areas suitable for each vector species, with a net increase for mosquitoes (*Anopheles gambiae*), a net decrease for tsetse flies (*Glossina morsitans*), but no net change for the ticks. The reasons for the different simulation results need to be explored, but they appear to hinge on the central importance of rainfall (and temperature) for mosquitoes, temperature (and atmospheric dryness) for tsetse flies, and temperature (and a variety of other environmental conditions) for ticks.

An important objective of such work is to map the risk of human disease using meteorological and environmental variables. However, the relationship between vector-borne disease incidence and climate variables is complicated by many socio-economic and environmental factors. Some progress has been made: for example, Hay *et al.* (1998) have successfully mapped malaria seasonality in the Gambia using satellite (NDVI) data.

Statistical-empirical models are based on the experience of mapping habitats, vectors, and disease, whether via remote sensing or other data. Such models are useful for the short- and long-term forecasting of vector species distributions. However, such models provide little or no information about the underlying mechanisms behind such changes in distribution. The additional use of process-based models of vector population dynamics (e.g. Randolph and Rogers 1997) can provide important information about the nature of the observed changes in vector abundance.

25.3.3   Mapping the risk of human disease

There is a long history of using mathematical models to understand the transmission of vector-borne infections like malaria in humans. Classical epidemiological models of infectious disease use the basic reproduction rate, R_0, defined as the number of new cases of a disease that will arise from one current case when introduced into a non-immune host population during a single transmission cycle (Rogers and Packer 1993). Predicting changes in the value of R_0 (which provides a direct index of public health impact) is far more difficult than predicting changes in the geographical range of vectors, as described above. The determinants of R_0 which are sensitive to temperature include: mosquito density, feeding frequency, survival, and extrinsic incubation period (Bradley 1993; Massad and Forattini 1998). The extrinsic incubation period (i.e. the duration of the development of the parasite in the mosquito) is particularly important. The minimum temperature for parasite development is the limiting factor for malaria transmission in many areas.

The formula for the basic reproduction rate and the directly related vectorial capacity allows calculation of the *critical density threshold* for a vector population (i.e. the minimum mosquito density needed to maintain disease transmission in a given area). The *epidemic* or *transmission potential* of malaria is then defined as the reciprocal of the mosquito critical density threshold (for a more detailed explanation of the epidemic potential see Martens 1998). Transmission potential is a summary parameter that has been widely used as a comparative index to estimate the effect of changes in ambient temperature on the population at risk of malaria. A high transmission potential indicates that, even if the vector population were to become smaller or less efficient, a given degree of endemicity may be maintained in a given area.

On a global scale, predictive modelling results have shown a projected increase of the populations at risk of malaria using a climate change scenario derived from a global climate model (see Box 1). Malaria is the world's most prevalent vectorborne disease—at present some 2400 million people are at risk of infection and an estimated 400 million cases occur annually (WHO data).

Global models entail aggregated inputs in both time and space. For example, such a model may assume that altitude or the characteristics of surface water are uniform over a large area. Most of the models used to date to estimate future changes in malaria have also used a composite measure of different species of *Anopheles* mosquitoes. A study by Martens *et al.* (1999) incorporated parameter values for 18 regionally dominant mosquito vector species. On the basis of a mid-range population growth scenario, this model estimates an additional 260–320 million people at risk of malaria by 2080. Globally, aggregated models often assume that there are universal relationships that are sufficiently dominant to yield a valid approximate overall forecast. Even so, the equations within a global model may well be inappropriate for particular local conditions. There is clearly a need for cross-validation of large- and small-scale studies (Root and Schneider 1995). Some recent attempts to apply these integrated modelling techniques to smaller-scale regional conditions have endeavoured to take account of local/regional conditions.

The regions with the greatest risk of increased malaria under future climate change are in present-day regions with unstable epidemic malaria currently on the altitude and latitude fringes of disease transmission. Plates 7 and 8 illustrate calculations of transmission potential for Africa. The largest changes in transmission potential are forecast at the fringes, both latitude and altitude, of current risk areas (Lindsay and Martens 1998). In highland areas, populations have little or no immunity to malaria, and epidemics in these regions are characterized by high morbidity and mortality in both children and adults.

The validation of predictive models using independent historical data is an important part of the modelling process. The potential risk maps in Plates 7 and 8 correspond well with the broad levels of endemicity that have been observed or estimated from field studies (Lysenko and Semashko 1968; WHO 1993). Unfortunately, historical data on vector and disease distribution are often not available, particularly in Africa (Snow *et al.* 1996). The model used by Lindsay and Martens (1998) fails to demonstrate malaria transmission in the Horn of Africa, however, which indicates current limitations in both data availability and the model itself.

25.3.4 Future food production and risk of hunger

Long-term changes in world climate would affect the foundations of public health: sufficient food and safe and adequate drinking water. Integrated assessment modelling studies have recently addressed the potential global impacts of climate change on water resources and food supply. Although it is not yet possible to forecast the direct and indirect impacts on human health, these assessments of food and water availability are important in identifying regional and local vulnerability.

There is an important difference between sensitivity and vulnerability to climate change. A given disease system may be particularly *sensitive* to the effects of climate change based on its biological or physiological characteristics. However, the actual *vulnerability* of a population to that particular disease may be considerably lessened by adaptive responses (Balbus 1998). Thus, population growth is likely to be the major driving cause of water stress in a number of countries (particularly in Africa, the Middle East and the Indian subcontinent) and this may be exacerbated by climate change (Arnell 1999).

An integrated assessment of the impact of climate change on global food production is described below (Parry *et al.* 1999). A population at 'risk of hunger', based upon methods developed by the Food and Agriculture Organisation (FAO) of the UN, is defined as a population with an income insufficient to either produce or buy their food requirements.

Integrated assessment has been used to link models together. In this case, all models have been individually peer-reviewed and separately validated with historical data. Regionally based crop yield models are first used to simulate the effects of climate change—a global climate model (GCM)-based scenario—and increased CO_2 (which has a fertilisation effect) on the yield of the major cereal crops. An established world food trade model (the Basic Linked System) is then used to simulate the economic consequences of yield changes; these include changes in world food output and in world food prices. Assuming no change in climate, the model estimates that world cereal production approximately doubles from about 1800 million metric tonnes (mmt) in 1990 to about 3500 mmt in 2050, matching global food requirements throughout the period. Food prices are estimated to rise but the relative risk of hunger will decrease. These projections are consistent with those of FAO (based on expert judgement). They assume a 50% liberalisation of trade by 2020 and an annual increase in cereal yields of just under 1%. Some consider these assumptions to be optimistic, but they are consensus-based estimates.

Worldwide, the additional number of people at risk of hunger due to climate change is projected to be about 36 million by the 2020s (533 million compared to 497 million projected without climate change). It is important to note that the direction and order of magnitude of the forecast changes are more important than the absolute quantitative estimates. These actual estimates are given here to indicate the relative importance of population growth, economic trends, and climate change on future estimates of populations at risk of hunger. Further, global estimates mask important regional and local differences. The integrated assessment estimated that yields would decrease in low latitude countries, in particular the arid and sub-humid tropics. These effects would be exacerbated where countries were unable to afford adaptive measures.

Note also that these assessments are long-term and focus on average effects over space and time. At the local level (e.g. in very vulnerable areas) and over short periods (e.g. in spells of drought or flooding) the effects of climate change may be more adverse. Ideally, such modelling should also take into account estimates of the impact of climate change on plant pests and pathogens, given changes in local ecological circumstances. However, such discontinuous, 'surprise' events or processes are usually not amenable to modelling.

25.3.5 Stratospheric ozone depletion, ultraviolet irradiation, and skin cancer incidence

Stratospheric ozone depletion is, strictly, a separate process from that of tropospheric accumulation of greenhouse gases and the resultant climate change. There are, however, some physical interactions between the two processes. The modelling of future changes in skin cancer incidence in response to stratospheric ozone depletion illustrates well the use of relatively clear-cut, linked process-based modelling.

Information on the general relationship between solar exposure and skin cancer is available from a large body of epidemiological research. It provides estimates of risk increments associated with different amounts of time, by life-stage, spent exposed to solar radiation. It has not been generally possible to measure (especially in retrospect) an individual's actual radiation exposure; rather, the exposure has been expressed in terms of indices such as person-time outdoors, frequency of severe exposure episodes, or category of occupation. Yet, in order to estimate how future changes in ultraviolet irradiance might alter the incidence of skin cancer, we require estimates of risk gradients associated with actual levels of ultraviolet radiation exposure. It has been necessary to glean these from broad-brush population-level epidemiological studies that describe the relationship between average ambient local exposure levels and local skin cancer rates.

A model developed by Martens, Slaper, and colleagues (Martens *et al.* 1996; Slaper *et al.* 1996) vertically integrates the dynamic aspects of the source-to-risk causal chain: from production and emission of ozone-depleting substances, through global strato-spheric chlorine concentrations, local depletion of stratospheric ozone, the resulting increases in ultraviolet-B radiation (UV-B) levels, and finally, to the effects on skin cancer rates. Several delay mechanisms in the effect of ozone depletion on skin cancer rates are important, such as tumour latency. In the case of ozone depletion, the separate scenarios modelled relate to various international agreements which restrict the production of ozone depleting substances. Thus, full compliance with the Copenhagen Amendments to the Montreal Protocol (the latest and most restrictive agreement) would lead to a peak in stratospheric chlorine concentration and ozone depletion in the first decade of the twenty-first century, and to a peak in excess skin cancer of around 5–10% by about 2050. The latter delay is mainly due to the fact that skin cancer incidence depends both on early-life exposure and on the cumulative UV-B exposure. Another factor described in the model is a 'lifestyle factor' because skin cancer rates are very sensitive to sun exposure habits. In addition, as skin cancer occurs primarily among the elderly, the changing age-profile of the population is modelled.

25.4   Conclusions: the way ahead

The anticipated range and magnitude of the potential health impacts of global climate change have prompted a rapid evolution of concepts and methods applicable to charac-terising and estimating those impacts. Some of the scientific tasks can be accomplished by the empirical study of analogue situations. However, many of them must be addressed via scenario-based risk assessment, using various types and levels of predictive modelling.

The piecemeal epidemiological evidence available to date provides an inadequate basis for predicting the full range, timing and magnitude of future health impacts of climate change and other global environmental changes (McMichael 1997) (Table 25.4). Further, the inevitable interaction between these global changes, both as processes and in their production of impacts, compounds the difficulty of predictive modelling. Considerable scientific effort is therefore now going into the development of integrated mathematical modelling, and into imbuing top-down models with the capacity for downscaled appli-cation to regions and countries that takes account of local physical, ecological, and demographic particulars.

Future health risk assessments of climate change will ultimately need to integrate the (global) climate change scenarios, with local socio-economic and environmental factors into an integrated (modelling) framework based on variables describing climate, vectors, parasites, human populations, and health impact. There has also been recent recognition of the need for integrated mathematical models to take account of feedback processes within and between linked systems. That is, complex systems may often need to be modelled as complex adaptive systems, displaying spontaneous or socially based adaptive responses. The use of genetic algorithms (Janssen and Martens 1997) and artificial neural networks (Sethi and Jain 1991), incorporating a capacity for adaptive change and 'learning' processes, holds promise for this purpose.

Table 25.4   Scenario-based health risk assessment: aspects and limitations (from McMichael *et al.* 1998)

- Exposures are drawn from plausible scenarios, including those projected by global climate models; they are not empirically observable realities. Such scenarios are inherently uncertain and this uncertainty increases markedly at higher geographical resolution.
- The scenarios include some exposure circumstances outside the range of documented human experience. Extrapolation of empirically documented health risks therefore requires caution.
- The exposure scenarios affect population health via diverse mechanisms—direct and indirect, immediate and delayed. Some health impacts would arise via demographic, infrastructural and economic disruption.
- Assessment of health impacts caused by perturbations of complex ecological systems (e.g. changes in the geography of infectious disease vectors) must address the dynamic, non-linear, stochastic behaviour of these systems.
- Realistic scenarios involve multiple coexistent, and often interacting, global changes. Many systems are changing simultaneously.
- The projection of scenarios many decades into the future means that they refer to human populations living in unspecifiable future circumstances. (Future eventualities—fertility rates, new energy technologies, vaccine development, trends in urbanisation, levels of poverty, etc.—would all affect the vulnerability and response of human populations to global changes. These future contextual changes add further uncertainty to the assessment of future health impacts.)

A satisfactory approach to health risk assessment should emphasise the continuing empirical study and monitoring of human diseases in relation to climate and environmental factors. Further, a major shortcoming of many climate change impact assessments has been the superficial treatment of the adaptive capacities and options of diverse populations (Parry and Carter 1998).

Strategies to enhance population adaptation should promote measures that are not only appropriate for current conditions but also build the capacity to identify and respond to unexpected future developments. The restoration and improvement of general public health infrastructure will reduce vulnerability to the health impacts of climate change (McMichael and Kovats 2000). In the longer-term, and more fundamentally, improvements in the social and material conditions of life and in the reduction of inequalities within and between populations are required for sustained reduction in vulnerability to global environmental change.

Above all, the major social purpose of the predictive assessment of risks to health posed by scenarios of future environmental change is to inform and facilitate policy discussion and decision-making. Where the future health impacts of climate and other environmental change are assessed as adverse and significant, the case for primary prevention via social, economic, and technological changes is strengthened.

References

Arnell, N. W. (1999). Climate change and global water resources. *Global Environmental Change*, **9**, (Special Issue), S31–S50.

Balbus, J. M. (1998). Human health. In *Handbook on methods of climate change impact assessment and adaptation strategies, Version 2.0.* (J. F. Feenstra, I. Burton, J. B. Smith, and R. S. J., Tol, ed.). UNEP, Nairobi/Institute for Environmental Studies, Amsterdam.

Barrow, E. M. and Hulme, M. (1996). The changing probabilities of daily temperature extremes in the UK related to future global warming and changes in climate variability. *Climate Research,* **6**, 21–31.

Bouma, M. J. and van der Kaay, H. J. (1996). The El Niño Southern Oscillation and the historic malaria epidemics on the Indian subcontinent and Sri Lanka: an early warning system for future epidemics? *Tropical Medicine and International Health,* **1**, 86–96.

Bouma, M. J., Sondorp, H. E., and van der Kaay, H. J. (1994). Health and climate change. *Lancet,* **343**, 302.

Bouma, M. J., Kovats, R. S., Goubet, S. A., Cox, J. StH., and Haines, A. (1997). Global assessment of El Niño disaster burden. *Lancet,* **350**, 1435–8.

Bradley, D. J. (1993). Human tropical diseases in a changing environment. In *Environmental change and human Ciba Foundation Symposium 175,* 147–70. Wiley, Chichester.

Bryan, J. H., Foley, D. H., and Sutherst, R. W. (1996). Malaria transmission and climate change in Australia. *Medical Journal of Australia,* **164**, 345–7.

Carter, T. R., Parry, M. L., Harasawa, H., and Nishioka, S. (1994). *IPCC Technical guidelines for assessing climate change impacts and adaptations.* University College London.

Clayton, D. and Kaldor, J. (1987). Empirical Bayes estimates of age-standardized relative risks for use in disease mapping. *Biometrics,* **43**, 671–81.

Cressie, N. A. C. (1993). *Stastistics for spatial data* (rev. edn). Wiley, New York.

Das, A., Lele, S., Glass, G. E., Shields, T., and Platz, J. (1998). *Spatial modeling of vector abundance using generalized linear models: application of Lyme disease.* Unpublished manuscript. Statistics Research Division, Research Triangle Institute, 6110 Executive Blvd., Rockville MD 20852, USA.

Davis, A. J., Jenkinson, L. S., Lawton, J. H., Shorrocks, B., and Wood, S. (1998). Making mistakes when predicting shifts in species range in response to global warming. *Nature,* **391**, 783–6.

Epstein, P. R., Diaz, H. F., Elias, S. A., Grabherr, G., Graham, N. E., Martens, P. *et al.* (1998). Biological and physical signs of climate change: focus on mosquito-borne diseases. *Bulletin of the American Meteorology Society,* **78**, 409–17.

Glass, G. E., Amerasinghe, F. P., Morgan, J. M., and Scott, T. W. (1994). Predicting *Ixodes scapularis* abundance on white tailed deer using geographical information systems. *American Journal of Tropical Medicine and Hygiene,* **51**, 538–44.

Hales, S., Weinstein P., and Woodward A. (1996). Dengue fever epidemics in the South Pacific: driven by El Niño Southern Oscillation? *Lancet,* **348**, 1664–5.

Hales, S., Weinstein P., Souares, Y., and Woodward A. (1999). El Niño and the dynamics of vectorborne disease transmission. *Environmental Health Perspectives,* **107**, 99–102.

Hay, S. I., Tucker, C. J., Rogers, D. J., and Packer, M. J. (1996). Remotely sensed surrogates of meteorological data for the study of the distribution and abundance of arthropod vectors of disease. *Annals of Tropical Medicine and Parasitology,* **90**, 1–19.

Hay, S. I., Snow, R. W., and Rogers, D. J. (1998). Prediction of malaria seasons using multi-temporal meteorological satellite sensor data. *Transactions of the Royal Society of Tropical Medicine and Hygiene,* **92**, 12–20.

Hulme, M. (ed.) (1996). *Climate change and Southern Africa: exploration of some potential impacts. Implications for the SADC region* 40–55. Report commissioned by WWF International, Climatic Research Unit, University of East Anglia, Norwich.

IPCC (1996). *Climate change 1995. The science of climate change.* Contribution of Working Group I to the Second Assessment Report of the Intergovermental Panel on Climate Change (J. T. Houghton *et al.* ed.), Cambridge University Press, New York.

Janssen, M. and Martens, P. (1997). Modelling malaria as a complex adaptive system. *Artificial Life,* **3**, 213–36.

Kovats, R. S., Bouma, M., and Haines, A. (1999). *El Niño and health.* World Health Organisation, Geneva (WHO/SDE/PHE/99.4).

Levin, S. A., Grenfell, B., Hastings, A., and Perelson, A. S. (1997). Mathematical and computational challenges in population biology and ecosystems science. *Science,* **275**, 334–43.

Lindsay, S. W. and Martens, P. (1998). Malaria in the African Highlands: past, present and future. *Bulletin of the World Health Organisation*. **76**, 33–45.

Lindsay, S. W., Parson, L., and Thomas, C. J. (1998). Mapping the ranges and relative abundance of the two principal African malaria vectors, *Anopheles gambiae sensu stricto* and *An. arabiensis*, using climate data. *Proceedings of the Royal Society of London B*, **265**, 847–54.

Lines, J. (1993). The effects of climate and land-use changes on the insect vectors of human disease. In *Insects a changing environment, 17th Symposium of the Royal Entomological Society of London* (R. Harrington and N. E. Stork ed.), 158–75. Academic Press, London.

Loevinsohn, M. (1994). Climatic warming and increased malaria incidence in Rwanda. *Lancet*, **343**, 714–18.

Lysenko, A. Y. and Semashko, I. N. (1968). Geography of malaria. In *Medical geography* (A. Lebedew ed.), Academy of Sciences USSR, Moscow, Cited in Molineaux, L. (1988). The epidemiology of human malaria as an explanation of its distribution, including some implications for its control. In *Malaria, principles and practice of malariology*, Vol. 2 (W. H. Wernsdorfer and I. McGregor ed.), 913–98. Churchill Livingstone, New York.

MacKenzie, W. R., Hoxie, N. J., Proctor, M. E., Gradus, M. S., Blair, K. A., Peterson, D. E. *et al.* (1994). A massive outbreak in Milwaukee of Cryptospiridium infection transmitted through the public water supply. *New England Journal of Medicine*, **331**, 161–7.

Mantel, N. (1967). The detection of disease clustering and a generalized regression approach. *Cancer Research*, **27**, 209–20.

Martens, P. (1998). *Health and climate change: modelling the impacts of global warming and ozone depletion*. Earthscan, London.

Martens, P., den Elzen, M. G. J., Slaper, H., Koken, P. J. M., and Willems, B. A. T. (1996). The impact of ozone depletion on skin cancer incidence: an assessment of the Netherlands and Australia. *Environmental Modelling and Assessment*, **1**, 229–40.

Martens, P., Kovats, R. S., Nihof, S., de Vries, P., Livermore, M. T. J., Bradley, D. *et al.* (1999). Climate change and future populations at risk of malaria. *Global Environmental Change*, **9**, (Special Issue), S89–S107.

Massad, E. and Forattini, O. P. (1998). Modelling the temperature sensitivity of some physiological parameters of epidemiologic significance. *Ecosystem Health*, **4**, 119–29.

McMichael, A. J. (1993). Global environmental change and human population health: a conceptual and scientific challenge for epidemiology. *International Journal of Epidemiology*, **22**, 1–8.

McMichael, A. J. (1997). Integrated assessment of potential health impact of global environmental change: prospects and limitations. *Environmental Modelling and Assessment*, **2**, 129–37.

McMichael, A. J. and Kovats, R. S. (2000). Climate change and climate variability: adaptations to reduce impacts. *Environmental Monitoring and Assessment*, **61**, 49–64.

McMichael, A. J. and Martens, P. (1995). The health impacts of global climate change: grappling with scenarios, predictive models and multiple uncertainties. *Ecosystem Health*, **1**, 23–33.

McMichael, A. J., Haines, A., Slooff, R., and Kovats, S. (ed.) (1996). *Climate change and human health*. (WHO/EHG/96.7). World Health Organisation, Geneva.

McMichael, A. J., Patz, J. A., and Kovats, S. (1998). Impacts of global environmental change on future health and health care in tropical countries. *British Medical Bulletin*, **54**, 475–88.

Noji, E. (1997). *The public health consequences of disasters*. Oxford University Press, New York.

Parry, M. L. and Carter, T. R. (1998). *Climate impact and adaptation assessment: a guide to the IPCC approach*. Earthscan, London.

Parry, M., Rosenzweig, C., Iglesias, A., Fischer, G., and Livermore, M. T. J. (1999). Climate change and world food security: a new assessment. *Global Environmental Change*, **9**, (Special Issue), S51–S68.

Randolph, S. E. and Rogers D. J. (1997). A generic model for the African tick *Rhipicephalus appendiculatus*. *Parasitology*, **115**, 265–79.

Reeves, W. C., Hardy, J. L., Reisen, W. K., and Milby, M. M. (1994). Potential effect of global warming on mosquito-borne arboviruses. *Journal of Medical Entomology*, **31**, 323–32.

Reisen, W. K., Meyer, R. P., Presser, S. B., and Hardy, J. L. (1993). Effect of temperature on the transmission of western equine encephalomyelitis and St Louis encephalitis viruses by *Culex tarsalis* (Diptera: Culicidae). *Journal of Medical Entomology* **30**, 151–60.

Rogers, D. J. and Packer, M. J. (1993). Vector-borne diseases, models and global change. *Lancet*, **342**, 1282–4.

Rogers, D. J., Hay, S., and Packer, M. J. (1996). Predicting the distribution of tsetse flies in West Africa using temporal Fourier processed meteorological satellite data. *Annals of Tropical Medicine and Parasitology*, **90**, 224–41.

Rogers, D. J. and Randolph, S. E. (1991). Mortality rates and population, density of tsetse flies correlated with satellite imagery. *Nature*, **351**, 739–41.

Rooney, C., McMichael, A. J., Kovats, R. S., and Coleman, M. (1998). Excess mortality in England and Wales, and in Greater London, during the 1995 heatwave. *Journal of Epidemiology and Community Health*, **52**, 482–6.

Root, T. L. and Schneider, S. H. (1995). Ecology and climate: research strategies and implications. *Science*, **269**, 334.

Rose, J., Daeschner, G., Curreiro, F. C., Patz, J. A., Lele, S., and Easterling, D. (2000). Applying a geographic information system (GIS) to assess the relationship between weather and water-borne diseases in the US: 1972–1994. *Journal of the American Water Works Association* (in press).

Rotmans, J., Dowlatabadi, H., and Parson, E. A. (1996). Integrated assessment of climate change: evaluation of methods and strategies. In *Human choice and climate change: an international social science assessment* (S. Rayner and E. Malone ed.). Cambridge University Press, New York.

Sethi, I. and Jain, A. K. (1991). *Artificial neural networks and pattern recognition: old and new connections.* Elsevier, Amsterdam.

Slaper, H., Velders, G. J. M., Daniel, J. S., de Gruijl, F. R., and van der Leun, J. C. (1996). Estimates of ozone depletion and skin cancer incidence to examine the Vienna Convention achievements. *Nature*, **384**, 256–8.

Smit, B., Burton, I., Klein, R. J. T., and Wandel, J. (2000). An anatomy of adaptation to climate change and variability. *Climate Change* (in press).

Snow, R. W., March, K., and LeSueur, D. (1996). The need for maps of transmission intensity to guide malaria control in Africa. *Parasitology Today*, **12**, 455–7.

Sutherst, R. W., Maywald, G. F., and Skarratt, D. B. (1995). Predicting insect distributions in a changed climate. In *Insects in a changing environment, 17th Symposium of the Royal Entomological Society of London*, 60–91. (R. Harrington and N. E. Stork ed.). Academic Press, London.

Tulu, A. (1996). Determinants of malaria transmission in the highlands of Ethiopia: the impact of global warming on morbidity and mortality ascribed to malaria [unpublished Ph.D. thesis]. London School of Hygiene and Tropical Medicine, University of London.

van Asselt, M. B. A. Beusen A. H. W., and Hilderink H. B. M. (1996). Uncertainty in integrated assessment: a social scientific perspective. *Environmental Modelling and Assessment*, **1**, 71–90.

WHO (World Health Organisation) (1993). *The situation of malaria and its control in the world: status and progress since 1992* (CTD/MAL/MIP/WP/93.1). WHO, Geneva.

Index